Percutaneous Penetration Enhancers

Edited by

Eric W. Smith
Howard I. Maibach

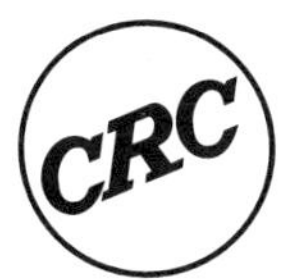

CRC Press
Boca Raton New York London Tokyo

Library of Congress Cataloging-in-Publication Data

Percutaneous penetration enhancers / edited by Eric W. Smith, Howard I. Maibach.
p. cm.
Includes bibliographical references and index.
ISBN 0–8493–2605–2
1. Transdermal medication. 2. Skin absorption. I. Smith, Eric W. II. Maibach, Howard I.
RM151.P474 1995
615′.6--dc20 95–7119
CIP

Direct all inquiries to CRC Press, Inc., 2000 Corporate Blvd., N.W., Boca Raton, Florida 33431.

International Standard Book Number 0-8493-2605-2
Library of Congress Card Number 95-7119
Printed in the United States of America 1 2 3 4 5 6 7 8 9 0
Printed on acid-free paper

PREFACE

One of the most exciting pharmaceutical areas that has developed in the past two decades is the transdermal delivery of drugs. The skin has classically been used only for localized drug delivery to the dermal strata; however, this route is now recognized as a valuable portal for the administration of cardioactive drugs, hormones, and some alkaloids to the systemic circulation. Transdermal administration avoids many of the bioavailability problems associated with oral drug administration and first-pass hepatic metabolism while producing zero-order delivery that can mimic intravenous drug administration. Unfortunately there are only a limited number of clinically useful drugs that have a sufficiently high skin permeability to be administered by this route because the inherent function of the skin is one of exclusion of external chemicals. In order for broader classes of drugs to be delivered across the stratum corneum, reversible methods of reducing the barrier potential of this tissue must be employed. This requisite has fostered the study of percutaneous penetration enhancers, both in the form of chemical entities and physical methods that will safely alter the permeability restrictions of the skin.

Many of the foremost researchers in the field of penetration enhancers have participated in the production of this volume. They have presented their latest research in the fields of chemical and physical enhancement methods, providing the most up-to-date theories on the mechanisms of action of each class of enhancer or technique. In addition, the latest analytical methods and tools that are available to the researcher for investigating penetration enhancement are described in detail with sample data from each method. Obviously a broad subject such as this cannot be covered completely in one text, however, we have attempted to present a representative picture of the topic based on the current literature, presented by researchers currently active in the field.

Howard I. Maibach
Eric W. Smith

THE EDITORS

Eric W. Smith, Ph.D., is a senior lecturer in Pharmaceutics in the School of Pharmaceutical Sciences, Rhodes University, Grahamstown, South Africa.

Dr. Smith received his Bachelor of Pharmacy Degree, with distinction, from Rhodes University in 1983, and, after a 12-month pharmacy internship, returned to his alma mater to read a Doctorate in the field of topical corticosteroid delivery, which he received in 1988. After a Post Doctoral Fellowship served under Dr. Maibach in San Francisco, Dr. Smith was appointed lecturer in Pharmaceutics at Rhodes University where he has recently been promoted to senior lecturer.

Dr. Smith is a member of the Academy of Pharmaceutical Sciences, the American Association of Pharmaceutical Scientists, and the American Pharmaceutical Association. Dr. Smith has been the recipient of various fellowship and research grants throughout his career from the Foundation for Research Development in South Africa. He, as author or co-author, has published and presented over 60 research papers on various aspects of transdermal drug delivery. His main current research interest is the *in vitro* and *in vivo* assessment of corticosteroid delivery from topical formulations.

Howard I. Maibach, M.D., is Professor of Dermatology at the School of Medicine, University of California, San Francisco, California.

Dr. Maibach is a graduate of Tulane University, and has served as Intern at the William Beaumont Army Hospital and as Fellow at the Hospital of the University of Pennsylvania. Dr. Maibach received his training in clinical dermatology at the University of Pennsylvania and, thereafter, embarked on a distinguished career at the University of California-San Francisco.

He has received numerous honors and awards including an honorary doctorate from the University of Paris-Sud and, recently, his peers, research fellows and students gathered at a conference in Basel specifically convened to celebrate Dr. Maibach's 65th birthday. His professional memberships are numerous and include the International, North American, and European Environmental Contact Dermatitis Research Groups. Dr. Maibach is the author, co-author, or editor of over 1000 research papers and 40 reference texts.

CONTRIBUTORS

William Abraham
Cygnus Therapeutic Systems
Redwood City, California

Geoffrey Allan
Insmed Pharmaceuticals
Richmond, Virginia

Takao Aoyagi
Institute of Biomedical Engineering
Tokyo Women's Medical College
Tokyo, Japan

Bruce J. Aungst
DuPont Merck Pharmaceutical
Wilmington, Delaware

Brian W. Barry
University of Bradford
School of Pharmacy
Bradford, West Yorkshire
United Kingdom

Barbara Bendas
Fachbereich Pharmazie der Martin-Luther-Universität
Halle, Germany

Bret Berner
Cygnus Therapeutic Systems
Redwood City, California

Harry E. Boddé
Centre for Bio-Pharmaceutical Sciences
Leiden, The Netherlands

Nicholas Bodor
College of Pharmacy
Hillis Health Center
University of Florida
Gainesville, Florida

Vanu G. Bose
Massachusetts Institute of Technology
Cambridge, Massachusetts

Joke A. Bouwstra
Centre for Bio-Pharmaceutical Sciences
Leiden, The Netherlands

Nadir Büyüktimkin
Pharmedic Company
Lake Forest, Illinois

Servet Büyüktimkin
School of Pharmacy
University of Kansas
Lawrence, Kansas

Etienne Camel
I.E.C.
Lyon, France

Sarat C. Chattaraj
School of Pharmaceutical Sciences
Rhodes University
Grahamstown, South Africa

Donald D. Chow
Center Laboratories, Inc.
Taipei, Taiwan

Owen I. Corrigan
Department of Pharmaceutics
School of Pharmacy
Trinity College
Dublin, Ireland

Peter A. D. Edwardson
ConvaTec WHRI
Deeside, Clwyd
United Kingdom

Thomas J. Franz
Dermatology Department
University of Arkansas for Medical Sciences
Little Rock, Arkansas

Kazuya Fukuda
Hisamitsu Pharmaceutical Company Inc.
Tokyo, Japan

John M. Haigh
School of Pharmaceutical Sciences
Rhodes University
Grahamstown, South Africa

Mitsuru Hashida
Faculty of Pharmaceutical Sciences
Kyoto University
Kyoto, Japan

Derek A. Hollingsbee
ConvaTec WHRI
Deeside, Clwyd
United Kingdom

Michael Jay
College of Pharmacy
University of Kentucky
Lexington, Kentucky

Matthew K. Kagy
Dermatology Department
University of Arkansas for Medical Sciences
Little Rock, Arkansas

Hans C. Korting
Dermatologische Klinik und Poliklinik, Ludwig-Maximilians Universität
München, Germany

Robert Langer
Massachusetts Institute of Technology
Cambridge, Massachusetts

Geoffrey Lee
Department of Pharmaceutical Technology
Erlangen University
Erlangen, Germany

Paul A. Lehman
Dermatology Department
University of Arkansas for Medical Sciences
Little Rock, Arkansas

Puchun Liu
Ciba
Suffern, New York

Thorsteinn Loftsson
Department of Pharmacy
University of Iceland
Reykjavik, Iceland

Fred Logan
Department of Dermatology
University of California
San Francisco, California

Philip S. Magee
BIOSAR Research Project
Vallejo, California

Howard I. Maibach
Department of Dermatology
University of California
San Francisco, California

Takafumi Manako
Hisamitsu Pharmaceutical Company Inc.
Tokyo, Japan

Sybille Matschiner
Fachbereich Pharmazie der Martin-Luther-Universität Halle
Germany

Joseph Melendres
Department of Dermatology
University of California
San Francisco, California

Efraim Menczel
Wolfson Holon Medical Center
Tel Aviv, Israel

Bozena B. Michniak
College of Pharmacy
University of South Carolina
Columbia, South Carolina

Yu Nagase
Sagami Chemical Research Centre
Sagamihara, Kanagawa
Japan

Junzo Nakamura
School of Pharmaceutical Sciences
Nagasaki University
Nagasaki, Japan

Reinhard Neubert
Fachbereich Pharmazie der
Martin-Luther-Universität Halle
Halle, Germany

Koyo Nishida
School of Pharmaceutical Sciences
Nagasaki University
Nagasaki, Japan

Kanji Noda
Hisamitsu Pharmaceutical Company Inc.
Tokyo, Japan

Mark R. Prausnitz
Massachusetts Institute of Technology
Cambridge, Massachusetts

Danyi Quan
Theratech Inc.
Research Park
Salt Lake City, Utah

J. David Robertson
Department of Chemistry
University of Kentucky
Lexington, Kentucky

Stephen B. Ruddy
Sterling Winthrop Inc.
Collegeville, Pennsylvania

J. Howard Rytting
School of Pharmacy
University of Kansas
Lawrence, Kansas

Burton H. Sage, Jr.
Becton Dickinson Research Center
Research Triangle Park, North Carolina

Hitoshi Sasaki
School of Pharmaceutical Sciences
Nagasaki University
Nagasaki, Japan

Monika-Hildegard Schmid
Dermatologische Klinik und Poliklinik,
Ludwig-Maximilians Universität
München, Germany

Yuji Shimozono
Hisamitsu Pharmaceutical
Company Inc.
Tokyo, Japan

Eric W. Smith
School of Pharmaceutical Sciences
Rhodes University
Grahamstown, South Africa

Elka Touitou
Department of Pharmacy
The Hebrew University of Jerusalem
Jerusalem, Israel

Roderick B. Walker
School of Pharmaceutical Sciences
Rhodes University
Grahamstown, South Africa

James C. Weaver
Massachusetts Institute of Technology
Cambridge, Massachusetts

Ronald C. Wester
Department of Dermatology
University of California
San Francisco, California

Richard J. White
ConvaTec Medical Department
Ickenham
United Kingdom

Johann W. Wiechers
Unilever Research
Colworth Laboratory
Sharnbrook, Bedford
United Kingdom

Adrian C. Williams
University of Bradford
School of Pharmacy
Bradford, West Yorkshire
United Kingdom

Wolfgang Wohlrab
Haut Klinic der
Martin-Luther-Universität Halle
Germany

Ooi Wong
Cygnus Therapeutic Systems
Redwood City, California

Shigenori Yahiro
Hisamitsu Pharmaceutical
Company Inc.
Tokyo, Japan

Fumiyoshi Yamashita
Faculty of Pharmaceutical Sciences
Kyoto University
Kyoto, Japan

Tadanori Yano
Hisamitsu Pharmaceutical Company Inc.
Tokyo, Japan

TABLE OF CONTENTS

Chapter 1.1

Percutaneous Penetration Enhancers: The Fundamentals

Eric W. Smith and Howard I. Maibach

CONTENTS

I. INTRODUCTION

Over the past few years major advances have been made in the field of transdermal drug delivery (TDD). Increasing numbers of drugs are being added to the list of therapeutic agents that can be delivered to the systemic circulation, in clinically effective concentrations, via the skin portal. This is in spite of the inherent protective function of the stratum corneum (SC), which is primarily one of excluding foreign substances from entering the body. Much of the recent success in the field of TDD is attributable to the rapidly expanding body of knowledge in the field of SC barrier structure and function. Modern concepts that have evolved in this discipline have dramatically changed the way scientists view the SC, which was once considered to be a simple, "dead" layer of cells.

The complexity of the biochemical environment which constitutes the dermal barrier to the ingress of chemicals is only now beginning to be comprehended by researchers. The bilayer domains of the intercellular lipid matrices within the SC,[1] coupled with its hydrophilic and lipophilic regions and the highly keratinized intracellular environment of the flattened corneocytes, form an excellent penetration barrier which must be breached if poorly penetrating drugs are to be administered at an appropriate rate. The first recognized penetration enhancers were simple disruptive, keratolytic agents that permanently destroyed the integrity of the SC and were generally nonspecific in the penetration enhancement of all chemicals. More recently it was found that diffusion barrier reduction may conveniently, and more elegantly, be achieved in a reversible manner via the use of chemical or physical enhancers.

II. OBJECTIVES

The objectives in TDD are simple to define, but are often very difficult to achieve in practice. The skin must be exposed to an appropriate delivery vehicle from which the drug can partition at an appropriate rate. Thereafter, the drug must diffuse through

0-8493-2605-2/95/$0.00+$.50

the skin strata to the dermis from which systemic absorption can take place. Partitioning between the vehicle and SC is dependent on the relative solubility of the drug in each environment. Often, it has been found that the composition of the topical vehicle greatly affects the rate and extent to which the drug penetrates the dermal barrier.[2,3] Postulating the effect that a particular topical delivery vehicle will have on the permeation process is not a simple matter because the dosage form in contact with the skin is seldom a simple solution; more often it is a complex mixture of several chemicals which may interact in several (often opposing) ways as far as penetration enhancement is concerned. The "leaving potential", or thermodynamic activity, of the drug in the vehicle is therefore a major factor in the delivery process.[4]

The partitioning behavior will determine the concentration of the drug achieved in the first lamina of the SC. As the diffusion process across the barrier is a passive one, theory would predict that the higher this superficial drug concentration, the greater the mass transfer across the skin. Some drugs have an inherently low affinity for, and therefore, low solubility in, the SC environment, with concomitantly low permeation potential. Once in solution in this domain, the permeant must then diffuse through the hydrophilic and/or lipophilic environment of the SC at an appropriate rate; this is often unattainable for many classes of drug without some modification of the structured barrier layer. The objectives for the use of a penetration enhancer may therefore be defined as the employment of an innocuous chemical or physical means to (reversibly) improve the solubility of the drug in the SC and facilitate diffusion of the drug through the barrier layer to the vasculature. These two parameters of the drug absorption process may be conveniently modified by the use of chemical or physical enhancement methods.

III. CHEMICAL ENHANCERS

Although the intercellular lipid environment and the intracellular protein environment may form potential routes for drug penetration, chemical enhancers are believed to operate mainly in the intercellular spaces of the SC, the major diffusion route for lipophilic moieties. The exact mechanisms by which many chemical penetration enhancers function have not been clearly elucidated; it is almost certain that they will have multiple effects once absorbed into the SC. Effects that have been documented include an alteration of the solvent potential of the SC biochemical environment and a disordering of the intercellular lipid matrix following insertion of the enhancer into the bilayer structure. In the former case the stabilized presence of the chemical within the lipid bilayers (consisting mainly of ceramides, sterols, triglycerides, free fatty acids, and phospho- and glycosphingolipids) will alter subtly the overall solvent potential of the entire matrix. If this matrix now exhibits a greater affinity for the topically administered drug then the latter has a greater potential to partition from the delivery vehicle and dissolve in the SC. Theoretically, a penetration enhancer which has a similar solubility to the drug and has a high affinity for the skin would tend to facilitate the dissolution of the coadministered drug. Once in the outermost laminae of the skin, the drug must still diffuse through the diverse biochemical environments of the intercellular domains, or through the proteinaceous intracellular matrices of the SC before the epidermis and the vasculature of the dermis are reached. The enhanced solubility of the diffusant in the chemically modified strata also may assist with this translocation process.

Modern investigative techniques have shown that many enhancers may operate via a disruption of the ordered structure of the intercellular lipid region of the SC.[5-7] The insertion of the enhancer molecule between the parallel carbon chains of the fatty acids is believed to enhance the fluidity of this environment, thereby facilitating the diffusion of the coadministered drug.[8,9] The fundamental parameter here is suggested to be one of viscosity; the ordered, bilayer lipid structure having a relatively high, gel-like viscosity which is reduced by the incorporation of elongated, alkyl chain enhancers between the lipid molecules. Research has also suggested that in some cases an association of the enhancer molecules may form separate domains within the bilayer structure,[10] which additionally contributes to increasing the fluidity of the matrix.

It is possible that both mechanisms may operate simultaneously; an additive effect on the overall rate of drug delivery may then be expected. If an enhancer, or combination of enhancers, affects both the solubility of the diffusant in the SC and reduces the rigidity of the lipid matrix, then the overall increase in the flux rate theoretically should approximate the product of the increases afforded by either enhancement method alone. This approach has been investigated.[11,12]

IV. PHYSICAL ENHANCERS

The uncertainty of chemical means of penetration enhancement makes the use of a specific physical technique attractive for certain drug classes. Ionized drugs, for example, and complex macromolecules such as proteins or peptides may be induced to permeate the SC at a faster rate than normal by the application of a small electrical current across the membrane.[13,14] The charged permeant is repelled from the electrode of similar polarity into the SC, which acts as the electrical conduit to the companion electrode. This type of iontophoretically enhanced permeation has one major advantage in that the flux of the permeant can be precisely controlled by varying the applied current, and thus the drug delivery therapy can be accurately tailored for the patient. A transient period occurs after termination of the current application during which the permeability of the skin remains at an elevated level before normal barrier function is restored. This suggests that some physical change takes place within the skin ducts or SC rather than a simple electrostatic driving force which would cease once the potential difference across the skin was removed.

The use of ultrasound, or phonophoresis, as a physical penetration enhancer also has been researched.[15,16] In this case the wave energy causes a decrease in the barrier potential, the cause of which is still to be clearly defined, but is thought to be associated with the conversion of the wave energy absorbed by the skin into mechanical energy and heat within the SC. The energy transfer in this process can be extensive and damaging to the skin if the incident frequency and intensity are relatively large. Presumably this absorbed energy would also increase the fluidity of the barrier domains and increase the kinetic energy of the molecules, both of which would increase mass transfer across the membrane.

V. CONCLUSIONS

In order for the transdermal route to be used for the delivery of drugs that are normally only poorly absorbed through the skin, some form of simultaneously applied penetration enhancer is required. Greater understanding of the biochemical composition and functioning of the SC barrier has facilitated the development and testing of chemical and physical penetration enhancers. Chemicals that enhance the absorption of coadministered drugs are currently believed to act via enhanced solubility or increased lipid fluidity mechanisms. Alternatively, physical enhancers rely on electrochemical or sonic energy potentials for facilitating drug diffusion. While all these mechanisms are still in their infancy, the groundwork has been established for delivering more drugs in a sustained release manner through the SC. The chapters that follow explore each of these concepts in greater detail and provide the current status and limitations of each topic.

REFERENCES

1. **Harada, K., Murakami, T., Yata, N., and Yamamoto, S.,** Role of intercellular lipids in stratum-corneum in the percutaneous permeation of drugs, *J. Invest. Dermatol.,* 99, 278, 1992.
2. **Bonina, F. P., Carelli, V., Di Colo, G., Montenegro, L., and Nannipieri, E.,** Vehicle effects on *in vitro* skin permeation of and SC affinity for model drugs caffeine and testosterone, *Int. J. Pharm.,* 100, 41, 1993.
3. **Smith, E. W., Meyer, E., and Haigh, J. M.,** Blanching activities of betamethasone formulations. The effect of dosage form on topical drug availability, *Drug Res.,* 40, 618, 1990.
4. **Davis, A. F. and Hadgraft, J.,** Effect of supersaturation on membrane transport. I. Hydrocortisone acetate, *Int. J. Pharm.,* 76, 1, 1991.
5. **Bouwstra, J. A., Gooris, G. S., Brussee, J., Salomons-de Vries, M. A., and Bras, W.,** The influence of alkyl-azones on the ordering of the lamellae in human SC, *Int. J. Pharm.,* 79, 141, 1992.
6. **Engblom, J. and Engstrom, S.,** Azone® and the formation of reversed monocontinuous and bicontinuous lipid-water phases, *Int. J. Pharm.,* 98, 173, 1993.
7. **Schuckler, F., Bouwstra, J. A., Gooris, G. S., and Lee, G.,** An X-ray diffraction study of some model stratum-corneum lipids containing azone and dodecyl-l-pyroglutamate, *J. Control. Rel.,* 23, 27, 1993.
8. **Golden, G. M., McKie, J. E., and Potts, R. O.,** Role of SC lipid fluidity in transdermal drug flux, *J. Pharm. Sci.,* 76, 25, 1987.
9. **Francoeur, M. L., Golden, G. M., and Potts, R. O.,** Oleic acid: its effects on SC in relation to (trans)dermal drug delivery, *Pharm. Res.,* 7, 621, 1990.
10. **Ongpipattanakul, B., Burnette, R. R., Potts, R. O., and Francoeur, M. L.,** Evidence that oleic acid exists in a separate phase within SC lipids, *Pharm. Res.,* 8, 350, 1991.
11. **Komata, Y., Kaneko, A., and Fujie, T.,** *In vitro* percutaneous absorption of thiamine disulphide through rat skin from a mixture of propylene glycol and fatty acid or its analog, *Chem. Pharm. Bull.,* 40, 2173, 1992.
12. **Williams, A. C. and Barry, B. W.,** Urea analogues in propylene glycol as penetration enhancers in human skin, *Int. J. Pharm.,* 36, 43, 1989.
13. **Singh, P. and Roberts, M. S.,** Iontophoretic transdermal delivery of salicylic acid and lidocaine to local subcutaneous structures, *J. Pharm. Sci.,* 2, 127, 1993.
14. **Heit, M. C., Williams, P. L., Jayes, F. L., and Chang, S. K.,** Transdermal iontophoretic peptide delivery: *in vitro* and *in vivo* studies with luteinizing hormone releasing hormone, *J. Pharm. Sci.,* 82, 554, 1993.
15. **Bommannan, D., Okuyama, H., Stauffer, P., and Guy, R. H.,** Sonophoresis. I. The use of high-frequency ultrasound to enhance transdermal drug delivery, *Pharm. Res.,* 9, 559, 1992.
16. **Tachibana, K.,** Transdermal delivery of insulin to alloxan-diabetic rabbits by ultrasound exposure, *Pharm. Res.,* 9, 952, 1992.

Chapter 1.2

Penetration Enhancer Classification

Sarat C. Chattaraj and Roderick B. Walker

CONTENTS

I. INTRODUCTION

Percutaneous absorption is the crux of transdermal drug delivery (TDD) and to a large degree determines the feasibility of the transdermal route of administration for most bioactive compounds. Of all barrier membranes the stratum corneum (SC) is recognized as the predominant diffusional barrier for drugs and other xenobiotics.[1] Drug permeation through the skin may be enhanced by physical (hydration,[2] iontophoresis,[3] phonophoresis,[4] heat enhancement,[5] and laser energy enhancement[6]), chemical (penetration-enhancing chemicals[7]), and biochemical means (prodrug molecules,[8] chemical modification,[9] enzyme inhibition,[10] and liposomal vesicles[11]).

One generalized approach to overcoming the barrier properties of the skin for drugs and biomolecules is the incorporation of suitable vehicles or other chemical compounds into transdermal delivery systems. Substances that help promote drug diffusion through the SC and epidermis are referred to as skin-penetration enhancers, accelerants, adjuvants, or sorption promoters.[12] These adjuvants may reduce the capacity for drug binding to the skin, thereby improving drug transport. Consequently, penetration enhancer use has become more prevalent and is a growing trend in TDD.

0-8493-2605-2/95/$0.00+$.50

Ideal penetration enhancers should have the following characteristics:[12]

1. Be both pharmacologically and chemically inert and chemically stable
2. A high degree of potency with specific activity and reversible effects on skin properties
3. Show compatibility with formulation and system components
4. Be nonirritant, nonsensitizing, nonphototoxic, and noncomedogenic
5. Be odorless, tasteless, colorless, and cosmetically acceptable
6. Have a solubility parameter approximating that of skin (i.e., 10.5 $cal^{1/2}cm^{3/2}$ [13]).

Lambert et al.[14] have graded most penetration enhancers into three classes: those that act primarily as solvents and hydrogen bond acceptors (e.g., dimethylsulfoxide, DMSO, dimethylacetamide, DMA, and dimethylformamide, DMF), simple fatty acids and alcohols, and weak surfactants containing a moderately sized polar group (e.g., Azone®, 1-dodecylazacycloheptan-2-one). Hori et al.[15] adapted the approach of Fujita[16] and reported a classification system for percutaneous penetration enhancers using a conceptual diagram for classification of compounds. They determined organic and inorganic values for permeation enhancers using Fujita's data,[16] and the resultant plot of organic vs. inorganic values showed two distinct areas on the diagram. Compounds such as DMSO, ethanol, propylene glycol, and *N*-methyl pyrrolidone are located in one area and compounds such as azone, oleic acid, and lauryl alcohol are in another area, suggesting that these chemicals may have different physicochemical properties. Pfister et al.[12] classified chemical penetration enhancers as either polar or nonpolar, according to the Hildebrand solubility parameter.

Many known and newly developed chemical entities have been investigated for their ability to enhance the percutaneous penetration of drugs. A simple, relevant classification system for these excipients is essential, and would be valuable in the development of transdermal dosage forms. This chapter focuses on the various chemicals which have been shown to enhance skin penetration.

II. CHEMICAL PENETRATION ENHANCERS

Perusal of the literature reveals that numerous classes of chemical compounds have been used or assessed for their ability to promote or enhance the permeation of biomolecules through the skin. Table 1 provides an overview of some of the different chemical classes that have been used and examples of materials within specific classes.

A. SULFOXIDES

Dimethylsulfoxide is probably the earliest used and most extensively studied penetration enhancer. It has a broad spectrum of activity, including the enhancement of penetration through both plant and animal membranes,[36] and is known to enhance the permeation of various chemical agents by acting directly on the barrier.[43] Solutions of DMSO in concentrations exceeding 60% are particularly useful for increasing skin penetration of a wide range of ionic and nonionic compounds of mol wt <3000.[7] The reported concentration-dependent behavior of DMSO suggests that this permeation enhancer may function by either reducing the resistance of the skin to the drug molecule or by promotion of drug partitioning from the dosage form.[44] Attempts to elucidate the manner in which DMSO promotes skin permeation have resulted in a

Table 1 Chemical Penetration Enhancers

Chemical Class	Examples	Ref.
Sulfoxides	Dimethylsulfoxide, decylmethylsulfoxide	17, 18
Alcohols	Alkanol: ethanol, propanol, butanol, pentanol, hexanol, octanol, nonanol, decanol, 2-butanol, 2-pentanol, benzyl alcohol	19, 20
	Fatty alcohol: caprylic, decyl, lauryl, 2-lauryl, myristyl, cetyl, stearyl, oleyl, linoleyl, linolenyl alcohol	21
Fatty acids	Linear: valeric, heptanoic, pelagonic, caproic, capric, lauric, myristic, stearic, oleic, caprylic	21, 22
	Branched: isovaleric, neopentanoic, neoheptanoic, neononanoic, trimethyl hexanoic, neodecanoic, isostearic	21, 22
Fatty acid esters	Aliphatic-isopropyl *n*-butyrate, isopropyl *n*-hexanoate, isopropyl *n*-decanoate, isopropyl myristate, isopropyl palmitate, octyldodecyl myristate	23
	Alkyl: ethyl acetate, butyl acetate, methyl acetate, methylvalerate, methylpropionate, diethyl sebacate, ethyl oleate	24
Polyols	Propylene glycol, polyethylene glycol, ethylene glycol, diethylene glycol, triethylene glycol, dipropylene glycol, glycerol, propanediol, butanediol, pentanediol, hexanetriol	25
Amides	Urea, dimethylacetamide, diethyltoluamide, dimethylformamide, dimethyloctamide, dimethyldecamide	21. 26
	Biodegradable cyclic urea: 1-alkyl-4-imidazolin-2-one	27
	Pyrrolidone derivatives: 1-methyl-2-pyrrolidone, 2-pyrrolidone, 1-lauryl-2-pyrrolidone, 1-methyl-4-carboxy-2-pyrrolidone, 1-hexyl-4-carboxy-2-pyrrolidone, 1-lauryl-4-carboxy-2-pyrrolidone, 1-methyl-4-methoxycarbonyl-2-pyrrolidone, 1-hexyl-4-methoxycarbonyl-2-pyrrolidone, 1-lauryl-4-methoxycarbonyl-2-pyrrolidone, N-cyclohexylpyrrolidone, *N*-dimethylaminopropylpyrrolidone, *N*-cocoalkypyrrolidone, *N*-tallowalkylpyrrolidone	21, 28
	Biodegradable pyrrolidone derivatives: Fatty acid esters of *N*-(2-hydroxyethyl)-2-pyrrolidone	14
	Cyclic amides: 1-dodecylazacycloheptane-2-one (Azone®), 1-geranylazacycloheptan-2-one, 1-farnesylazacycloheptan-2-one, 1-geranylgeranylazacycloheptan-2-one, 1-(3,7-dimethyloctyl)azacycloheptan-2-one, 1-(3,7,11-trimethyldodecyl)azacyclohaptan-2-one, 1-geranylazacyclohexane-2-one, 1-geranylazacyclopentan-2,5-dione, 1-farnesylazacyclopentan-2-one	29, 30
	Hexamethylenelauramide and its derivatives	31
	Diethanolamine, triethanolamine	25
Surfactants	Anionic: Sodium laurate, sodium lauryl sulfate	32, 33
	Cationic: Cetyltrimethyl ammonium bromide, tetradecyltrimethylammonium bromide, benzalkonium chloride, octadecyltrimethylammonium chloride, cetylpyridinium chloride, dodecyltrimethylammonium chloride, hexadecyltrimethylammonium chloride	33–35
	Nonionics: Poloxamer (231, 182, 184), Brij (30, 93, 96, 99), Span (20, 40, 60, 80, 85), Tween (20, 40, 60, 80), Myrj (45, 51, 52), Miglyol 840	21, 36, 37
	Bile salts: Sodium cholate, sodium salts of taurocholic, glycholic, desoxycholic acids	38
	Lecithin	39

Table 1 (continued) Chemical Penetration Enhancers

Chemical Class	Examples	Ref.
Terpenes	Hydrocarbons: D-Limonene, α-pinene, β-carene Alcohols: α-Terpineol, terpinen-4-ol, carvol Ketones: Carvone, pulegone, piperitone, menthone Oxides: Cyclohexene oxide, limonene oxide, α-pinene oxide, cyclopentene oxide, 1,8-cineole Oils: Ylang ylang, anise, chenopodium, eucalyptus	40, 41
Alkanones	*N*-heptane, *N*-octane, *N*-nonane, *N*-decane, *N*-undecane, *N*-dodecane, *N*-tridecane, *N*-tetradecane, *N*-hexadecane	41
Organic acids	Salicylic acid and salicylates (including their methyl, ethyl, and propyl glycol derivatives), citric and succinic acid	42

number of mechanisms of action being postulated, including elution of lipid, lipoprotein, and nucleoprotein structures of the SC,[45,46] denaturation of the structural proteins of the SC,[47] and delamination.[48] It was reported that DMSO increases lipid fluidity by disrupting tightly packed lipid chains, which resulted in an interaction between the polar head groups of the lipids via hydrogen bonding.[48] Dimethylsulfoxide enhanced the absorption of salicylic acid from hydrophillic ointment USP and hydrophillic petrolatum USP[49] and facilitated the transport of salicylic acid and sodium salicylate,[50] hydrocortisone and testosterone,[51] scopolamine,[48] antimycotics,[52] fluocinolone acetonide,[53] and flufenamic acid.[54]

Another important candidate in this group is decylmethylsulfoxide (DCMS). Cooper[55] extended earlier studies with *n*-decylmethylsulfoxide on penetration of both polar and nonpolar substances. Unlike DMSO, DCMS is effective at concentrations as low as 0.1% and is reported to enhance polar drug permeation more effectively than nonpolar drugs.[18,55] *In vitro* experiments demonstrated the influence of DCMS on the permeation of methotrexate,[56] naloxone,[21] pyridostigmine bromide,[57] hydrocortisone, and progesterone[58] through human skin and peptides through hairless mouse skin. Cooper[55] proposed that the permeation enhancing effect of DCMS occurs as a result of protein–DCMS interactions, resulting in a change in protein conformation, thus creating a passage of aqueous channels. Furthermore, the interaction between DCMS and lipids may play a significant role in DCMS activity. Sekura and Scala[18] reported that in the alkylsulfoxide series, $C_{10}MSO$ was a more effective enhancer of nicotinic acid skin penetration than DMSO, C_6MSO, $C_{12}MSO$, or $C_{14}MSO$.

B. ALCOHOLS

Several reports in the literature reveal that alkanols are capable of penetrating the skin.[59] To gain an understanding of the mechanism of skin permeation, the effects of a variation in alkyl chain length of alkanols on the skin permeation rate of indomethacin were investigated. Results of these studies showed that as the alkyl chain length of alkanols increased, the transdermal permeation rate of indomethacin increased to a maximum, and then decreased as the number of methylene groups in the alkyl chain increased to six and eight.[60] It was postulated that the low molecular weight alkanols ($C \leq 6$) may act as solubilizing agents, thereby enhancing the solubility of indomethacin in the fatty matrix of the SC, thus promoting permeation.[59,60] Ethanol has been used as a solubilizer and enhancer for estradiol[61] and fentanyl[62] and showed a 4.3-fold higher cumulative amount absorbed than in a control experiment without enhancer. The *in vitro* steady-state flux of levonorgestrel through rat skin using the alkanols also was reported.[2] The enhancement effect diminished as the alkyl chain length increased beyond C_4. The mechanism of action of the alkanols[20] may be explained to some degree by assuming that increased partitioning of levonorgestrel into viable epidermal cells limits transdermal flux, and the more hydrophobic alkanols may extract lipids from the SC, leading to increased diffusion through this part of the skin.

C. POLYOLS

Propylene glycol (PG) is widely used in dermatological[63] and topical pharmaceutical products,[64] and has been shown to effectively increase the skin penetration of various topical drugs.[65] Undiluted PG enhanced the *in vitro* skin permeation of estradiol,[25] metronidazole,[66,67] and trifluorothymidine.[68] Propylene glycol, with other cosolvents, enhanced the skin permeation of steroids,[69] methotrexate,[70] midazolam maleate, and diazepam.[71] A 43-fold enhancement of diazepam and 86-fold enhancement of midazolam maleate transport was observed when used with 5% azone in a PG:ethanol:water (2:2:1) vehicle. The penetration of betamethasone 17-benzoate in human volunteers was investigated[58] in a nonoccluded vasoconstrictor test using drug solutions at 10% saturation. Vehicles containing 90% PG resulted in borderline improvement of steroid bioavailability when compared to a nonpenetration enhancer, dimethylisosorbide. However, the study showed that inclusion of 2% Azone® or 5% oleic acid to the PG produced a more bioactive formulation.

Møllgaard and Hoelgaard[66] evaluated the effects of 21 different organic solvents (including different glycols such as ethylene glycol, diethylene glycol, triethylene glycol, and polyethylene glycol) on the *in vitro* estradiol permeation through human skin. The results indicated that an increased number of ethylene oxide groups in the molecules led to the steady-state flux becoming smaller and the lag time increasing. Compounds such as 1,2-ethanediol, 1,3-propanediol, 1,4-butanediol and 1,5-pentanediol showed similar results as the number of alkyl groups increased. Barry[44] reported that PG may solvate α-keratin and occupy hydrogen bonding sites, thus reducing drug-tissue binding and promoting permeation.

D. ALKANES

Hori et al.[41] studied the absorption of both diazepam and propranolol across rat and mouse skin using straight-chain alkanes (C_7 to C_{16}). All were found to enhance propranolol and diazepam flux across rat and mouse skin *in vitro* except in the case of diazepam flux, which was not enhanced by heptane. These results were confirmed by Melendres et al.,[72] who investigated propranolol hydrochloride penetration *in vitro* and *in vivo* through human skin by using nonane as a permeation enhancer. Their results showed that nonane can increase propranolol hydrochloride bioavailability by enhanced penetration through human skin. Nonane-enhanced penetration was thought to occur by extensive barrier alteration of the SC and epidermis. In addition, the irritant properties of the enhancer decreased the barrier properties of the skin without destroying it.

E. FATTY ACIDS

Long-chain fatty acids have been shown to be effective penetrant enhancers *in vitro* for a variety of coapplied drugs.[64,73] Drugs that have shown increased skin permeability in the presence of fatty acids include naloxone,[21] betamethasone 17-benzoate,[58] mannitol and hydrocortisone,[74] nitroglycerin,[75] and acyclovir.[76] The importance of selected fatty acids as topical penetration enhancers for pharmaceuticals was reviewed recently.[77] Most reported studies on fatty acid penetration enhancers have focused on oleic acid. Aungst et al.[21] investigated the effects of linear and branched fatty acids of various chain lengths on skin permeation expecting branched isomers to disrupt membrane lipid packing. The ability of certain fatty acids to increase permeability of the skin appears to be related to a selective perturbation of the intercellular lipid bilayers present in the SC.[77] Different penetration-enhancing effects have been observed for various octadecanoic acids (C_{18}) with respect to the number of double bonds, position of double bonds, and *cis/trans* configuration of the fatty acid isomers. Among stearic, oleic, and linolenic acids, maximum enhancement was observed with linoleic acid.[21] Oleic acid treatment of the SC decreased the phase transition temperatures of the lipids, as shown by differential scanning calorimetry (DSC) and infrared spectroscopy, indicating increased motional freedom or fluidity of the lipids.[77]

F. ESTERS

Ethyl acetate[24] has been used as a permeation enhancer with drugs such as levonorgestrel, 17β-estradiol, hydrocortisone, 5-fluorouracil, and nifedipine. Methyl propionate and butyl acetate also were reported to act as permeation enhancers. The mechanism of action of ethyl acetate is unknown, however, predictions on its mechanism of permeation enhancement can be reconciled in terms of the physicochemical properties of the compound. Ethyl acetate is a polar, hydrogen-bonding compound that has a degree of water solubility, which suggests that it may act in a similar manner to the smaller polar enhancers such as DMSO and DMF.[24] These chemicals penetrate the SC and increase the lipid fluidity by forming a solvation shell around polar head groups, which leads to a disruption of lipid packing. Isopropyl myristate (IPM) has a direct action on the SC, permeating into the liposomal bilayers of the membrane. The effect was to increase fluidity of the membranes, promoting permeation of the biomolecules.[23] Aliphatic esters act mainly on lipids in the SC, increasing diffusivity in the SC and/or the partition coefficient between the SC and vehicle of both the drug and solvent.

G. AMINES AND AMIDES

1. Urea

Urea was used successfully as a penetration enhancer for several drugs. Urea is able to moisturize the skin (by hydration of the SC) and to function as a mild keratolytic after prolonged contact with the skin, possibly through an ability to split hydrogen bonds between cells in the SC.[78] Kim et al.[79] reported that hydration and pretreatment with urea in solution resulted in a greater permeability of ketoprofen, indicating that hydrophillic diffusion channels are important for ketoprofen penetration through rat skin. Urea analogues in PG enhanced the permeability of 5-fluorouracil sixfold by increasing the diffusivity of the SC in human skin.[80] A cream with 10% urea increased the water retention capacity of the SC by 100% and had little effect on the epidermal water barrier.[78] The moisturizing and keratolytic effects of urea were shown to increase the activity and bioavailability of hydrocortisone from Alphaderm® cream.[81] Wong et al.[27] reported a series of new biodegradable transdermal penetration enhancers known as cyclic ureas. Their investigations were designed to produce penetration enhancers that maintained their excellent penetration-enhancing effects with reduced toxicity. This type of penetration enhancer consists of two parts: a highly polar parent moiety that is an unsaturated cyclic urea, such as (1-alkyl-4-imidazolin-2-one)[27] and a long-chain alkyl ester group. Wong et al.[82] evaluated the penetration-enhancing effects of these substances on the transport of indomethacin in petrolatum ointment, through shed skin of the black rat snake, and reported penetration enhancement of indomethacin with three of these analogues to be comparable to or better than Azone®.

2. Dimethylacetamide and Dimethylformamide

Dimethylacetamide and DMF have been used as less potent but more acceptable alternatives to DMSO. Both DMA and DMF accelerated the skin permeation of griseofulvin,[83] betamethasone 17-benzoate in human,[58] and caffeine through isolated human SC.[84] At lower concentrations, they appear to partition preferentially into the keratin regions. At higher concentrations, they affect the lipid domains, and it has been proposed that these enhancers increase lipid fluidity.[85] In addition, at high concentrations, their mode of action may include the formation of a solvation shell around the polar head groups of lipids, thus disrupting lipid packing. Small amides such as *N,N*-DMF and *N,N*-DMA showed substantial penetration enhancement at high concentrations. Longer chain amides appear to be active at much smaller concentrations and include Azone®. A series of *n*-alkanoic *N,N*-diethylamides were used to promote the percutaneous absorption of ibuprofen and naproxen with some success.[86]

3. Pyrrolidones

Pyrrolidones are dipolar and aprotic in nature, factors of importance in their mode of action.[87] Sasaki et al.[88] reported 1-methyl-2-pyrrolidone to be a potential enhancer and have investigated various derivatized lipophilic and hydrophilic forms of 1-methyl 2-pyrrolidone with respect to their absorption enhancement and transdermal penetration of phenosulfonpthalein (phenol red) as a model (unabsorbable) drug. 1-methyl-2-pyrrolidone was used to promote penetration and to develop a reservoir of drug in the SC[1,58,89] of a variety of compounds including griseofulvin, theophylline, tetracycline, ibuprofen, and betamethasone 17-benzoate. Lambert et al.[14] presented a novel class of penetration enhancers based on fatty acid esters of *N*-(2-hydroxyethyl)-2-pyrrolidone. These derivatives represent varied lipophilicity due to the introduction of a range of functional groups. Elongation of the alkyl side chain increased the lipophilicity of pyrrolidone, and introduction of carboxy groups decreased the non-polar nature of the compound. Seki et al.[90] reported the *in vitro* permeation of azidothymidine through rat skin from an IPM solution and found a significant enhancement of permeation by adding *N*-methyl-2-pyrrolidone to the formulation. Pyrrolidone derivatives reportedly interact with both keratin in the SC[91] and with lipids in the skin structure.[92]

4. Azone®

If DMSO is considered the most extensively studied accelerant of the 1970s, Azone® was the most extensively studied of the 1980s.[7] Azone® is a novel percutaneous penetration enhancer that effectively promotes the absorption of certain drugs.[29] Azone® is a chemical combination of pyrrolidone and DCMS. It is a colorless and relatively odorless compound that causes minimal irritation to human skin. The major advantage of this compound is that it can be incorporated into a variety of topical preparations at low concentrations (in most cases, Azone® is used at a concentration of 1 to 5%) with significant accelerant effects. Azone® was reported to enhance the diffusivity of drugs such as 5-fluorouracil,[93] antibiotics, and glucocorticoids and peptides[94] through the skin. Stoughton[95] reported that Azone® can be applied undiluted to skin without significant discomfort. The safety of Azone® has been studied by Stoughton and McClure[29] and by Stoughton,[95] and elimination of Azone® from the human body appears to be safe.[96] Azone® is an effective permeation enhancer for both hydrophilic and hydrophobic drugs.[29,95] Barry and Bennett[74] suggested that Azone® is likely to be more useful for enhancing the permeability of hydrophilic compounds than for increasing the permeability of lipophilic drugs. However, Azone® did enhance skin penetration and retention of a steroid to a significant degree ($p < 0.05$).[97] Studies designed to consider the interplay of Azone®, PG, and other glycols[67,68] showed the importance of differentiating between the effect of accelerants on physicochemical factors of the formulation and the permeability characteristics of the skin. Moreover, enhancement properties can be increased further by the use of a cosolvent such as PG. Hoelgaard and Møllgaard[98] reported that Azone® enhanced the permeation of PG itself, indicating that the two components may be transported through the same pathways within the skin membrane. Differential scanning calorimetry data showed that Azone® dramatically affected the lipid structure of the SC and, being more soluble in PG than in water, was able to partition easily into the intercellular domain.[44] Beastall et al.[99] reported that the incorporation of Azone® into lipid bilayers decreased the transition temperature within the lipid bilayer, which induced the formation of a liquid phase, with a resultant increase in membrane fluidity.

Okamoto et al.[30] compared the effect of nine azacycloalkanone (five-, six-, or seven-member ring) derivatives with an alkyl or alkenyl (terpene) chain (10, 15, or 20 carbons) as potential penetration enhancers for 6-mercaptopurine (6-MP) through guinea pig skin. They found that the optimal tail chain length of an effective penetration enhancer is C_{12}. The size of the azacyclo ring had less effect on the enhancing activity than did the tail chain length. Tail chain length (C_{10} to C_{20}) has important effects on enhancing activity. This study also showed that the unsaturated tail chain has *trans* double bonds,[100] and that the enhancing effect was nearly equivalent to a saturated tail chain. *Trans* double bonds in the tail chain appear to cause less skin irritancy. Reller[101] reported that compounds with double bonds were more irritating than those with a saturated alkyl chain. The number of carbonyl groups greatly affected the enhancing activity. In addition, compounds with two carbonyl groups in the azacyclopentane ring were far less effective than the other enhancers.

Several amides and cyclic amines were prepared and investigated as *in vitro* penetration enhancers for diffusion of hydrocortisone, griseofulvin, and erythromycin through hairless mouse skin.[31] Experimental results demonstrated that extensive drug penetration can be enhanced by compounds such as hexamethylenelauramide and 1-dodecylhexahydro-2-azepin-2-one.[31]

H. TERPENES

Terpene compounds found in essential oils such as orange oil are well-established penetration enhancers for compounds into human skin.[102] A series of terpenes was assessed as skin penetration enhancers for 5-fluorouracil as a model polar drug. It was shown that both mono- and sesquiterpenes increase the percutaneous absorption of the compound, primarily by increasing drug diffusivity of the drug within the SC.[103] Differential scanning calorimetry studies indicate that increased diffusivity occurs due to disruption of the intercellular lipid barrier.[104,105] Cornwell and Barry[105] reported that treatment of human epidermis tissue with terpenoid penetration enhancers increased the electrical conductivity of the tissue, suggesting the opening of new polar pathways within and across the SC. Williams and Barry[40] studied the permeation enhancement of 5-fluorouracil in the presence of different classes of cyclic terpenes. Of the terpenes evaluated, the hydrocarbon terpenoids were least effective, oxides moderately effective, and the alcohols, ketones, and cyclic ethers most effective accelerants of 5-fluorouracil permeation.

I. SURFACE-ACTIVE AGENTS

Surfactants are frequently used in the formulation of topical products to impart improved stability and an elegance to these preparations. Surfactants adsorb at interfaces and interact with biological membranes which may contribute to the overall penetration enhancement of compounds.[106] Reports in the literature reveal that sodium lauryl sulfate (SLS) decreases the barrier function of the skin[32,33] for some permeants and various surfactants, thereby enhancing the penetration of compounds across biological membranes.[107,108]

In general, cationic surfactants are more destructive to skin tissues, causing greater increases in flux than anionic surfactants. Cationic surfactants showed a remarkable ability to increase the flux of lidocaine from saturated systems in PG–water mixtures through excised human skin *in vitro.*[109] Stoughton[95] reported greater damage and permeation enhancement with anionic surfactants than with nonionic surfactants. Gershbein[33] confirmed that cetyltrimethyl ammonium bromide (CTAB, cationic) and SLS (anionic) cause extensive damage to skin, resulting in a large increase in transdermal flux. Aoyagi et al.[34] postulated that polymerization of the surfactant, which creates a macromolecule, may reduce the irritancy potential of the enhancer by reducing its permeability. Middleton[110] proposed that anionic surfactants alter the barrier function of the SC, allowing the removal of water-soluble agents that normally act as plasticizers.

Of the three major classes of surface-active agents, nonionic surfactants are able to emulsify sebum, thereby enhancing the thermodynamic activity coefficients of drugs,[36,111] and permitting drug molecules to penetrate more effectively into the cells. Their effect on drug penetration is, in part, dependent on the ability of drug molecules to partition between the bulk phase (free form) and the micelle phase (bound form). Sarpotdar and Jatz[112] investigated the effect of two nonionic surfactants, polysorbate 20 and polysorbate 60, on the permeation of lidocaine[13] and found an increase in lidocaine penetration flux in the presence of PG concentrations up to an optimum level. Shen et al.[36] investigated the effect of 15 nonionic surfactants on the percutaneous absorption of salicylic acid and sodium salicylate in the presence of DMSO. Preparations containing 1% (w/w) of each surfactant were incorporated into white petrolatum ointment base USP containing 10% (w/w) DMSO and 10% (w/w) salicylic acid or 11.6% (w/w) sodium salicylate. The results of the study indicate that percutaneous absorption of salicylic acid was significantly enhanced by the incorporation of surfactants such as sorbitan monopalmitate, sorbitan trioleate, poloxamer 231, poloxamer 182, polyoxyethylene-4-lauryl ether, polyoxyethylene-2-oleyl ether, and polyoxyl-8-stearate into the ointment.

Bile salts such as sodium cholate and combinations of taurocholate and glycocholate recently were found to enhance the percutaneous penetration of indomethacin and the hypocalcemic peptide, elcatonin.[113,114]

J. BIODEGRADABLE PENETRATION ENHANCERS

In order to reduce both local and systemic toxicity, biodegradable penetration enhancers that have reversible action within the skin and that produce safe degradation products have been synthesized.[105] Dodecyl *N,N*-dimethylamino acetate (DDAA) is degraded by esterase catalyzed hydrolysis to *N,N*-dimethylglycine and *n*-dodecanol.[115] The presence of esterases in the epidermis and dermis of the skin ensure that local biodegradation can occur. *In vitro* diffusion studies[116,117] using human, shed snake, and rabbit pinna (ear) skin show increased permeability of these membranes to many drugs. However, the duration and extent of penetration enhancement and possible irritation of DDAA have not been studied *in vivo*. Turunen et al.[118] compared the enhancement effects of dodecyl *N,N*-dimethylamino isopropionate (DDAIP),[6] a methylated derivative of DDAA, to DDAA, oleic acid, lauryl alcohol, and Azone® with 5-fluorouracil as a model drug. Results of this study show DDAIP to be more effective as a penetration enhancer in shed snake skin than DDAA, Azone®, and other enhancers tested.

K. CYCLODEXTRINS

Several papers discuss the influence of β-cyclodextrin on the drug permeation through membranes.[119,120] Cyclodextrins are biocompatible substances consisting of cyclic oligosaccharides of six, seven, or eight glucose units: α-, β-, and γ-cyclodextrin, respectively. They are able to form inclusion complexes with lipophilic drugs and by this mechanism increase the solubility of these drugs in aqueous solutions.[121] Vollmer et al.[122] studied the effect of different concentrations of 2-hydroxypropyl-β-cyclodextrin (HPβCD) and 2,6-dimethyl-β-cyclodextrin (DIMEB) on the transdermal absorption of liarazole using an *in vivo* model. They found the concentration of liarzole in the skin to be low in a formulation containing 20% HPβCD at pH 7, whereas the concentration in the skin on application of liarzole with DIMEB and PG/oleic acid was higher.

III. CONCLUSION

The physicochemical diversity and variation in mechanisms of action of compounds investigated for their penetration enhancement effects make a simple classification scheme for percutaneous penetration enhancers difficult to set up. Perhaps a comprehensive understanding of the mechanisms by which these agents enhance drug permeation, in conjunction with their physicochemical parameters, hold the key to the development of a useful classification system.

ACKNOWLEDGMENT

The authors would like to express their gratitude to Prof. Isadore Kanfer and Dr. Eric Smith for their suggestions and ideas during editing and preparation of this manuscript.

REFERENCES

1. **Barry, B. W.,** *Dermatological Formulations: Percutaneous Absorption,* Marcel Dekker, New York, 1983, 33 and 160.
2. **Sznitowska, M., Berner, B., and Maibach, H. I.,** *In vitro* permeation of human skin by multipolar ions, *Int. J. Pharm.,* 99, 43, 1993.
3. **Banga, A. K., and Chien, Y. W.,** Iontophoretic delivery of drugs: fundamentals, developments and biomedical applications, *J. Control. Rel.,* 7, 1, 1988.
4. **Starr, C.,** Special delivery: new systems send drugs on their way, *Drug Topics,* 18, 36, 1988.
5. **Kuratomi, Y. and Miyauchi, K.,** Methods and instruments of moxibustion, U.S. Patent 4,747,841, 1988.
6. **Jacques, S. L.,** Controlled removal of human SC by pulsed laser to enhance percutaneous transport, U.S. Patent 4,775,361, 1988.
7. **Woodford, R.,** Topical penetration enhancers, *Manuf. Chem.,* 58, 49, 1987.
8. **Sloan, K. B. and Bodor, N.,** Hydroxymethyl and acyloxymethyl prodrugs of theophylline: enhanced delivery of polar drugs through skin, *Int. J. Pharm.,* 12, 299, 1982.
9. **Choi, H. K., Flynn, G. L., and Amidon, G. L.,** Transdermal delivery of bioactive peptides: the effect of N-decylmethyl sulfoxide, pH, and inhibitor on enkephalin metabolism and transport, *Pharm. Res.,* 7, 1099, 1990.
10. **Morimoto, K., Iwakura, Y., Miyazaki, M., and Nakatami, E.,** Effects of proteolytic enzyme inhibitors on enhancement of transdermal iontophoretic delivery of vasopressin and analogue in rats, *Int. J. Pharm.,* 81, 119, 1992.
11. **Mezei, M. and Gulasekharam, V.,** Liposomes — a selective drug delivery system for the topical route of administration. I. Lotion dosage form, *Life Sci.,* 26, 1473, 1980.
12. **Pfister, W. R., Dean, S., and Hsieh, S. T.,** Permeation enhancers compatible with transdermal drug delivery systems. I. Selection and formulation considerations, *Pharm. Tech.,* 8, 132, 1990.
13. **Sloan, K. B., Siver, K. G., and Koch, S. A. M.,** The effect of vehicle on the diffusion of salicylic acid through hairless mouse skin, *J. Pharm. Sci.,* 75, 744, 1986.
14. **Lambert, W. J., Kudlar, R. J., Hollard, J. M., and Curry, J. T.,** A biodegradable transdermal penetration enhancer based on N-(2-hydroxyethyl)-2-pyrrolidone. I. Synthesis and characterization, *Int. J. Pharm.,* 45, 181, 1993.
15. **Hori, M., Satoh, S., and Maibach, H. I.,** Classification of penetration enhancers: a conceptual diagram, *J. Pharm. Pharmacol.,* 42, 71, 1990.
16. **Fujita, A.,** Prediction of organic compounds by a conceptual diagram, *Chem. Pharm. Bull.,* 2, 163, 1954.
17. **Scheuplein, R. J. and Blank, I. H.,** Permeability of the skin, *Physiol. Rev.,* 51, 702, 1971.
18. **Sekura, D. L. and Scala, J.,** The percutaneous absorption of alkyl methylsulfoxides, *Adv. Biol. Skin,* 12, 257, 1988.
19. **Tsuzuki, N., Wong, O., and Higuchi, T.,** Effect of primary alcohols on percutaneous absorption, *Int. J. Pharm.,* 46, 19, 1988.
20. **Friend, D., Catz, P., Heller, J., Reid, J., and Baker, R.,** Transdermal delivery of levonorgestrel. I. Alkanols as permeation enhancers *in vitro, J. Control. Rel.,* 7, 243, 1988.

21. **Aungst, B. J., Rogers, N. J., and Shefter, E.,** Enhancement of naloxone penetration through human skin *in vitro* using fatty acids, fatty alcohols, surfactants, sulfoxides and amines, *Int. J. Pharm.*, 33, 225, 1986.
22. **Aungst, B. J.,** Structure/effect studies of fatty acid isomers as skin penetration enhancers and skin irritants, *Pharm. Res.*, 6, 244, 1989.
23. **Sato, K., Sugibayashi, K., and Morimoto, Y.,** Effect and mode of action of aliphatic esters on *in vitro* skin permeation of nicorandil, *Int. J. Pharm.*, 43, 31, 1988.
24. **Friend, D., Catz, P., Heller, J., Reid, J., and Baker, R.,** Simple alkyl esters as skin permeation enhancers, *J. Control. Rel.*, 9, 33, 1989.
25. **Møllgaard, B. and Hoelgaard, A.,** Permeation of estradiol through the skin — effect of vehicles, *Int. J. Pharm.*, 15, 185, 1983.
26. **Feldman, R. J. and Maibach, H. I.,** Percutaneous penetration, *Arch. Dermatol.*, 109, 58, 1974.
27. **Wong, O., Huntington, J., Konishi, R., Rytting, J. H., and Higuchi, T.,** Unsaturated cyclic ureas as new non-toxic biodegradable penetration transdermal penetration enhancers. I. Synthesis, *J. Pharm. Sci.*, 77, 967, 1988.
28. **Sasaki, H., Kojima, M., Mori, Y., Nakamura, J., and Shibasaki, J.,** Enhancing effects of pyrrolidone derivatives on the transdermal penetration of 5-fluorouracil, triamcinolone acetonide, indomethacin and flurbiprofen, *J. Pharm. Sci.*, 80, 533, 1991.
29. **Stoughton, R. B. and McClure, W. D.,** Azone®: a new non-toxic enhancer of percutaneous penetration, *Drug Dev. Ind. Pharm.*, 9, 725, 1983.
30. **Okamoto, H., Hashida, M., and Sezaki, H.,** Structure-activity relationship of 1-alkyl or 1-alkenylazacycloalkanone derivatives as percutaneous penetration enhancers, *J. Pharm. Sci.*, 77, 418, 1988.
31. **Mirejovsky, D. and Takruri, H.,** Dermal penetration enhancement profile of hexamethylenelauramide and its homologues: *in vitro* versus *in vivo* behaviour of enhancers in the penetration of hydrocortisone, *J. Pharm. Sci.*, 75, 1089, 1986.
32. **Chowhan, Z. T. and Pritchard, R.,** Effect of surfactants on the percutaneous absorption of naproxen. I. Comparison of rabbit, rat and human excised skin, *J. Pharm. Sci.*, 67, 1272, 1978.
33. **Gershbein, L. L.,** Percutaneous toxicity of thioglycate mixtures in rabbits, *J. Pharm. Sci.*, 68, 1230, 1979.
34. **Aoyagi, T., Terashima, O., Suzuki, N., Matsui, K., and Nagase, Y.,** Polymerization of benzalkonium chloride type monomers and application to percutaneous drug absorption enhancers, *J. Control. Rel.*, 13, 63, 1990.
35. **Tan, E. L., Liu, J. C., and Chien, Y. W.,** Effect of cationic surfactants on the transdermal permeation of ionized indomethacin, *Drug Dev. Ind. Pharm.*, 19, 685, 1993.
36. **Shen, W. W., Danti, A. G., and Bruscato, F. N.,** Effect of nonionic surfactants on percutaneous absorption of salicylic acid and sodium salicylate in the presence of dimethylsulfoxide, *J. Pharm. Sci.*, 65, 1780, 1976.
37. **Mahajour, M., Mauser, B. K., Rashidbaigi, Z. A., and Fauzi, M. B.,** Effect of propylene glycol diesters of caprylic and capric acids (Miglyol 840) and ethanol binary systems on *in vitro* skin permeation of drugs, *Int. J. Pharm.*, 95, 161, 1993.
38. **Carelli, V., Colo, D. G., Nannipieri, E., and Serafini, M. F.,** Bile acids as enhancers of steroid penetration through excised hairless mouse skin, *Int. J. Pharm.*, 89, 81, 1993.
39. **Kato, A., Ishibashi, Y., and Miyake, Y.,** Effect of egg yolk on transdermal delivery of bunazosin hydrochloride, *J. Pharm. Pharmacol.*, 39, 399, 1987.
40. **Williams, A. C. and Barry, B. W.,** Terpenes and the lipid-protein-partitioning theory of skin penetration enhancement, *Pharm. Res.*, 8, 17, 1991.
41. **Hori, M., Satoh, S., Maibach, H. I., and Guy, R. H.,** Enhancement of propranolol hydrochloride and diazepam skin absorption *in vitro:* effect of enhancer lipophilicity, *J. Pharm. Sci.*, 80, 32, 1991.
42. **Sugibayashi, K., Nemoto, M., and Morimoto, Y.,** Effect of several penetration enhancers on the percutaneous absorption of indomethacin in hairless rats, *Chem. Pharm. Bull.*, 36, 1519, 1988.
43. **Chanderasekharan, S. K. and Shaw, J. E.,** Factors influencing the percutaneous absorption of drugs, *Curr. Problems Dermatol.*, 7, 142, 1978.
44. **Barry, B. W.,** Mode of action of penetration enhancers in human skin, *J. Control. Rel.*, 6, 85, 1987.
45. **Embery, G. and Dugrad, P. H.,** The isolation of DMSO soluble components from human epidermis preparations: a possible mechanism of action of dimethylsulfoxide in effecting percutaneous migration phenomena, *J. Invest. Dermatol.*, 57, 308, 1971.

46. **Allenby, A. C., Creasy, N. H., Edington, J. A. G., Fletcher, J. A., and Schock, C.,** Mechanism of action of accelerants on skin penetration, *Br. J. Dermatol.,* 81, 47, 1969.
47. **Montes, L. F., Day, J. L., Wand, C. J., and Kennedy, L.,** Ultrastructural changes in the horny layer following local application of DMSO to guinea pig skin, *J. Invest. Dermatol.,* 48, 184, 1967.
48. **Chandrasekharan, S. K., Campbell, P. S., and Michaels, A. S.,** Effect of dimethylsulfoxide on drug permeation through human skin, *AIChE J.,* 23, 810, 1977.
49. **Stelzer, J. M., Colaizzi, J. L., and Wurdack, P. J.,** Influence of dimethylsulfoxide on the percutaneous absorption of salicylic acid and sodium salicylate from ointments, *J. Pharm. Sci.,* 57, 1732, 1968.
50. **Marcus, F., Colaizzi, J. L., and Barry, H.,** pH effects on salicylate absorption from hydrophillic ointment, *J. Pharm. Sci.,* 59, 1616, 1970.
51. **Maibach, H. I. and Feldman, R. J.,** The effect of DMSO on the percutaneous penetration of hydrocortisone and testosterone in man, *Ann. N.Y. Acad. Sci.,* 141, 423, 1967.
52. **Stuttgen, G. and Baner, E.,** Bioavailability, skin and nail penetration of topically applied antimycotics, *Mykosen,* 25, 74, 1982.
53. **Stoughton, R. B. and Fritsch, W.,** The influence of dimethylsulfoxide on human percutaneous absorption, *Arch. Dermatol.,* 90, 512, 1964.
54. **Hwang, C. C. and Danti, A. G.,** Percutaneous absorption of flufenamic acid in rabbits: effect of dimethylsulfoxide and various non-ionic surface active agents, *J. Pharm. Sci.,* 72, 857, 1983.
55. **Cooper, E. R.,** Effect of decylmethyl sulfoxide on skin penetration, in *Solution Behaviour of Surfactants,* Vol. 2, Mittal, K. L., and Fendler, J. H., Eds., Plenum Press, New York, 1982, 1505.
56. **McCullough, J. L., Snyder, D. S., Weinstein, G. D., Stein, B., and Friendland, A.,** Factors affecting human percutaneous penetration of methotrexate and its analogues *in vitro, J. Invest. Dermatol.,* 66, 103, 1976.
57. **Mitra, A. K. and Wirtanen, D. J.,** The effect of skin permeation enhancers on the transdermal delivery of pyridostigmine bromide, *Drug Dev. Ind. Pharm.,* 15, 1855, 1989.
58. **Bennett, S. L. B., Barry, B. W., and Woodford, R.,** Optimization of bioavailability of topical steroids: non-occluded penetration enhancers under thermodynamic control, *J. Pharm. Pharmacol.,* 37, 298, 1984.
59. **Durreheim, H., Flynn, G. L., Higuchi, W. I., and Behl, C. R.,** Permeation of hairless mouse skin. I. Experimental methods and comparison with human epidermal permeation by alkanols, *J. Pharm. Sci.,* 69, 781, 1980.
60. **Chien, Y. W., Xu, H., Chiang, C. C., and Hung, Y. C.,** Transdermal controlled administration of indomethacin. I. Enhancement of skin permeability, *Pharm. Res.,* 5, 103, 1988.
61. **William, R. G., Marilou, S. P., Patricia, C., and Lotte, S. A.,** New transdermal delivery system for estradiol, *J. Control. Rel.,* 2, 89, 1985.
62. **Gale, R. M., Lee, E. S., Taskovich, L. T., and Yum, S. I.,** U.S. Patent 4,588,580, 1986.
63. **Ghosh, T. K. and Banga, A. K.,** Methods of enhancement of transdermal drug delivery. IIA. Chemical permeation enhancers, *Pharm. Tech.,* 17, 62, 1993.
64. **Cooper, E. R.,** Increased skin permeability for lipophilic molecules, *J. Pharm. Sci.,* 73, 1153, 1984.
65. **Lorenzetti, O. J.,** Propylene glycol gel vehicles, *Cutis,* 23, 747, 1979.
66. **Møllgaard, B. and Hoelgaard, A.,** Vehicle effect on topical drug delivery. I. Influence of glycols and drug concentrations on skin transport, *Acta Pharm. Suec.,* 20, 433, 1983.
67. **Wotton, P. K., Møllgaard, B., Hadgraft, J., and Hoelgaard, A.,** Vehicle effect on topical drug delivery. II. Effect of azone on the cutaneous permeation of metronidazole and propylene glycol, *Int. J. Pharm.,* 24, 19, 1985.
68. **Seth, N. V., Freedman, D. J., Higuchi, W. I., and Spruance, S. L.,** The influence of azone, propylene glycol, and polyethylene glycol on *in vitro* skin penetration of trifluorothymidine, *Int. J. Pharm.,* 28, 201, 1986.
69. **Woodford, R. and Barry, B. W.,** Optimization of bioavailability of topical steroids: thermodynamic control, *J. Invest. Dermatol.,* 79, 388, 1982.
70. **Vaidyanathan, R., Chaubl, M. G., and Vasavada, R. C.,** Effect of pH and solubility on *in vitro,* skin penetration of methotrexate from a 50% v/v propylene glycol-water vehicle, *Int. J. Pharm.,* 25, 85, 1985.
71. **Touitou, E.,** Transdermal delivery of anxiolytics: *in vitro* skin permeation of midazolam maleate and diazepam, *Int. J. Pharm.,* 33, 37, 1986.

72. **Melendres, J. L., Nangia, A., Sedik, A., Hori, M., and Maibach, H. I.,** Nonane enhancers propranolol hydrochloride penetration in human skin, *Int. J. Pharm.,* 92, 243, 1993.
73. **Akhter, S. A. and Barry, B. W.,** Penetration enhancers in human skin: effect of oleic acid and azone on flurbiprofen permeation, *J. Pharm. Pharmacol.,* 36, 7, 1984.
74. **Barry, B. W. and Bennett, S. L.,** Effect of penetration enhancers on the permeation of mannitol, hydrocortisone and progesterone through human skin, *J. Pharm. Pharmacol.,* 39, 535, 1987.
75. **Loftsson, T., Gildersleeve, N., and Bodor, N.,** The effect of vehicle additives on the transdermal delivery of nitroglycerin, *Pharm. Res.,* 4, 436, 1987.
76. **Cooper, E. R., Merritt, E. W., and Smith, R. L.,** The effect of fatty acids and alcohols on the penetration of acyclovir, *J. Pharm. Sci.,* 74, 688, 1985.
77. **Golden, G. M., McKie, J. E., and Potts, R. O.,** Role of *SC,* lipid fluidity in transdermal drug flux, *J. Pharm. Sci.,* 76, 25, 1987.
78. **Grice, K., Sattar, H., and Baker, H.,** Urea and retinoic acid in icthyosis and their effect on transepidermal water loss and water holding capacity of *SC, Acta Dermatol.,* 53, 114, 1973.
79. **Kim, C. K., Kim, J. J., Chi, S. C., and Shim, C. K.,** Effect of fatty acids and urea on the penetration of ketoprofen through rat skin, *Int. J. Pharm.,* 99, 109, 1993.
80. **Williams, A. C. and Barry, B. W.,** Urea analogues in propylene glycol as penetration enhancers in human skin, *Int. J. Pharm.,* 36, 43, 1989.
81. **Woodford, R. and Barry, B. W.,** Alphaderm cream (1% hydrocortisone plus 10% urea). I. Investigation of vasoconstrictor activity, bioavailability and application regimens in human volunteers, *Curr. Ther. Res.,* 35, 759, 1984.
82. **Wong, O., Tsuziki, N., Nghiem, B., Kuehnhoff, J., Itoh, T., Masaki, K., Huntington, J., Konish, R., Rytting, J. H., and Higuchi, T.,** Unsaturated cyclic ureas as new non-toxic biodegradable transdermal penetration enhancers. II. Evaluation study, *Int. J. Pharm.,* 52, 191, 1989.
83. **Monro, D. D. and Stoughton, R. B.,** Dimethylacetamide (DMAC) and dimethylformamide (DMFA): effect on percutaneous absorption, *Arch. Dermatol.,* 92, 585, 1965.
84. **Southwell, D. and Barry, B. W.,** Penetration enhancers for human skin: mode of action of 2-pyrrolidone and dimethylformamide on partition and diffusion of model compounds water, n-alcohols and caffeine, *J. Invest. Dermatol.,* 80, 507, 1983.
85. **Barry, B. W.,** Mode of action of penetration enhancers on the kinetics of percutaneous absorption, *J. Control. Rel.,* 5, 43, 1987.
86. **Irwin, W. J., Sanderson, F. D., and Wan Po, A. L.,** Percutaneous absorption of ibuprofen and naproxen: effect of amide enhancers on transport through rat skin, *Int. J. Pharm.,* 66, 243, 1990.
87. **Hadgraft, J.,** Penetration enhancers in percutaneous absorption, *Pharm. Int.,* 17, 252, 1984.
88. **Sasaki, H., Kojima, M., Mori, Y., Nakamura, J., and Shibasaki, J.,** Enhancing effect of pyrrolidine derivatives on transdermal drug delivery. I., *Int. J. Pharm.,* 44, 15, 1988.
89. **Akhter, S. A. and Barry, B. W.,** Absorption through human skin of ibuprofen and flurbiprofen: effect of dose variation, deposited drug films, occlusion and the penetration enhancer N-methyl-2-pyrrolidone, *J. Pharm. Pharmacol.,* 37, 27, 1985.
90. **Seki, T., Kawaguchi, T., Sugibayashi, K., Juni, K., and Morimoto, Y.,** Percutaneous absorption of azidothymidine in rats, *Int. J. Pharm.,* 57, 73, 1989.
91. **Barry, B. W.,** Transdermal drug delivery, in *Drug Delivery Systems: Fundamentals and Techniques,* Johnson, P. and Lloyd-Jones, J. G., Eds., Ellis Horwood, Chichester, U.K., 1987, 200.
92. **Kim, C. K., Hong, M. S., Kim, Y. B., and Han, S. K.,** Effect of penetration enhancers (pyrrolidone derivatives) on multilamellar liposomes of *SC* lipids: a study by UV spectroscopy and differential scanning calorimetry, *Int. J. Pharm.,* 95, 43, 1993.
93. **Stoughton, R. B.,** Enhanced percutaneous penetration with 1-dodecylazocycloheptan-2-one, *Arch. Dermatol.,* 118, 474, 1982.
94. **Bodde, H. E., Verhoef, J. C., and Ponec, M.,** Transdermal peptide delivery, *Biochem. Soc. Trans.,* 17, 943, 1980.
95. **Stoughton, R. B.,** Azone® (1-dodecylazacycloheptan-2-one) enhances percutaneous penetration, in *Psoriasis,* Faber, E. M., Ed., Grune & Stratton, Orlando, FL, 1982, 346.
96. **Wiechers, J. W., Drenth, B. F. H., Jonkman, J. H. G., and De Zeeuw, R. A.,** Percutaneous absorption and elimination of the penetration enhancer Azone® in humans, *Pharm. Res.,* 4, 519, 1987.

97. **Michniak, B. B., Chapman, J. M., and Seyda, K. L.,** Facilitated transport of two model steroids by esters and amides of clofibric acid, *J. Pharm. Sci.,* 82, 214, 1993.
98. **Hoelgaard, A., and Møllgaard, B.,** Dermal drug delivery — improvement by choice of vehicle or drug derivative, *J. Control. Rel.,* 2, 111, 1985.
99. **Beastall, J. C., Hadgraft, J., and Washington, C.,** Mechanism of action of azone as a percutaneous penetration enhancer: lipid bilayer fluidity and transition temperature effects, *Int. J. Pharm.,* 43, 207, 1988.
100. **Okamoto, H., Makiko, O., Hashida, M., and Sezaki, H.,** Enhanced penetration of mitomycin-c through hairless mouse and rat skin by enhancers with terpene moieties, *J. Pharm. Pharmacol.,* 39, 531, 1987.
101. **Reller, H. H.,** in *Safety and Efficacy of Topical Drugs and Cosmetics,* Kligman, A. M. and Leyden, J. J., Eds., Grune & Stratton, New York, 1982, 311.
102. **Cornwell, P. A. and Barry, B. W.,** The routes of penetration of ions and 5-fluorouracil across human skin and the mechanisms of action of terpene skin penetration enhancers, *Int. J. Pharm.,* 94, 189, 1993.
103. **Cornwell, P. A. and Barry, B. W.,** The mechanism of action of sesquiterpene skin penetration enhancers, *J. Pharm. Pharmacol.,* 43, 56, 1991.
104. **Williams, A. C. and Barry, B. W.,** Differential scanning calorimetry does not predict the activity of terpene penetration enhancers in human skin, *J. Pharm. Pharmacol.,* 42, 156, 1990.
105. **Cornwell, P. A. and Barry, B. W.,** The effects of a series of homologous terpene alcohols on the lipid structure of human *SC* as assessed by differential scanning calorimetry, in *Prediction of Percutaneous Absorption,* Vol. 2, Scott, R. C., Guy, R. H., Hadgraft, J., and Boddé, H. E., Eds., IBC Technical Services, London, 1992, 394.
106. **Ashton, P., Hadgraft, J., Brian, K. R., Miller, T. A., and Walters, K. A.,** Surfactant effects in topical drug availability, *Int. J. Pharm.,* 41, 189, 1988.
107. **Riegelman, S. and Crowell, W. J.,** Kinetics of rectal absorption. I. Preliminary investigation into absorption rate processes, *Am. J. Pharm. Assoc. Sci. Ed.,* 47, 115, 1958.
108. **Riegelman, S. and Crowell, W. J.,** Kinetics of rectal absorption. II. The absorption of anions, *Am. J. Pharm. Assoc. Sci. Ed.,* 47, 123, 1958.
109. **Kushla, G. P., Zatz, J. L., Mills, O. H., Jr., and Berger, R. S.,** Non-invasive assessment of anaesthetic activity of topical lidocaine formulations, *J. Pharm. Sci.,* 82, 1118, 1993.
110. **Middleton, J. D.,** Mechanism of action of surfactants on water binding properties of isolated *SC, J. Soc. Cosmet. Chem.,* 20, 399, 1969.
111. **Higuchi, T.,** Physical Chemical Analysis of Percutaneous Absorption Processes from Creams and Ointments, presented at The Society of Cosmetic Chemists Seminar, New York, September 1959.
112. **Sarpotdar, P. P. and Jatz, J. L.,** Evaluation of penetration enhancement of lidocaine by non-ionic surfactants through hairless mouse skin *in vitro, J. Pharm. Sci.,* 72, 176, 1986.
113. **Chiang, C. H., Lai, J. S., and Yang, K. H.,** The effects of pH and chemical enhancers on the percutaneous absorption of indomethacin, *Drug Dev. Ind. Pharm.,* 17, 91, 1991.
114. **Ogiso, T., Iwaki, M., Yoneda, I., Horinouchi, M., and Yamashita, K.,** Percutaneous absorption of elcatonin and hypocalcemic effect in rat, *Chem. Pharm. Bull.,* 39, 449, 1991.
115. **Buyuktimkin, N., Buyuktimkin, S., and Rytting, J. H.,** Stability of several alkyl N,N-dimethylamino acetates having potential as biodegradable transdermal penetration enhancers, *Pharm. Res. (Suppl.),* 8, S-139, 1991.
116. **Martin, R. J., Denyer, S. P., and Hadgraft, J.,** Skin metabolism of topically applied compounds, *Int. J. Pharm.,* 39, 23, 1987.
117. **Hirvonen, J., Rytting, J. H., and Paronen, P.,** Dodecyl N,N-dimethylamino acetate and azone enhances drug penetration across human, snake and rabbit skin, *Pharm. Res.,* 8, 933, 1991.
118. **Turunen, T. M., Buyuktimkin, S., Buyktimkin, N., Urtti, A., Paronen, P., and Rytting, J. H.,** Enhanced delivery of 5-fluorouracil through shed snake skin by two new transdermal penetration enhancers, *Int. J. Pharm.,* 92, 89, 1993.
119. **Uekama, K., Otagiri, M., Sakai, A., Irie, T., Matsuo, N., and Matsuoka, Y.,** Improvement in the percutaneous absorption of beclomethasone dipropionate by γ-cyclodextrin complexation, *J. Pharm. Pharmacol.,* 37, 532, 1985.

120. **Frijlink, H. W., Schoonen, A. J. M., and Lerk, C. F.,** The effect of cyclodextrins on drug absorption. I. *In vitro* observations, *J. Pharm. Sci.,* 65, 709, 1976.
121. **Uekama, K., Fujinaga, T., Hirayama, F., Otagiri, M., and Yamasaki, M.,** Inclusion complexations of steroid hormones with cyclodextrins in water and in solid phase, *Int. J. Pharm.,* 10, 1, 1982.
122. **Vollmer, U., Muller, B. W., Mesens, J., Wilffert, B., and Peters, T.,** *In vivo* skin pharmacokinetics of liarozole: percutaneous absorption studies with different formulations of cyclodextrin derivatives in rats, *Int. J. Pharm.,* 99, 51, 1993.

Chapter 2.1

Penetration Enhancement by Skin Hydration

Ronald C. Wester and Howard I. Maibach

CONTENTS

"All day I faced the barren waste without the taste of water, cool clear water — water."

I. INTRODUCTION

Evolution has created a highly specialized skin in animals and humans, whose fluids and precious chemicals are reasonably retained within the body. Skin also is sufficiently flexible and elastic to permit freedom of movement. However, the skin is not a perfect barrier to the environment. *In vivo* a continuous diffusion of water occurs from within the body through the stratum corneum (SC) and into the environment, the transepidermal water loss. This is passive diffusion, and it occurs because of the water concentration gradient in the SC. At any one relative humidity, a water concentration gradient is established *in vivo* such that the concentrations of water in the various layers of the SC differ, but each remains relatively constant. Because of the gradient, water will still move through the tissue and into the environment.[1] The reverse procedure also occurs in that water applied to the environment side of skin can be absorbed through skin into the body. The average permeability coefficient for water is 1.55×10^{-3} cm/h.[2]

Thus, skin is a hydrated tissue with passive but continual water diffusion dependent upon water concentration gradient. This water concentration gradient can be influenced. The question we will try to answer is: can this water system be sufficiently influenced such that water can be classified as an "enhancer" of percutaneous absorption? Discrimination should be made as to whether the test study results are due to skin damage or if the tissue remains intact.

A. INFLUENCE OF HYDRATION

Water plays an extremely important role in the rate of absorption of materials through the skin and can act as a common vehicle and the endogenous plasticizer of the SC. Under normal conditions the SC is always partially hydrated. A gradient in water

0-8493-2605-2/95/$0.00+$.50

concentration exists through the tissue corresponding to an average water concentration of approximately 0.9 g/g dry tissue weight. This amount of water in *in vitro* studies increases the rate of absorption of the SC approximately tenfold over its value when perfectly dry.[3] Upon additional contact with liquid water, the SC can ultimately absorb three to five times its own weight in water. This further hydration results in an additional approximate two- to threefold increase in the rate of absorption to water and other polar molecules. The increase in steroid absorption is observed *in vitro* when water vapor is allowed to come into contact with dry SC having a surface deposit of cortisone. The initial rate of absorption (J_s) with "dry" SC was 2.64×10^{-11}.[3] The introduction of water vapor increased the rate to 3.62×10^{-10}, a logarithmic increase in rate of absorption. The reintroduction of drierite and subsequent decrease in water content decreased the rate to 2.7×10^{-11}.

Stoughton[4] studied the *in vivo* and *in vitro* rates of absorption of ethyl nicotinate for skin hydrated by warm or cold water immersion. Excised human skin was mounted over a well containing saline and the SC of the epidermis remained exposed to the air. Ethyl nicotinate labeled with ^{14}C was applied to the epidermal surface and the rate of appearance of radioactivity in the saline below was taken as the rate of absorption of ethyl nicotinate. Table 1 indicates that hydrated skin allowed about five times as much ethyl nicotinate to pass through skin not previously hydrated. Table 2 expresses results obtained when determining the minimum concentration of ethyl nicotinate necessary to produce erythema on the forearms of human volunteers. One forearm was previously soaked in warm or cool water for 30 min before the application of graded concentrations of ethyl nicotinate. The nonhydrated arm required about five to ten times the concentration of ethyl nicotinate to reproduce erythema as did the hydrated arm. Stoughton concluded that the increased rate of absorption with hydration caused the clinical changes in the epidermis.

Piotrowski[5] studied the effects of temperature and humidity on the rate of absorption of nitrobenzene vapor through skin. Table 3 shows the influence of humidity on the rate of absorption of nitrobenzene. With the temperature kept constant at 25°C, a 35 to 67% increase in humidity increased the rate of absorption of nitrobenzene through human skin from 0.25 to 0.38 mg/h. Thus, the humidity (water vapor) increased the rate of absorption of nitrobenzene.

Wurster and Kramer[6] measured the rate of absorption of acetylsalicylic acid through skin. When the tissue was hydrated, the rate of absorption of the most water-soluble ester increased more than that of the other esters studied. This work was extended by Fritz and Stoughton.[7] Full hydration of the keratin (accomplished by layering water over acetylsalicylic acid on the epidermal surface) dramatically increased the rate of absorption when compared to conditions of lower humidity at the same temperature.

The early work of McKenzie and Stoughton[8] show the importance of hydration on skin by employing occlusive plastic film in corticosteroid therapy. They showed that the degree of vasoconstriction of corticoids could be increased substantially by occluding the site of application. This prevents the loss of water vapor from the skin and thus hydrates the SC. Vehicles may also affect skin penetration by their ability to reduce water vapor loss from the skin surface. Of the common vehicles, paraffin bases have shown the greatest effect on suppressing a transepidermal water diffusion.

Table 1 Percent Penetration of Ethyl Nicotinate Following Hydration of the Skin (30-min period for penetration)

	No.	Penetration Average (%)
Warm water	4	5.80
Cold water	4	5.88
Control	8	0.98

Table 2 *In Vivo* Hydration of Human Skin Factor Difference in Endpoint Concentrations of Ethyl Nicotinate Giving Erythema on Hydrated vs. Nonhydrated Arm

Warm Water Hydration (30 min; *n* = 22)		
Hydrated arm average	0.0017	Factor difference = 12
Nonhydrated arm average	0.02	
Cool Water Hydration (30 min; *n* = 15)		
Hydrated arm average	0.003	Factor difference = 6
Nonhydrated arm average	0.02	

Note: Endpoint pharmacodynamic data must not be assumed to directly equate to penetration.

Table 3 Effects of Temperature and Humidity on the Absorption of Nitrobenzene Vapor Through the Skin

No. of experiments	Temperature (°C)	Humidity (%)	Absorbed rate/ U conc (mg/h:μg/l)
3	25	35	0.25
3	30	25	0.22
4	25	67	0.38

Most vehicles develop a high degree of occlusion and thus increase the rate of absorption of materials.

Behl and co-workers[9] studied the influence of hydration on alkanol permeation through hairless mouse skin. The skin was immersed in saline for up to 30 h and a steady-state rate permeation was established in several minutes. These circumstances allowed multiple sequential runs over a period in which the permeability coefficients of some chemicals were gradually changing. The permeability of water, methanol, and ethanol was slightly affected by hydration. However, the permeability coefficient of butanol and hexanol doubled during the first 10 h of immersion. More hydrophobic alkanols seem to be less sensitive to the aqueous conditioning.

Behl and Barrett[10] examined the possible effects of hydration on the barrier integrity of Swiss mouse skin using water, methanol, ethanol, and butanol as permeants, and the previously described procedure involving multiple sequential permeation

Table 4 Diffusivity of Water in SC as a Function of Its Water Content

Relative humidity (%)	Water content, c_m (g/cm^3)	Diffusivity, D ($\times 10^{10}$ cm^2/s)		
		Subject A	Subject B	Subject C
46	0.096	3.19	3.19	2.50
62	0.127	4.30	3.52	2.93
81	0.194	9.26	9.57	4.01
93	0.358	8.11	8.34	3.77

runs on skin. The permeation rate of water increased almost linearly up to 30 h of hydration, then tended to level off. Transport rates of methanol and ethanol increased, and then plateaued at about 15 h. These results conflict with the earlier findings of hairless mouse skin, in which the permeability of these three compounds was unaffected by aqueous immersion. The permeation rate of butanol also increased during the first 15 h of hydration, then gradually declined over the next 25 h. The results again conflict with the hairless mouse species in which butanol permeability doubled in 10 h and then plateaued.

The diffusivity of water in the SC is a function of its water content, which is related to relative humidity (and by extension to water content in the environment). This is shown by Blank[1] in Table 4. Note the simple elegance of relating *in vivo* the external environment (humidity) with water SC content and diffusivity. This contrasts to the previous studies of Behl et al.,[9,10] in which skin is subjected to water for 30 h or more, which questions the integrity of the skin during these studies.

Table 5 is from Barry,[11] which puts skin hydration and skin permeability in terms of pharmaceutical usage. Transdermal patches and occlusive dressings fully hydrate skin and show marked increases in permeability. This simply underlines how skin hydration is manipulated pharmaceutically to produce enhanced skin permeability. The pharmaceutical endpoint is to produce these positive drug delivery effects without risk of injury to skin (and a poor product).

B. WATER PERMEABILITY AND HAZARDOUS METALS

Table 6 gives the *in vitro* percutaneous absorption of cadmium from water through human skin. At the lower water vehicle volume of 2.5 μl/cm^2 the plasma receptor fluid accumulation (absorbed dose) was 0.1 to 0.2% dose, and the skin content was 2.4 to 3.2% dose. When the water vehicle volume was increased to 5 μl/cm^2 the plasma receptor fluid accumulation increased to 0.5 to 0.6% dose and skin content increased to 8.8 to 12.7% dose. This suggests that percutaneous absorption of cadmium may be dependent on water volume, and, as an extension in logic, to a dependency on water movement within skin.[12]

Figure 1 gives receptor fluid accumulation of mercury during *in vitro* percutaneous absorption with human skin. Topical treatments include increasing volumes of surface water (10, 100, and 1000 μl) and the amount of mercury was constant for each dosing (micrograms per square centimeter). Thus, the only variable was the volume of water, and higher water volume gave the higher amount of mercury skin absorption.

Table 5 Usual Effects of Common Vehicles on Skin Hydration and Skin Permeability, in Order of Decreasing Hydration

Vehicle	Examples/constituents	Effect on skin hydration	Effect on skin permeability
Transdermal patch	Impermeable backing layer	Prevents water loss; full hydration	Marked increase
Occlusive dressing	Plastic film, unperforated waterproof plaster	Prevents water loss, full hydration	Marked increase
Lipophilic	Paraffins, oils, fats, waxes, fatty acids, alcohols, esters	Prevents water loss, may produce full hydration	Marked increase
Absorption base	Anhydrous lipid material plus water/oil emulsifiers	Prevents water loss; marked hydration	Marked increased
Emulsifying base	Anhydrous lipid material plus oil/water emulsifiers	Prevents water loss; marked hydration	Marked increase
Water-in-oil emulsion	Oily creams	Retards water loss; raised hydration	Increase
Oil-in-water emulsion	Aqueous creams	May donate water; slight hydration increase	Slight increase?
Humectant	Water-soluble bases, glycerol, glycols	May withdraw water; decrease hydration	Can decrease or act as penetration enhancer
Powder	Clays, organics, inorganics, "shake" lotions	Aid water evaporation; decreased excess hydration	Little effect on SC

Table 6 *In Vitro* Percutaneous Absorption of Cadmium from Water through Human Skin

Skin source	Human plasma receptor fluid	Skin	Surface wash	Total
	Percentage applied dose			
	Water, 5 μl/cm²			
1	0.5 ± 0.2	8.8 ± 0.6	93 ± 3	103 ± 3
2	0.6 ± 0.6	12.7 ± 11.7	74 ± 11	88 ± 20
	Water, 2.5 μl/cm²			
3	0.2 ± 0.2	2.4 ± 1.6	86 ± 3	89 ± 3
4	0.1 ± 0.04	3.2 ± 4.4	88 ± 13	92 ± 12

Note: $n = 3$ replicates per skin source. Exposure time, 16 h. Cadmium as 116 ppb in water.

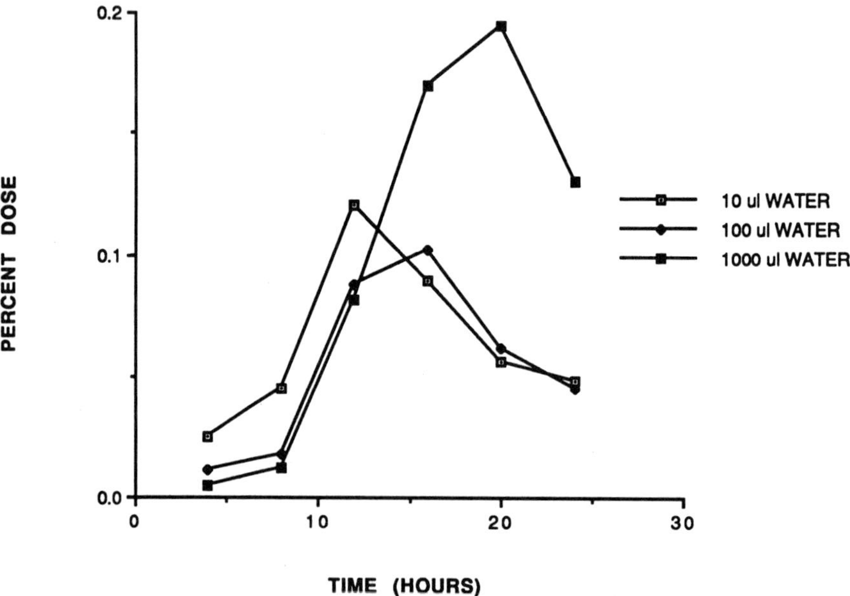

Figure 1 With mercury dose concentration equal per unit of skin area, an increase in surface water volume per unit of skin area caused an increase in mercury percutaneous absorption through human skin. It is hypothesized that water acts as a solvent to mercury.

Thus, with both cadmium and mercury, indications are dependent on surface water volume. The larger surface water volume probably shifts the direction of water movement and the metal follows the water. Here, water acts as a solvent.

C. WATER AND PERCUTANEOUS ABSORPTION FROM CLOTH

Table 7 shows part of a study to determine percutaneous absorption of chemicals from cloth into and through human skin. Glyphosate as a 1% water solution was

Table 7 Percutaneous Absorption of Glyphosate from Cotton Cloth into Human Skin: Influence of Water

Donor conditions	Treatment	Dose absorbed (%)
1% solution	None	1.4 ± 0.2
Cotton–solution	0 d	0.7 ± 0.3
Cotton–solution	1 d	0.08 ± 0.01
Cotton–solution	Add water	0.4 ± 0.1

dosed on human skin and percutaneous absorption was 1.4 ± 0.2% dose absorbed. When the glyphosate was dosed on cotton sheets and the dosed cotton sheet was placed on skin, absorption decreased to 0.7 ± 0.3%. Letting the cotton/glyphosate air dry for 1 d further reduced absorption to 0.08 ± 0.01%. Adding water to the dried cotton/glyphosate sheet "activated" the glyphosate and increased absorption back to 0.4 ± 0.1%. Here, water appears to be acting as an external solvent and as a solvent it influences the percutaneous absorption.

II. OCCLUSION

The early work of Feldmann and Maibach conclusively showed that occlusion enhances percutaneous absorption, and that this enhanced absorption was in part due to increased humidity under the occluding cover. This dogma was accepted universally until Bucks[14] showed that this may not apply to all compounds in all situations. In the Bucks study occlusion significantly enhanced the percutaneous absorption of estradiol, testosterone, and progesterone, but not that of hydrocortisone (the Feldmann-Maibach study showed enhanced hydrocortisone absorption with occlusion). The only known difference in study design was that in the Bucks study occlusion was for 24 h, while in the Feldmann-Maibach study occlusion was for many days.

Twenty-four hour occlusion would be more typical in clinical utilization in dermatologic therapy. We suspect that the biology and biophysics of occlusion have not been fully defined. Perhaps the dramatic enhancement noted with vasoconstriction of corticoids and occlusion could be related to shunts in skin activated by occlusion, but not of sufficient bulk to provide increased urinary excretion (where endpoint analysis takes place to determine *in vivo* bioavailability).

III. DISCUSSION

Water-soluble extractive substances compromise 20 to 42% of normal SC by weight. The strongly hydroscopic properties of these water-soluble compounds suggest a prominent role for them in regulating the water content of SC cells. The removal of some of the substances following excessive exposure to water may compromise barrier cell permeability. Excessive water uptake may further impede barrier function in the SC by facilitating intracellular passage through otherwise tightly packed keratin and perhaps by inducing swelling or even bursting of cell membranes. Also, the enhanced water content of extracellular nucleopolysaccharide substances might impair intracellular adhesiveness. Certainly the gross irritability of the SC is significantly increased by excessive hydration.[13]

Our definition of the function of an enhancer is that (A) the chemical acts as a solvent, or (B) the chemical causes a physical change within skin, or a combination of A and B. Water certainly acts as a solvent, and water occupies a unique situation in which this solvent already exists within the skin where transport takes place. Thus, the enhancement occurs by altering the water concentration gradient that exists between the skin and the environment. As to water causing physical changes to skin, the system certainly can be pushed *in vitro* (studies over periods of days) and *in vivo* (excessive occlusion) where at least the physical appearance of skin is changed. This seems to be due more to extreme external or study conditions; the system fails as would be expected for any living tissue. Thus, water can be classified as an enhancer with solvent function, which retains the natural integrity of the skin within a "normal" use system.

During the Vietnam War, great morbidity occurred in booted soldiers' feet ("paddy foot"). Although a booted foot involves a complex interaction of more substances than just water, the latter has been considered critical in initiating this form of damage. Much of the U.S. Army's studies in this area were not published, yet it is clear that a reasonable model exists, i.e., the patch chamber with excess water for a week or so induces frank dermatitis. The implication for water-percutaneous penetration studies appears obvious.

REFERENCES

1. **Blank, I. H.,** The effect of hydration on the permeability of the skin, in *Percutaneous Absorption,* 1st ed., Bronaugh, and Maibach, H. I., Eds., Marcel Dekker, New York, 1985, 97.
2. Dermal Exposure Assessment: Principles and Applications, EPA/600/8–91/011B, 1992, Environmental Protection Agency, Washington, D.C., 97.
3. **Scheuplein, R. J.,** Site variations and permeability, in *The Physiology and Pathophysiology of the Skin,* Vol. 5, Jarrett, A. Ed., Academic Press, New York, 1978, 1731.
4. **Stoughton, R. B.,** Percutaneous absorption, *Arch. Environ. Health,* 11, 551, 1965.
5. **Piotrowski, J.,** Further investigations on the evaluation of exposure to nitrobenzene, *Br. J. Ind. Med.,* 24, 60, 1967.
6. **Wurster, D. E. and Kramer, S. F.,** Investigation of some factors influencing percutaneous absorption, *J. Pharm. Sci.,* 50, 288, 1961.
7. **Fritz, W. C. and Stoughton, R. B.,** The effect of temperature and humidity on the penetration of acetylsalicylic acid in excised human skin, *J. Invest. Dermatol.,* 41, 307, 1963.
8. **McKenzie, A. W. and Stoughton, R. B.,** Method for comparing percutaneous absorption of steroids, *Arch. Dermatol.,* 86, 608, 1962.
9. **Behl, C. R., Flynn, G. L., Kurihara, T., Harper, N., Smith, W., Higushi, W. I., Ho, N. F. H., and Pierson, C. L.,** Hydration and percutaneous absorption. I. Influence of hydration on alkanol permeation through hairless mouse skin, *J. Invest. Dermatol.,* 75, 346, 1980.
10. **Behl, C. R. and Barrett, M.,** Hydration and percutaneous absorption. II. Influence of hydration on water and alkanol permeation through Swiss mouse skin; comparison with hairless mouse, *J. Pharm. Sci.,* 10, 1212, 1981.
11. **Barry, B. W.,** Vehicle effect: what is an enhancer?, in *Topical Drug Bioavailability, Bioequivalence, and Penetration,* Shah, and Maibach, H. I., Eds., Plenum Press, New York, 1993, 261.
12. **Wester, R. C., Maibach, H. I., Sedik, L., Melendres, J., DiZio, S., and Wade, M.,** *In vitro* percutaneous absorption of cadmium from water and soil into human skin, *Fund. Appl. Toxicol.,* 19, 1, 1992.
13. **Malkinson, F. D.,** Industrial problems relating to the SC, *Arch. Environ. Health,* 11, 538, 1965.
14. **Bucks, D. A. W.,** Predictive approaches. II. Mass balance procedure, in *Topical Drug Bioavailability, Bioequivalence and Penetration,* Shah, and Maibach, H. I., Eds., Plenum Press, New York, 1993, 183.

Chapter 2.2

Hydration and Topical Corticosteroid Absorption

John M. Haigh and Eric W. Smith

CONTENTS

I. INTRODUCTION

It has been known for many years that increasing the permeability of the stratum corneum (SC) may be achieved by simply increasing the water content of this tissue.[1,2] Although the precise mechanism by which penetration is improved is still unclear, hydration by occlusion is known to cause a swelling of the corneocytes, to increase the amount of water associated with the intercellular lipid domains, and to increase the temperature of the occlusion site. Of all the methods of enhancing the penetration of corticosteroids, hydration of the skin (by preventing transepidermal water loss) is by far the most innocuous and the most physiological that causes minimal toxicity or irritancy under normal circumstances. Hydration is totally and rapidly reversible and thus has no prolonged effects on the barrier condition of the skin. These features make simple occlusion an attractive and safe method of enhancing the transdermal delivery of drugs. In cases in which increasing the water content of the SC will not sufficiently improve the transdermal delivery of the corticoid to achieve therapeutic concentrations, other methods of percutaneous penetration enhancement, often in addition to the hydration, are necessary.[3]

II. STRATUM CORNEUM HYDRATION AND TRANSDERMAL DIFFUSION

The precise effects that hypernormal hydration states have on the barrier structure of the SC have been the focus of much recent research.[4,5] It is now understood that the principal route of chemical penetration is through the lamellar interkeratinocyte lipid matrix and that the biochemistry of this domain controls the magnitude of the barrier to penetration.[6,7] The SC is always partially hydrated *in vivo* (5 to 15%), the degree of hydration being dependent on the composition of the lipoprotein environment and on the ambient conditions. The water content of the SC may be increased up to 50% with impervious occlusion. Although it was initially thought that additional water may simply increase the size of pores in the membrane,[8] recent research has shown that a more complex relationship may exist between the water content of the

0-8493-2605-2/95/$0.00+$.50

intercellular lipid bilayers and their resultant fluidity or disorder,[9] the latter directly influencing the ease with which drugs can permeate the skin. Alternatively, it was suggested that hydration may induce lipid phase separation, or that the influence of water on other structures within the SC (such as the intracellular keratin) may be more influential in enhancing penetration.[10] It should be mentioned that occlusion of the application sites will also prevent accidental removal of the applied drug by abrasion or exfoliation, and may thereby assist in improving drug delivery to the skin by maintaining a maximal concentration gradient across the tissue.

A. CORTICOSTEROID ABSORPTION *IN VIVO*

Occlusion has been used for almost 4 decades to enhance the absorption of anti-inflammatory corticosteroids from topical delivery vehicles.[11] This nonphysiological hydration was easily induced by employing occluding vehicles, such as ointments, which prevent the evaporation of transpirational moisture from the skin due to their lipophilic nature.[12] Simple plastic wrap or more sophisticated hydrocolloid dressings applied over the corticosteroid formulation appear to be even more successful in trapping water under the application site, and thereby enhancing penetration of the corticosteroid.[13–15]

McKenzie and Stoughton[16] investigated the effect of occlusion on corticosteroid absorption by using their early version of the human skin blanching (or vasoconstriction) assay. They showed that the concentrations of corticoid required to induce topical skin blanching were 100 times smaller when external occlusion was used as compared to nonoccluded application. It was also found that some agents would only demonstrate vasoactive properties when occlusion was used.[17] It appears that a minimum occlusion time of 3 h is required for skin blanching[18] and that maximum blanching is observed after a 10-h occlusion period.[19] Furthermore, Feldmann and Maibach[20] showed that percutaneous hydrocortisone penetration into systemic circulation increased tenfold under occlusion. These observations serve to emphasize the magnitude of the effect that hydration can have on corticosteroid absorption. In contrast, Bucks et al.[21] reported a number of experiments that demonstrate no enhanced absorption of hydrocortisone caused by different occlusion methods and application regimens. These results reinforce the effect that different experimental protocols may have on the results obtained and the interpretations made from these data.

In spite of the latter results, scientists still regard hydration as a convenient, facile, and relatively safe method of enhancing transdermal corticosteroid delivery. This belief has been validated by the superior clinical results obtained up to now by occluding corticosteroid application sites in routine dermatotherapy. These observations also were corroborated by the *in vivo* bioassays for corticosteroids using healthy human volunteers that were conducted by several laboratories worldwide.

The optimized human skin blanching assay[22,23] for assessing topical corticosteroid availability has been practiced in our laboratories for several years. The results of several thousand observations[24,25] have repeatedly demonstrated greater skin blanching in the occluded application mode as compared to the unoccluded application procedure. The interpretation of these results is fairly simple: in almost every case in which the drug and delivery vehicle is occluded, the enhanced hydration of the SC facilitates greater penetration of corticosteroid into and through this tissue when

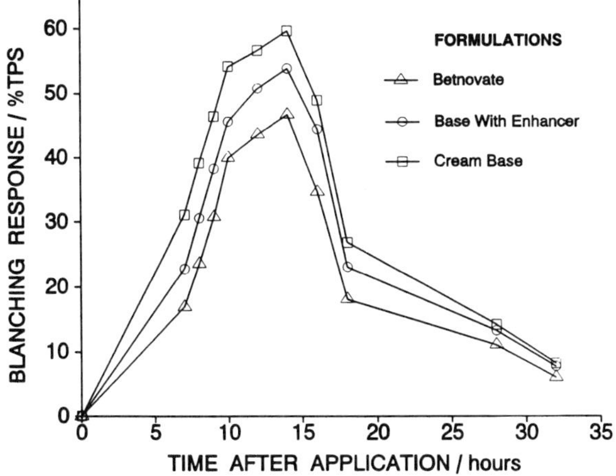

Figure 1 Skin blanching profiles of Betnovate cream, base formulation, and base formulation plus penetration enhancer applied with occlusive cover for 6 h.

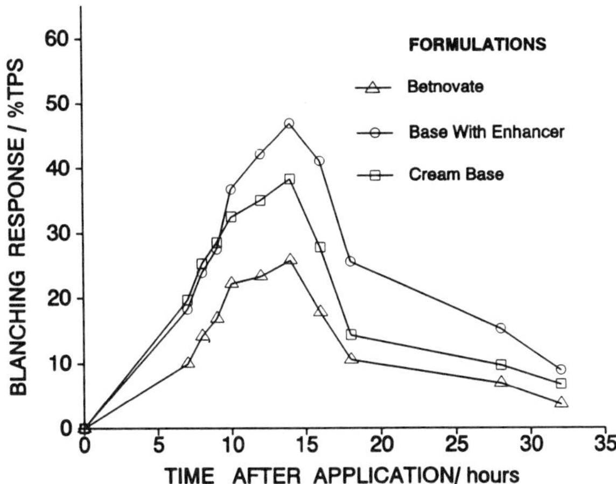

Figure 2 Skin blanching profiles of Betnovate cream, base formulation, and base formulation plus penetration enhancer applied without occlusion.

compared directly to application sites that are unoccluded. Typical results from a topical equivalence skin blanching assessment are depicted in Figures 1 and 2 for occluded and nonoccluded application modes, respectively. These trials were mounted to compare the delivery of betamethasone 17-valerate from two experimental cream formulations (one containing propylene glycol as the enhancer and one containing no enhancer) and commercial Betnovate cream (Glaxo, South Africa), all formulations containing the drug at 0.12% concentration. These results clearly indicate the greater skin blanching observed and, by inference, greater topical drug availability produced by 6-h impervious occlusion of the application sites for all three formulations. The results of this study are also interesting in that occlusion tends to enhance the delivery of drug from the cream base to a greater extent than it does the delivery from the base containing enhancer. In the occluded mode the drug availability is greatest from the cream base, whereas in the unoccluded mode drug availability is greatest from the formulation containing the enhancer. Studies such as these may help to provide some insight into the mode of action of delivery vehicles and the *in vivo* interactions between penetration enhancers and water.

Exceptions to this universal trend of greater topical corticosteroid availability from occluded vehicles are rare in the literature.[26,27] The skin blanching induced by Topilar cream (Syntex, United Kingdom), which contains fluclorolone acetonide, and Eumovate ointment (Glaxo, South Africa), which contains clobetasone butyrate, appear to show greater topical availability in the nonoccluded mode than when applied under occlusion. The reasons are unexplained. This phenomenon must be associated with a decrease in the partitioning potential between vehicle and hydrated SC.

B. CORTICOSTEROID PENETRATION *IN VITRO*

The use of *in vitro* permeation cell systems to augment topical corticosteroid delivery studies is now commonplace in dermatopharmaceutical research. When using animal membranes for this research the question of nonphysiological hydration of the tissue may pose problems in interpreting the data generated from these systems.[28,29] Hydration of biological membranes may be induced by harvesting techniques[30] that require immersion in water, by the experimental protocol which may require both sides of the membrane to be bathed by aqueous solvents, or by the application of relatively infinite amounts of donor vehicle that would occlude the surface of the tissue and allow full hydration from the distal receptor fluid. Flux measurements obtained under these circumstances would be expected to be greater than if the experiments were carried out under more physiological conditions, and several experimental protocols have attempted to overcome these problems.[31,32] This aspect may also contribute to the relatively poor general correlation of *in vitro* with *in vivo* results obtained from these experiments. One should obviously strive to duplicate physiological hydration conditions as much as possible in permeation cell experiments if correlation with *in vivo* flux data is the objective.

III. SUMMARY

Hydration of the SC to hyperphysiological conditions is possible by impervious occlusion of the skin surface. This prevents evaporation of transpirational moisture, increases the temperature of the site, causes a swelling of the keratinocytes, and alters the equilibrium interaction between water and the intercellular lipid domains. The net effect of this hydration is a reduction in the barrier properties of the SC, which may be utilized beneficially in clinical practice for enhancing the delivery of anti-inflammatory corticosteroids to the epidermis. The enhanced topical corticosteroid availability that can be induced by occlusion is clearly and reproducibly evident *in vivo* when utilizing the optimized human skin blanching bioassay. This method allows an assessment to be made of the degree of improved delivery that can be expected from a particular delivery vehicle when applied to the skin with and without occlusion. Full hydration of biological membranes has posed some problems *in vitro* when laboratory permeation cell systems are used to assess drug delivery from topical vehicles. Current *in vitro* protocols attempt to limit membrane hydration to as near-physiological conditions as possible.

Hydration of the skin by occlusion of the application site is still the most facile manner of increasing the mass of drug that can be delivered to and through the skin. The hydration is rapidly reversible and generally causes no other effects, although occlusion for prolonged periods can increase the microbial count on the skin and can lead to irritancy reactions, as is often experienced with patch delivery systems. The only drawback to the use of hydration as a penetration enhancer appears to be the limited percutaneous enhancement demonstrated by occlusion alone for certain classes of drug. In these cases more rigorous chemical or physical means of penetration enhancement are necessary.

REFERENCES

1. **Blank, I. H. and Scheuplein, R. J.,** Transport into and within the skin, *Br. J. Dermatol.,* 81(Suppl. 4), 4, 1969.
2. **Idson, B.,** Percutaneous absorption, *J. Pharm. Sci.,* 64, 901, 1975.
3. **Barry, B. W., Southwell, D., and Woodford, R.,** Optimization of bioavailability of topical steroids: penetration enhancers under occlusion, *J. Invest. Dermatol.,* 82, 49, 1984.
4. **Potts, R. O.,** SC hydration: experimental techniques and interpretations of results, *J. Soc. Cosmet. Chem.,* 37, 9, 1986.
5. **Wiedmann, T.,** Application of solid-state nuclear magnetic resonance (NMR) to the study of skin hydration, *Pharm. Res.,* 5, 611, 1988.
6. **Elias, P. M.,** Epidermal lipids, barrier function, and desquamation, *J. Invest. Dermatol.,* 80, 44, 1983.
7. **Elias, P. M. and Menon, G. K.,** Structural and lipid biochemical correlates of the epidermal permeability barrier, *Adv. Lipid Res.,* 24, 1, 1991.
8. **Shelmire, J. B.,** Factors determining the skin-drug vehicle relationship, *Arch. Dermatol.,* 82, 24, 1960.
9. **Potts, R. O. and Francoeur, M. L.,** The influence of SC morphology on water permeability, *J. Invest. Dermatol.,* 96, 459, 1991.
10. **Mak, V. H., Potts, R. O., and Guy, R. H.,** Does hydration affect intercellular lipid organization in the SC?, *Pharm. Res.,* 8, 1071, 1991.
11. **Neering, H., Van Der Kroon, H. V. M., and Roeleveld, C. G.,** Treatment of localized skin lesions with betamethasone 17-valerate and triamcinolone acetonide in alcoholic solution under occlusive dressing, *Dermatologica,* 145, 395, 1972.
12. **Dempski, R. E., De Marco, J. D., and Marcus, A. D.,** An *in vitro* study of the relative moisture occlusive properties of several topical vehicles and Saran Wrap, *J. Invest. Dermatol.,* 44, 361, 1965.
13. **Kragballe, K. and Larsen, F. G.,** A hydrocolloid occlusive dressing plus triamcinolone acetonide cream is superior to clobetasol cream in palmo-planter pustulosis, *Acta Dermatol. Venereol.,* 71, 540, 1991.
14. **Neering, H., Van Der Kroon, H. V. M., and Roeleveld, C. G.,** Treatment of localized skin lesions with betamethasone 17-valerate and triamcinolone acetonide in alcoholic solution under occlusive dressing, *Dermatologica,* 145, 395, 1972.
15. **Berardesca, E., Vignoli, G. P., Fideli, D., and Maibach, H.,** Effect of occlusive dressings on the stratum-corneum water holding capacity, *Am. J. Med. Sci.,* 304, 25, 1992.
16. **McKenzie, A. W. and Stoughton, R. B.,** Method for comparing percutaneous absorption of steroids, *Arch. Dermatol.,* 86, 608, 1962.
17. **McKenzie, A. W.,** Percutaneous absorption of steroids, *Arch. Dermatol.,* 86, 611, 1962.
18. **Szadurski, J., Renz, R., and Gasser, D.,** Onset of the vasoconstrictor effect of diflucortolone valerate, betamethasone valerate, and fluocinolone acetonide ointments applied for varying periods under occlusive dressings, *Dermatologica,* 153, 236, 1976.

19. **Magnus, A. D., Haigh, J. M., and Kanfer, I.,** Assessment of some variables affecting the blanching activity of betamethasone 17-valerate cream, *Dermatologica,* 160, 321, 1980.
20. **Feldmann, R. J. and Maibach, H. I.,** Penetration of ^{14}C hydrocortisone through normal skin, *Arch. Dermatol.,* 91, 661, 1965.
21. **Bucks, D. A. W., Maibach, H. I., and Guy, R. H.,** Occlusion does not uniformly enhance penetration *in vivo,* in *Percutaneous Absorption. Mechanisms - Methodology - Drug Delivery,* Bronaugh, R. L. and Maibach, H. I., Eds., Marcel Dekker, New York, 1989, chap. 5.
22. **Haigh, J. M. and Kanfer, I.,** Assessment of topical corticosteroid preparations: the human skin blanching assay, *Int. J. Pharm.,* 19, 245, 1984.
23. **Smith, E. W., Meyer, E., Haigh, J. M., and Maibach, H. I.,** The human skin blanching assay as an indicator of topical corticosteroid bioavailability and potency: an update, in *Percutaneous Absorption. Mechanisms - Methodology - Drug Delivery,* Bronaugh, R. L. and Maibach, H. I., Eds., Marcel Dekker, New York, 1989, 443.
24. **Smith, E. W., Meyer, E., and Haigh, J. M.,** Accuracy and reproducibility of the multiple-reading skin blanching assay, in *Topical Corticosteroids,* Maibach, H. I. and Surber, C., Eds., S. Karger, Basel, 1992, 65.
25. **Smith, E. W., Meyer, E., Haigh, J. M., and Maibach, H. I.,** The human skin blanching assay for comparing topical corticosteroid availability, *J. Dermatol. Treat.,* 2, 69, 1991.
26. **Barry, B. W. and Woodford, R.,** Comparative bio-availability of proprietary topical corticosteroid preparations; vasoconstrictor assays on thirty creams and gels, *Br. J. Dermatol.,* 91, 323, 1974.
27. **Meyer, E., Magnus, A. D., Haigh, J. M., and Kanfer, I.,** Comparison of the blanching activities of Dermovate, Betnovate and Eumovate creams and ointments, *Int. J. Pharm.,* 41, 63, 1988.
28. **Foreman, M. I.,** SC hydration; consequences for skin permeation experiments, *Drug Dev. Ind. Pharm.,* 12, 461, 1986.
29. **Rolland, A., Demichelis, G., Jamoulle, J. C., and Shroot, B.,** Influence of formulation, receptor fluid, and occlusion, on *in vitro* drug release from topical dosage forms, using an automated flow-through diffusion cell, *Pharm. Res.,* 9, 82, 1992.
30. **Rietschel, R. L. and Akers, W. A.,** Effects of harvesting techniques on hydration dynamics: gravimetric studies of SC, *J. Soc. Cosmet. Chem.,* 29, 777, 1978.
31. **Franz, T. J.,** The finite dose technique as a valid *in vitro* model for the study of percutaneous absorption in man, *Curr. Problems Dermatol.,* 7, 58, 1978.
32. **Bucks, D. A. W., Maibach, H. I., and Guy, R. H.,** Mass balance and dose accountability in percutaneous absorption studies: development of a nonocclusive application system, *Pharm. Res.,* 5, 313, 1988.

Chapter 2.3

Use of Occluding Hydrocolloid Patches

Derek A. Hollingsbee, Richard J. White, and Peter A. D. Edwardson

CONTENTS

I. INTRODUCTION

Skin occlusion, typically with plastic films, has been used in dermatology for many years to increase the efficacy of topical corticosteroids.[1,2] Enhancement of the bioavailability of corticosteroids and mobilization of drug reservoirs that develop in the skin on initial application have been demonstrated by skin blanching studies.[3,4]

The use of plastic occlusive films is not without adverse side effects. Side effects resulting from corticosteroid overloading, such as skin thinning and adrenal suppression, can be controlled by appropriate dosing. Condensed moisture from transepidermal water loss (TEWL) and sweat which accumulate under the film with prolonged occlusion can cause skin maceration and irritation, proliferation of skin microflora, and an increase in the pH of the microenvironment.[5]

The experience gained by ConvaTec (a Bristol-Myers Squibb Company) with continuous use of hydrocolloid ostomy and wound dressings led to the development of a specific, self-adhesive hydrocolloid patch (Actiderm*) for use in combination with topical corticosteroids to enhance steroid delivery.[6] The hydrocolloids present absorb the excess TEWL and allow for prolonged application (typically 2 to 7 d) without discomfort. Actiderm has a number of other characteristics that make it more advantageous than plastic film occlusion (Table 1).

II. EFFECT OF HYDROCOLLOID PATCHES ON SKIN HYDRATION

Occlusion of the skin with an impermeable or a semipermeable cover increases stratum corneum (SC) hydration. This is the predominating influence on increasing skin permeability to topically applied agents. Vasoconstriction studies in which betamethasone valerate cream was occluded with films of varying water vapor transmissions demonstrated that the bioavailability of the corticosteroid is related to,

* Actiderm is a trademark of Bristol-Myers Squibb.

0-8493-2605-2/95/$0.00+$.50

Table 1 Comparison of the Use Characteristics of Actiderm with Saran® Wrap as Occlusive Dressings in Dermatology

	Actiderm	Saran Wrap
Hydration level under patch	Controlled	Uncontrolled, TEWL condensation leads to maceration
Effect on skin flora	Very little effect	Rapid proliferation
Surface contact with skin	Excellent	Poor, constantly changes with movement
Fixation	Self-adhesive	External fixation required
Wearability	Good, even on elbows and knees	Easily creased and torn
Cosmetic appearance	Good	Poor

and can be controlled to some extent by, the degree of occlusivity, which in turn modulates SC hydration. Hydrocolloid patches do not transmit water vapor to any significant extent, however, they do absorb transepidermal water and therefore also influence the degree of SC hydration.

Hydrocolloid patches absorb water in both liquid and vapor form. The rate of uptake is largely dependent on the water-absorptive properties of the hydrocolloids contained and their concentration, although the hydrophilic/hydrophobic nature of the adhesive matrix also plays a part. The thickness of the adhesive has only a small influence on liquid water uptake rates; on the other hand, water vapor uptake (which is much slower) is very dependent (Figures 1 and 2). Scanning electron microscopy (SEM) studies of hydrated, freeze-fractured hydrocolloid adhesives have shown that in the case of vapor absorption hydrocolloid particles throughout the entire adhesive mass increasingly swell with time, while in the case of liquid absorption the predominant effect of uptake is surface swelling and disruption.

Studies of a range of hydrocolloid patches demonstrated a direct correlation between *in vitro* water vapor absorption and rate of patch hydration *in vivo* (Figure 3) on forearm skin. Mean absorption rate for Actiderm over a 96-h period was determined

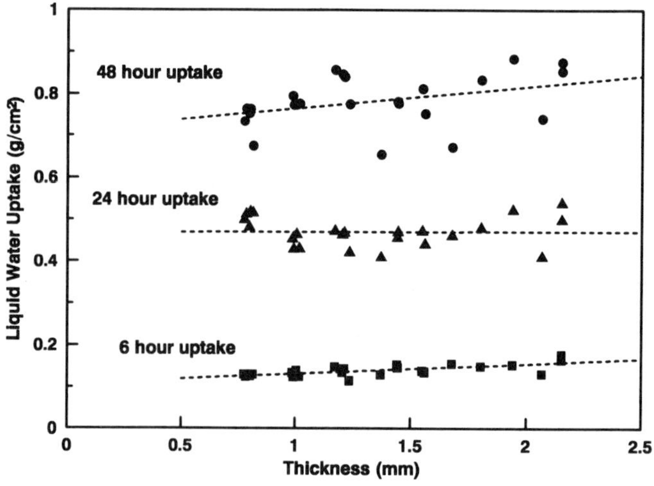

Figure 1 The effect of adhesive thickness on the liquid water uptake of a hydrocolloid patch.

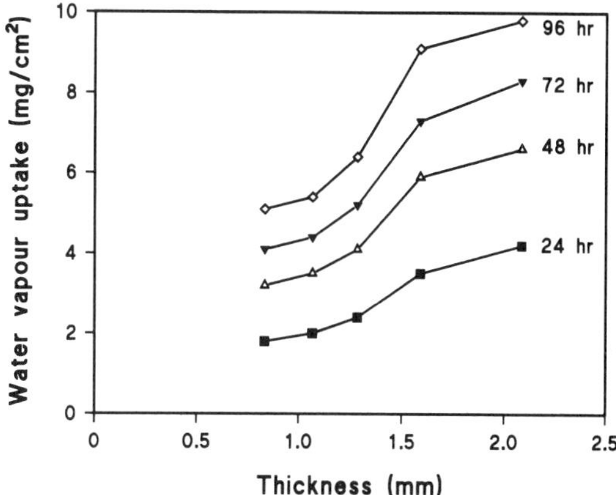

Figure 2 The effect of adhesive thickness on the water vapor uptake of a hydrocolloid patch.

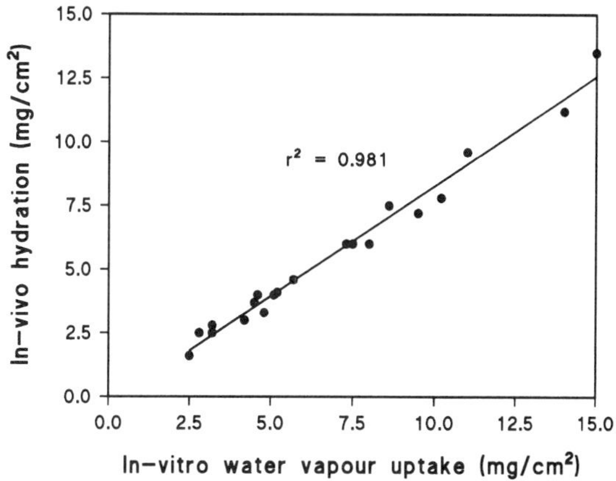

Figure 3 The correlation of water vapor absorption of a hydrocolloid patch *in vitro* with hydration *in vivo* when applied to forearm skin.

as 1.16 $g/m^2/h^1$, with the rate declining from 1.66 to 0.49 $g/m^2/h^1$ from day 1 to day 4.[7] This rate, being below the normal range of TEWL (2 to 7 $g/m^2/h^1$),[8] guarantees hydration of the skin.

A noninvasive infrared (FTIR) skin reflectance method was developed and utilized for the purpose of monitoring the degree of skin hydration after removal of adhesive patches and tapes.[9,10] The method employs attenuated total reflectance infrared (ATR-IR) spectroscopy to measure weak O-H stretch in the infrared spectrum of the skin formed by the presence of water at 2100 cm. This absorbance is distant from interference due to skin and most topically applied substances and therefore may be used to quantify skin water content (hydration). Excised human skin at increasing levels of hydration was used to validate the assay, the method giving a linear response of SC water concentration from 0.05 to 0.60 g/cm^3. The resting level of the SC is around 0.08 to 0.10 g/cm^3. On occlusion with an absorptive dressing such

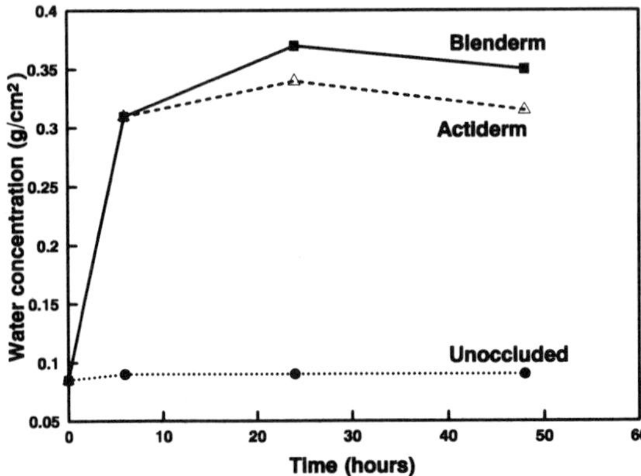

Figure 4 The change in water concentration of the skin with time under occlusion with Actiderm and Blenderm.

as Actiderm or nonabsorptive occlusive tapes such as Blenderm* this level quickly increased over a 6-h period to approximately 0.32 g/cm^3 and plateaus to around 0.3 to 0.4 g/cm^3 within 24 h. Studies conducted over a 48-h period demonstrated that the skin under Actiderm is only slightly less hydrated than Blenderm (Figure 4).

The rapid removal of liquid water (condensed TEWL or from sweat) from the surface of the skin and subsequent dissipation throughout the adhesive mass reduces the potential for maceration. Utilizing SEMs of skin replicas, skin microtopography has shown the skin surface structure virtually unchanged under Actiderm even after 110 h (Figure 5), in contrast to Saran** Wrap occlusion, which ablated the skin microtopography through maceration by excessive hydration in only 16 h.

In vivo skin microbiology studies also showed that despite the skin hydrating under Actiderm, the proliferation of commensal and colonizing bacteria is minimal in comparison to plastic film occlusion.[11] Problems of skin irritation and microbial accumulation were observed with transdermal patch delivery systems.[12] Hydrocolloid adhesive-based delivery systems is an approach that can be used to obviate such problems.

III. ENHANCEMENT OF PERCUTANEOUS ABSORPTION

The occlusion of topically applied drugs and chemicals generally results in increased rates of skin penetration. This effect is attributed mainly to the increase in SC permeability resulting from its hydration. In the case of hydrocolloid patches the absorption of water into the adhesive mass will lessen this to some extent. Additionally, when applied over topical preparations, interaction with or absorption into the patch may reduce the thermodynamic activity of the penetrating agent at the skin surface, resulting in a reduced penetration rate.

A. *IN VITRO* SKIN PENETRATION

In vitro skin penetration studies, using isolated human epidermis or epidermal membranes, of triamcinolone acetonide (TACA) applied as a cream[16] or an alcoholic

* Blenderm is a trademark of 3M Healthcare.

** Saran is a trademark of Dow Chemical.

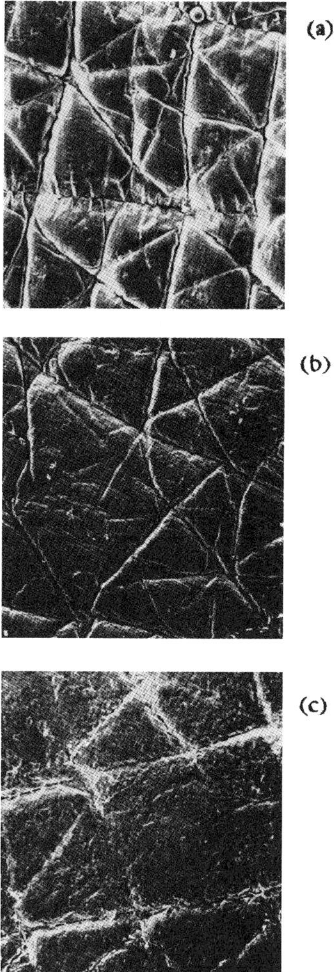

Figure 5 EMs of normal skin, skin occluded by Actiderm for 110 h, and skin occluded by Saran Wrap for 16 h. (a) Normal, untreated human volar forearm (× 50). (b) Adjacent site to (a), occluded with Actiderm for 110 h (× 50). (c) Adjacent site to (a), occluded with Saran Wrap for 16 h (× 50).

solution[13] indicate that the overall effect of Actiderm is to markedly increase and prolong absorption, even if the fluxes achieved are not as high as with plastic film occlusion.

B. SKIN BLANCHING STUDIES

Skin blanching (vasoconstriction) studies have been used extensively to indicate *in vivo* the bioavailability of topical steroid preparations applied under Actiderm. The technique of Barry and Woodford[14] has been adapted for these studies to generate a series of blanching response time curves throughout a treatment regime, as exemplified in Figure 6 for the application of betamethasone valerate 0.1% cream under Actiderm.

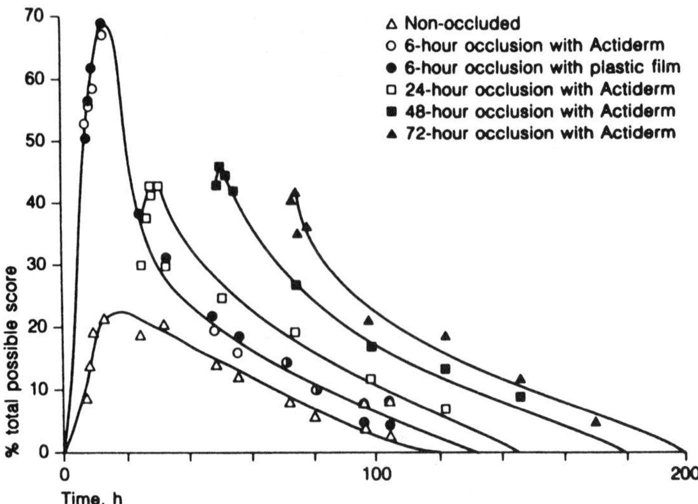

Figure 6 Skin blanching induced by the application of 0.1% betamethasone valerate cream applied unoccluded or under occlusion.

The potential of Actiderm to provide high blanching activity for prolonged periods from a single application has been demonstrated with a wide range of low to high potency corticosteroid creams.[15] In all cases the degree of enhancement, assessed as the ratio of response under Actiderm to the response unoccluded, is approximately 2- to 3-fold for both the peak response and 'area under the curve.' Improved bioavailability with increasing application time, as assessed by AUC, is also indicated.[16]

A single application of TACA 0.1% cream applied under Actiderm provides a blanching profile very similar to that of Saran Wrap when applied for times up to and including 48 h.[17] The apparent contradiction between this result and the difference in skin penetration rates seen between Saran Wrap and Actiderm *in vitro* is probably an indication that sufficient steroid is delivered under Actiderm to fully saturate cell receptors, giving a maximum response with less in excess. Actiderm was shown to produce greater activity than twice-daily applications of unoccluded TACA 0.1% cream and similar or greater activity than that of highly potent clobetasol propionate 0.05% cream.[18]

Studies on the effect of TACA dosage (both by reducing the concentration of drug and quantity of cream applied) have shown that although a dose response relationship exists, the dose can be reduced considerably without compromising the blanching response.[18]

Enhancement of blanching activity, similar to that seen with steroid creams, was also demonstrated with the occlusion of alcoholic solutions and sprays using Actiderm. Such nongreasy preparations offer an advantage over creams in that they provide better adhesion between patch and skin. Although some enhancement of penetration was demonstrated with TACA 0.1% ointment, the extent was not comparable to that achieved for Saran Wrap occlusion or for the application of a cream of similar strength under Actiderm; absorption of the oily vehicle into the adhesive of the hydrocolloid patch is the likely cause.[18]

IV. CLINICAL STUDIES

Although occlusion has been used extensively to increase the skin penetration of topically applied corticosteroids in clinical practice, occlusion alone has an inherent biological propensity to improve psoriasis and to break the scratch–itch cycle in chronic eczema.[19–22]

Friedman[23] found that Duoderm,* a hydrocolloid patch used as a wound dressing, was active as a treatment for plaque psoriasis, and reported that it was as effective as topical 0.025% fluocinolone acetonide cream in a 10-week study. Actiderm monotherapy, in a large, multicenter study, showed complete clearance of psoriatic lesions in 17 of 69 patients studied over a 10-week period.[24]

In clinical practice a synergistic effect is derived from the combination of hydrocolloid patches and topical corticosteroids. Studies in which hydrocolloid patches were applied over topical corticosteroids confirmed the results of skin blanching studies by consistently demonstrating apparent increased steroid potency.

A comparative study between TACA 0.1% lotion applied under Duoderm E (a hydrocolloid wound dressing patch) or under a plastic film (Opsite** IV 3000) applied weekly and twice-daily unoccluded TACA cream showed a marked improvement for the hydrocolloid patch–steroid combination therapy.[25] The lack of effectiveness of the plastic film suggests occlusive conditions were not achieved due to its high water vapor transmission rate and lack of close contact with the skin.

David and Lowe[26] compared Actiderm alone to Actiderm applied over TACA 0.1% cream replaced every 48 h, to Saran wrap applied over TACA 0.1% cream replaced every 12 h, and to TACA 0.1% cream applied twice daily unoccluded in 38 patients with stable psoriasis vulgaris. Best results were obtained for the steroid–Actiderm combination.

Bagatell[27] compared Actiderm over hydrocortisone valerate 0.2% cream, replaced every 48 h, to unoccluded betamethasone dipropionate 0.05% cream applied twice daily in 31 patients with stable plaque psoriasis. After 3 weeks, 55% of lesions treated with Actiderm combination and 26% treated with the betamethasone dipropionate cream had achieved a "good" or "clear" response.

Other trials comparing Actiderm–steroid therapy to orthodox topical steroids in psoriasis have consistently demonstrated the advantages of hydrocolloid patch–dressing combination therapy, particularly with regard to more rapid reduction of scaling and pruritus.[28–31] Actiderm over TACA 0.1% cream was compared against twice-daily treatment of clobetasol propionate 0.05% cream for the treatment of palmo-plantar pustulosis and was shown to be clinically superior, with 63% of Actiderm-treated lesions having cleared at the end of treatment as compared to 16% for the superpotent steroid monotherapy.[32] Actiderm applied over betamethasone valerate 0.1% cream proved superior to the unoccluded ointment for the treatment of lichen simplex chronicus over a 4-week trial period,[33] while in another study Actiderm applied over halcinonide 0.1% cream every 7 d was found to be equipotent to twice-daily unoccluded application of betamethasone dipropionate 0.05% cream.[34] Clinical experience with the Actiderm patch, when used over a variety of topical steroids, shows it to be well accepted by patients because it is easy to apply and comfortable to wear.

---

* Duoderm is a trademark of Bristol-Myers Squibb.

** Opsite is a trademark of Smith and Nephew.

V. CONCLUSIONS

Hydrocolloid patches such as Actiderm and Duoderm provide an acceptable form of skin occlusion to hydrate the skin and enhance the absorption of topical corticosteroids applied under them. Their water-absorptive properties are such that condensed moisture and sweat is rapidly removed from the surface of the skin, preventing the undesirable side effects of skin maceration and bacterial proliferation. Therapeutically, the hydrocolloid patches act to provide a synergistic combination of the benefits of occlusion and enhanced corticosteroid absorption to accelerate healing of steroid-responsive dermatoses.

REFERENCES

1. **Scholtz, J. R.,** Topical therapy of psoriasis with fluocinolone acetonide, *Arch. Dermatol.,* 84, 1029, 1961.
2. **Sulzberger, M. B. and Witten, V. H.,** Thin pliable plastic films in topical dermatological therapy, *Arch. Dermatol.,* 84, 1027, 1961.
3. **McKenzie, A. W. and Stoughton, R. B.,** Method for comparing percutaneous absorption of steroids, *Arch. Dermatol.,* 86, 88, 1962.
4. **Vickers, C. F. H.,** Existence of a reservoir in the SC, *Arch. Dermatol.,* 88, 20, 1963.
5. **Aly, R., Shirley, C., Cunico, B., and Maibach, H.,** Effect of prolonged occlusion on the microbial flora, pH, carbon dioxide and transepidermal water loss on human skin, *J. Invest. Dermatol.,* 71, 378, 1978.
6. **Hollingsbee, D. A. and Timmins, P.,** Topical adhesive systems, in *Bioadhesion — Possibilities and Future Trends,* Gurny, R. and Junginger, H. E., Eds., Wissenschaften Verlag Gesellschaft, Stuttgart, 1990.
7. **Ladenheim, D.,** Some Factors Affecting the Properties and Performance of Dermatological Patches, Ph.D. thesis, Brighton Polytechnic, Brighton, U.K., 1991.
8. **Roskos, K. V. and Guy, R. H.,** Assessment of skin barrier function using transepidermal water loss: the effects of age, *Pharm. Res.,* 6, 949, 1989.
9. **Edwardson, P. A. D., Walker, M., Gardner, R. S., and Jacques, E.,** The use of FTIR for the determination of SC hydration *in vitro* and *in vivo, J. Pharm. Biomed. Anal.,* 9, 1089, 1991.
10. **Edwardson, P. A. D., Walker, M., and Breheny, C.,** Quantitative FTIR determination of skin hydration following occlusion with hydrocolloid containing adhesive dressings, *Int. J. Pharm.,* 91, 51, 1993.
11. **Lilly, H. A. and Lawrence, J. C.,** The effect of Actiderm dermatological patch and Saran wrap on the bacteriological flora of skin in *Beyond Occlusion: Dermatology Proceedings,* Ryan T. J., Ed., Royal Society of Medicine Services International Congress and Symp. Ser. No. 137, Royal Society of Medicine Services Limited, London, 1988.
12. **Van Doorne, H. and Junginger, H. E.,** Skin irritation caused by transdermal drug delivery systems during long-term (5 days) application, *Br. J. Dermatol.,* 112, 461, 1985.
13. **Kadir, R., Barry, B. W., Fairbrother, J. E., and Hollingsbee, D. A.,** Delivery of triamcinolone acetonide through human epidermis: effect of Actiderm, a new hydrocolloid dermatological patch, *Int. J. Pharm.,* 60, 139, 1990.
14. **Barry, B. and Woodford, R.,** Comparative bio-availability of proprietary topical corticosteroid preparations; vasoconstrictor assays on thirty creams and gels, *Br. J. Dermatol.,* 91, 343, 1974.
15. **Martin, G. P. and Marriott, C.,** The influence of a new hydrocolloid dermatological patch on the blanching response induced by topical corticosteroid formulations, *Curr. Ther. Res.,* 46, 828, 1989.
16. **Fairbrother, J. E., Hollingsbee, D. A., and White, R. J.,** Hydrocolloid dermatological patches–corticosteroid combinations, in *Topical Corticosteroids,* Maibach, H. I. and Surber, C. S., S. Karger, Basel, 1992, 503.
17. **Queen, D., Martin, G. P., Marriott, C., and Fairbrother, J. E.,** Assessment of the potential of a new hydrocolloid dermatological patch Actiderm[R] in the treatment of steroid responsive dermatoses, *Int. J. Pharm.,* 44, 25, 1988.

18. **Hollingsbee, D. A., Fairbrother, J. E., Marriott, C., Martin, G., and Monger, L.,** The effect of a hydrocolloid dermatological patch (Actiderm) in potentiating the skin blanching activity of triamcinolone acetonide, *Int. J. Pharm.,* 77, 199, 1991.
19. **Fry, L., Almeyda, J., and McMinn, R.,** Effect of plastic occlusive dressings on psoriatic epidermis, *Br. J. Dermatol.,* 82, 458, 1970.
20. **Fisher, L. B. and Maibach, H. I.,** Physical occlusion controlling epidermal mitosis, *J. Invest. Dermatol.,* 59, 106, 1972.
21. **Shore, R. N.,** Treatment of psoriasis with prolonged application of tape, *J. Am. Acad. Dermatol.,* 15, 540, 1986.
22. **Fisher, L. B., Maibach, H. I., and Trancik, R. J.,** Effects of occlusive tape systems on the mitotic activity of epidermis, *Arch. Dermatol.,* 114, 384, 1978.
23. **Friedman, S. J.,** Management of psoriasis vulgaris with a hydrocolloid occlusive dressing, *Arch. Dermatol.,* 123, 1046, 1987.
24. **Telfer, N. R., Ryan, T. J., Blanc, D., Merk, H., Lotti, T., Juhlin, L., and Cherry, C. A.,** Results of a multicentre trial of Actiderm in the treatment of plaque psoriasis, in *Beyond Occlusion: Dermatology Proceedings,* Ryan, T. J., Ed., Royal Society of Medicine Services International Congress and Symp. Ser. No. 137, Royal Society of Medicine Services Limited, London, 1988.
25. **van de Kerkhof, P. C. M., van der Walle, H. B., Bollyut, A., Vlijmen-Willems, I. M. J. J., Chang, A., and Boezeman, J. B. M.,** Weekly treatment of psoriasis with a hydrocolloid dressing (DuoDerm E) in combination with triamcinolone acetonide: a controlled, comparative study, in press.
26. **David, M. and Lowe, N. J.,** Psoriasis therapy: comparative studies with a hydrocolloid dressing, plastic film occlusion, and triamcinolone acetonide cream, *J. Am. Acad. Dermatol.,* 21, 511, 1989.
27. **Bagatell, F. K.,** Management of psoriasis: a clinical evaluation of the dermatological patch, Actiderm^R, over a topical steroid, *Adv. Ther.,* 5, 291, 1988.
28. **Raymond, G. P.,** Hydrocolloid dermatological patch over a corticosteroid cream in the treatment of psoriasis, *Curr. Ther. Res.,* 5(45), 767, 1989.
29. The Actiderm Multi-Center Study Group, A trial of the Actiderm dermatological patch and topical corticosteroids in the treatment of psoriasis vulgaris, *Cutis,* 46, 84, 1990.
30. **Gonzalez, J. R. and Caban, F.,** Treatment of psoriasis with triamcinolone acetonide 0.1% under occlusion: a comparison of two hydrocolloid dressings, *Bol. Assoc. Med. P.R.,* 82(7), 288, 1990.
31. **Wilkinson, R. D. and Ohayon, M.,** Therapeutic response to a dermatologic patch and betamethasone valerate 0.1% cream in the management of chronic plaques in psoriasis, *Cutis,* 45(6), 468, 1990.
32. **Kragballe, K. and Larsen, F.,** A hydrocolloid occlusive dressing plus triamcinolone acetonide cream is superior to clobetasol cream in palmo-plantar pustulosis, *Acta Derm. Venereol. (Stockholm),* 71, 540, 1991.
33. **Ilchyshyn, A. and Mortimer, P.,** Final Report of Two Clinical Trials Comparing Actiderm Over 0.1% Betamethasone Valerate Cream with 0.1% Betamethasone Valerate Ointment in the Treatment of Lichen Simplex, unpublished ConvaTec data on file.
34. Actiderm Dermatological Patch Over Halcinonide Cream 0.1% versus Betamethasone Dipropionate Ointment 0.05% in the Management of Lichen Simplex Chronicus, unpublished ConvaTec data on file.

Chapter 3.1

Alcohols

Bret Berner and Puchun Liu

CONTENTS

I. INTRODUCTION

The simple term, alcohols, refers to monohydric alcohols as distinguished from glycols (dihydric alcohols) and glycerols (trihydric alcohols). Ethanol, with its history as a cosolvent and its well-established systemic toxicology and local tolerability, was the clear choice for the first enhancer to be incorporated into transdermal drug delivery (TDD) systems. It is currently contained in commercial TDD systems for estradiol[1] and fentanyl.[2] The interactions of ethanol with skin in terms of its permeation, primary irritation, and cutaneous metabolism are probably better characterized than any other enhancer. This chapter summarizes this characterization along with information concerning isopropanol.

Examples of aqueous ethanol or isopropanol as enhancers with different permeants are summarized in Table 1. More applications may be found in the patent literature.[3] For most of the lipophilic and hydrophilic permeants, the maximum enhancement of flux across skin was observed from 25 to 75% alcohol.

The flux enhancement may be synergistically increased by adding a nonpolar long-chain enhancer to polar ethanol or isopropanol. While the polar enhancers traverse the skin, nonpolar enhancers are largely retained in the stratum corneum (SC); both aspects make the combination a superior enhancer system to the individual enhancers. The mixtures of the polar and nonpolar enhancers were found to work particularly well with lipophilic permeants such as steroids. Table 2 presents examples of such enhancing mixtures with ethanol or isopropanol.

0-8493-2605-2/95/$0.00+$.50

Table 1 Examples of Hydroalcoholic Enhancers of Ethanol or Isopropanol

Alcohol	Permeant	Skin	Ref.
Ethanol	Testosterone	Human, *in vivo*	17
	Estradiol	Human, *in vitro* and *in vivo*	4–6, 30, 42–43
	Nitroglycerin	Human, *in vitro* and *in vivo*	15, 34
	Salicylate	Human, *in vitro*	44
	Ibuprofen	Hairless rat, *in vitro*	45
	Flurbiprofen		
	Indomethacin		
	Isosorbide dinitrate		
	Cyclobarbital		
	Aminopyrine		
	5-Fluorouracil		
	Diclofenac sodium		
	Nicorandil		
	Antipyrine		
	Morphine hydrochloride		
	Isoproterenol hydrochloride		
	Dopamine hydrochloride		
	Diclofenac	Hairless rat, *in vitro*	27
	Nicotinamide	Hairless mouse, *in vitro*	46
	Nicardipine	Rhesus monkey, *in vivo*	47
	Ketorolac		
	Fentanyl	Human, *in vitro* and *in vivo*	17
	Propranolol	Human, *in vitro*	17
Ethanol, isopropanol	Acyclovir	Hairless mouse and rat, *in vitro*	48
	Hydrocortisone	Hairless mouse, *in vitro*	6, 43, 49
	Tetraethylammonium		
	Estradiol		
	Estrone		
	Mannitol		
	Levonorgestrel	Rat, *in vitro*	50
Isopropanol	Terbutaline sulfate	Human, *in vitro*	25, 28

II. ACTION OF ALCOHOLS ON THE STRATUM CORNEUM BARRIER

A. ENHANCEMENT FACTOR

The flux of drug delivered transdermally is proportional to the thermodynamic activity of the drug and inversely proportional to the resistance of the SC. The enhancement factor *(E)* is a measure of the reduction in this resistance by an enhancer in terms of membrane-related properties, i.e., diffusion coefficient *(D),* activity coefficient in SC (γ_m), and diffusion path length *(h).* These membrane properties are compared to permeation from an infinitely dilute solution of the enhancer (i.e., water) as a reference state (superscript *o*), with any change in these properties in the presence of a significant activity of the enhancer (superscript *) as:[4]

$$E = \frac{\left(\dfrac{D}{\gamma_m h}\right)^*}{\left(\dfrac{D}{\gamma_m h}\right)^o} = \frac{\left(\dfrac{P}{\gamma_v}\right)^*}{\left(\dfrac{P}{\gamma_v}\right)^o} = \frac{\left(\dfrac{J}{a_d}\right)^*}{\left(\dfrac{J}{a_d}\right)^o} \tag{1}$$

Table 2 Examples of Combination Enhancers of Ethanol or Isopropanol

Mixtures				
Alcohol	**Others**	**Permeant**	**Skin**	**Ref.**
Ethanol	Cyclic monoterpenes	Diclofenac sodium	Rat, *in vivo*	51
	Miglyol® 840	Tetrahydroaminoacridine	Human, *in vitro*	52
		Diltiazem	Hairless mouse, *in vitro*	
		Atenolol		
		Tazifylline		
		Hydrocortisone		
	Ethyl acetate, oleic acid	Levonorgestrel	Hairless mouse, *in vitro*	53
	1-Menthol	Morphine hydrochloride	Hairless rat, *in vitro*	54
	Urea	Indomethacin	Rat, *in vitro*	55
	Glycerides	Ketoprofen	Hairless mouse, *in vitro*	56
	Panasate® 800	Ketoprofen	Hairless mouse, *in vitro*	56
	Propylene glycol, urea, water	Ketoprofen	Rat, *in vitro*	57
Isopropanol	Tween® 80	Hydrocortisone	Mouse, *in vitro*	49
	Isopropyl myristate	Physostigmine	Human, *in vitro*	58
	Isopropyl myristate	Estradiol	Human, *in vitro*	59
	Lauric acid	Naloxone	Human, *in vitro*	60
	Lauryl alcohol			
	Na lauryl sulfate			

where J, P, γ_v, and a_d are the steady-state flux, the permeability coefficient, activity coefficient in the vehicle, and the activity on the skin surface, respectively.

Accounting for both thermodynamic and kinetic factors, the enhancement factor (E) may be mechanistically described by two simple theoretical limits: the thermodynamic model ($E = \gamma_m^o/\gamma_m^*$ with constant D and h), where the solubility parameter (e.g., polarity) of the lipoidal barrier is altered by the enhancer, and the kinetic model [$E = (D^*/D^o)/(h^*/h^o)$ with constant γ_m], where the lipoidal barrier is physically altered (e.g., disorder and/or change in the path length) in the presence of the enhancer.

In principle, determination of the enhancement factor (E) by Equation 1 should be only for the experiments with the same solvent compositions on both sides of the skin. In practice, the receptor component is usually saline or water. For the solvent or dilute solutions of the drug, the enhancement factor is the ratio of permeability coefficients normalized by the ratio of the activity coefficients in the vehicles. The latter is obtained either from the partial vapor pressure of the solvent or from the solubility of drugs.[4,5] When using saturated solutions of drug with the same thermodynamic activity of unity, the enhancement factor is simply the ratio of the flux of drug in the presence of enhancers to that from water. Figure 1 summarizes the enhancement factors as a function of ethanol activity for both estradiol and ethanol itself across human skin. Similar results were obtained for hairless mouse skin.[5,6]

B. SPECTROSCOPIC STUDIES OF ALCOHOLIC EFFECTS ON THE STRATUM CORNEUM

A variety of spectroscopic tools used to probe lipids[7,8] have elucidated the interaction of alcohols with SC.[9,10] At high concentrations of ethanol or isopropanol and with longer chain length alcohols, the extraction of lipids and proteins was noted.[9] In Fourier transform infrared spectroscopy decreased absorbance of the alkyl chains of the lipid and of the amide I band of the SC proteins was observed after exposure to

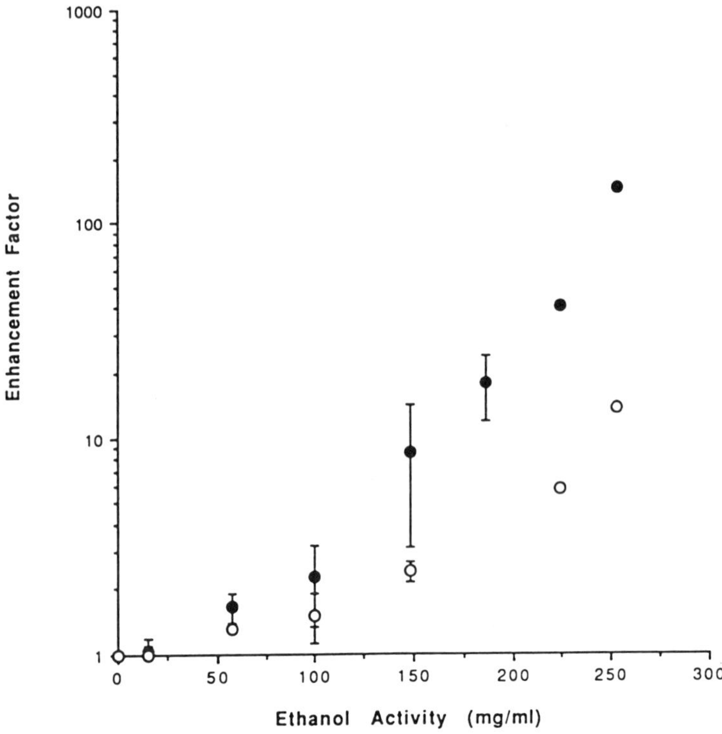

Figure 1 Enhancement factors (*E*) of estradiol (filled circles) and ethanol itself (open circles) in human epidermal membrane as a function of aqueous ethanol activity in both sides of the skin at 32°C ($n = 3$ to 6 for each point). (Data from Liu, P., Kurihara-Bergstrom, T., and Good, W. R., *Pharm. Res.,* 8, 938, 1991.)

alcohols. These effects tended to increase with increasing chain length of the alcohol. Short-chain alcohols did not alter the order or mobility of the SC lipids. Lipid extraction was noted with alcohols and was sufficiently extensive with octanol that this effect could not be evaluated.[10] For polar solutes some evidence exists that increases in permeation with alcohols correlate with this extraction.[9] Recent studies of the impedance of skin indicated that ions traverse skin through pores with a mean 25 Å pore radius and –0.05 C/m^2 surface charge.[11] The change after treatment with aqueous ethanol in the impedance of skin relative to its initial value in saline suggests increased porosity after exposure to even 50% (v/v) ethanol for 16 h.[12] Reversibility and whether the source of the change in porosity is from the area fraction or the pore radius was not discussed.

III. A SIMPLE MODEL FOR ALCOHOLIC ENHANCERS

Substantial insight can be gained about skin permeation by considering the lipophilic ($K \gg 1$, where K is partition coefficient) and the hydrophilic ($K \ll 1$) limits for permeants.

When $K \gg 1$, the hydrophobic permeant traverses the SC through a tortuous route by dissolving in the fluid lipidic regions of the SC. While much of the SC lipid is in a solid phase, a small portion of fluid lipids exist.[13] Dissolution in these fluid lipids is comparable to solubility in oils and is governed by the ideal solution theory.[14] The primary action of ethanol may be to dissolve in these fluid lipidic regions and increase the solubility of these lipophilic drugs.[13] The three key features of this effect of ethanol are[15]

1. The flux of drug across SC is linear with the flux of ethanol.
2. The enhancement is reversible.
3. The diffusion constant of drug in the SC is unchanged, and therefore, the enhancement is independent of the molecular weight of the drug.

When $K \ll 1$, in particular, for ionic permeants, permeation through rare pores predominates.[11] The extraction of lipophilic and peptidic solutes to increase the porosity of the SC is the major effect of ethanol for hydrophilic permeants. Competing with this effect, the solubility of ionized drugs may decrease with increasing alcoholic content of the donor solution, and consequently, the concentration within the pore (the driving force for permeation across the pore) may decrease. The three key features of these effects of ethanol on very hydrophilic permeants are[16]

1. The flux of drug across the SC is not linear with the flux of ethanol.
2. The enhancement is, at most, in part reversible.
3. For compounds that are more soluble in water, a substantial concentration of water is required for optimal enhancement.

A. ETHANOL AND LIPOPHILIC PERMEANTS

The solubility of lipophilic drugs, e.g., nitroglycerin,[15] estradiol,[1] and fentanyl,[17] in the SC is linear with the concentration of ethanol in the SC. This linear behavior of the cosolvency of ethanol with the SC is the focal point for understanding ethanol as an enhancer for skin permeation of lipophilic drugs. For these solutes, this linear behavior contrasts with a porous model of solubilities in the SC, which would have predicted a nonlinear dependence because ethanol increases the porosity of skin and the solubility of these drugs in aqueous ethanol increases faster than exponentially with ethanol concentration (v/v).

Within the model for lipophilic permeants, the ethanol dissolves in the fluid lipids of the SC. Using triolein as a single phase model of these lipids, the solubilities of model compounds in ethanol:triolein mixtures are linear with the concentration of ethanol. For the solubility of progesterone, this linearity with ethanol concentration may be explained by the low molecular weight of ethanol. As ethanol is added to the cosolvent, the moles of cosolvent per volume of cosolvent increase, and therefore, the solubility of drug, calculated on a weight per volume basis, increases linearly with ethanol concentration.[13] Analogous linear behavior was reported for the solubilization of hydrocarbons by alcohols, amines, and mercaptans,[18] as well as for triglyceride:aqueous ethanol:butanol microemulsions.[13] This linearity of the concentration of permeant in dilute solutions of ethanol in weak nonionic surfactants, such as triolein, leads to the key observations concerning the skin permeation of ethanol.

The first prediction of this model is the reversibility of the enhancement. Because the enhancement is related to the increased solubility of the drug in the SC resulting from increased ethanol, removal of the ethanol causes cessation of the increased solubility and skin permeation. This reversibility has been demonstrated for nitroglycerin.[15]

For dilute solutions of ethanol in triolein and presumably in "fluid SC lipids", the change in the viscosity is small.[13] Consequently, to a first approximation the diffusion constant of the permeant in the SC is constant. For several test compounds, it was observed that ethanol did not influence the time lag for skin permeation.[15,17] While the time lag is most sensitive to changes in the diffusion constant and the path length, ethanol may affect the time lag through the solubility, and an expression for this effect of ethanol on the time lag has been derived.[15] Because the diffusion constant of the permeant is constant, and depends exponentially on the molecular volume for a free volume mechanism,[14] the enhancement by ethanol should be independent of molecular volume, or to a good approximation, molecular weight.[15] For nitroglycerin (mol wt = 227), estradiol (mol wt = 278), progesterone (mol wt = 314), salicylic acid (mol wt = 138), fentanyl (mol wt = 336), and propranolol (mol wt = 259), the enhancement factors, which range from 5 to 20, do not vary systematically with molecular weight.[15,17] This constant diffusion coefficient is in contrast to the predictions of a model in which ethanol "fluidizes lipids".

Provided (1) the solubility of drug in the SC is linear with the ethanol content in SC, (2) the diffusion coefficient in the SC is independent of the ethanol concentration, and (3) the activity of the drug is proportional to that of ethanol throughout the SC (the drug follows the ethanol through the SC), the flux of the drug through the skin will be linear with the flux of ethanol.[1,15] This linear dependence of the fluxes (Figure 2) was observed for estradiol,[1,17] nitroglycerin,[15] fentanyl,[17] and progesterone.[19] In Figure 3, the enhancement factor, *E,* is plotted against ethanol concentration. Note that linearity with the concentration of ethanol is also a good approximation for concentrations of ethanol of <0.4. This linear dependence of TDD on the delivery of ethanol is the basis of the design of membrane-controlled transdermal systems containing ethanol.[20] To control the entry of the drug into the body through the skin, control the delivery of ethanol.

Interactions of ethanol with skin as an enhancer should result in a decreased activation energy for skin permeation of the drug in the presence of ethanol.[15] While the activation energy for skin permeation of progesterone from water is 19 kcal/mol,[19] the activation energy for skin permeation of progesterone (Table 3) from aqueous ethanol (70% v/v) is 11 kcal/mol. This activation energy for permeation in the presence of ethanol is typical for a change in solubility in a liquid; in particular, the activation energy for the solubility of progesterone in aqueous ethanol (7:3 v/v) is 10.2 kcal/mol (Table 3). These results are consistent with models of diffusion in either fluid lipid regions or in liquid-filled pores.

To complete our simple model of aqueous ethanol and SC, the role of water must be considered. Water is the only known plasticizer for skin or keratins.[21] At low water content, the keratins shrink and the epidermis becomes more impermeable.[21] For ethanol concentrations of <70% (v/v), the activity of water is still quite close to unity.[22] At higher concentrations of ethanol, the SC dehydrates. Consequently, the uptake of ethanol into the SC or the delipidized SC is optimal[13] at approximately 70%

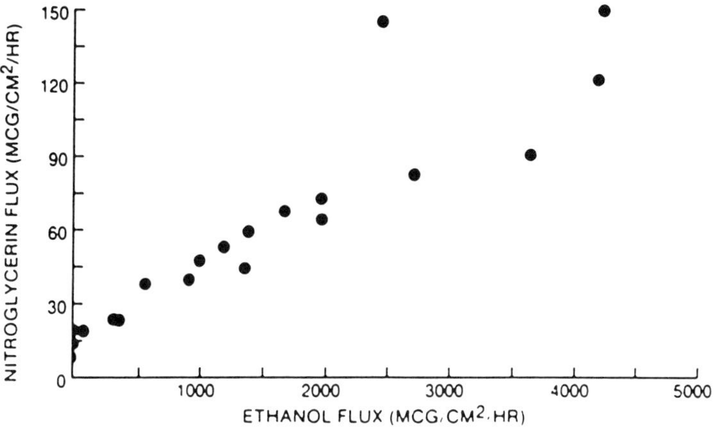

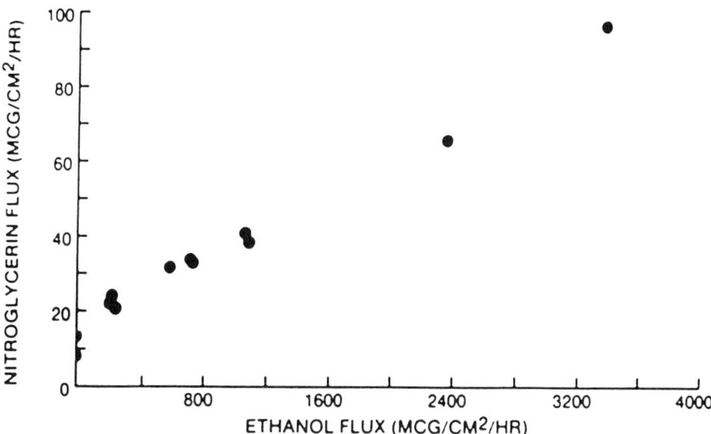

Figure 2 The skin permeation of nitroglycerin vs. ethanol flux (μg/cm²/h) at 32°C for individual skin samples for six different skin donors (A) and for an individual donor (B). Note the linearity. (Data taken from Berner, B. et al., *J. Pharm. Sci.*, 78, 402, 1989.)

ethanol (v/v). This optimum in the uptake of ethanol into the SC produces optima in the fluxes of ethanol and drug across the SC at approximately 70% ethanol (v/v). Such optima are shown for nitroglycerin and ethanol in Figure 4.

B. POLAR AND IONIZABLE PERMEANTS

Permeation of polar compounds through a porous pathway depends on a balance of increased permeability due to extraction of lipidic and peptidic substances by the alcohols and decreased driving force due to decreased solubility in alcoholic solvents with lower dielectric constants. For certain rather lipophilic ionized compounds, i.e., buprenorphine, their solubility in aqueous ethanol is greater than in water, and consequently, the flux of buprenorphine from aqueous ethanol (50% v/v) across the

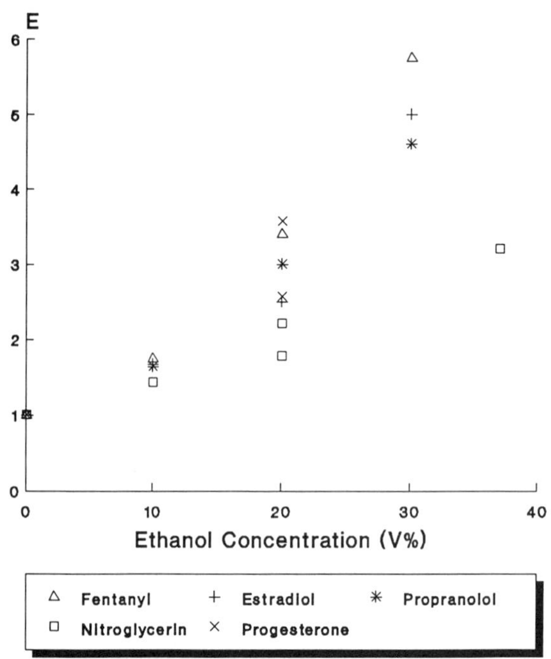

Figure 3 The enhancement factor, *E*, under solvent gradient conditions for five drugs vs. ethanol concentration. Note the linearity for ethanol concentrations <40% (v/v). (Data for nitroglycerin are from Reference 15, for progesterone from Reference 19, and for estradiol, fentanyl, and propranolol from Reference 17.)

Table 3 Temperature Dependence of the Solubility in and Skin Permeation of Progesterone from Aqueous Ethanol (70% v/v)

Temperature (°C)	Solubility (mg/ml)	Steady-State Flux (μg/cm²/h)
25	28.6	
32	36.6	11.9 ± 1.4
38	58.0	18.2 ± 2.2
45	81.6	26.6 ± 4.2

Data taken from Berner, B., Juang, R. H., and Rosen, R., Report BPR 86082, Ciba-Geigy, 1986.

skin is approximately fivefold greater than from aqueous solution.[23] For zwitterionic permeants such as the active metabolites of the angiotensin-converting enzyme inhibitors, benazeprilat and CGS 16617,[16] the solubility decreases rapidly with the addition of alcohols to water. Skin permeation is highly variable, but is probably optimized at about 20% ethanol (v/v).

For the series of 75% (v/v) alcohols (methanol, ethanol, and isopropanol), only the flux of mannitol from isopropanol[9] across the skin increased as compared to a saline donor (Table 4). The similarity of the fluxes from methanol and ethanol to saline

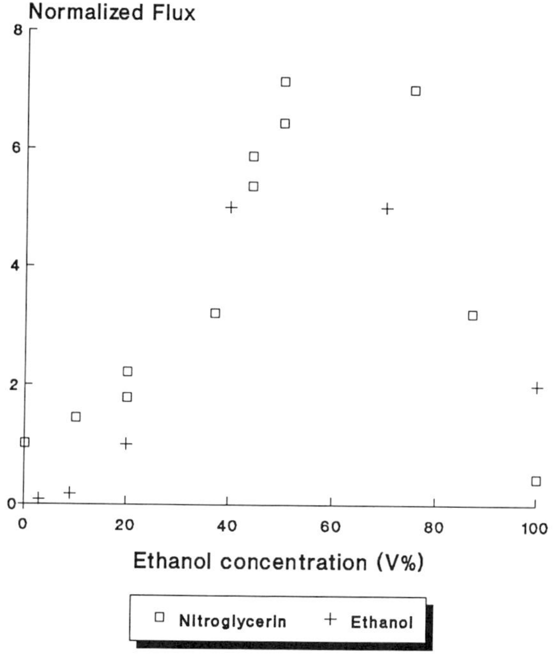

Figure 4 The normalized fluxes through skin of nitroglycerin (normalized to flux from water) and ethanol (normalized to flux from 20% v/v ethanol) at 32°C vs. ethanol concentration. Note the optima. (Data taken from Berner, B. et al., *J. Pharm. Sci.,* 78, 402, 1989.)

Table 4 Skin Permeation of Mannitol from Alcoholic Solutions

Solvent	Solubility (μg/ml)	Flux across Epidermis (μg/cm²/h)	Permeability (cm/s × 10⁸)
Saline	185	1.7 ± 2.3	0.54
Methanol (75% v/v)	11.7	0.77 ± 0.23	3.9
Ethanol (75% v/v)	10.6	2.98 ± 1.56	15.2
Isopropanol (75% v/v)	11.7	26.2 ± 15.3	93.4

Note: Error bars are S.D.

Data taken from Goates, C. Y. and Knutson, K., *Biochim. Biophys. Acta.,* in press.

results in part from the decreased solubility in alcohols (10 to 11 μg/ml) as compared to saline (185 μg/ml). The permeability of human epidermis to mannitol increases with the chain length of the alcohol (Table 4). Permeability ranks these solvents in the same order as the decreased infrared absorbance of the alkyl chains and the amide I band, measures of the extraction of lipids and proteins or peptides from the SC.[9]

For ionizable permeants, the process of skin permeation is complicated by the simultaneous presence of both ionized and nonionized species in solution, each of which permeates through the skin at different rates. The permeability for the nonionized species is much greater than for the ionized species. In aqueous solution the total flux of drug can be maximized by adjusting the pH of the solution to balance the concentrations of the nonionized fraction and the total solubility of the drug.

The addition of alcohols to water alters both the pH of the solution and the pK_a of the drug. The ionization equilibrium of the drug species depends on the solvent, which functions both as a dielectric medium and a proton acceptor/donor.[24] Increasing the concentration of alcohol in water decreases the dielectric constant of the medium from 78.5 in water to 24 in ethanol or 18 in isopropanol. As a result of lowering the dielectric constant, a larger effect on the electrostatic part of the free energy change is expected with a weak acid than a weak base. In the weak acid case dissociation involves the creation of electric charges, whereas the latter is an isoelectric process. For example, in water[25] terbutaline is a weak base (β-hydroyethylamine, $pK_a = 8.6$) and even a weaker acid (phenol, $pK_a = 9.4$). With increasing isopropanol concentration up to 60% (v/v), its amine pK_a value was lowered slightly, and the phenolic pK_a was raised to 10.5. Conductivity results also suggested an increased fraction of uncharged or zwitterionic species at higher concentrations of isopropanol.[25] Similar phenomena were reported for benzoic acid in aqueous isopropanol[26] and diclofenac in aqueous ethanol.[27]

Furthermore, lowering the dielectric constant of the medium enhances ionic association. ^{15}N-nuclear magnetic resonance studies in 60 to 80% (v/v) isopropanol[25] were consistent with significant ion–pair and ion–triplet formations between the protonated terbutaline and its counterion sulfate anion. As a result, the total flux of terbutaline across the skin was greatly increased in comparison to permeation from water.[25,28]

IV. A COMPREHENSIVE MODEL FOR ALCOHOL/PERMEANT COTRANSPORT

A more complete diffusion model was presented recently for the correlation of steady-state fluxes of estradiol with ethanol from aqueous ethanol solutions saturated with estradiol.[4] Assuming that transport of estradiol and ethanol across the SC occurs through the same lipoidal pathway/mechanism, this model accounts for the following important facts:

1. The enhancement factors for both estradiol and ethanol itself are ethanol concentration-dependent as shown in Figure 1.
2. An ethanol gradient exists across the skin during cotransport of estradiol and ethanol; thus, the enhancement factors are position-dependent in SC.
3. Regardless of ethanol concentration at the surface of the SC, saturated estradiol maintains a constant unit thermodynamic activity, while ethanol does not.

Based on this model, the fluxes of estradiol and ethanol can be predicted with the donor ethanol activity and the enhancement factors of both permeants. Another prediction from the model is that the flux from the saturated estradiol solution is not linearly correlated with ethanol flux for the full range of ethanol concentrations. However, an approximate linear estradiol–ethanol flux relationship can be achieved at the higher ethanol concentration range, where ethanol activity in the donor solution is less dependent on its concentration. Finally, a complex flux correlation is expected when the permeant and solvent enhancer traverse the SC through different pathway(s)/mechanism(s).

Table 5 Incidence of Erythema after Wearing Placebo Transdermal Estradiol Systems Containing Ethanol

Score	Abdomen	Back
0	972	1019
1	196	151
2	45	29
3	2	2
4	2	3
Total	1217	1204

V. PRIMARY SKIN IRRITATION OF ALCOHOLS

In terms of toxicology, ethanol and isopropanol are the most acceptable of the short-chain alkanols. The primary skin irritation of ethanol under occlusion has been well characterized for the transdermal estradiol system, which contains ethanol USP. As discussed earlier, ethanol is delivered to the skin from an ethanolic drug reservoir across a laminate consisting of membrane and adhesive layers in series. As a result, the ethanol concentration at the skin surface is about 40 to 60%. In a study of over 1200 postmenopausal women (Table 5) who wore placebo transdermal estradiol systems on the back and on the abdomen for 3½ d, the incidence of erythema observed 24 h after removal of the placebo transdermal system was 18%. Mild erythema or scores of grade 1, which is primarily of cosmetic significance, accounted for 81% of the incidence of erythema. In clinical studies patient discontinuation for reasons associated with skin irritation occurred in approximately 2% of the subjects.[29] The incidence of erythema is statistically lower on the back than on the abdomen. Similar reduced irritation scores were reported for the application of placebo transdermal estradiol systems to buttocks. To reduce irritation, the buttocks may be substituted for the abdomen as the site of application for transdermal estradiol systems.

The primary skin irritation of isopropanolic solutions in rabbits was assessed following a 24-h application under occlusion (Table 6). Because the mean score after both neat and 60% isopropanol indicates that moderate erythema and edema occurred at 1 h after removal, the level of irritation in actual usage may be unacceptable. Lower concentrations of isopropanol should be better tolerated. This would have to be confirmed in both pilot and clinical studies. However, as a comparison to the primary irritation index of 2.5 for isopropanol, the primary irritation index in rabbits for 24-h application of the placebo transdermal estradiol system was 0.9. Given the disappearance of the erythema and edema by 48 h and the use of different trained graders in the tests for ethanol and isopropanol, the comparison may not be strictly valid.

VI. EFFECT OF ETHANOL ON CUTANEOUS METABOLISM

In addition to enhancing the transport of estradiol across the SC, ethanol at low levels ($\leq$25% v/v) acts as an inhibitor of the metabolism of estradiol to estrone in fresh hairless mouse skin *in vitro*.[30,31] The metabolic conversion and the ethanol inhibition occurs in the basal layer of the viable epidermis, where 17β-hydroxysteroid dehydrogenase,

Table 6 Primary Skin Irritation from Isopropanol in Rabbits Following a 24-h Dermal Application

Skin Condition	Time after Removal (h)	Isopropanol (60%)		Isopropanol	
		Erythema	Edema	Erythema	Edema
Intact	1	1.67	2.67	1.67	2.67
	48	0.33	0.00	0.33	0.17
Abraded	0.5	1.83	2.33	2.00	2.67
	48	0.83	0.00	0.67	0.00
Primary irritation index		2.4		2.5	

Note: $n = 6$.

an enzyme located in skin microsomes, that has a preference for NADP as a cofactor.[32] Even at a local concentration of ethanol of 2% in the basal layer, ethanol retards the metabolism of estradiol to estrone by a factor of 10, based upon the flux of the metabolite, estrone.[30] The decrease in the apparent first-order enzyme rate constant as a function of ethanol concentration was consistent with the kinetics of competitive inhibition. It had been hypothesized that the enzyme inhibition may be partly related to the lowering of the chemical potential of estradiol by ethanol. However, with increasing ethanol concentration from 0 to 25%, a 20-fold increase in estradiol solubility is not sufficient to account for the more than 200-fold decrease in the enzyme rate constant.[30] Interestingly, acute ethanol exposure was also reported to inhibit competitively the action of mixed function oxidase in rat hepatic microsomes.[33]

The effect of ethanol on cutaneous metabolism also has been studied *in vivo* in humans to some extent. In a study in healthy volunteers of an administered transdermal nitroglycerin dose with a simultaneous infusion of ^{15}N-nitroglycerin,[34] the absolute bioavailability of transdermal nitroglycerin was 71 ± 14%, with a ratio of 0.94 ± 0.73 of 1,2:1,3 glycerol dinitrates produced.[35] The intravenous infusion produced a ratio of 18 ± 20 dinitrate metabolites. For a transdermal nitroglycerin system containing ethanol, the absolute bioavailability was 92 ± 13%, with a ratio of dinitrate metabolites of 1.7 ± 1.5. It appears that ethanol dramatically suppressed the cutaneous metabolism of nitroglycerin. However, the flux of nitroglycerin from the ethanol-enhanced transdermal system was two- to threefold greater than from the system without ethanol, and the possibility of saturable enzyme kinetics should be considered.

Transdermal delivery of testosterone across scrotal skin may lead to elevated levels of dihydrotestosterone, and cutaneous metabolism has been cited as the cause.[36] However, delivery of testosterone from a transdermal system containing the combined enhancers ethanol, triolein, and oleic acid[37] across nonscrotal skin resulted in dihydrotestosterone levels comparable to healthy men.[38] While Mazer et al.[38] attributed this difference to differences in regional cutaneous metabolism, suppression of metabolism by the enhancing mixture containing ethanol or differences in fluxes also may account for these observations.

VII. DESIGN OF TRANSDERMAL SYSTEMS WITH ETHANOL

Two principles have been used to design transdermal systems containing ethanol. In the commercial transdermal estradiol system the delivery of estradiol to the skin is controlled by a membrane-adhesive laminate that determines the rate of delivery of ethanol to the skin. In a transdermal testosterone system undergoing clinical trials a composition of mixed enhancers including ethanol must be delivered to the surface of the skin, and this mixture flows through a microporous membrane.[38]

For membrane-controlled transdermal systems, system design relies upon the skin permeation of the drug being linear with the skin transport of ethanol, and the membrane-adhesive laminate is selected to control the delivery of ethanol to the skin. For ethylene vinyl acetate membranes, the relationship is simplified further because the steady-state flux of ethanol across the membrane-adhesive laminate is linear, with the concentration of ethanol in the drug reservoir.[39] Thus, the enhancement factor for the drug across skin from such membrane-controlled systems is linear with the concentration of ethanol in the reservoir.[40] The enhancement factors observed in *in vitro* skin permeation studies[40] and in an absolute bioavailability study in six healthy volunteers[34] were 2.2 and 2.3, respectively. Moreover, presumably as a result of controlling the delivery of ethanol, the intersubject variation in the *in vivo* transdermal delivery rate of nitroglycerin for this ethanol-enhanced membrane-controlled system was reduced 57% as compared to the system without ethanol.[34]

When more than one solvent is present in the enhancing mixture, a monolithic system is the simplest way to ensure that the appropriate composition is delivered to the surface of the skin. A gel on a microporous membrane is one method of achieving delivery of the appropriate composition.[41]

REFERENCES

1. **Good, W. R., Powers, M. S., Campbell, P., and Schenkel, L.,** A new transdermal delivery system for estradiol, *J. Control. Rel.,* 2, 28, 1985.
2. **Gale, R. M., Goetz, V., Lee, E. S., Taskovich, L. T., and Yum, S. I.,** Device for Delivering Fentanyl Across the Skin at a Constant Rate to Maintain Analgesia over a Long Period, U.S. Patent 4,588,580, 1986.
3. **Santus, G. C. and Baker, R. W.,** Transdermal enhancer patent literature, *J. Control. Rel.,* 25, 1, 1993.
4. **Liu, P., Kurihara-Bergstrom, T., and Good, W. R.,** Cotransport of estradiol and ethanol through human skin *in vitro:* understanding the permeant/enhancer flux relationship, *Pharm. Res.,* 8, 938, 1991.
5. **Ghanem, A., Mahmoud, H., Higuchi, W. I., Rohr, U. D., Borsadia, S., Liu, P., Fox, J. L., and Good, W. R.,** The effects of ethanol on the transport of β-estradiol and other permeants in hairless mouse skin. II. A new quantitative approach, *J. Control. Rel.,* 6, 75, 1987.
6. **Ghanem, A., Mahmoud, H., Higuchi, W. I., Liu, P., and Good, W. R.,** The effects of ethanol on the transport of lipophilic and polar permeants across hairless mouse skin: methods/validation of a novel approach, *Int. J. Pharm.,* 78, 137, 1992.
7. **Devaux, P. F. and Seigneuret, M.,** Specificity of lipid-protein interactions as determined by spectroscopic techniques, *Biochim. Biophys. Acta,* 822, 463, 1985.
8. **Cherry, R. J.,** Rotational and lateral diffusion of membrane proteins. *Biochim. Biophys. Acta,* 559, 289, 1979.

9. **Goates, C. Y. and Knutson, K.,** Enhanced permeation of polar compounds through human epidermis. I. Permeability and membrane structural changes in the presence of short-chain alcohols, *Biochim. Biophys. Acta,* in press.
10. **Guy, R. H., Mak, V. H. W., Kai, T., Bommannan, D., and Potts, R. O.,** Percutaneous penetration enhancers: mode of action, in *Prediction of Percutaneous Penetration,* Scott, R. C., Guy, R. H., and Hadgraft, J., Eds., IBC Technical Services, London, 1990, 215.
11. **Dinh, S. M., Luo, C. W., and Berner, B.,** Upper and lower limits of human skin electrical resistance in iontophoresis, *AIChE J.,* 39, 2011, 1993.
12. **Dinh, S. M. and Kachmar, D. A.,** Salt concentration and solvent effects on the *in vitro* electrical resistance of human skin, *Proc. ACS,* 207, PMSE, 43, March 13 to 17, 1994.
13. **Berner, B., Juang, R. H., and Mazzenga, G. C.,** Ethanol and water sorption into SC and model systems, *J. Pharm. Sci.,* 78, 472, 1989.
14. **Kasting, G. B., Smith, R. L., and Cooper, E. R.,** Effect of lipid solubility and molecular size on percutaneous absorption, *Pharmacol. Skin,* 1, 138, 1987.
15. **Berner, B., Mazzenga, G. C., Otte, J. H., Steffens, R. J., Juang, R. H., and Ebert, C. D.,** Ethanol-water mutually enhanced transdermal therapeutic systems. II. Skin permeation of ethanol and nitroglycerin, *J. Pharm. Sci.,* 78, 402, 1989.
16. **Mazzenga, G. C., Berner, B., and Jordan, F.,** The transdermal delivery of zwitterionic drugs. II. The flux of zwitterion salts, *J. Control. Rel.,* 20, 163, 1992.
17. **Yum, S., Lee, E., Taskovich, L., and Theeuwes, F.,** Permeation enhancement with ethanol: mechanism of action through skin, in *Drug Permeation Enhancement,* Hsieh, D. S., Ed., Marcel Dekker, New York, 1994, chap. 8.
18. **Shinoda, K.,** *Principles of Solution and Solubility,* Marcel Dekker, New York, 1978, 183.
19. **Berner, B., Juang, R. H., and Rosen, R.,** Report BPR 86082, Ciba-Geigy, Ardsley, NY, 1986.
20. **Comfort, A., Dinh, S. M., Otte, J., Shevchuk, I., and Berner, B.,** Enhanced transport in a therapeutic system, *Biomaterials,* 11, 729, 1990.
21. **Blank, I. H., Maloney, J., Emslie, A. G., and Simon, I.,** The diffusion of water across the SC as a function of its water content, *J. Invest. Dermatol.,* 82, 188, 1984.
22. **Berner, B., Otte, J. H., Mazzenga, G. C., Steffens, R. J., and Ebert, C. D.,** Ethanol-water mutually enhanced transdermal therapeutic system. I. Nitroglycerin solution properties and membrane transport, *J. Pharm. Sci.,* 78, 314, 1989.
23. **Nightingale, J., Kurihara-Bergstrom, T., Mirley, C., Signor, C., and DeNoble, L.,** *In vitro* transdermal delivery of buprenorphine HCl, *Proc. Int. Symp. Control. Rel. Bioact. Mater.,* 19, 246, 1992.
24. **Bockris, J. O'M. and Reddy, A. K. N.,** *Modern Electrochemistry,* Vol. 1, Plenum Press, New York, 1970, chap. 5.
25. **Liu, P., Kurihara-Bergstrom, T., Clarke, F. H., Gonnella, N., and Good, W. R.,** Quantitative evaluation of aqueous isopropanol enhancement on skin flux of terbutaline (sulfate). I. Ion associations and species equilibria in the formulation, *Pharm. Res.,* 9, 1035, 1992.
26. **Pal, A. and Lahiri, S. C.,** Conductometric studies on the dissolution constants of benzoic acid in 2-propanol + water mixtures, *Z. Phys. Leipzig,* 268, s378, 1987.
27. **Obata, Y., Takayama, K., Maitani, Y., Machida, Y., and Nagai, T.,** Effect of ethanol on skin permeation of nonionized and ionized diclofenac, *Int. J. Pharm.,* 89, 191, 1993.
28. **Kurihara-Bergstrom, T. and Liu, P.,** Enhanced *in vitro* skin transport of ionized terbutaline using its sulfate salt form in aqueous isopropanol, *S.T.P. Pharm. Sci.,* 1, 52, 1991.
29. *Physician's Desk Reference,* 47th ed., Medical Economics Data, Oradell, NJ, 1993, 895.
30. **Liu, P., Higuchi, W. I., Song, W., Kurihara-Bergstrom, T., and Good, W. R.,** Quantitative evaluation of ethanol effects on diffusion and metabolism of β-estradiol in hairless mouse skin, *Pharm. Res.,* 8, 865, 1991.
31. **Liu, P., Higuchi, W. I., Ghanem, A., Kurihara-Bergstrom, T., and Good, W. R.,** Assessing the influence of ethanol on simultaneous diffusion and metabolism of β-estradiol in hairless mouse skin for the 'asymmetric' situation *in vitro, Int. J. Pharm.,* 78, 123, 1992.
32. **Davis, B. P., Rampini, E., and Hsia, S. L.,** 17β-Hydroxysteroid dehydrogenase of rat skin. Substrate specificity and inhibitors, *J. Biol. Chem.,* 247, 1407, 1972.
33. **Rubin, E., Gang, H., Misra, P. S., and Liever, C. S.,** Inhibition of drug metabolism by acute ethanol intoxication. A hepatic microsomal mechanism, *Am. J. Med.,* 49, 801, 1970.

34. **Kochak, G. M., Berner, B., DeWitte, W., Leal, M., and Sambol, N. C.,** Variational analysis of the transdermal delivery rate from two prototypical ethanol-water nitroglycerin TTS devices and Transderm Nitro-10 in the normal population, *J. Pharmacokin. Biopharm.*, 20, 443, 1992.
35. **Steffens, R. J., Hayes, M. J., Powell, M., Berner, B., Morgan, J., Joshi, J., Guernsey, K., and Good, W. R.,** The cutaneous metabolism of nitroglycerin, *Proc. Int. Symp. Control. Rel. Bioact. Mater.*, 19, 236, 1992.
36. **Ahmed, S. R., Boucher, A. E., Manni, A., Santen, R. J., Bartholomew, M., and Demars, L. M.,** Transdermal testosterone therapy in the treatment of male hypogonadism, *J. Clin. Endocrinol. Metab.*, 66, 546, 1988.
37. **Patel, D. C. and Chang, Y.,** Penetration Enhancement with Binary Systems of Oleic Acid, Oleins, and Oleyl Alcohol with Lower Alcohols, U.S. Patent 4,863,970, 1989.
38. **Mazer, N. A., Heiber, W. E., Moellmer, J. F., Meikle, A. W., Stringham, J. D., Sanders, S. W., Tolman, K. G., and Odell, W. D.,** Enhanced transdermal delivery of testosterone: a new physiological approach for androgen replacement in hypogonadal men, *J. Control. Rel.*, 19, 347, 1992.
39. **Dinh, S. M., Berner, B., Sun, Y. M., and Lee, P. I.,** Sorption and transport of ethanol and water in poly(ethylene-co-vinyl acetate) membrane, *J. Membr. Sci.*, 69, 223, 1992.
40. **Comfort, A., Dinh, S. M., Otte, J. H., Shevchuk, I., Kochak, G., and Berner, B.,** *In vitro* and *in vivo* correlation of ethanol-enhanced nitroglycerin TTS, *Proc. Int. Symp. Control. Rel. Bioact. Mater.* 19, 244, 1992.
41. **Chang, Y., Patel, D. C., and Ebert, C. D.,** Device for Administering an Active Agent to the Skin or Mucosa, U.S. Patent 4,849,224, 1989.
42. **Pershing, L. K., Lambert, L. D., and Knutson, K.,** Mechanism of ethanol-enhanced permeation across human skin *in vivo, Pharm. Res.*, 7, 170, 1990.
43. **Kim, Y., Ghanem, A., Mahmoud, H., and Higuchi, W. I.,** Short chain alkanols as transport enhancers for lipophilic and polar/ionic permeants in hairless mouse skin: mechanism(s) of action, *Int. J. Pharm.*, 80, 17, 1992.
44. **Kurihara-Bergstrom, T., Knutson, K., DeNoble, L., and Goates, C.,** Percutaneous absorption enhancement of an ionic molecule by ethanol-water systems in human skin, *Pharm. Res.*, 7, 762, 1990.
45. **Hatanaka, T., Shimoyama, M., Sujibayashi, K., and Morimoto, Y.,** Effect of vehicle on the skin permeability of drugs: polyethylene glycol 400-water and ethanol-water binary solvents, *J. Control. Rel.*, 23, 247, 1993.
46. **Kai, T., Mak, V. H. W., Potts, R. O., and Guy, R. H.,** Mechanism of percutaneous penetration enhancement: effect of n-alkanols on the permeability barrier of hairless mouse skin, *J. Control. Rel.*, 12, 103, 1990.
47. **Yu, D., Sanders, L. M., Davidson, G. W. R., III, Marvin, M. J., and Ling, T.,** Percutaneous absorption of nicardipine and ketorolac in rhesus monkeys, *Pharm. Res.*, 5, 457, 1988.
48. **Okamoto, H., Muta, K., Hashida, M., and Sezaki, H.,** Percutaneous penetration of acyclovir through excised hairless mouse and rat skin: effect of vehicle and percutaneous penetration enhancer, *Pharm. Res.*, 7, 64, 1990.
49. **Shahi, V. and Zatz, J. L.,** Effect of formulation factors on penetration of hydrocortisone through mouse skin, *J. Pharm. Sci.*, 67, 789, 1978.
50. **Friend, D., Catz, P., Heller, J., Reid, J., and Baker, R.,** Transdermal delivery of levonorgestrel. I. Alkanols as permeation enhancers *in vitro*, *J. Control. Rel.*, 7, 243, 1988.
51. **Obata, Y., Takayama, K., Machida, Y., and Nagai, T.,** Combined effect of cyclic monoterpenes and ethanol on percutaneous absorption of diclofenac sodium, *Drug Design Discovery*, 8, 137, 1991.
52. **Mahjour, M., Mauser, B. E., Rashidbaigi, Z. A., and Fawzi, M. B.,** Effects of propylene glycol diesters of caprylic and capric acids (Miglyol® 840) and ethanol binary systems on *in vitro* skin permeation of drugs, *Int. J. Pharm.*, 95, 161, 1993.
53. **Catz, P. and Friend, D. R.,** Effect of cosolvents on ethyl acetate enhanced percutaneous absorption of levonorgestrel, *J. Control. Rel.*, 12, 171, 1990.
54. **Morimoto, Y., Sugibayashi, K., Kobayashi, K., Shoji, H., Yamazaki, J., and Kimura, M.,** A new enhancer-coenhancer system to increase skin permeation of morphine hydrochloride *in vitro*, *Int. J. Pharm.*, 91, 9, 1993.

55. **Nishihata, T., Rytting, J. H., Kamada, A., Matsumoto, K., and Takahashi, K.,** Combined effect of alcohol and urea on the *in vitro* transport of indomethacin across rat dorsal skin, *J. Pharm. Sci.,* 79, 487, 1990.
56. **Goto, S., Uchida, T., Lee, C. K., Yasutake, T., and Zhang, J.,** Effect of various vehicles on ketoprofen permeation across excised hairless mouse skin, *J. Pharm. Sci.,* 82, 959, 1993.
57. **Kim, C. K., Kim, J., Chi, S., and Shim, C.,** Effect of fatty acids and urea on the penetration of ketoprofen through rat skin, *Int. J. Pharm.,* 99, 109, 1993.
58. **Pardo, A., Shiri, Y., and Cohen, S.,** Percutaneous absorption of physostigmine: optimization of delivery from a binary solvent by thermodynamic control, *J. Pharm. Sci.,* 79, 573, 1991.
59. **Goldberg-Cettina, M., Liu, P., Nightingale, J., and Kurihara-Bergstrom, T.,** Enhanced transdermal delivery of estradiol *in vitro* using binary vehicles of isopropyl myristate and short-chain alkanols, *Int. J. Pharm.,* submitted.
60. **Aungst, B. J., Rogers, N. J., and Shefter, E.,** Enhancement of naloxone penetration through human skin *in vitro* using fatty acids, fatty alcohols, surfactants, sulfoxides and amides, *Int. J. Pharm.,* 33, 225, 1986.

Chapter 3.2

Propylene Glycol

Barbara Bendas, Reinhard Neubert, and Wolfgang Wohlrab

CONTENTS

I. INTRODUCTION

Propylene glycol (PG) is used widely as a constituent in dermatological formulations. Its importance as a cosolvent for lipophilic drugs and potential enhancers such as Azone®, fatty a cids, or fatty alcohols is recognized, but the literature provides conflicting results as to whether this molecule is able to increase skin permeability. The alteration of the barrier function includes affecting the bilayer structure of the intercellular lipids and/or the keratinocytes, especially the α-keratin structure.[1,2] It is questionable whether increased drug uptake, based on higher partitioning into the stratum corneum (SC) as a consequence of solvent penetration, could be considered to be an enhancer action because the intact skin structure is not changed. This effect, directed at the increase of the solution capacity within the SC, is supposed to be the action of PG.[1,3] However, it is unlikely that only one mechanism is responsible for the enhancement of drug penetration, particularly for small solvent molecules such as short-chain alcohols and glycols, without specific structure elements in the molecule.

Based on numerous experiments, the action of solvents such as PG was attributed to a pure cosolvent effect.[4] Maximizing the thermodynamic activity of a drug in the vehicle PG contributes to increased drug uptake into the skin. The permeation of many drugs, especially of very lipophilic molecules, was shown to be unaffected when they were applied in PG as compared to a standard vehicle. Therefore, the effects of PG were explained by differences in drug solubility on the donor side.

According to Hadgraft,[5] the decrease in barrier function and the effect on the thermodynamic activity of the drug in the vehicle are difficult to separate because

0-8493-2605-2/95/$0.00+$.50

they are complementary. Walters[6] emphasized that PG acts only as a cosolvent, producing saturated or nearly saturated solutions of the permeant. However, he included results of experiments that were conducted under thermodynamic control, and therefore, an enhancement effect should be detected.

Many efforts have been made to clarify the way in which PG acts to promote drug penetration into or permeation through the skin. *In vitro* permeation studies and *in vivo* investigations on its influence showed that the results depend strongly on the experimental conditions. Therefore, the interpretation of the results is heterogeneous. Important support to understanding the mechanisms by which PG acts is provided by biophysical investigations that employed differential scanning calorimetry (DSC), small-angle X-ray scattering (SAXS), or Fourier transform infrared attenuated total reflection spectroscopy (FTIR/ATR). With these methods it seems possible to look inside the arrangement of SC structure at the molecular level and explain why the permeation of some drugs is enhanced by PG, whereas the permeation of other drugs is not influenced.

II. *IN VITRO* STUDIES

A. USING RELEASE MODELS

In 1968 Poulsen and co-workers[7] published results from studies on the *in vitro* release of two topical steroids, fluocinolone acetonide and its acetate ester from binary PG–water mixtures used as gels with carbopol 934. The release studies were carried out without a separating membrane between the donor and acceptor phases. Isopropyl myristate (IPM) was used as the acceptor. It was shown that the release of steroid depends directly on the physicochemical properties of the drugs in the vehicle and on the relation to the acceptor. The determining properties are solubility in the vehicle and partition behavior. Over the range of various PG contents a maximum of released drug occurs. Using the partition coefficients *(K)* between IPM and the PG–water mixtures as an index of the relative thermodynamic activity of the two steroids in the vehicles, it was pointed out that the drugs were delivered according to their affinity to the gels (Figure 1). This implies that a releasing maximum exists for PG contents, which provides the fully solubilized drug in the vehicle in order to maximize thermodynamic activity. For PG contents below this limit, the release rate is determined by the dissolution process.

This work shows the action of PG as a cosolvent. Steroid uptake into the receptor phase is controlled by the vehicle. Studies on the permeation of drugs through human abdominal skin and the vasoconstrictor assay confirmed the results obtained from the release studies.[8]

Miller et al.[9] presented studies in which the soluble local anesthetic tetracaine (free base and acid salt) in PG–saline mixtures was used as the basic to gain an understanding of the factors affecting percutaneous absorption. The physicochemical data were compared to the fluxes obtained from permeation studies that used a synthetic polycarbonate membrane and hairless mouse skin. The fluxes through both membranes were in agreement. An optimal PG content for the permeation rate of the tetracaine mixture did exist. According to the theory, the flux maximum, indicating a maximum thermodynamic activity, is related to the poorest solvent of the drug. However, in this study the highest fluxes were measured at a solubility of the

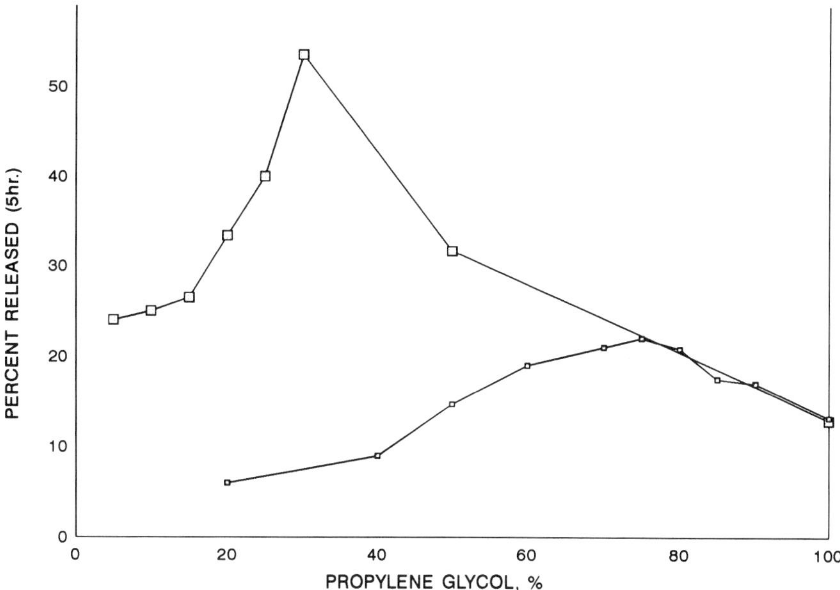

Figure 1 Release profile for 0.025% fluocinolone acetonide (□) and 0.025% fluocinonide (▫) at 25°C (PG-water gels). (From Ostrenga et al., *J. Pharm. Sci.*, 60, 1175, 1971. With permission.)

tetracaine mixture near its maximum. Therefore, the partition seems not to be the permeation controlling factor. Two possible explanations were given for this problem: either the solution is micellar, and therefore no relation exists between solubility and thermodynamic activity, or a significant solvent velocity is created, carrying the drug through the membrane. However, the latter would not explain the decreased permeability beyond the maximum.

The topic of our investigations was the penetration mechanism of topical steroids with differing physicochemical properties caused by PG. PG was applied as binary aqueous mixtures. A multilayer membrane system consisting of a collodium matrix in which dodecanol is immobilized was used as acceptor.[10] We showed that PG has a dual action on the penetration of lipophilic drugs, which were applied as saturated solutions under finite dose conditions. Here, solubility seems to be the most important factor because it "decides" whether the penetration is thermodynamically controlled or whether an enhancement effect of PG dominates. The most lipophilic drug, betamethasone 17-valerate, showing the lowest solubilities in PG–water mixtures, penetrates as predicted from the physicochemical parameters (thermodynamic control) (Figure 2).

The same is true for hydrocortisone 17-butyrate (HCB) up to a PG content of 40%. The thermodynamically determined maximum of penetration is shifted to 20% PG. This is explained by the higher solubilities of HCB in PG–water mixtures and the corresponding lower partition coefficients. For PG contents >40% PG enhances HCB penetration. The penetrated amount increases with increasing PG content. This enhancement of PG dominates for hydrocortisone uptake into the acceptor, although it provides the highest affinities for PG–water mixtures (Figure 2). This effect can be

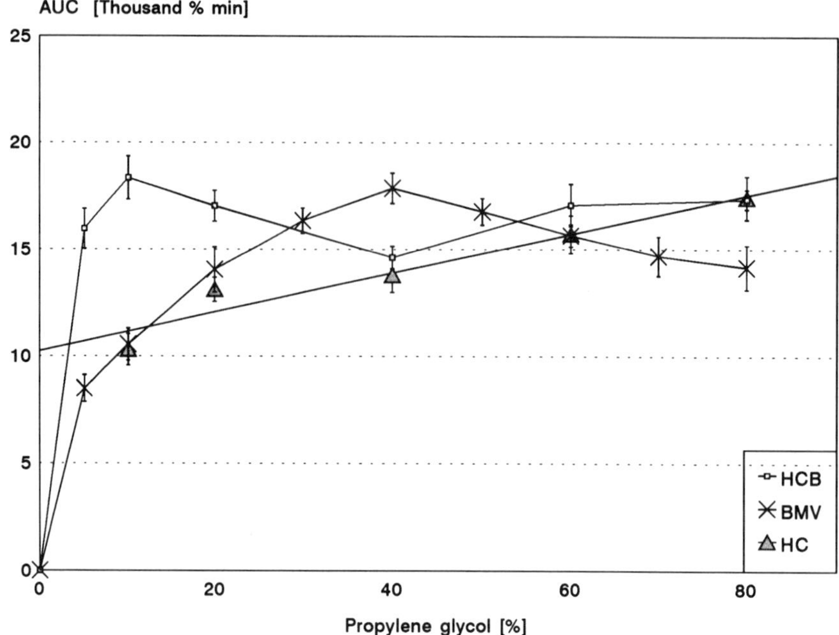

Figure 2 Penetration behavior of betamethasone-17-valerate (BMV) and hydrocortisone-17-butyrate (HCB) and hydrocortisone (HC) from propyleneglycol-water mixtures into the multilayer artificial acceptor system. (From Bendas, B., Doctoral thesis, Martin Luther Universität, Halle, 1993).

explained only by increased drug solubility and partition within the acceptor due to PG penetration. Propylene glycol penetrates rapidly and to a large extent into the acceptor membranes. The acceptor solubility of all compounds is shown to be improved by this process. Only hydrocortisone penetration is enhanced by PG, however. Comparison of the initial PG and drug penetration indicates that all compounds are enhanced by PG in this time interval. Additionally, the extent of drug penetration can be correlated to the solubility of the drugs in the corresponding PG–water mixtures. Extrapolating from the results it is supposed that the major effect of PG arises from a solvent drag effect for hydrocortisone and from the thermodynamic control for betamethasone 17-valerate.

B. USING MODELS WITH NATURAL MEMBRANES

Although it was shown that when using animal skin it is not possible to predict penetration enhancement effects for human skin treatment without restrictions, many studies on accelerant actions have been carried out in this field.[11] However, animal skin seems to be an alternative in screening whether an accelerant can exert an effect. On this basis, the flux of diflorasone diacetate through hairless mouse skin was studied using both a PG vehicle and a PG–water mixture.[12] Turi et al. discussed their results with respect to the solubility profile and skin–vehicle partitioning as the function of the solvent concentration. The flux data confirmed that the permeation was dependent on partition, as predicted from the physicochemical parameters. Additionally, a rather easy permeation was observed for PG. The resistance of the skin to PG declined as the weight fraction of PG was increased. Pretreating the skin with PG for 18 h led to permeation values of the drug twice those obtained without pretreatment. On the one hand, these results show a thermodynamic, controlled permeation profile of the drug. On the other hand, PG pretreatment increases the permeated drug, indicating that the solvent acts as an enhancer.

Sarpotdar and Zatz[13,14] studied the influence of PG from binary PG–water mixtures on lidocaine and hydrocortisone flux and permeated amounts following application under infinite dose conditions. In both cases decreasing values were measured with increasing PG content, indicating that derived from Fick's law, the thermodynamic activity declines as the affinity of the drug to the vehicle rises. Therefore, no evidence exists for an enhancing effect of PG. Similar results were obtained if the finite dose technique was applied. However, other studies showed that an enhancing effect of PG for hydrocortisone does exist.[10,24] Because PG penetration and the increased solubilizing capacity of the SC for hydrocortisone are evident, one should take into account the possibility that PG establishes a reservoir of hydrocortisone into the SC. The amount of hydrocortisone that permeates into the acceptor compartment will then be determined by the partition between the skin and the acceptor medium. Therefore, an enhancement of PG can be covered.

In contrast, Kaiho et al.[15] showed that the uptake of a drug (indomethacin) applied transdermally into the systemic circulation is directly related to the permeation of PG, even if one or two accelerants are added to the PG base. The percutaneous absorption profiles of indomethacin and PG were almost the same and did not differ significantly when the vehicle contained PG and stearyl alcohol or stearic acid. The authors proposed as a possible mechanism that the drug uptake into the skin takes place together with PG. Later results confirmed this dependence on the content of oleic acid in the formulation.[16]

The importance of the established experimental conditions was emphasized by the studies of Goodman and Barry.[17] The permeation of the polar 5-fluorouracil (5-FU) and the more nonpolar estradiol was measured using fully hydrated human epidermal membranes applying infinite dose conditions. Propylene glycol was ineffective for 5-FU as a vehicle. The results of a finite dose study using a dried film of the drug indicated an enhanced 5-FU permeation if the permeation was not measured at steady state.[17,18]

Tiemessen and co-workers[19] studied the influence of various enhancers on the skin barrier. To divide enhancer effects in dependence on controlled hydration, isolated human SC was placed between two silicone membranes, which allows hydration to the desired degree. The results obtained from the steady-state fluxes of the lipophilic nitroglycerine indicate an increased permeability of the SC with an increasing of its water content of the SC. Under both fully hydrated SC (70 to 80%) and controlled hydrated SC (57% water), the PG treatment did not cause any increase in the SC permeability of the lipophilic model drug.

Other results[20] were obtained from studies concerning the dependence of steroid penetration on PG. Polano and Ponec used sheets of human abdominal epidermis and showed that penetration of HCB exceeds the level of penetration from an oil-in-water cream or plastibase if PG is added to the formulation. The penetration rate does not level out when the saturated vehicle is diluted by increasing the PG content. PG penetrated readily through the epidermis, and the maximum penetration rate of PG

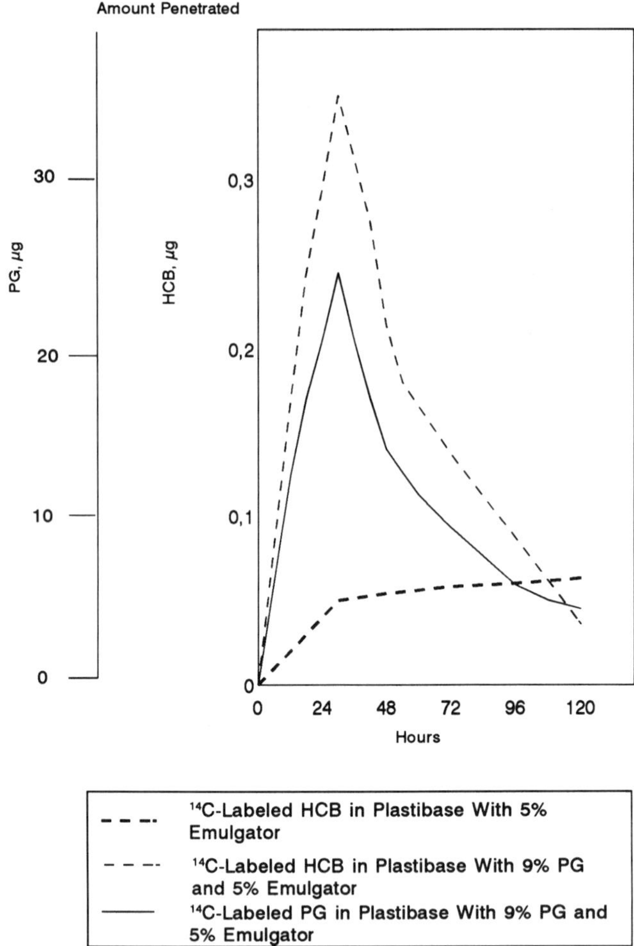

Figure 3 Penetration of hydrocortisone 17-butyrate from two different vehicles and of PG from plastibase with emulgator. (From Polano, M. K. and Ponec, M., *Arch. Dermatol.*, 112, 675, 1976. With permission.)

and HCB occurred simultaneously (Figure 3). Therefore, the authors speculated that PG and HCB penetrate together into the epidermis. Furthermore, it was shown that by creating a dry atmosphere, despite the absence of hydration, PG is able to enhance penetration of HCB, whereas in creams without PG the opposite effect occurred. Even more HCB penetrated in the dry atmosphere. In our opinion this observation confirms the hypothesis that the solvent PG is able to carry the lipophilic drug through the interface of the vehicle–epidermis membrane.

The effect of PG applied in a binary mixture with glycerol on the steady-state flux of estradiol and metronidazole through excised human skin was the topic of the studies offered by Mølgaard and Hoelgaard.[21] Two principal results were pointed out. On the one hand, estradiol and metronidazole fluxes increase with increasing weight fractions of PG in PG–glycerol mixtures. On the other hand, the effect of PG on flux

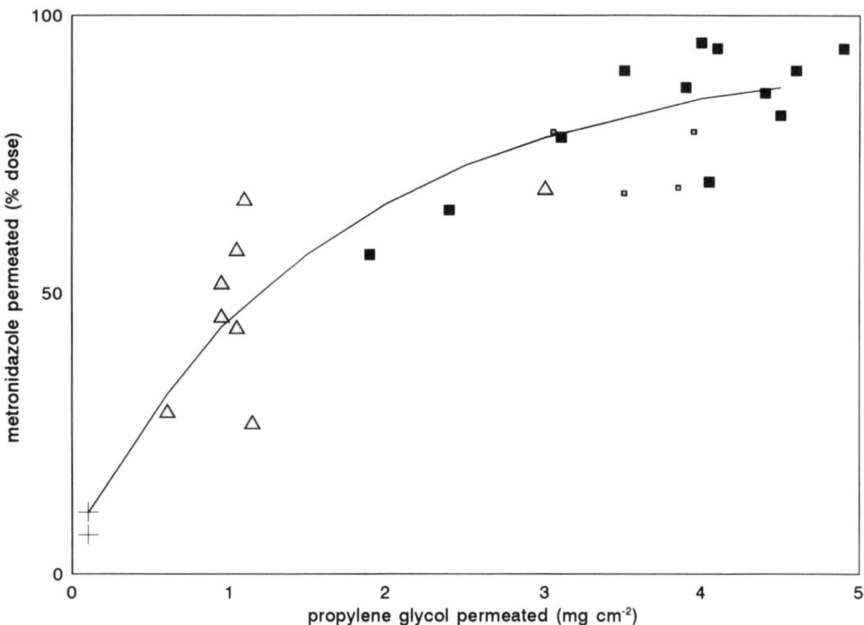

Figure 4 Comparison of 90-h permeation of metronidazole and PG from various PG vehicles through human skin *in vitro*. □: PG, pure state, +: PG–glycerol mixtures, Δ: PG–water gels, ■: PG–alkanol mixtures. (From Mølgaard, B. and Hoelgaard, A., *Acta Pharm. Suec.*, 20, 443, 1983. With permission.)

is nearly linearly dependent on the concentrations of both drugs in the vehicle. The investigators concluded that the vehicle effect can be related mainly to the action of PG on the skin membrane and less so to the drug–vehicle interaction.

Extended studies showed that a simultaneous permeation of estradiol, metronidazole, and PG through human SC exists.[22] The results indicate that altering the barrier permeability for metronidazole is associated with the amount of PG that permeates the skin. Furthermore, the flux of PG and the drug increases with higher PG content on the donor side. Because the permeation rates of PG, estradiol, and metronidazole are unaffected by the aqueous phase in binary PG–water mixtures and by the varying degree of drug saturation (from 0.8 to 100%), the thermodynamic activity of drugs in the vehicles seems not to determine the permeation behavior. It is obvious that the degree of PG permeation plays an important role in drug transport through the skin. A positive correlation between metronidazole and PG permeation is given in Figure 4. It is supposed that the drug is kept dissolved in PG while permeating the SC. On the other hand, the phenomenon is less significant and unexplained for estradiol. The importance of other vehicle components for the extent of PG permeation is emphasized. Whereas glycerol decreases PG permeation, medium chain length alcohols favor PG diffusion into the skin. Furthermore, the solubility of metronidazole in PG–water mixtures increases much more (from 10 to 22 mg/ml) than the solubility of estradiol (from 0.002 to 2.8 mg/ml) when the PG content was increased from 20 to 80%. This result supports the theory of the significance of "carrying through" of the solubilized drug by PG. (The importance of the solubility in PG was also discussed for the differing penetration behavior of betamethasone 17-valerate and hydrocortisone, which are from 0.016 to 2.1 mg/ml and from 0.68 to 10.5 mg/ml soluble in PG–water mixtures.[10])

An extensive study demonstrating that drug solubilization in the vehicle, partitioning, solvent penetration, and barrier disruption can contribute to increased skin permeation of drugs from PG–enhancer mixtures was undertaken by Aungst et al.[23] The drugs investigated differed in their polarities, providing solubilities in PG ranging from ≈3 to 250 mg/ml. Only saturated solutions were used for the diffusion studies. The authors showed that PG permeation was affected by adding fatty acids and dodecylamine. All of the additives increased the PG flux as compared to PG alone. Furthermore, lag time was decreased, but not to the same extent found for the flux.

Comparison between changes in permeability and partitioning enables investigators to decide whether a barrier disruption is involved in the increased permeability. The results indicate that the relative contributions of the factors vary from drug to drug. For instance, in a combination of indomethacin and dodecylamine in PG, increasing solubility is mainly responsible for the increased flux, and the permeability coefficient was thus unchanged.

Barry and Bennett[24] were concerned with the mode of action of potential penetration enhancers in human skin. They selected three model compounds as penetrants, mannitol, hydrocortisone, and progesterone, with widely differing physicochemical properties. The permeation studies were carried out after a dry film of the vehicle composition with acetone was deposited on the skin surface. Flux time curves were recorded which illustrate that the flux of the drugs peaks after the enhancer composition was applied. Two further acetone applications were made to prove whether a drug reservoir in the SC was established. Whereas PG has no influence on the permeation of the hydrophilic mannitol and has a poor effect on the lipophilic progesterone, the permeation of hydrocortisone increased 30-fold as compared to the control. The maximum flux is increased by a factor of 50. Progesterone, which is a more nonpolar steroid than hydrocortisone, offers high partition coefficients into the SC. The rate-limiting step is assumed to be the diffusion out of the SC. Therefore, enhancer effects should be less dramatic. Taking the experimental data and theoreticals into consideration, the authors concluded further that enhancement of PG occurs when the penetrant is more soluble in the solvent than in the water.

Kastings and co-workers[25] observed an enhanced permeation of tripolidine through excised human skin. The amount permeated from the PG base is nearly four times higher than that from oily vehicles, although only the oily vehicles provide the maximum thermodynamic activity. The authors explained the effect as a combined action of PG and water. When both solvents are sufficiently incorporated into the SC they may modify the solubility of the permeant in the tissue. Because of its high solubility in PG tripolidine is assumed to undergo this mechanism.

III. *IN VIVO* INVESTIGATIONS

A. PHARMACODYNAMIC EFFECTS

For some drugs it is possible to draw conclusions from the intrinsic activity of skin penetrability. This procedure is very well assessed for topical glucocorticoids, which produce a skin blanching of induced erythema due to their vasconstrictory effect. Results derived from formulations with and without added enhancers, providing the same thermodynamic activity for the investigated glucocorticoid, can be estimated by the inset, intensity, and duration of the skin blanching response.

The influence of PG on the bioavailability of betamethasone 17-benzoate was compared to the basic vehicle dimethylisosorbide by Barry et al.[26,27] The experimental arrangement was given by the standard occluded vasoconstrictor assay without thermodynamic control. From numerous studied enhancers only *N*-methyl-2-pyrrolidone (NMP) was more effective than the standard. The bioavailability of the applied PG vehicle was less than the dimethylisosorbide application. In contrast, using the nonoccluded blanching assay and maintaining constant thermodynamic activity at 10% saturation, quite different results were obtained.[26,28] For example, the pyrrolidones offered increased bioavailability. Furthermore, the bioavailability of betamethasone 17-benzoate was enhanced by azone (2%) and oleic acid (1.5 and 5%), applied with PG, providing maximum thermodynamic activity of the enhancers. Oleic acid dissolved in dimethylisosorbide provides no enhancement. With PG alone, the bioavailability of betamethasone 17-benzoate is slightly increased by a factor of 0.5, which is estimated to be a "borderline improvement".

By using different experimental arrangements different results can be obtained which can determine whether a chemical is regarded as an enhancer for a special drug. Both the differences in thermodynamic activity and the occlusion are supposed to be involved in the negative enhancement for betamethasone 17-benzoate in the case described first. It is known that the hydration of the SC enhances the permeability for especially hydrophilic or polar drugs; however, betamethasone 17-benzoate is a very lipophilic compound ($K_{oct/water}$>12,000). On the one hand, if a transcellular pathway is taken into account for drug diffusion, occlusion could lead to the swelling of the corneocytes. The SC will be more permeable, but it does not provide a better diffusion medium for lipophilic compounds. On the other hand, the maximized hydration of the polar head groups of the intercellular lipids, which may increase their fluidity, may provide the same problems to overcome the aqueous layers.

Induced erythema caused by the vasodilation of nicotinates was taken as the basis of further evaluations of *in vivo* penetration.[29] Benzylnicotinate was applied in a solution-type ointment at different concentrations after pretreating volunteers' forearms with either moisturizers or PG in aqueous solutions. The time between application and the appearance of a visible erythema was measured. The concentration-response curves obtained after pretreatment with the moisturizer or PG along with water (standard) are shifted parallel to lower concentrations when the penetration of benzylnicotinate is enhanced. The bioavailability factor (*f*) is then given by the horizontal distance between standard and test with medium response level. The tested moisturizers decreased *f* compared to the standard. Only PG enhanced significantly the penetration of benzylnicotinate. Two possible directions of the action of PG were discussed. PG may act as a cosolvent in the skin followed by an increase in the partition coefficient of the drug for SC–vehicle. Additionally, favored hydration of the α-keratin and the lipid bilayers was taken into account. The negative effect of the moisturizers was explained by the competition of the moisturizers with water for bonding sites in the corneocytes and polar regions of the lipid bilayers, which reduced the hydration grade. The structuring of water via some moisturizers, which is responsible for decreased diffusion coefficients of drugs *in vitro,* is possibly involved. However, it is likely that for the lipophilic benzylnicotinate ($K_{oct/water} = 211$) an increased hydration may hinder the diffusion much as it does for betamethasone 17-benzoate. Therefore, it is not expected that moisturizers would promote the penetration of lipophilic compounds. In contrast, PG is known to displace water from the bonding sites. The changed environment for the diffusing drug molecule probably favors its entrance and facilitates the transfer through the SC.

IV. ENHANCEMENT SYNERGISM OF PROPYLENE GLYCOL IN COMBINATION WITH A POTENTIAL PENETRATION ENHANCER

Propylene glycol has a greater effect on the penetration of drugs when it is applied together with different enhancers than each vehicle alone. Numerous papers describe this synergism in Table 1. Aungst et al.[29] showed that the effectiveness of an enhancer depends directly on the vehicle. Propylene glycol seems to be the best vehicle for the enhancers tested as compared to isopropanol, polyethylene glycol 400, mineral oil, or isopropyl myristate (IPM).

The effect of the vehicle (PG, ethanol, IPM, isopropanol) on the enhancement of acyclovir using terpene enhancers and azone was investigated by Okamoto et al.[30] Based on the solubility parameters, the authors postulated that the highest effect should be obtained using a mixture of a lipophilic vehicle and a hydrophilic enhancer. The results confirmed that on the one hand, the permeation of acyclovir is decreased if the solubility parameters of PG and the enhancer approximate. On the other hand, maximum enhancement was achieved with azone and PG, and it is for these that the solubility parameters differ mostly.

The enhancers are also able to increase the penetration of PG. This effect was pointed out by a number of researchers.[15,16,23] Mahjour et al.[34] investigated the permeability of narcotic analgesics using linoleic acid or azone in combination with PG. They estimated that the mixture of PG and linoleic acid or azone not only favors the penetration of the enhancers, but also the influx of PG into the skin. Due to similar effects of the mixtures on permeation of drugs, the authors suggested a nonspecific enhancement effect based on PG uptake into the skin.

The enhancement synergism is emphasized by studies on the effect of the terpene bisalbolol, PG, and their mixture on the 5-FU penetration presented by Kadir and Barry.[35] The enhancer combination provides a 16.9-fold increased flux of 5-FU. At the end of the experiment the flux difference between application of terpene and that of the mixture was diminished. A "washout" of PG from the SC was assumed to be responsible for this effect. The improvement in permeation is maintained if PG is continuously added to the application site. These results provide an argument that PG does not only mediate the transfer of the enhancer into the lipid bilayer of the SC, but also actively takes part in the enhancement effect. Therefore, it can be supposed that a "solvent drag effect" due to PG also exists for the potential enhancers.[16,22,37] In this case the effect of a "hydrophobic" enhancer is less determined by the activity in the vehicle, but depends on the solubility of the enhancer in PG.

Thus, it can be summarized that besides a special action of PG, the composition of the total vehicle determines the thermodynamic activity of the single components and their ability to diffuse out of the vehicle and the activity gradient to the SC.[17,30–32]

Table 1 Enhancement Synergism of Propylene Glycol and Potential Penetration Enhancers

	PG/Azones®	PG/Decyl-MSO	PG/Fatty Acids, Alcohols, Amides	PG/Pyrrolidones	Pg/*n*-Tensides	PG/Terpenes
Morphine derivatives	+ [35]		+ [35]			
Hydrocortisone 21-acetate	+ [34]			+ [34]		
Hydrocortisone	+ [24]	+ [24]	+ [24]	+ [24]	+ [14]	
5-Fluorouracil	+ [17], [18]	+ [17], [18], [39]	+ [17], [23] – [40]			+ [31], [36]
Acyclovir	+ [31]		+ [38]			+ [31]
Triamcinolone acetonide	+ [41]		+ [33]			+ [36]
Lidocaine					+ [13]	
Indomethacin			+ [15], [16], [23]			
Estradiol	+ [17], [18]	+/– [17] + [18]	+ [17], [18]			
Betamethasone 17-valerate	+ [28]		+ [28]	+ [27]		

Note: + enhancement effect; – no enhancement.

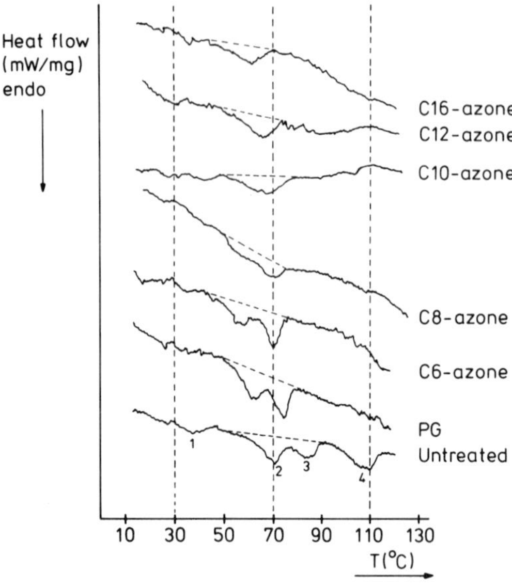

Figure 5 Thermal behavior of the SC after thermal treatment for 10 h at 320 K. Pretreatment with c_h-Azones® in combination with PG. (From Bouwstra, J. A. et al., *J. Control. Rel.*, 15, 209, 1991. With permission.)

V. BIOPHYSICAL INVESTIGATIONS ON THERMODYNAMIC AND STRUCTURAL ASPECTS OF THE STRATUM SORNEUM BARRIER

Changes in the phase transition temperatures of the intercellular lipids should refer one to an incorporation of enhancer molecules into the SC. Goodman and Barry[41] used the DSC technique to obtain further information on the action of PG. For this purpose SC samples were treated with PG–water solutions for an appropriate time. PG affects the phase transition temperatures T2/T3 (associated with lipid melting) only slightly. A decrease in transition temperature from 87°C of the control to 82°C of pure PG was detectable only for T3. Propylene glycol did not affect the T4 transition temperature (protein denaturation), but the peak shape was broadened. Although the change in T2/T3 is too small to explain the increased permeability of some drugs described in previous chapters, the alteration of T4 is associated with changes occurring in dehydrated SC sheets. Concerning the known competition of PG with water for the hydrogen bonding sites, it seems possible that either PG penetrates into the corneocytes or that PG, staying in the intercellular spaces, dehydrates the intracellular protein structures due to its hygroscopicity. However, the authors conclude from the T4 changes that PG solvates the keratinocytes and, therefore, transcellular drug transport becomes more imaginable.

Bouwstra et al.[42] studied the effect of PG on the physicochemical properties of the human SC by combining SAXS with differential thermoanalysis.[42] The 24-h pretreatment of the SC sample with pure PG shows that the T2/T3 transitions were shifted 10°C to lower transition temperatures (Figure 5). The shapes of the peaks remained unaffected, as detected by Goodman and Barry. The temperature shift indicates an

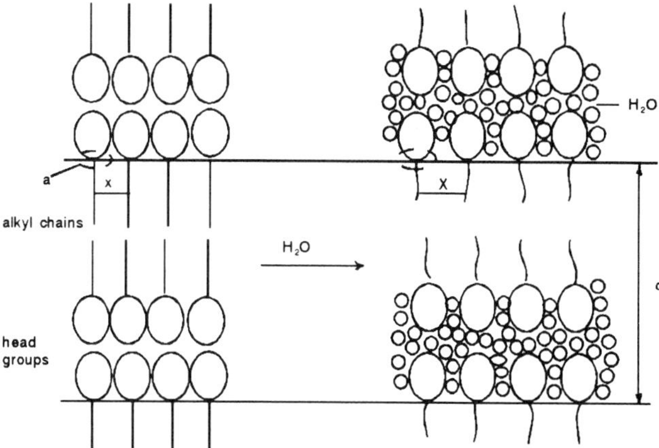

Figure 6 Uptake of water in a bilayer: a possible mechanism. a, Interfacial area per molecule; d, repeat distance; x, distance between two alkyl chains. (From Bouwstra, J. A. et al., *J. Control. Rel.*, 15, 209, 1991. With permission.)

interaction of PG with the SC lipids. In contrast, the results obtained from SAXS indicate that pretreating the SC with PG does not affect the lamellar distance of the bilayers, suggesting that no swelling of the lipid bilayers occurred. The main peak position of the scattering curve is independent of the water content, implying that the repeated distance between the lamellae is not affected by the degree of the hydration of the SC. An intercalation of PG may provide the explanation for the obtained results; the gel–liquid transition is determined not only by the alkyl chain length and the degree of saturation but also by the nature of the head groups. When small amounts of PG intercalate between the lipid layers in the head group regions the interfacial area per liquid molecule rises. The increase of this area can lead to an lateral swelling of the lipid alkyl chains. This should be compensated for by a minor shortening of the mean alkyl chain length in the lipid layers. This agrees with the results obtained from both methods (Figure 6).

Degree and recovery of structural changes of the SC caused by an enhancer are detectible using the FTIR/ATR. Takeuchi et al. reported extended studies of the influence of PG on the molecular mobility of the SC lipids and keratinized proteins for the hydrophobic penetrant, indomethacin, and a hydrophilic penetrant, 6-carboxyfluorescin.[43] The frequency changes due to the CH_2 C-H antisymmetric stretching band near 2920/cm in the SC lipids were used as an index by which to evaluate enhancer action. Frequency changes of the amide I region near 1640/cm, which were sensitive to the conformation of proteins, were used as an index for 6-carboxyfluorescin. The treatment of the skin with the enhancers resulted in a significant C-H antisymmetric stretching band. Whereas shift and broadening indicate a lipid disordering, no similar shift was observed with PG (Figure 7). The FTIR/ATR spectrum of the amide I region illustrates changes in all cases with respect to the untreated skin. A protein conformational change was detected even if the influence of PG alone was studied. Thus, the authors suggest that PG is able to change the conformation of α- to β-keratin. Furthermore, PG causes the polar solute 6-carboxyfluorescin to accumulate. This suggests the alteration of the conformation of

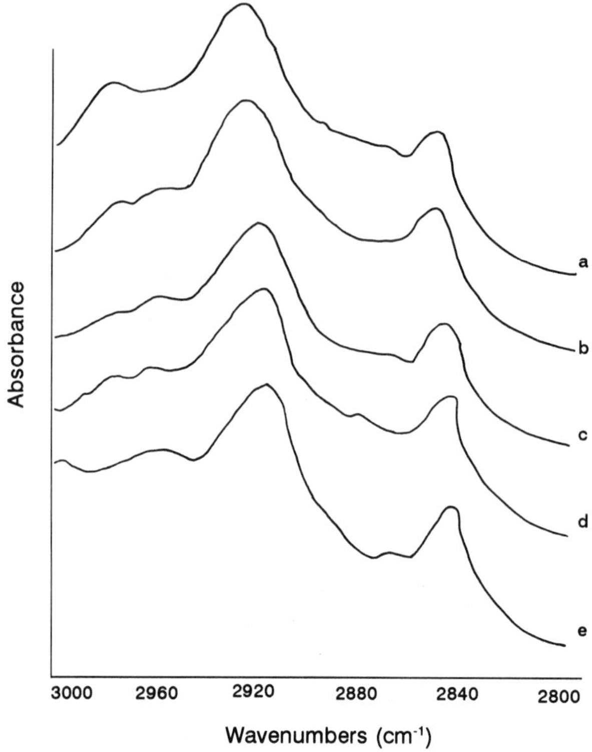

Figure 7 Representative FTIR/ATR spectra of rat abdominal SC in the CH_2 C-H asymmetric stretching region following 2 h of pretreatment with (a) 0.15 *M* oleylamine acid in PG, (b) 0.15 *M* oleic acid in PG, (c) 1% indomethacin in PG, (d) PG alone, and (e) without treatment. (From Takeuchi, Y. et al., *Chem. Pharm. Bull.,* 40, 1887, 1992. With permission.)

the SC proteins. However, electron microscopic photographs do not support this assumption.[44]

PG-pretreated skin samples show a corneocyte with intact lipid multilamellar stacks still attached. The isotropic granular structures indicate that the cell is surrounded by PG. Propylene glycol possibly infiltrates the outermost layers of the intercellular spaces. No interaction with the lamellar lipid structures or uptake into the corneocytes can be proven. Concerning the assumed dehydration of the SC due to PG, the authors explained the action of PG as follows. Because most of the water is accumulated within the corneocytes and because PG does not penetrate into the cells it seems to be likely that PG withdraws water from the cells due to its hygroscopicity. This fact agrees with the results obtained from the DSC studies by Bouwstra et al.[42] that the thermal denaturation peak of the protein (T4) disappears in the dried SC because higher temperatures are necessary for its denaturation.

VI. CONCLUSIONS

The results obtained from the transport studies emphasize that PG is able to enhance the permeation of lipophilic, polar drugs. The penetration of PG into the SC contributes to a favored partitioning of drug molecules due to changed activity gradients.

The solubilizing capacity of the aqueous sites of the SC is increased. The accumulation of PG may cause the establishment of a drug reservoir. On the other hand, only drugs that are highly soluble in PG offer enhanced penetration behavior. Therefore, it seems likely that the sorption promoting effect is related mainly to a solvent drag effect of PG. Simultaneous permeation profiles of several compounds and PG indicate that drug transport is directly linked to the solvent flow into and through the SC. Thus, the solubility is the most important factor because it determines whether the solvent drag effect or the thermodynamic control on the donor side dominate for drug transport.

Propylene glycol replaces water from its bonding sites in the intercellular space. Therefore, the incorporation of lipophilic, polar molecules must be improved. Although conformational changes of the keratin structure of the corneocytes were detected using the infrared technique electron microscopy pictures showed that PG does not infiltrate into the cells. Changes of the peak shape detected by DSC confirm that PG withdraws water from the cells.

Thus, the action site of PG is fixed on the bilayer structures of the intercellular lipids. However, SAXS studies could not prove changes in the lamellar distance. Phase-transition temperatures associated with the lipid melting of PG-pretreated SC samples are slightly decreased. Therefore, it must be assumed that the hydration spheres of the lipid head groups are disturbed without a measurable influence on the alkyl chain position of the lipids.

REFERENCES

1. **Barry, B. W.,** Mode of action of penetration enhancers in human skin, *J. Control. Rel.,* 6, 85, 1987.
2. **Barry, B. W.,** Lipid-protein-partitioning theory of skin penetration enhancement, *J. Control. Rel.,* 15, 237, 1991.
3. **Barry, B. W.,** Action of skin penetration enhancers-lipid protein partitioning theory, *Int. J. Cosmet. Sci.,* 10, 281, 1988.
4. **Ritschel, V. A. and Sprockel, O. L.,** Sorption promoters for topically applied substances, *Drugs Today,* 24, 613, 1988.
5. **Hadgraft, J.,** Penetration enhancers in percutaneous absorption, *Pharm. Int.,* 5, 252, 1984.
6. **Walters, K. A.,** Penetration enhancers and their use, in *Transdermal Therapeutic Systems,* Hadgraft, J. and Guy, R., H., Eds., Marcel Dekker, New York, 1989, chap. 10.
7. **Poulsen, B. J., Young, E., Coquilla, V., and Katz, M.,** Effect of topical vehicle composition on the *in vitro* release of fluocinolone acetonide and its acetate ester, *J. Pharm. Sci.,* 57, 928, 1968.
8. **Ostrenga, J., Steinmetz, C., and Poulsen, B.,** Significance of vehicle composition. I. Relationship between topical vehicle composition, skin penetrability, and clinical efficacy, *J. Pharm. Sci.,* 60, 1175, 1971.
9. **Miller, K. J., II, Rao, Y. K., Goodwin, S. R., Westermann-Clark, G. B., and Shah, D. O.,** Solubility and *in vitro* percutaneous absorption of tetracaine from solvents of propylene glycol and saline, *Int. J. Pharm.,* 98, 101, 1993.
10. **Bendas, B., Neubert, R., and Wohlrab, W.,** Mechanisms of Penetration of Glucocorticoids from Hydrogels into Various Acceptor Systems, presented at 40th Ann. Congr. of APV, Mainz, Germany, March 9 to 12, 1994.
11. **Bond, J. R. and Barry, B. W.,** Hairless mouse skin is limited as a model for assessing the effects of penetration enhancers in human skin, *J. Invest. Dermatol.,* 90, 810, 1988.
12. **Turi, J. S., Danielson, D., and Woltersom, J. W.,** Effects of polyoxypropylene 15 stearyl ether and propylene glycol on percutaneous penetration rate of diflorasone diacetate, *J. Pharm. Sci.,* 68, 275, 1979.
13. **Sarpotdar, P. P. and Zatz, J. L.,** Evaluation of penetration enhancement of lidocaine by nonionic surfactants through hairless mouse skin *in vitro, J. Pharm. Sci.,* 75, 176, 1986.

14. **Sarpotdar, P. P. and Zatz, J. L.,** Percutaneous absorption enhancement by nonionic surfactants, *Drug Dev. Ind. Pharm.,* 12, 1625, 1987.
15. **Kaiho, F., Nomura, H., Makabe, E., and Kato, Y.,** Percutaneous absorption of indomethacin from mixtures of fatty alcohol and propylene glycol (FAPG bases) through rat skin: effects of fatty acid added to FAPG base, *Chem. Pharm. Bull.,* 35, 2928, 1987.
16. **Nomura, H., Kaiho, F., Sugimoto, Y., Miyashita, Y., Dohi, M., and Kato, Y.,** Percutaneous absorption of indomethacin from mixtures of fatty alcohol and propylene glycol (FAPG bases) through rat skin: effects of oleic acid added to FAPG base, *Chem. Pharm. Bull.,* 38, 1421, 1990.
17. **Goodman, M. and Barry, B. W.,** Action of penetration enhancers on human skin as assessed by the permeation of model 5-FU and estradiol. I. Infinite dose technique, *J. Invest. Dermatol.,* 91, 223, 1988.
18. **Goodman, M. and Barry, B. W.,** Lipid-protein-partitioning (LPP) theory of skin enhancer activity: finite dose technique, *Int. J. Pharm.,* 57, 29, 1989.
19. **Tiemessen, H. L. G. M., Bodde, H. E., de Ligt, F., and Junginger, H. E.,** Enhanced Nitroglycerine Permeation through SC under Controlled Hydration Conditions, presented at 15th Symp. Control. Rel. Biol. Mater., Basel, 1988.
20. **Polano, M. K. and Ponec, M.,** Dependence of corticosteroid penetration on the vehicle, *Arch. Dermatol.,* 112, 675, 1976.
21. **Mølgaard, B. and Hoelgaard, A.,** Vehicle effect on topical drug delivery. I. Influence of glycol and drug concentration on skin transport, *Acta Pharm. Suec.,* 20, 433, 1983.
22. **Mølgaard, B. and Hoelgaard, A.,** Vehicle effect on topical drug delivery. II. Concurrent skin transport of drugs and vehicle components, *Acta Pharm. Suec.,* 20, 443, 1983.
23. **Aungst, B. J., Blake, J. A., and Hussain, M. A.,** Contributions of drug solubilization, partitioning, barrier disruption, and solvent permeation to the enhancement of skin permeation of various compounds with fatty acids and amines, *Pharm. Res.,* 7, 712, 1990.
24. **Barry, B. W. and Bennett, S. L.,** Effect of penetration enhancers on the permeation of mannitol, hydrocortisone and progesterone through human skin, *J. Pharm. Pharmacol.,* 39, 535, 1985.
25. **Kastings, G. B., Francis, W. R. and Roberts, G. E.,** Skin penetration enhancement of tripolidine base by propylene glycol, *J. Pharm. Sci.,* 82, 551, 1993.
26. **Barry, B. W., Southwell, D., and Woodford, R.,** Optimization of bioavailability of topical steroids: penetration enhancers under occlusion, *J. Invest. Dermatol.,* 82, 49, 1984.
27. **Bennett, S. L., Barry, B. W., and Woodford, R.,** Optimization of bioavailability of topical steroids: non-occluded penetration enhancers under thermodynamic control, *J. Pharm. Pharmacol.,* 37, 298, 1985.
28. **Lippold, B. C. and Hackemüller, D.,** The influence of skin moisturizers on drug penetration *in vivo, Int. J. Pharm.,* 61, 205, 1990.
29. **Aungst, B. J., Rogers, N. J., and Shefter, E.,** Enhancement of naloxone penetration through human skin *in vitro* using fatty acids, fatty alcohols, surfactants, sulfoxides and amides, *Int. J. Pharm.,* 33, 225, 1986.
30. **Okamoto, H., Muta, K., Hashida, M., and Sezaki, H.,** Percutaneous penetration of acyclovir through excised hairless mouse and rat skin: effect of vehicle and percutaneous penetration enhancer, *Pharm. Res.,* 7, 64, 1990.
31. **Sheth, N. V., Freeman, D. J., Higuchi, W. I., and Spruance, S. L.,** The influence of azone, propylene glycol and polyethylene glycolon *in vitro* skin penetration of trifluorothymidine, *Int. J. Pharm.,* 28, 201, 1986.
32. **Loftsson, T., Gildersleeve, N., Soliman, R., and Bodor, N.,** Effect of oleic acid on diffusion of drugs through hairless mouse skin, *Acta Pharm. Nord.,* 1, 17, 1989.
33. **Michiniak, B. B., Player, M. R., Chapman, J. M., and Sowell, J. W.,** *In vitro* evaluation of a series of azone analogs as dermal penetration enhancers. I., *Int. J. Pharm.,* 91, 85, 1993.
34. **Mahjour, M., Mauser, B. E., and Fawzi, M. B.,** Skin permeation enhancement: effects of linoleic acid and azone on narcotic analgesies, *Int. J. Pharm.,* 1, 56, 1989.
35. **Kadir, R. and Barry, B. W.,** α-Bisalbolol, a possible safe penetration enhancer for dermal and transdermal therapeutics, *Int. J. Pharm.,* 70, 87, 1991.
36. **Yamada, M., Uda, Y., and Tanigawara, Y.,** Mechanism of enhancement of percutaneous absorption of molsidomine by oleic acid, *Chem. Pharm. Bull.,* 35, 3399, 1987.

37. **Cooper, E. R., Merrit, E. W., and Smith, R. L.,** Effect of fatty acids and alcohols on the penetration of acyclovir across human skin *in vitro*, *J. Pharm. Sci.,* 74, 688, 1985.
38. **Touitou, E.,** Skin permeation enhancement by n-decylmethyl sulfoxide: effect of solvent systems and insights on mechanism of action, *Int. J. Pharm.,* 43, 1, 1988.
39. **Katz, M. and Poulsen, B. J.,** Corticoid, vehicle and skin interaction in percutaneous absorption, *J. Soc. Cosmet. Chem.,* 23, 565, 1972.
40. **Chow, A. S. L., Kaka, J., and Wang, T. S.,** Concentration dependent enhancement of 1-dodecylazacycloheptan-2-one on the percutaneous penetration kinetics of triamcinolone acetonide, *J. Pharm. Sci.,* 73, 1794, 1984.
41. **Goodman, M. and Barry, B. W.,** Action of penetration enhancers on human SC as assessed by Differential Scanning Calorimetry, in *Percutaneous Absorption,* Bronaugh, R. L. and Maibach, H. I., Eds., Marcel Dekker, New York, 1989, chap. 33.
42. **Bouwstra, J. A., de Vries, M. A., Gooris, G. S., Bras, W., Brussee, J., and Ponec, M.,** Thermodynamic and structural aspects of the skin barrier, *J. Control. Rel.,* 15, 209, 1991.
43. **Takeuchi, Y., Yasukawa, H., Yamaoka, Y., Kato, Y., Morimoto, Y., Fukumori, Y., and Fukuda, T.,** Effects of fatty acids, fatty amines and propylene glycol on rat SC lipids and proteins *in vitro* measured by Fourier Transform Infrared/Attenuated Total Reflection (FT-IR/ATR) Spectroscopy, *Chem. Pharm. Bull.,* 40, 1887, 1992.
44. **Hoogstraate, A. J., Verhoef, J., Brussee, J., Ijzerman, A. P., Spies, F., and Bodde, H. E.,** Kinetics, ultrastructural aspects and molecular modelling of transdermal peptide flux enhancement by n-alkylazacycloheptanones, *Int. J. Pharm.,* 76, 37, 1991.

Chapter 4.1

Amines and Amides as Penetration Enhancers

Bozena B. Michniak

CONTENTS

I. INTRODUCTION

The reports are numerous on methods of augmenting the penetration of molecules across the skin from various species. Many deal with enhancers, otherwise known as accelerants or sorption promoters. These are agents whose ideal properties were outlined by Katz and Poulsen[1] in 1971, and concern aspects such as pharmacological inertness, nontoxicity, compatibility, etc. Unfortunately, no compound studied thus far exhibits all these ideal attributes, however, many show sufficient promise to justify further research.

II. DIMETHYLACETAMIDE AND DIMETHYLFORMAMIDE

Dimethylsulfoxide (DMSO) was one of the earliest enhancers tested (see Chapter 5.2).[2,3] Later, *N,N*-dimethylacetamide (DMA) and *N,N*-dimethylformamide (DMF) were reported as effective in addition to decylmethylsulfoxide (see Chapter 5.1)[4,5] (Figure 1). Both DMA and DMF were found to increase transepidermal water loss, but were less effective than DMSO. The authors concluded that DMSO, DMF, and DMA exerted a direct effect on the stratum corneum (SC). Patients were reported to tolerate DMA and DMF better than DMSO and did not experience the unpleasant taste and mouth odor which follows the topical application of DMSO. This phenomenon is caused by dimethylsulfide, a metabolite of DMSO. Aungst et al.[6] studied naloxone penetration through human cadaver skin. Enhancers tested included 10% v/v Azone® and DMA in propylene glycol (PG). Naloxone base was added in excess of its solubility to this formulation. Control naloxone flux was 1.6 ± 0.4 µg/cm²/h ($n = 10$) which increased to 2.0 ± 0.3 ($n = 3$) with DMA and 25.2 ± 5.4 ($n = 3$) with Azone®. With dodecylamine, the naloxone flux was 25.1 ± 0.9 µg/cm²/h ($n = 3$) and with DMSO 1.7 ± 0.9 µg/cm²/h ($n = 3$). Bennett et al.[7] assessed 0.1% betamethasone 17-benzoate bioavailability using a nonoccluded blanching assay and several enhancers, including Azone® and DMF. The test maintained the thermodynamic activity of the steroid approximately constant (10% saturation). *N,N*-Dimethylformamide provided slightly less enhancement than Azone®, however, Azone® was effective

0-8493-2605-2/95/$0.00+$.50

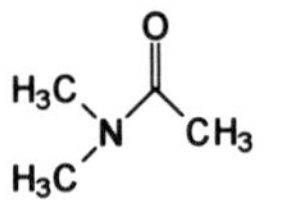

$$\text{Dimethylacetamide: } (H_3C)_2N\text{–}C(=O)\text{–}CH_3$$

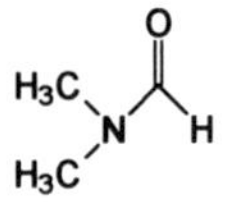

$$\text{Dimethylformamide: } (H_3C)_2N\text{–}C(=O)\text{–}H$$

Figure 1 Structures of DMA and DMF.

only in combination with PG. It was suggested by Sharata and Burnette[8] that dipolar aprotic solvents such as DMSO, DMF, and DMA cause swelling of the cells within the SC, thereby disrupting the barrier property of the skin. However, the exact mechanism by which these organic solvents enhance percutaneous penetration has not been fully elucidated. The properties and potential toxicity of DMA were discussed by Spiegel and Noseworthy.[9]

In summary, DMSO DMF, and DMA have been shown to be effective dermal enhancers for a variety of drugs, and are often used as standards for comparison when newer agents are being investigated.

III. AMINES

Several potential enhancers, including diphenhydramine base, chlorpheniramine base, and nicotine, were tested using procaterol base and hairless mouse skin *in vitro*.[10] The highest permeability coefficient for the drug was obtained from chlorpheniramine base > diphenhydramine base > nicotine. Flux, however, was highest from nicotine > chlorpheniramine base > diphenhydramine base, due mostly to differences in drug solubilities. All three enhancers had sufficient water solubility to partition from the skin into the receptor solution. Highest enhancer flux and permeability coefficients were reported for nicotine > chlorpheniramine base > diphenhydramine base.

Bachman and Hofmann[11] reported the use of three alkanolamines (diethanolamine, choline, and dimethylaminoethanol) to increase the percutaneous permeability of tenoxicam. It was reported that good penetration properties were obtained by using tenoxicam salts (such as its diethanolammonium salt) with water and gel-forming agents.

Several fatty amines were tested as possible enhancers, in addition to a series of fatty acids.[12] Fatty acids are discussed in more detail in Chapter 9.1. The amines studied in human cadaver skin included dodecylamine, triethylamine, phenylethylamine, and stearylamine (all 0.5 *M* in PG), with two model drugs, indomethacin and fluorouracil. For indomethacin, the highest flux was observed with triethylamine (40.7 ± 21.8 $\mu g/cm^2/h$). The lowest flux was reported for stearylamine (0.7 ± 0.06 $\mu g/cm^2/h$) and phenylethylamine (0.4 ± 0.2 $\mu g/cm^2/h$). Using fluorouracil, the highest flux was seen with dodecylamine (527.6 ± 30 $\mu g/cm^2/h$) and the lowest with phenylethylamine (9.7 ± 2.2 $\mu g/cm^2/h$) and triethylamine (10.4 ± 1.2 $\mu g/cm^2/h$). Control fluxes for PG alone were 0.5 ± 0.05 $\mu g/cm^2/h$ for indomethacin and 1.9 ± 0.5 $\mu g/cm^2/h$ for fluorouracil.

Creasey et al.[13,14] reported the use of di-2-ethylhexylamine as an enhancer using human SC.

IV. OTHER AMIDES

A series of *N,N*-dimethylalkylamides [$(CH_3)_2N–CO–(CH_2)_nCH_3$] were evaluated as enhancers using rat skin.[15] These were added into 50% PG in aqueous buffer (pH 5.5) together with either ibuprofen or naproxen. C_8 or C_{10} (1%), C_{12} (0.145%), and C_{14} (0.034%) were present in each formulation. These compounds were reported to possess insecticidal and antimicrobial activity in addition to their enhancing properties in skin.[16,17] With ibuprofen, the highest flux was obtained with C_8 amide (159.2 $\pm$ 7.3 $\times$ 10^{-3} μmol/cm²/h and the lowest with C_{12} (107.5 $\pm$ 18.0 $\times$ 10^{-3} μmol/cm²/h. With naproxen, the order was changed; the C_{10} amide produced the highest flux and C_6 the lowest (C_6 flux was not reported for ibuprofen) (Table 1).

Michniak et al.[18] tested several clofibric acid amides (Figure 2) using male athymic nude mouse skin *in vitro* and hydrocortisone 21-acetate and betamethasone 17-valerate as model drugs (Tables 2 and 3). In these tables enhancers were applied in PG at 0.4 *M* together with excess steroid. Enhancer pretreatment for 1 h and 6-h post-treatment were examined with enhancer **4.** Control enhancers included Azone®, isopropyl myristate, and dimethyllauramide.

Transdermal penetration with compounds **1** through **3** was not significantly different from that of control. Compound **4,** however, showed a relatively large enhancement with drugs for flux, receptor concentrations at 24 h, and skin steroid contents as compared to controls and other enhancers tested. One-hour pretreatment increased flux and decreased the skin content of drug. Six-hour post-treatment with enhancer showed an elevation of all parameters over control, but the values (excluding flux) were lower than those for coadministration and pretreatment. As the alkyl chain length of the amide series increased, the concentration in the receptor phase at 24 h initially increased, then peaked and decreased. This parabolic phenomenon was observed with other enhancer series.[19,20] It is important to note that 1-h pretreatment with enhancer increased receptor concentrations at 24 h 2.54-fold, however, steroid skin content decreased (with hydrocortisone 21-acetate). When screening enhancers, it is important to examine the concentrations obtained transdermally as well as the skin content of drug; i.e., mass balance data on both enhancer and drug will yield significant information on how the two agents are distributed in the system. Some enhancers we have tested yielded high skin contents, but did not increase flux significantly.[21] This may be important when selecting an enhancer for topical/local use or for transdermal use only.

Sugibayashi et al.[22] suggested that the lipophilicity of enhancers may be an important factor for their activity. Some of the enhancers tested against indomethacin suspensions were *N,N*-diethyl-3-methylbenzamide, (Deet, *N-N*-diethyl-*m*-toluamide) (Figure 3), urea, Azone®, DMSO, and diethylsebacate (all at 10%), using hairless rat skin *in vitro.* Ethanol aqueous solution (40% ethanol) was used as the donor solution. Deet was found to be less effective than DMSO and took some time to affect the skin barrier. The difference in the cumulative amount of indomethacin penetrated from control (40% ethanol only) for Deet was about 2-fold in 12 h and 3-fold at 24 h. Urea showed no significant enhancement over control values. Azone® markedly enhanced

Table 1 Flux, Permeability Coefficients (K_p) for Ibuprofen (A) and Naproxen (B) from Suspensions in 50% PG

A	Vehicle	Flux (×10³) (μmol/cm²/h)	K_p (×10³) (cm/h)
	Aqueous buffer	25.2 (5.9)	11.27 (2.64)
	50% PG[a]	70.1 (4.4)	4.69 (0.29)
	1% C_8, 50% PG	159.2 (7.3)	9.03 (0.43)
	1% C_{10}, 50% PG	135.6 (8.6)	8.32 (0.53)
	0.145% C_{12}, 50% PG	107.5 (18.0)	7.32 (1.23)
	0.034% C_{14}, 50% PG	114.6 (5.8)	7.87 (0.40)
	0.025% Azone®, 50% PG	65.9 (8.5)	4.40 (0.57)
B	**Vehicle**	**Flux (×10³) (μmol/cm²/h)**	**K_p (×10³) (cm/h)**
	Aqueous buffer	23.3 (1.0)	19.24 (0.83)
	50% PG[a]	13.1 (2.1)	1.57 (0.25)
	1% C_6, 50% PG	19.8 (7.0)	1.68 (0.59)
	1% C_8, 50% PG	93.4 (13.7)	7.12 (1.04)
	1% C_{10}, 50% PG	131.3 (11.1)	12.10 (1.02)
	0.145% C_{12}, 50% PG	42.4 (2.5)	5.81 (0.34)
	0.034% C_{14}, 50% PG	68.2 (5.0)	7.17 (0.53)
	0.025% Azone®, 50% PG	2.89 (0.22)	4.26 (0.23)

[a] Control; C_6, dimethylhexanamide; C_8, dimethyloctanamide; C_{10}, dimethyldecanamide; C_{12}, dimethyldodecanamide; C_{14}, dimethyltetradecanamide. Figures in parentheses are standard errors.

From Irwin, W. J., Sanderson, F. D., and Li Wan Po, A., *Int. J. Pharm.*, 66, 243, 1990. With permission.

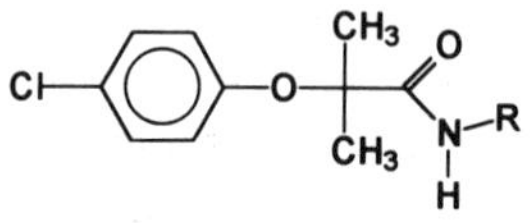

R	
H	1
CH_2CH_3	2
$(CH_2)_3CH_3$	3
$(CH_2)_7CH_3$	4
$(CH_2)_9CH_3$	5
$(CH_2)_{11}CH_3$	6
$(CH_2)_{13}CH_3$	7
$(CH_2)_{15}CH_3$	8

Figure 2 Clofibric acid amides tested as penetration enhancers.

Table 2 Penetration Experiments with Hydrocortisone 21-Acetate[a]

Enhancer +PG	n	J_{max} (μ*M*/cm²/h¹)	*C* of HC (μ*M*)	SC (μg/g) Main Drug (HCA)	SC (μg/g) Metabolite (HC)
None	6	0.04 ± 0.01	0.62 ± 0.09	281.0 ± 17.2	178.0 ± 3.1
IPM	6	0.20 ± 0.02	2.28 ± 0.14	381.0 ± 16.9	18.3 ± 0.6
DML	5	0.68 ± 0.08	8.86 ± 1.00	356.0 ± 5.5	6.3 ± 0.8
Azone	6	0.81 ± 0.09	10.90 ± 1.02	341.0 ± 9.7	6.4 ± 2.0
4	6	0.33 ± 0.05	12.60 ± 2.71	1530.0 ± 30.4	69.4 ± 3.2
4 (1-h pretreatment)	5	1.09 ± 0.17	32.00 ± 8.14	376.0 ± 8.7	120.0 ± 1.9
4 (6-h pretreatment)	6	0.60 ± 0.01	1.44 ± 1.11	433.0 ± 41.9	56.0 ± 10.0
5	5	0.26 ± 0.01	9.14 ± 0.49	675.1 ± 30.1	5.9 ± 0.3
6	5	0.62 ± 0.02	7.26 ± 1.06	487.1 ± 20.8	115.0 ± 8.6
7	5	0.18 ± 0.02	7.37 ± 0.94	553.0 ± 10.5	5.7 ± 0.1
8	5	0.18 ± 0.01	9.14 ± 0.68	515.0 ± 9.9	2.1 ± 0.1

[a] Results are expressed as mean ± standard deviation. J_{max}, maximum flux at initial steady state; *C*, concentration in receptor after 24 h; SC, concentration of drug in whole skin after 24 h; PG, propylene glycol; IPM, isopropyl myristate; DML, dimethyllauramide; HCA, hydrocortisone 21-acetate; HC, hydrocortisone.

From Michniak, B.B., Chapman, J.M., Jr., and Sowell, J.W., Sr., *J. Pharm. Sci.*, 82, 214, 1993. Reproduced with permission of the American Pharmaceutical Association.

Table 3 Penetration Experiments With Betamethasone 17-Valerate[a]

Enhancer +PG	n	J_{max} (μ*M*/cm²/h)	*C* of BMV (μ*M*)	*C* of BM (μ*M*)	SC of BMV (μg/g)
None	8	0.12 ± 0.01	5.94 ± 0.33	0.73 ± 0.11	863.9 ± 12.1
IPM	6	0.26 ± 0.02	17.61 ± 0.82	2.11 ± 0.35	707.9 ± 51.3
DML	5	0.31 ± 0.06	17.91 ± 3.34	1.89 ± 0.22	895.3 ± 53.7
Azone	5	0.16 ± 0.03	9.48 ± 1.21	1.64 ± 0.21	1028.0 ± 42.9
4	12	0.19 ± 0.01	12.21 ± 0.34	1.55 ± 0.24	2490.0 ± 20.5
4 (1-h pretreatment)	5	1.28 ± 0.31	56.61 ± 12.30	12.20 ± 1.61	1228.0 ± 37.6
4 (6-h pretreatment)	6	0.23 ± 0.02	10.60 ± 2.09	1.25 ± 0.40	825.0 ± 16.0
5	5	0.50 ± 0.10	22.61 ± 2.19	5.32 ± 1.08	588.0 ± 20.2
6	6	0.25 ± 0.03	13.72 ± 1.52	6.35 ± 2.05	547.0 ± 8.6
7	5	0.35 ± 0.03	15.80 ± 1.86	4.99 ± 2.59	677.0 ± 13.6
8	5	0.22 ± 0.05	13.00 ± 1.56	2.36 ± 0.97	794.0 ± 10.6

[a] Results are expressed as mean ± standard deviation. J_{max}, maximum flux at initial steady state; *C*, concentration in receptor after 24 h; SC, concentration of drug in whole skin after 24 h; PG, propylene glycol; IPM, isopropyl myristate; DML, dimethyllauramide; BMV, betamethasone 17-valerate, BM, betamethasone.

From Michniak, B.B., Chapman, J.M., Jr., and Sowell, J.W., Sr., *J. Pharm. Sci.*, 82, 214, 1993. Reproduced with permission of the American Pharmaceutical Association.

skin permeation of the drug and was slightly more effective than DMSO (the cumulative amount of indomethacin penetrated was approximately 1.6 mg/cm² over a 32-h period). Diethylsebacate showed a similar drug penetration profile, however, the enhancement was approximately 50% of that of Azone®.

Windheuser et al.[23] tested Deet against a wide variety of model drugs including hydrocortisone, hydrocortisone acetate, hydrocortisone 17-butyrate, hydrocortisone

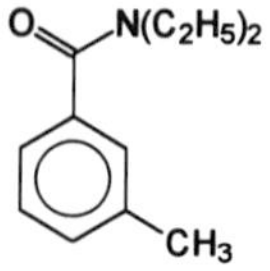

O N(C2H5)2

CH3

Figure 3 Chemical structure of *N,N*-diethyl-*m*-toluamide.

17-valerate, dibucaine, benzocaine, indomethacin, ibuprofen, erythromycin, tetracycline hydrochloride, griseofulvin, myco-21-phenolic acid, and methylsalicylate. All experiments were performed *in vitro* using hairless mouse skin. It was apparent that Deet caused dramatic enhancements of drug delivery for all drugs tested (Table 4). Ibuprofen and methylsalicylate were found to dissolve in the petrolatum base, while the other drugs were suspensions. Other authors using an *in vivo* rat model and nifedipine found that Deet was far less effective than Azone®.[24] This apparent lack of activity of Deet was also reported by Barry et al.[25]

Deet-based compounds have been used extensively as insect repellants, and skin penetration of Deet has been measured *in vivo* in humans as well as in rats, rabbits, beagles, hairless dogs, and rhesus monkeys.[26–30] Dermal absorption over 24 h of ^{14}C-labeled Deet in acetone was examined.[30] Rats dosed mid-dorsally showed absorption of 36 ± 8%, with a urinary excretion half-life of 20 h. Amounts and rate of absorption in monkeys was site dependent, with the lowest being on the forearm, 14 ± 5% ($t^1/_2$ = 4 h), and the highest on the ventral forepaw, 68 ± 9% ($t^1/_2$ = 8 h). The forehead and dorsal forepaw were the two other sites tested.

In another study Michniak et al.[31] tested 14 novel acyclic amides using *in vitro* diffusion cell techniques (Figure 4). Hydrocortisone 21-acetate was used as the permeant (a saturated solution with excess solid in PG) and fluxes and full-thickness hairless mouse skin steroid contents were recorded (Table 5). Enhancer **13** showed the highest activity for flux (35.22-fold over control with no enhancer) and for skin drug content (4.3-fold over control). These values were higher than those for Azone®, which were 19.51 and 1.5 over control, respectively. Enhancers **12, 18,** and **19** were similar to Azone® and **11, 17,** and **18** increased skin drug content to a greater degree than Azone®. Other authors such as Miniskanian and Peck[32,33] already tested and patented several open ring amide-containing enhancers. Wong et al.[34] reported that several dimethylaminoacetates had higher enhancing activity as compared to Azone®. Indomethacin was used as the model drug and shed snake skin as the membrane. Using Azone® as the standard, dodecyl *N,N*-dimethylaminoacetate, decyl *N,N*-dimethylaminoacetate, and octyl *N,N*-dimethylaminoacetate produced relative enhancements of 2.0, 3.8, and 2.5 times those of Azone®, respectively.

In conclusion, several amines and amides show promise as potential dermal penetration enhancers.[35] Further studies need to be performed to evaluate toxicities, appropriate enhancer concentrations, vehicle(s), and other model drugs which can be utilized with these enhancers in topical or transdermal systems.

ACKNOWLEDGMENT

The author wishes to thank Mark Player, M.D., for helpful discussions and for the preparation of figures, and Emily Willingham for typing the manuscript.

Table 4 Diffusion Of Various Drugs Through Hairless Mouse Skin

Drug	Formulations	Applied Drug Delivered (%)
Hydrocortisone	Hydrocortisone cream[a] 1% vs. 1% drug in Deet	1.6 vs. 35.0
Hydrocortisone acetate	Hydrocortisone acetate cream[b] 1% vs. 1% drug in Deet	0.67 vs. 27.6
Hydrocortisone 17-butyrate	Hydrocortisone 17-butyrate cream[c] 0.1% vs. 0.1% drug in Deet	4.7 vs. 63.1
	Hydrocortisone 17-butyrate ointment[b] 0.1% vs. 0.1% drug in Deet	2.0 vs. 63.1
Hydrocortisone 17-valerate	Hydrocortisone 17-valerate cream[d] 0.2% vs. 0.2% drug in Deet	6.1 vs. 40.8
Dibucaine	Dibucaine cream[e] 0.5% vs. 0.5% drug in Deet	15.0 vs. 82.0
Benzocaine	Benzocaine cream[f] 1% vs. 1% drug in Deet	12.3 vs. 35.7
Indomethacin	1% drug in petrolatum vs. 1% drug in Deet	0.9 vs. 37.6
Ibuprofen	1% drug in petrolatum vs. 1% drug in Deet	63.5 vs. ≃100
Erythromycin	1% drug in petrolatum vs. 1% drug in Deet	Not detectable vs. 83.4
Tetracycline hydrochloride	Tetracycline lotion[g] vs. 0.22% drug in Deet	Not detectable vs. ≃100
Griseofulvin	0.5% drug in petrolatum vs. 0.5% drug in Deet	0.4 vs. 29
Mycophenolic acid	1% drug in petrolatum vs. 1% drug in Deet	Not detectable vs. 42
Methylsalicylate	5% drug in petrolatum vs. 5% drug in Deet	Not detectable vs. 9
Triethanolamine salicylate	Triethanolamine salicylate lotion[h] 10% vs. 1% drug in Deet	16 vs. 89

[a] Hytone Cream, Dermik Laboratories, Inc., Fort Washington, PA 19034.

[b] Carmol Cream and Locoid Ointment, respectively, Ingram Pharmaceutical Co., San Francisco, CA 94111.

[c] Locoid Cream, Torii Pharmaceutical Co., Tokyo, Japan.

[d] Westcort Cream, Westwood Pharmaceuticals, Inc., Buffalo, NY 14213.

[e] Nupercainal Cream, Ciba Pharmaceuticals, Summit, NJ 07901.

[f] Solarcaine Cream, Plough, Inc., Memphis, TN 38151.

[g] Topicycline Lotion, Proctor and Gamble, Cincinnati, OH 45202.

[h] Asper Lotion, Thompson Medical Co., Inc., New York, NY 10022.

From Windheuser, J.J., Haslan, J.L., Caldwell, L., and Shaffer, R.D., *J. Pharm. Sci.,* 71, 1211, 1982. Reproduced with permission of the American Pharmaceutical Association.

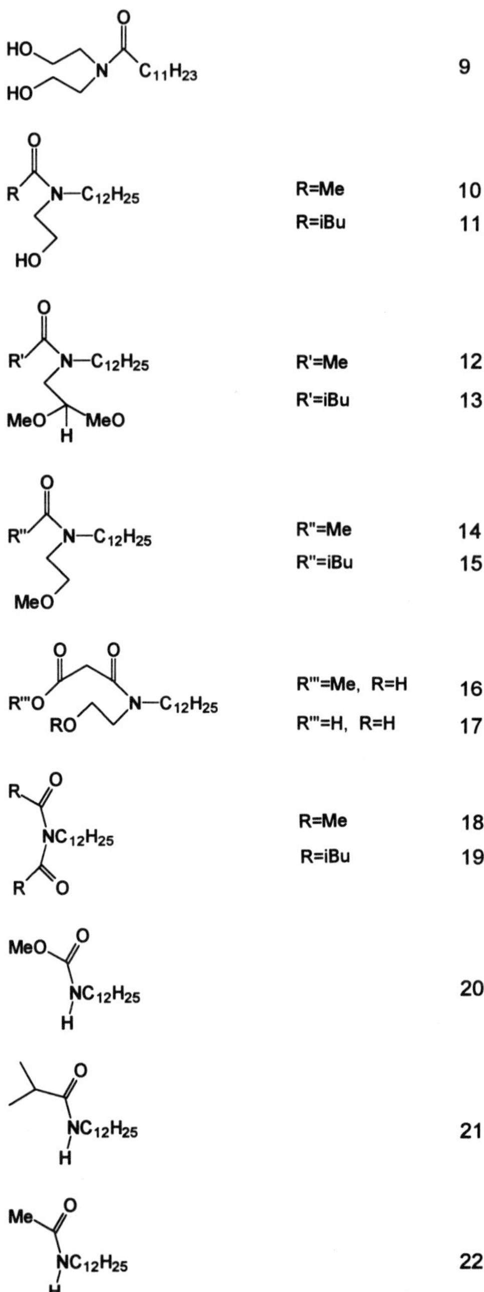

Figure 4 Open ring amides tested for percutaneous absorption enhancement.

Table 5 Effect Of Enhancers **9** Through **22** On The Percutaneous Penetration And Skin Retention Of Hydrocortisone 21-Acetate In Hairless Mouse Skin

Enhancer in PG[a,f]	m.p. (°C)	L[b](h)	Flux (μM/cm²/h)	$E.R._{flux}$[e]	Q^{c}_{24}(μM)	$E.R._{Q24}$[e]	SC (HCA)[d] (µg/g)	SC (HC)[d] (µg/g)	$E.R._{SC}$[e] (HCA & HC)
None (n = 8)[g]	—	1.16 ± 0.32	0.045 ± 0.016	1.00	0.751 ± 0.250	1.00	285.2 ± 21.6	ND[h]	1.0
Azone® (n = 5)	—	0.73 ± 0.09	0.878 ± 0.251	19.51	28.760 ± 4.624	38.30	410.6 ± 34.4	9.9 ± 34.4	1.5
9 (n = 5)	—	0.84 ± 0.21	0.613 ± 0.212	13.62	9.353 ± 2.288	12.45	185.2 ± 65.2	ND	0.7
10 (n = 5)	—	0.30 ± 0.10	0.936 ± 0.129	20.80	9.474 ± 2.499	12.62	343.4 ± 132.1	ND	1.2
11 (n = 5)	—	0.10 ± 0.02	0.901 ± 0.206	20.02	6.253 ± 2.268	8.33	577.2 ± 81.1	4.6 ± 3.1	2.0
12 (n = 5)	39–41	3.03 ± 1.24	1.160 ± 0.156	25.78	27.185 ± 5.695	36.20	477.1 ± 40.7	2.9 ± 0.9	1.7
13 (n = 5)	26.5	0.60 ± 0.29	1.585 ± 0.294	35.22	59.973 ± 6.999	79.86	1219.3 ± 281.5	4.1 ± 1.9	4.3
14 (n = 5)	—	0.62 ± 0.15	1.104 ± 0.632	24.53	13.618 ± 5.968	18.13	508.9 ± 101.2	ND	1.8
15 (n = 5)	82–83	0.99 ± 0.19	0.255 ± 0.089	5.67	2.560 ± 0.894	3.41	126.7 ± 22.9	ND	0.4
16 (n = 5)	—	1.74 ± 0.84	0.640 ± 0.105	14.22	5.329 ± 1.266	7.10	70.2 ± 17.2	ND	0.3
17 (n = 5)	—	0.84 ± 0.32	0.264 ± 0.088	5.87	3.868 ± 1.944	5.15	625.3 ± 123.5	11.3 ± 2.4	2.2
18 (n = 5)	20–25	2.96 ± 1.01	0.641 ± 0.194	14.24	28.762 ± 6.299	38.30	741.5 ± 50.6	4.8 ± 1.9	2.6
19 (n = 5)	54–54.5	0.69 ± 0.25	2.582 ± 0.846	57.38	28.024 ± 8.397	37.32	260.2 ± 106.8	ND	0.9
20 (n = 5)	55–55.5	0.87 ± 0.20	1.322 ± 0.255	29.38	12.293 ± 2.404	16.37	265.6 ± 58.1	ND	0.9
21 (n = 5)	48	0.73 ± 0.14	0.293 ± 0.099	6.51	4.849 ± 1.463	6.46	293.7 ± 88.5	ND	1.0
22 (n = 5)	42.5–43	1.50 ± 0.56	0.451 ± 0.102	10.02	7.463 ± 2.946	9.94	289.6 ± 50.4	3.3 ± 0.9	1.0

[a] PG, propyleneglycol.
[b] L, lag time.
[c] Q_{24}, receptor concentration after 24 h.
[d] SC, skin content of hydrocortisone 21-acetate (HCA) and hydrocortisone (HC) (metabolite).
[e] E.R., enhancement ratio compared to control (control = 1.00).
[f] Saturation solubilities (M) at 32 ± 0.5°C.
[g] *n*, PG of **15** = 0.274; **19** = 0.226; **21** = 0.293 (although **12, 20,** and **22** were solids, they were soluble at 0.4 *M*).
[h] ND, not detected.

From Michniak, B.B., Player, M.R., Fuhrman, L.C., Christensen, C.A., Chapman, J.M., Jr., and Sowell, J.W., Sr., *Int. J. Pharm.*, 110, 231, 1994.

REFERENCES

1. **Katz, M. and Poulsen, B. J.,** Absorption of drugs through the skin, in *Handbook of Experimental Pharmacology,* Brodie, B. B. and Gilette, J., Eds., Springer-Verlag, New York, 1971, 103.
2. **Stoughton, R. B.,** Dimethylsulfoxide (DMSO) induction of a steroid reservoir in human skin, *Arch. Dermatol.,* 91, 657, 1965.
3. **Stoughton, R. B. and Fritsch, W. E.,** Influence of dimethylsulfoxide (DMSO) on human percutaneous absorption, *Arch. Dermatol.,* 90, 512, 1964.
4. **Munro, D. D. and Stoughton, R. B.,** Dimethylacetamide (DMAC) and dimethylformamide (DMFA) effect on percutaneous absorption, *Arch. Dermatol.,* 92, 585, 1965.
5. **Baker, H. J.,** The effects of dimethylsulfoxide, dimethylformamide, and dimethylacetamide on the cutaneous barrier to water in human skin, *J. Invest. Dermatol.,* 50, 283, 1968.
6. **Aungst, B. J., Rogers, N. J., and Shefter, E.,** Enhancement of naloxone penetration through human skin *in vitro* using fatty acids, fatty alcohols, surfactants, sulfoxides, and amides, *Int. J. Pharm.,* 33, 225, 1986.
7. **Bennett, S. L., Barry, B. W., and Woodford, R.,** Optimization of bioavailability of topical steroids: non-occluded penetration enhancers under thermodynamic control, *J. Pharm. Pharmacol.,* 57, 570, 1985.
8. **Sharata, H. H. and Burnette, R. R.,** Effect of dipolar aprotic permeability enhancers on the basal SC, *J. Pharm. Sci.,* 77, 27, 1988.
9. **Spiegel, A. J. and Noseworthy, M. M.,** Use of non-aqueous solvents in parenteral products, *J. Pharm. Sci.,* 52, 917, 1963.
10. **Mauser, B. E., Majhour, M., and Fawzi, M. B.,** Cholesterol solubility and skin penetration enhancement, *Proc. Int. Symp. Control. Rel. Bioact. Mater.,* 16, 302, 1989.
11. **Bachmann, H. and Hofmann, P.,** Tenoxicam: a non-steroidal anti-inflammatory drug for topical application, in *Skin Pharmacokinetics,* Schroot, B. and Schaefer, H., Eds., S. Karger, Basel, 1987, 256.
12. **Aungst, B. J., Blake, J. A., and Hussain, M. A.,** Contributions of drug solubilization, partitioning, barrier disruption, and solvent permeation to the enhancement of skin permeation of various compounds with fatty acids and amines, *Pharm. Res.,* 7, 712, 1990.
13. **Allenby, A. C., Creasey, N. H., Edginton, J. A. G., Fletcher, J. A., and Schock, C.,** Mechanism of action of accelerants on skin penetration, *Br. J. Dermatol.,* 81, 47, 1969.
14. **Creasey, N. H., Battensby, J., and Fletcher, J. A.,** Factors affecting the permeability of skin. The relation between *in vivo* and *in vitro* observations, *Curr. Problems Dermatol.,* 7, 95, 1978.
15. **Irwin, W. J., Sanderson, F. D., and Li Wan Po, A.,** Percutaneous absorption of ibuprofen and naproxen: effect of amide enhancers on transport through rat skin, *Int. J. Pharm.,* 66, 243, 1990.
16. **Hwang, Y. S. and Mulla, M. S.,** Insecticidal activity of alkanamides against immature mosquitoes, *J. Agric. Food Chem.,* 28, 1118, 1980.
17. **Bistline, R. G., Maurer, E. W., Smith, F. D., and Linfield, W. M.,** Fatty acids, amides, and anilides. Synthesis and antimicrobial properties, *J. Am. Oil Chem. Soc.,* 57, 98, 1980.
18. **Michniak, B. B., Chapman, J. M., and Seyda, K. L.,** Facilitated transport of two model steroids by esters and amides of clofibric acid, *J. Pharm. Sci.,* 82, 214, 1993.
19. **Tsuzuki, N., Wong, O., and Higuchi, T.,** Effect of primary alcohols on percutaneous absorption, *Int. J. Pharm.,* 46, 19, 1988.
20. **Golden, G. M., McKie, J. E., and Potts, R. O.,** Role of the SC lipid fluidity in transdermal drug flux, *J. Pharm. Sci.,* 76, 25, 1987.
21. **Michniak, B. B., Player, M. R., Chapman, J. M., Jr., and Sowell J. W., Sr.,** *In vitro* evaluation of a series of Azone® analogs as dermal penetration enhancers. I., *Int. J. Pharm.,* 91, 85, 1993.
22. **Sugibayashi, K., Nemoto, M., and Morimoto, Y.,** Effect of several penetration enhancers on the percutaneous absorption of indomethacin in hairless rats, *Chem. Pharm. Bull.,* 36, 1519, 1988.
23. **Windheuser, J. J., Haslam, J. L., Caldwell, L., and Shaffer, R. D.,** The use of *N,N*-diethyl-m-toluamide to enhance dermal and transdermal delivery of drugs, *J. Pharm. Sci.,* 71, 1211, 1982.
24. **Kondo, S., Mizuno, T., and Sugimoto, I.,** Effects of penetration enhancers on percutaneous absorption of nifedipine. Comparison between Deet and Azone®, *J. Pharmacobio-Dyn.,* 11, 88, 1988.

25. **Barry, B. W., Southwell, D., and Woodford, R.,** Optimization of bioavailability of topical steroids. Penetration enhancers under occlusion, *J. Invest. Dermatol.,* 82, 49, 1984.
26. **Feldmann, R. J. and Maibach, H. I.,** Absorption of some organic compounds through skin in man, *J. Invest. Dermatol.,* 54, 339, 1970.
27. **Reifenrath, W. G., Robinson, P. B., Bolton, V. D., and Aliff, R. E.,** Percutaneous penetration of mosquito repellents in the hairless dog: effect of dose on percentage penetration, *Food Cosmet. Toxicol.,* 19, 195, 1981.
28. **Snodgrass, H. L., Nelson, D. C., and Weeks, M. H.,** Dermal penetration and potential for placental transfer of the insect repellent, *N,N*-diethyl-m-toluamide, *Am. Ind. Hyg. Assoc. J.,* 43, 747, 1982.
29. **Moody, R. P., Riedel, D., Ritter, L., and Franklin, C. A.,** The effect of DEET (*N,N*-diethyl-m-toluamide) on dermal persistence and absorption of the insecticide fenitrothion in rats and monkeys, *J. Toxicol. Environ. Health,* 22, 51, 1987.
30. **Moody, R. P., Benoit, F. M., Riedel, D., and Ritter, L.,** Dermal absorption of the insect repellent DEET (*N,N*-diethyl-m-toluamide) in rats and monkeys: effect of anatomical site and multiple exposure, *J. Toxicol. Environ. Health,* 26, 137, 1989.
31. **Michniak, B. B., Player, M. R., Fuhrman, L. C., Christensen, C. A., Chapman, J. M., Jr., and Sowell, J. W., Sr.,** *In vitro* evaluation of a series of Azone® analogs as dermal penetration enhancers. III. Acyclic amides, *Int. J. Pharm.,* 110, 231, 1994.
32. **Miniskanian, G. and Peck, J. V.,** U.S. Patent Application 199,801, 1988, *Chem. Abstr.,* 113, 1990, 15862k.
33. **Peck, J. V. and Miniskanian, G.,** U.S. Patent Application 179,144, 1988, *Chem. Abstr.,* 113, 1990, 103387n.
34. **Wong, O., Huntington, J., Nishihata, T., and Rytting, J. H.,** New alkyl *N,N*-dialkyl-substituted aminoacetates as transdermal penetration enhancers, *Pharm. Res.,* 6, 286, 1989.
35. **Ghosh, T. K. and Banga, A. K.,** Methods of enhancement of transdermal drug delivery. IIB. Chemical penetration enhancers, *Pharm. Tech.,* 17, 68, 1993.

Chapter 4.2

Alkyl *N,N*-Disubstituted-Amino Acetates

Nadir Büyüktimkin, Servet Büyüktimkin, and J. Howard Rytting

CONTENTS

I. INTRODUCTION

Transdermal drug delivery (TDD) is an approach to drug administration which may reduce the incidence of adverse effects, avoid first-pass metabolism in the liver and gastrointestinal system, and encourage better patient compliance. Due to the formidable barrier effect of the outermost layer of human skin, the stratum corneum (SC), TDD is usually restricted to drugs that are effective at low levels and have suitable permeability characteristics. Therefore, this route is generally available only to a limited number of drugs. To overcome this problem, many methods have been attempted. An interesting and useful approach is the use of chemical penetration enhancers.

By definition a desirable enhancer is a chemical whose primary property in relation to skin is to reversibly reduce the barrier resistance of the SC without damaging any viable cells.[1] Many compounds have been evaluated for their possible penetration-enhancing effects. However, the majority of them have not been marketed due to their toxicity, side effects, low permeation-enhancing properties, or a lack of understanding of their mode of action. Some excellent reviews related to enhancers and their modes of action have been published.[2–7]

II. BIODEGRADABLE PENETRATION ENHANCERS

In TDD the safety and the toxicity of enhancers is an important issue. For example, Ibuki[8] reported that the LD_{50} value of Azone®, a well-known enhancer, is 232 mg/kg when given intraperitoneally to mice. Development of biodegradable enhancers was undertaken to reduce toxicity and to introduce a temporal character to enhancers. Wong et al.[9,10] prepared some 1-alkyl-4-imidazolin-2-ones containing ester and

0-8493-2605-2/95/$0.00+$.50

Table 1 Some Possible Biodegradable Penetration Enhancers with Ester Structure

Chemical Class	Date	Biodegradability demonstrated	Ref.
L-Lysine esters	1985		14
Proline esters	1987		15
4-Imidazolin-2-ones	1988	+	9, 10, 16
	1989		
	1989		
Alkyl *N,N*-dialkylamino acetates	1989	+	17–20
	1989		
	1990		
	1992		
Methyl esters of *n*-alkyl fatty acids	1989		21
Pyroglutamic acids esters	1989	+	22, 23
	1990		
ε-Amino caproic acid esters	1989		24, 25
	1993		
Short-chain alkyl esters	1989		26, 27
	1989		
Alkyl *N,N*-dialkyl amino alkanoates	1991	+	28–30
	1992		
	1993		
Clofibric acid esters and amides	1990	+	31, 32
	1993		
Lactic acid esters	1992		33
N-(2-hydroxyethyl)-2-pyrrolidones	1993	+	34

carbonate moieties. A primary reason for the preparation of these types of enhancers was to allow them to exert their penetration-enhancing effects on drug transport and to be fragmented by enzymes in the skin to nontoxic compounds while passing through the skin where esterase activity is known to exist, and therefore to limit in time their activity.[11–13]

A survey of the literature related to biodegradable or possibly biodegradable transdermal permeation enhancers is given in Table 1. Except for L-lysine esters, which were designed for gastrointestinal absorption, and L-proline esters, pioneering work was started by Higuchi's group.

III. ALKYL *N,N*-DISUBSTITUTED AMINO ACETATES AS PENETRATION ENHANCERS

A. RATIONALE

The idea of alkyl *N,N*-disubstituted amino acetates being good enhancers was initiated by the fact that long-chain alcohols are known to enhance the transdermal delivery of several compounds. Therefore, ester derivatives of alcohols may exhibit good enhancing properties and also may be cleaved into substituted amino acids and alcohols. These compounds were first developed by modifying the alkyl chain length and alkyl substituents on the amine group which led to straight chain amino acetates.[17]

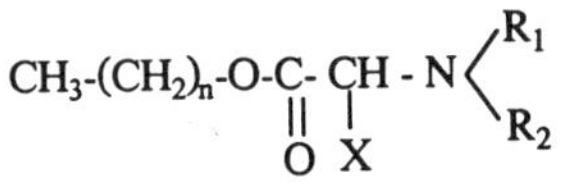

$$CH_3\text{-}(CH_2)_n\text{-}O\text{-}\underset{\underset{O}{\|}}{C}\text{-}\underset{\underset{X}{|}}{CH}\text{-}N\begin{matrix} R_1 \\ R_2 \end{matrix}$$

Alkyl (N,N-disubstitutedamino)-acetates

n=11	X=H	$R_1,R_2=CH_3$	DDAA (straight chain)
n=11	$X=CH_3$	$R_1,R_2=CH_3$	DDAIP (branched)

Figure 1 Chemical structures of alkyl (*N,N*-disubstituted amino)-acetates.

A later approach was based on an evaluation of alkyl or aryl substitutions of the carbon atom in the acetate moiety together with variation in alkyl chain length which gave branched derivatives.[28] Typical structures are shown in Figure 1.

B. SYNTHESIS AND PROPERTIES

Substituted amino acetates are generally synthesized by reacting an alkyl 2-bromo- or chloro-alkanoate, obtained by the reaction of the corresponding *n*-alkanol with the appropriate 2-bromo- or chloroalkanoyl halogenide, with disubstituted amines followed by extensive silica gel column chromatography using ethyl acetate as eluent.[17,28]

Alkyl *N,N*-disubstituted amino acetates are liquid at room temperature and have a pleasant odor. They are not soluble in water, but are soluble in ethanol–water mixtures. They are miscible with most organic solvents. They are highly soluble in acids, but are decomposed in the presence of alkalies.

C. PENETRATION PROFILES

Alkyl *N,N*-disubstituted amino acetates are useful in the transdermal permeation of a variety of compounds. Several drugs that have been studied include indomethacin, 5-fluorouracil, clonidine, hydrocortisone, diltiazem, minoxidil, sotalol, propranolol, and timolol. In their first paper Wong et al.[17] reported the synthesis and the permeation characteristics of some alkyl *N,N*-disubstituted amino acetates and compared the penetration enhancement of indomethacin in formulations using shed snake skin as a model membrane. Azone® was taken as a reference enhancer. According to their permeation data most of these enhancers were at least equal to or more active than Azone®. Wong and co-workers also showed that an increase in the chain length of thc *N,N*-dialkyl group decreases the activity. For example, the substitution of a methyl group with an ethyl or methyl piperazine group in this moiety reduces the permeation enhancement considerably. In these series the compound with a decyl group as the alkyl moiety in the ester group was shown to be the lead structure.

Further studies were also conducted to evaluate the permeation characteristics of ionized and nonionized species of indomethacin and clonidine (acidic and basic drugs) in the presence of dodecyl-*N,N*-dimethylamino acetate (DDAA) as the model enhancer.[18] The total penetration fluxes at pH 7.0 for both drugs using skins pretreated with DDAA were at least 11 times higher than those found for controls without enhancer treatment. Based on studies conducted at pH 4.6 and 7.0, the permeability coefficient of nonionized clonidine was found to be 2.5×10^{-3} cm/h, whereas that of the ionized form was 2.4×10^{-4} cm/h, confirming that the nonionized form penetrates the skin better than the ionized form. The nonionized form of indomethacin in the presence of enhancers penetrated the skin five times faster than the ionized form. However, the permeability coefficients K_{HA} for the nonionized species during enhanced and control experiments are identical, indicating that the enhancer had little effect on the permeability of the nonionized species of the drug. Permeability coefficients of the ionized species (K_{A-}) for enhanced and control experiments were 7.97×10^{-4} and 2.19×10^{-5} cm/h, with a ratio of 36.4.

Büyüktimkin et al.[28–30] made further modifications at the carbon atom of the acetate moiety of the molecule. The substitution of one hydrogen atom of DDAA with a methyl group gives dodecyl 2-(*N,N*-dimethylamino) propionate (or dodecyl 2-methyl-2-(*N,N*-dimethylamino) acetate) (DDAIP). The enhancing activity of DDAIP was evaluated by examining the permeation enhancements of model acidic, basic, and neutral drugs, i.e., indomethacin, clonidine, and hydrocortisone, from aqueous suspensions or solutions using shed snake skin as the model membrane. To demonstrate that the enhancing effect of DDAIP is due to DDAIP molecule, and not primarily to a decomposition product, *n*-dodecanol, which shows some penetration enhancement for various drugs,[35,36] was also included in the penetration experiments. After pretreating the skin for 2 h the absorption promoting effect of *n*-dodecanol was very small as compared to DDAIP, suggesting that for significant penetration enhancement, the intact enhancer is important. For comparison purposes, Azone® was also included in the experiments. The lag times of all three drugs were between 0.5 and 1.5 h. Sample penetration profiles for indomethacin are given in Figure 2. Compared to Azone®, the absorption promoting activity of DDAIP was substantial. After 28 h, ~70% of the indomethacin was transported into the receptor phase. For Azone® this amount was ~13% of the applied drug. It also was shown that DDAIP exhibits at least twice the enhancement activity of DDAA for several drugs.

In another set of experiments penetration-enhancing activities of DDAIP and other branched compounds such as decyl 2-(*N,N* dimethylamino)-propionate (I) and dodecyl 2-(*N,N*-dimethylamino)-butyrate (II) were evaluated using indomethacin and clonidine as model drugs and shed snake skin as the model membrane. For these drugs average penetration expressed in terms of flux were 7.2, 4.03, 4.14, and 28.05, 26.21, 18.09 μg/h/cm², respectively.[29]

The effectiveness of this class of enhancers was confirmed by the preparation and the evaluation of octyl 2-(*N,N* dimethylamino)-propionate (III), tetradecyl 2-(*N,N*-dimethylamino)-propionate (IV), and dodecyl *N,N*-dimethylamino-phenyl acetate (V) using Azone® as control.[30] For indomethacin and clonidine the average penetration in terms of flux with shed snake skin pretreated with them and Azone® were 5.3, 9.7, 2.4, 2.0 and 30.0, 54.0, 27.0, 22.2 μg/h/cm², respectively. In the hydrocortisone experiments the fluxes obtained with I, III, IV, V, and Azone® were calculated as 4.2, 1.1, 3.0, 1.4, and 1.8 μg/h/cm².

Turunen et al.[37] reported enhanced delivery of 5-fluorouracil (5-FU), a drug with poor cutaneous permeability, using DDAIP and DDAA. Oleic acid, *n*-dodecanol, and Azone® were used for comparison. The permeability enhancement of DDAA and Azone® was observed to be approximately equal. However, DDAIP increased the skin permeability of 5-FU significantly more than DDAA or Azone®. For DDAA the drug flux increased constantly as more enhancer was applied to the skin during

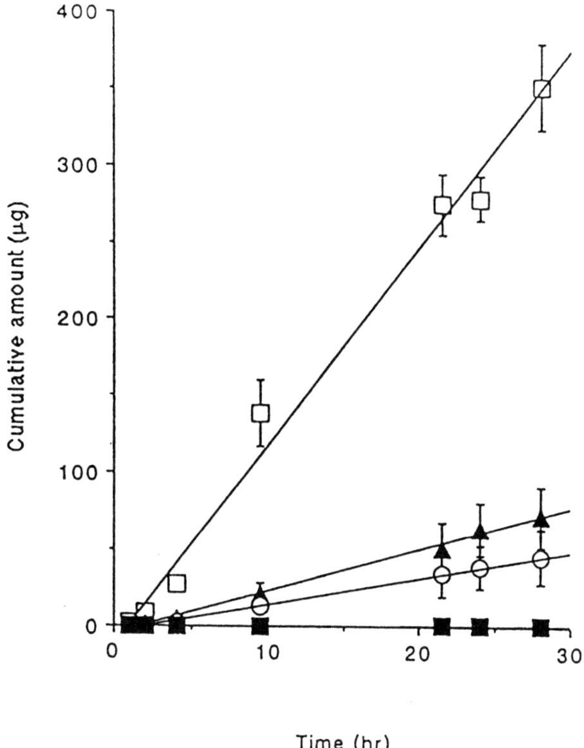

Figure 2 The penetration profiles of indomethacin in the presence of DDAIP (□), Azone® (▲), lauryl alcohol (○), and control (■). Each point and bar shows the mean and standard deviation of 20 experiments performed in 4 different shed snake skin. (From Büyüktimkin, S., Büyüktimkin, N., and Rytting, J. H., *Pharm. Res.,* 10, 1632, 1993. With permission.)

pretreatment. For DDAIP, 5-FU flux increased initially more steeply, but amounts of 10 µl or more did not markedly increase the flux further. The difference between these two enhancers was greatest at 10 µl (~4.0-fold).

In a comparative evaluation study Wongpayapkul and Chow[38] examined the permeation of propranolol hydrochloride through human cadaver skin. Saturated solutions of the drug with or without enhancers was used as the test solutions in an equimolecular ratio of propranolol and enhancer. Azone®, dodecane, *n*-dodecanoic acid, *n*-dodecanol, DDAA, and decyl *N,N*-dimethylamino acetate were used as enhancers. The flux obtained using DDAA was about three times higher than that obtained with Azone®, lauric acid, or *n*-dodecanol.

Using human skin, shed snake skin, and rabbit pinna skin as *in vitro* model membranes, Hirvonen et al.[39] compared the fluxes of 5-FU, propranolol, and indomethacin (hydrophilic to lipophilic drugs) after pretreating the skin with DDAA and Azone®. The enhancer DDAA was found to increase drug permeability at least as well as Azone®, and in most cases it was a more effective penetration enhancer.

Using 5% hydroxypropylmethyl cellulose gels of propranolol and timolol, the permeation-enhancing effects of DDAA, *n*-dodecanol, and Azone® through rabbit pinna skin were compared.[40] The results confirm that DDAA is a better penetration enhancer than Azone® and *n*-dodecanol for the delivery of propranolol in this model. For timolol both enhancers performed equally well. *In vivo* studies with propranolol, DDAA, and Azone® showed similar enhancement, whereas in the case of timolol, Azone® was the more effective promoter.

The permeability of sotalol and ^3H_2O after pretreatment with enhancer was also examined using human and shed snake skin in an *in vitro* passive diffusion cell and after pretreatment using iontophoresis.[41] The results showed that DDAA was a better enhancer than Azone® for the delivery of sotalol and ^3H_2O. However, combinations of iontophoresis and penetration enhancers did not further increase the permeation.

The effect of concentration on drug permeability for the enhancers DDAA, Azone®, and *n*-dodecanol was also examined by Hirvonen et al.[42] They found that permeability generally increased with enhancer concentration up to a point after which no further increase was observed. Although it was not the most potent, DDAA was found to be the most efficient enhancer of the three enhancers studied.

Also, DDAA was found to be useful in the delivery of the tetrapeptide, hisetal, from propylene glycol and pH 7.0 phosphate buffer formulations using hairless mouse skin as the model membrane. The activity of DDAA was found to increase the permeation of hisetal at a concentration of 3% to a greater extent (1.5-fold) than Azone® at the same concentration.[43] Under these experimental conditions its activity was not reversible within 12 h. These findings led to the conclusion that DDAA induces its permeability enhancing effect through changes in the lipid structure of the SC similarly to Azone® and oleic acid. The same workers also confirmed these results using the same formulations on human skin as the model membrane.[44]

D. BIODEGRADABILITY

Büyüktimkin et al.[45] evaluated the biodegradability of amino acetate enhancers such as octyl, decyl, dodecyl (DDAA), and tetradecyl *N,N*-dimethylamino acetates. They selected porcine esterase for *in vitro* biodegradability studies. Using this model they found that all of the enhancers were converted to degradation products, for example, *N,N*-dimethylglycine and the corresponding *n*-alkanol, with half-lives ranging from 3.55 to 8.02 min, respectively. Confirmation that these enhancers may be biodegraded in the presence of skin esterases is illustrated in Figure 3. Decomposition products of the enhancers were isolated and identified by physicochemical and spectrophotometric methods and compared to reference samples.

Another indication of the biodegradability of DDAA was shown by Hirvonen et al.[40] using rabbit pinna SC and shed snake skin as model membranes. They found that the enhancer effect of DDAA was reversed within 4 d, whereas the effects of Azone® and *n*-dodecanol, taken as model enhancers, lasted considerably longer. In later differential scanning calorimetry (DSC) studies[46] using human, rabbit pinna, and shed snake skin, the reversibility of action of the penetration enhancer DDAA was shown. Four days after pretreatment with DDAA, lipid endotherms returned, while in the case of Azone® and *n*-dodecanol, they remained absent.

Biodegradability of DDAIP was also proven using *in vitro* porcine esterase hydrolysis.[28] The compound showed a half-life of 18.5 min. Its decomposition products *N,N*-dimethyl-β-alanine and *n*-dodecanol were isolated and identified.

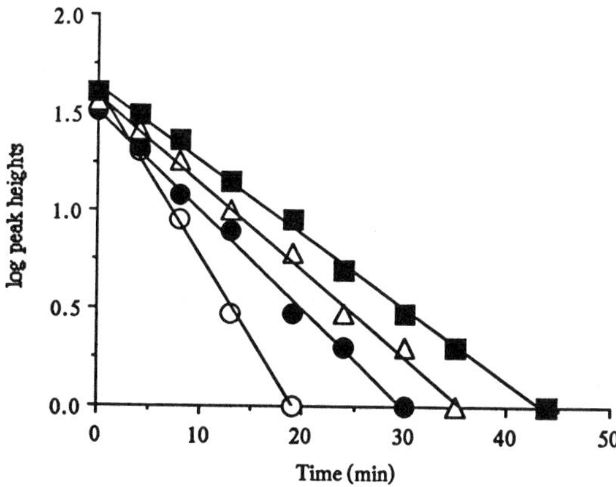

Figure 3 Degradation profiles of alkyl *N,N*-dimethylamino acetates in the presence of porcine esterase; (○) octyl, (●) decyl, (□) dodecyl (DDAA), and tetradecyl (■) substituted enhancers.[45]

E. MECHANISM OF ACTION OF ALKYL *N,N*-DISUBSTITUTED-AMINO ACETATES

In order to understand the mechanism for the activity of the penetration enhancer DDAA, enhancer pretreated human SC, rabbit pinna SC, and shed snake skin samples were compared using DSC.[46] The lipoidal components of rabbit skin were extracted and their DSC endotherms were compared to the endotherms of the entire SC. The mechanism of action of DDAA was found to be based mainly on the disruption of the lipoidal bilayer of the SC. Characteristic lipid endotherms of the skin disappeared within 1, 3.5, 48, and 96 h after pretreatment with DDAA, but the protein endotherms at 90°C remained unaffected.

Electrochemical characterization of human skin pretreated with DDAA by impedance spectroscopy shows that DDAA increases the heterogeneity of skin by opening new penetration routes and increasing the disorder of the lipoidal matrix.[47] As a consequence, the ohmic resistance, capacitive properties, and fractal dimension of the skin increased.

An examination of the differences in permeability of 5-FU suggests that the mode of action may be different between the two penetration enhancers, DDAA and DDAIP.[37] A dramatic increase in enhancement is seen in DDAIP, which differs from DDAA by one methyl group. An examination of R_m values as an expression of lipophilicity shows that DDAIP is more lipophilic than DDAA (0.194 and 0.061, respectively). Half-lives of these enhancers in the presence of esterase are 6.8 and 18.5 min. However, in the skin the half-lives of both enhancers may be considerably longer because the concentration of the enhancer in the skin after the application of pure enhancer may exceed the V_{max} values of the enzyme systems substantially. The difference in the effectiveness of the two enhancers may be due to (1) different solubilities in the skin, (2) a different concentration activity relationship in the skin, (3) different degrees of degradation in the skin, and (4) different rates of elimination from the skin. Lipophilicity of DDAIP may not be the only reason for its good enhancing properties because Azone® is an even more lipophilic enhancer. These data suggest that more than one mechanism of action may be involved.

The effect of DDAA, Azone®, oleic acid, *n*-dodecanol, and DDAIP on the lipid domain of the SC also was examined by fluorescence spectroscopy,[48] using buccal epithelial cell preparations in which epithelial barrier properties and lipid composition were shown to closely resemble that of the skin. After labeling the cells with 1,6-diphenyl-1,3,5-hexatriene, 1-(4(trimethylammonio)-phenyl)6-phenyl-1,3,5-hexatriene, and 8-anilino-1-naphthalene sulfonic acid fluorophores, enhancer-induced changes in the deep regions of the lipid domain, in the polar head groups of the lipid bilayer, and in the membrane surface were evaluated. All of the enhancers studied were found to decrease to some extent the lipid membrane packing order in a deep bilayer region in a concentration-dependent manner. DDAA was also shown to alter molecular movement on the surface of the bilayers. However, the lipid distribution of DDAIP was found to be surprisingly different than that of DDAA, which strongly suggests that other mechanisms of action such as interactions with membrane keratins or with the applied drugs may contribute significantly to the permeation-enhancing activity of DDAIP.

The possibility of interaction of DDAIP with drugs was confirmed by Büyüktimkin et al.[49] using indomethacin as the model drug. This interaction was examined using ultraviolet, infrared, ^{1}H and ^{13}C-nuclear magnetic resonance (NMR) spectrometry and Differential Scanning Calorimetry (DSC) studies. The existence of preferential hydrogen bonding between the carboxylic acid group of indomethacin and the tertiary amino group of DDAIP was observed. A dipole–dipole interaction was especially demonstrated by enhanced shifts of these protons in ^{1}H- and ^{13}C-NMR spectra. However, during high-performance liquid chromatography analysis (HPLC) of indomethacin flux samples, no peak retention shifts or changes in peak shape were observed, which also confirms that only transient complexes were formed. After passage through the skin the complexes probably dissociate into the parent compounds.

Further information with respect to the mode of action of DDAIP was obtained through delipidization studies using shed snake skin as a model membrane.[50] The permeation of clonidine, hydrocortisone, and indomethacin was examined in the presence of DDAIP and Azone® pretreated delipidized and natural shed snake skins. High penetration of clonidine and hydrocortisone after delipidization in the presence or absence of enhancers suggests that the lipid layer is the most important barrier for these drugs. Enhanced transport of hydrocortisone after delipidization in the presence of the enhancers may be due to the solubilization effect of both enhancers. Pretreatment of delipidized and natural shed snake skin using DDAIP gave similar enhancements for indomethacin. However, this enhancement was always higher than delipidized control or Azone-pretreated shed snake skin, which strongly suggests the existence of an interaction between DDAIP and the drug and with the lipid portion of the SC. To confirm the possible interaction of DDAIP with the keratin layer, the amount of free thiol groups leached from the SC was measured after pretreating the skin with the enhancers. Ethanol, which affects the protein domain of the human skin, also was used for comparison. Azone® pretreatment does not significantly influence the leaching of thiol groups which precludes significant interaction with the protein domain. However, ethanol and DDAIP similarly enhanced the amount of free thiol groups of keratin in the SC, which suggests some interaction with the proteins. It was shown that the liberation of thiol groups of protein may increase the hydration

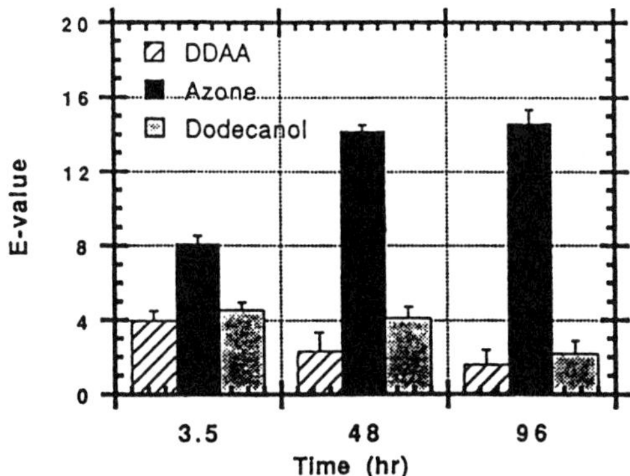

Figure 4 Development of skin irritation (chromametric *E* values) in rabbit pinna skin after single applications of 55 μl of pure liquid enhancers. Control value = 0 Mean ± SE, *n* = 3. (From Hirvonen, J., Sutinen, R., Paronen, P., and Urtti, A., *Int. J. Pharm.*, 99, 253, 1993. With permission.)

capability of the SC.[51] Water was shown to possess good permeation-enhancing characteristics. Consequently, water also may act as an enhancer through increased hydration of the skin after pretreatment with DDAIP.

F. TOXICITY STUDIES

Preliminary chronic toxicity studies on DDAA indicates that the compound has a low toxicity.[17] Subcutaneous application of 10% (w/w) DDAA dispersed in saline with 2% Tween® 80 to seven mice at a dose of 1 g/kg for 7 d shows that all animals survived a total dosage of 7 g/kg. However, they lost weight after the third day of injection. They regained normal weight during the postinjection period.

The irritation potential of DDAA was checked by spreading ~25 to 35 mg of petrolatum ointment made of 5% DDAA, 1% indomethacin, and 94% petrolatum base on a dorsal site of a hairless mouse up to nine doses over a period of 12 d. The low irritation of DDAA was confirmed by the absence of redness on the skin.[17]

The reversibility, the extent of penetration enhancement, and skin irritation by DDAA, Azone®, and *n*-dodecanol using timolol and propranolol as permeants and rabbit pinna skin as the model membrane were studied by Hirvonen et al.[40] Skin irritation was measured with a Minolta® CR 200 chromameter. After measuring rabbit pinna skin irritation by placing the chromameter vertically onto the test site, skin irritation *E* values were determined. As shown in Figure 4, Azone® was found to be the most irritating enhancer *in vivo* and this skin irritation increased with time. However, with DDAA irritation was much lower and decreased with time.

IV. SUMMARY

All of the *in vivo* and *in vitro* data collected clearly shows that alkyl *N,N*-dialkylamino acetates, especially DDAA and DDAIP, have significant transdermal penetration enhancing properties for the delivery of various drugs. They are at least equal to, or in the majority of cases more effective than, Azone®. The biodegradability of these compounds has been shown. Chromameter-aided irritation and primary chronic irritation studies confirm that these enhancers are less irritating than Azone®. The interaction studies show that with some drugs transient complexes which considerably improve penetration are formed. It was found that various enhancers may exhibit their mode of action through different mechanisms. The results of the present studies clearly demonstrate that alkyl *N,N*-disubstituted amino acetates may be useful in the transdermal delivery of many compounds.

REFERENCES

1. **Barry, B. W.,** Vehicle effect: what is an enhancer?, in *Topical Drug Bioavailability, Bioequivalence, and Penetration,* Shah, V. P. and Maibach, H. I., Eds., Plenum Press, New York, 1993, chap. 14.
2. **Ghosh, T. K. and Banga, A. K.,** Methods of enhancement of transdermal drug delivery. I. Physical and biochemical approaches, *Pharm. Technol.,* 17(3), 72, 1993.
3. **Ghosh, T. K. and Banga, A. K.,** Methods of enhancement of transdermal drug delivery. IIA. Chemical penetration enhancers, *Pharm. Technol.,* 17(4), 62, 1993.
4. **Ghosh, T. K. and Banga, A. K.,** Methods of enhancement of transdermal drug delivery. IIB. Chemical penetration enhancers, *Pharm. Technol.,* 17(5), 68, 1993.
5. **Santus, G. C. and Baker, R. W.,** Transdermal enhancer patent literature, *J. Control. Rel.,* 25, 1, 1993.
6. **Hirvonen, J.,** Enhancement of Transdermal Drug Penetration with Dodecyl *N,N*-Dimethylamino Acetate and Iontophoresis, Ph.D. thesis, Kuopio University, Kuopio, Finland, 1994, A.11.
7. **Franz, T. J., Tojo, K., Shah, K. R., and Kydonieus, A.,** Transdermal delivery, in *Treatise on Controlled Drug Delivery,* Kydonieus, A., Ed., Marcel Dekker, New York, 1992, 341.
8. **Ibuki, R.,** Use of Snake Skin as Model Membrane for Percutaneous Absorption Studies. Behavior of Several Penetration Enhancers in the System, Ph.D. thesis, University of Kansas, Lawrence, 1985.
9. **Wong, O., Huntington, J., Konishi, R., Rytting, J. H., and Higuchi, T.,** Unsaturated cyclic ureas as new non-toxic biodegradable transdermal penetration enhancers. I. Synthesis, *J. Pharm. Sci.,* 77, 967, 1988.
10. **Wong, O., Tsuzuki, N., Nghiem, B., Kuenhoff, J., Itoh, T., Masaki, K., Huntington, J., Konishi, R., Rytting, J. H., and Higuchi, T.,** Unsaturated cyclic ureas as new non-toxic biodegradable penetration enhancers. II. Evaluation study, *Int. J. Pharm.,* 52, 191, 1989.
11. **Nghiem, B. T. and Higuchi, T.,** Esterase activity in snake skin, *Int. J. Pharm.,* 44, 125, 1988.
12. **Tauber, U. and Rost, K. L.,** Esterase activity of the skin including species variations, in *Pharmacology of the Skin, Vol. I., Skin Pharmacokinetics,* Shroot, B. and Schaefer, H., Eds., S. Karger, Basel, 1987, 170.
13. **Fort, J. J. and Mitra, A. K.,** Effects of epidermal/dermal separation methods and ester chain configuration on the bioconversion of a homologous series of methotrexate dialkyl esters in dermal and epidermal homogenates of hairless mouse skin, *Int. J. Pharm.,* 102, 241, 1994.
14. **Fix, J. A. and Pogany, S. A.,** European Patent 85400771.3, 1985.
15. **Tsuda, Y., Sato, S., and Komata, T.,** Japanese Patent 62,226,930, 1987.
16. **Higuchi, T. and Wong, O.,** U.S. Patent 4,845,233, 1989.
17. **Wong, O., Huntington, J., Nishihata, T., and Rytting, J. H.,** New alkyl N,N-dialkyl-substituted amino acetates as transdermal penetration enhancers, *Pharm. Res.,* 6, 286, 1989.
18. **Fleeker, C., Wong, O., and Rytting, J. H.,** Facilitated transport of basic and acidic drugs in solutions through snakeskin by a new enhancer — dodecyl N,N-dimethylamino acetate, *Pharm. Res.,* 6, 443, 1989.
19. **Wong, O., Nishihata, T., and Rytting, J. H.,** U.S. Patent 4,980,378, 1990.
20. **Wong, O., Nishihata, T., and Rytting, J. H.,** U.S. Patent 5,082,866, 1992.
21. **Chukwumerije, O., Nash, R. A., Matias, J. R., and Orentreich, N.,** Studies on the efficiency of methyl esters of n-alkyl fatty acids as penetration enhancers, *J. Invest. Dermatol.,* 93, 349, 1989.
22. **Alexander, J. and Higuchi, T.,** U.S. Patent 4,847,250, 1989.
23. **Alexander, J. and Higuchi, T.,** U.S. Patent 4,970,206, 1990.

24. **Dolezal, P., Hrabalek, A., Mericka, P., Klimesova, V., Klimes, J., and Semecky, V.**, Czechoslovakian Patent PV 4278–89, 1989.
25. **Dolezal, P., Hrabalek, A., and Semecky, V.**, ε-Aminocaproic acid esters as transdermal penetration enhancing agents, *Pharm. Res.*, 10, 1015, 1993.
26. **Catz, P. and Friend, D. R.**, Alkyl esters as skin permeation enhancers for indomethacin, *Int. J. Pharm.*, 55, 17, 1989.
27. **Friend, D. R., Catz, P. and Heller, J.**, Simple alkyl esters as skin permeation enhancers, *J. Control. Rel.*, 9, 33, 1989.
28. **Büyüktimkin, S., Büyüktimkin, N., and Rytting, J. H.**, Synthesis and enhancing effect of dodecyl 2-(N,N-dimethylamino)-propionate (DDAIP) on the transepidermal delivery of indomethacin, clonidine, and hydrocortisone, *Pharm. Res.*, 10, 1632, 1993.
29. **Büyüktimkin, S., Büyüktimkin, N., and Rytting, J. H.**, New Alkyl α-(N,N-Dimethylamino)-Alkanoates as Transdermal Penetration Enhancers, Paper PDD 7049, American Association of Pharmaceutical Sciences (AAPS) 6th Annu. Meet., Washington, D.C., 1991.
30. **Büyüktimkin, S., Büyüktimkin, N., and Rytting, J. H.**, Penetration Enhancement of Indomethacin, Clonidine and Hydrocortisone by Some New Alkyl α-(N,N-Dimethylamino) Alkanoates, Paper PDD 7344, AAPS 7th Annu. Meet. San Antonio, TX, 1992.
31. **Michniak, B. B., Chapman, J. M., and Seyda, K. L.**, Clofibric Acid Amide Derivatives as Enhancers of Dermal Delivery of Indomethacin: Effect of Carbon Chain Length, Paper PDD 7265, AAPS 5th Annu. Meet., Las Vegas, 1990.
32. **Michniak, B. B., Chapman, J. M., and Seyda, K. L.**, Facilitated transport of two model steroids by esters and amides of clofibric acid, *J. Pharm. Sci.*, 82, 214, 1993.
33. **Saito, K., Heller, J., and Skinner, W. A.**, U.S. Patent 5,128,376, 1992.
34. **Lambert, W. J., Kudla, R. J., Holland, J. M., and Curry, J. T.**, A biodegradable transdermal penetration enhancer based on N-(2-hydroxyethyl)-2-pyrrolidone. I. Synthesis and characterization, *Int. J. Pharm.*, 95, 181, 1993.
35. **Bhatt, P. P., Rytting, J. H., and Topp, E. M.**, Influence of Azone® and lauryl alcohol on the transport of acetaminophen and ibuprofen through shed snake skin, *Int. J. Pharm.*, 72, 219, 1991.
36. **Chien, Y. W., Xu, H., Chiang, C., and Huang, Y.**, Transdermal controlled administration of indomethacin. I. Enhancement of skin permeability, *Pharm. Res.*, 5, 103, 1988.
37. **Turunen, T. M., Büyüktimkin, S., Büyüktimkin, N., Urtti, A., Paronen, P., and Rytting, J. H.**, Enhanced delivery of 5-fluorouracil through shed snake skin by two new transdermal penetration enhancers, *Int. J. Pharm.*, 92, 89, 1993.
38. **Wongpayapkul, L. and Chow, D.**, Comparative Evaluation of Various Enhancers on the Transdermal Permeation of Propranolol Hydrochloride, Paper PDD 7053, APPS 6th Annu. Meet. Washington, D.C., 1991.
39. **Hirvonen, J., Rytting, J. H., Paronen, P., and Urtti, A.**, Dodecyl N,N-dimethylamino acetate and Azone® enhance drug penetration across human, snake, and rabbit skin, *Pharm. Res.*, 8, 933, 1991.
40. **Hirvonen, J., Sutinen, R., Paronen, P., and Urtti, A.**, Transdermal penetration enhancers in rabbit pinna skin: duration of action, skin irritation, and *in vivo/in vitro* comparison, *Int. J. Pharm.*, 99, 253, 1993.
41. **Hirvonen, J., Kontturi, K., Murtomaki, L., Paronen, P., and Urtti, A.**, Transdermal iontophoresis of sotalol and salicylate; the effect of skin charge and penetration enhancers, *J. Control. Rel.*, 26, 109, 1993.
42. **Hirvonen, J., Paronen, P., and Urtti, A.**, Concentration-effect relationships of transdermal penetration enhancers, *Proc. Int. Symp. Control. Rel. Bioact. Mater.*, 20, 408, 1993.
43. **Ruland, A., Kreuter, J., and Rytting, J. H.**, Transdermal delivery of the tetrapeptide hisetal [melanotropin (6–9)]. I. Effect of various penetration enhancers: *in vitro* study across hairless mouse skin, *Int. J. Pharm.*, 101, 57, 1994.
44. **Ruland, A., Kreuter, J., and Rytting, J. H.**, Transdermal delivery of the tetrapeptide hisetal [melanotropin (6–9)]. II. Effect of various penetration enhancers: *in vitro* study across human skin, *Int. J. Pharm.*, 103, 77, 1994.
45. **Büyüktimkin, N., Büyüktimkin, S., and Rytting, J. H.**, Stability of Several Alkyl N,N-Dimethylamino Acetates Having Potential as Biodegradable Transdermal Penetration Enhancers, Paper PDD 7050, AAPS 6th Annu. Meet., Washington, D.C., 1991.

46. **Hirvonen, J., Rajala, R., Vihervaara, P., Laine, E., Paronen, P., and Urtti, A.,** Mechanism and reversibility of penetration enhancer action in the skin — a DSC study, *Eur. J. Pharm. Biopharm.,* in press.
47. **Kontturi, K., Murtomaki, L., Hirvonen, J., Paronen, P., and Urtti, A.,** Electrochemical characterization of human skin, by impedance spectroscopy: the effect of penetration enhancers, *Pharm. Res.,* 10, 381, 1993.
48. **Turunen, T. M., Urtti, A., Paronen, P., Audus, K. L., and Rytting, J. H.,** Effect of some penetration enhancers on epithelial membrane lipid domains: evidence from fluorescence spectroscopy studies, *Pharm. Res.,* 11, 288, 1994.
49. **Büyüktimkin, S., Büyüktimkin, N., and Rytting, J. H.,** Studies on the Interaction between Indomethacin and a New Penetration Enhancer Dodecyl 2-(N,N-Dimethylamino)-Propionate (DDAIP) and an Evaluation of Its Effect on Transdermal Delivery, Paper PDD 7266, AAPS 8th Annu. Meet., Orlando, FL, 1993.
50. **Büyüktimkin, N., Büyüktimkin, S., and Rytting, J. H.,** The Effect of Delipidization on the Penetration Enhancement of Indomethacin, Clonidine and Hydrocortisone through Shed Snake Skin in the Presence of Azone® and DDAIP (Dodecyl N,N-Dimethylamino Isopropionate), Paper PDD 7261, AAPS 7th Annu. Meet., San Antonio, TX, 1992.
51. **Nishihata, T., Suzuka, T., Yata, N., and Sakai, K.,** Protective effect of salicylate against 2,4-dinitrophenol-induced protein loss in the small intestine of rats, *J. Pharm. Pharmacol.,* 40, 516, 1988.

Chapter 5.1

Decylmethylsulfoxide

Elka Touitou and Donald D. Chow*

CONTENTS

I. INTRODUCTION

Dimethylsulfoxide (DMSO) has been known for many years as a skin penetrant and as a penetration enhancer for other compounds.[1] Due to a number of drawbacks such as the high concentration needed, skin irritation, and malodorous breakdown products, various derivatives of this molecule with potentially fewer side effects and more effective enhancing ability were sought.

Sekura and Scala[2] found that replacement of one methyl group of DMSO by long aliphatic chains resulted in a homologous series of nonionic amphiphilic molecules (Figure 1) which penetrate the skin and enhance penetration of other molecules. Degradation products of these substances are less volatile and less odoriferous than those of DMSO. The permeability constants for the penetration of this homologous series of alkyl methyl sulfoxides through guinea pig skin were determined *in vitro.* The results were further correlated with *in vivo* penetration and distribution of the sulfoxides in various tissues and their permeation-enhancing ability on two model, small molecules: polar thiourea and ionic nicotinate. The *in vitro* results indicated that the length of the alkyl chain affects the skin penetration of the sulfoxide derivative. Permeation of decylmethylsulfoxide (decyl-MSO) was 4.6 times greater than that of DMSO. Either longer or shorter chains exhibited lower permeation, with C_6 having a permeability of only 2.6 times that of DMSO.

When the authors[2] treated albino rabbits topically with aqueous solutions of radiolabeled alkyl sulfoxides, the amount of radioactivity accumulated in various tissues after 5 h showed a similar pattern to their ability to penetrate skin *in vitro;* in all tissues examined, decyl-MSO was found in the highest concentrations of all six sulfoxides tested. The greatest concentration difference between the derivatives was seen in the kidneys, which were established as the major pathway of elimination of DMSO in rabbits.[3] Here the concentration of decyl-MSO was found to be 11 μg/g, as opposed to only 2 μg/g for the C_6 derivative.

Sekura and Scala[2] showed that the greater capacity of decyl-MSO to penetrate the skin is well correlated with the ability of sulfoxide to enhance skin permeation of

* Work for this chapter was done while Dr. Chow was at American Cyanamid Company.

0-8493-2605-2/95/$0.00+$.50

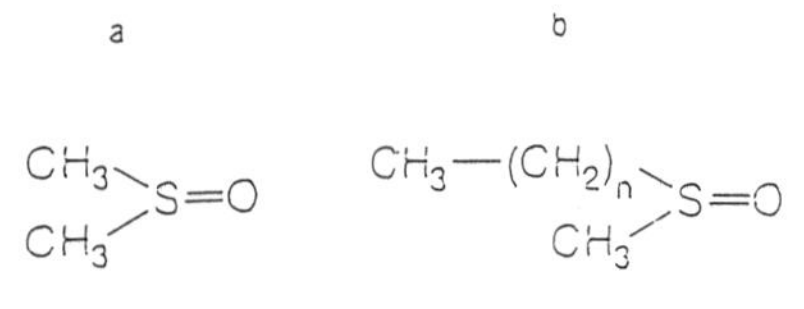

a

CH_3 \
S=O
CH_3 /

b

$CH_3—(CH_2)_n$ \
S=O
CH_3 /

Figure 1 The chemical structures of (a) DMSO and (b) Alkyl-DMSO.

other molecules. A 10% aqueous solution of this derivative was the most efficient of the six compounds tested in enhancing permeation of sodium nicotinate and thiourea through guinea pig skin.

Since its synthesis and first reports on its skin permeation enhancement properties, the effect of decyl-MSO on the skin permeation of a number of molecules has been investigated (Table 1). Enhanced permeation *in vitro* through excised skin was achieved for nicotinate,[2] methotrexate,[4] naproxen,[5] urea and salicylic acid (ionized),[6] naloxone,[7] mannitol,[8] somatostatin,[9] idoxyuridine (IDU),[10] 5-fluorouracil (5-FU),[10,11,29] pyridostigmine bromide,[12] oxymorphone,[13] enkephalin,[14] azidothymidine (AZT),[15] propanolamine,[16] acyclovir,[16] hydrocortisone,[16] and propranolol.[16] In addition, a number of patents[17–23] have been issued for compositions using decyl-MSO as a skin permeation enhancer (Table 2). It is interesting to note, however, that the number of reports of *in vivo* studies undertaken with decyl-MSO as a skin permeation enhancer is relatively small.[9,24–26]

A tetracycline topical dosage form containing 0.125% decyl-MSO in an aqueous ethanol solution was effective in the treatment of acne vulgaris when tested by seven groups of investigators on 300 patients in a 13-week clinical study.[25] In another clinical study on 135 patients with acne the same topical tetracycline formulation containing decyl-MSO was compared to an oral dose of 0.5 g/d tetracycline and to placebo.[26] It was found that the topical preparation produced statistically significant improvement of acne as compared to placebo after 7, 10, and 12 weeks of treatment. Decyl-MSO was first approved by the U.S. Food and Drug Administration in a topical preparation of tetracycline for the treatment of acne.

II. EFFECT OF DECYL-MSO ON SKIN PERMEATION OF DRUGS

Touitou and Abed[27] investigated the concentration-dependent penetration enhancement of 5-FU by decyl-MSO in propylene glycol (PG)-aqueous carriers. In these systems the enhancing effect was observed only at concentrations higher than 5% sulfoxide. At 15% enhancer, only a twofold increase was measured and the greatest effect, an increase of 72-fold over the control, was achieved at 40% enhancer concentration. Decyl-MSO likewise increased the concentration of drug retained in the skin. However, it is noteworthy that from a PG/H_2O pH 9 system a higher permeability and a smaller reservoir were obtained than from buffer pH 9 alone. This behavior was explained by the authors as due to transport of the fluorouracil anion by the glycol at pH 9.

In further studies Touitou[10,28] investigated the enhancing effect of decyl-MSO on molecules with different lyophilic characteristics: 5-FU, IDU and tetrahydrocannabinol (THC); the partitioning coefficients (octanol/water) of the three drugs were 0.01, 0.3, and 6000, respectively.

Table 1 Systems Containing Decyl-MSO and Various Drugs Tested for Skin Permeation *In Vitro*

Drug	Decyl-MSO Conc. (%)	Vehicle	Skin Type	Ref.
Acyclovir	0.189	H_2O	Hairless mouse	16
Azidothymidine	10	Buffer, pH 5	Hairless rat and human	15
5-Fluorouracil	1	PG-EtOH-H_2O	Hairless mouse	28
	1	H_2O	Hairless mouse	10
	15	PG	Hairless mouse	10
	4	H_2O	Human	11
	15	PG	Human	11
Hydrocortisone	0.189	H_2O	Hairless mouse	16
Idoxyuridine	1	H_2O	Hairless mouse	10
	15	PG	Hairless mouse	10
Mannitol	15	PG	Human	8
Methotrexate	2.5	H_2O	Human	4
Naloxone	10	PG, mineral oil	Human	7
Nicotinate	10	H_2O	Guinea pig	2
Oxymorphone HCl	5	EtOH	Human, hairless guinea pig	13
Peptides (dipeptides, enkephalin and amino acids)	10 m*M*	H_2O	Hairless mouse	14
Pyridostigmine bromide	0.1–2	H_2O	Human	12
Salicylic acid	0.1	H_2O, pH 9.9	Human	6
Somatostatin analogue	1	H_2O	Human, hairless mouse	9
Thiourea	10	H_2O	Guinea pig	2
Urea	0.06	H_2O	Human	6

Table 2 Patents with Decyl-MSO as an Enhancer for Delivery of Drugs through the Skin

Drug	Decyl-MSO Conc. (%)	Carrier	Dosage Form	Patent	Ref.
Dobutamine	0.9		Transdermal formulation	EP 492930 A2 (1992)	17
Hydrocortisone-acetate	0.1–10	PG	Topical application	US 3839566 (1974)	18
Insulin	33 or 50	Hydroxypropyl methylcellulose (HPMC)	Patch	WO 8505036 A1 (1985)	19
Methapyrilene-HCl	0.1–10	PG	Topical application	US 3839566 (1974)	18
Naloxone	50	poly (ethylene-vinyl-acetate) (PEVA)	Enhancer reservoir patch	DE 3614843 A1 (1986)	20
Organophosphates	10	EtOH	Local topical application	DE 2731366 (1978)	21
Pencyclovir	0.1–10	PG	Topical formulation	CA 2022632 AA (1991)	22
Tetracycline-HCl	0.125	Sucrose-monooleate EtOH	Topical composition	US 4046886 (1977)	23

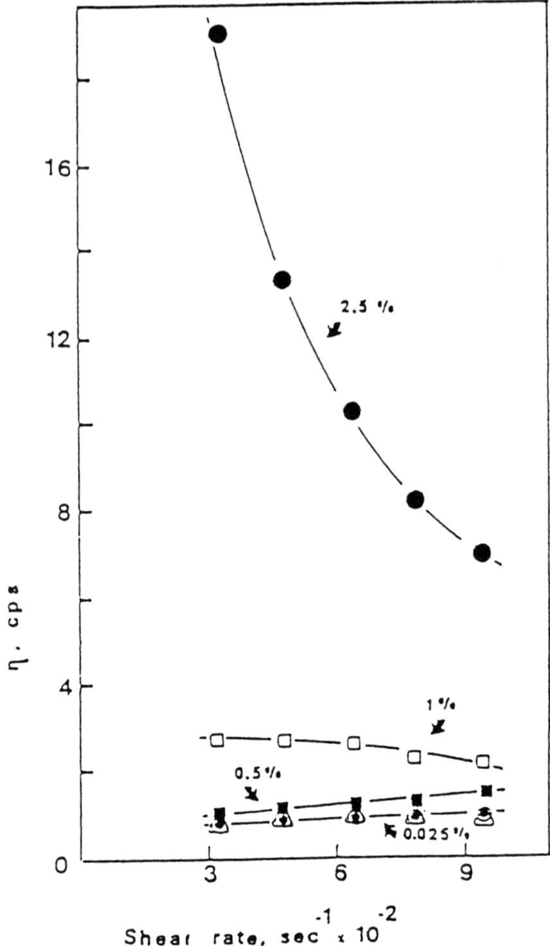

Figure 2 Rheograms of aqueous solutions containing various concentrations (0.025 to 2.5% w/v) of decyl-MSO tested at 23°C.

The permeation profiles of these drugs were measured in the presence of various concentrations of enhancer in aqueous, ethanolic, or PG carriers through hairless mouse skin. In aqueous solution a concentration-dependent enhancement of 5-FU by decyl-MSO was seen;[10] the enhancer was effective at concentrations as low as 0.1%. Maximum enhancement, 200-fold over that obtained for a system with no enhancer, was measured at 1% decyl-MSO. For IDU 1% decyl-MSO gave only a 44-fold permeation enhancement over control (no enhancer), this being the highest enhancement achieved in the concentration range of 0.1 to 15% decyl-MSO.[10] On closer examination of the decyl-MSO concentration effect in aqueous solution, a decrease in enhancing activity with concentrations over 5% decyl-MSO was observed. This is clearly explained by the increased viscosity of the solution with increasing enhancer concentration, as illustrated in Figures 2 and 3. The rheograms of viscosity vs. concentration show that at values >1% a drastic increase occurs in viscosity of the solution, which is highly affected by the shear rate.

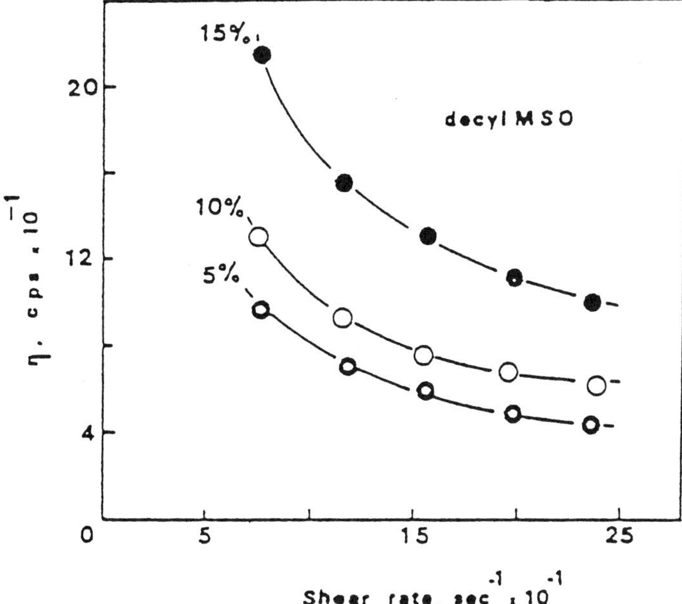

Figure 3 Rheograms of aqueous solutions containing various concentrations (5 to 15% w/v) of decyl-MSO tested at 23°C.

The permeation enhancement of both compounds, 5-FU and IDU, from PG carriers was significantly smaller than from aqueous systems.[10] In PG systems enhanced permeation was observed only at enhancer concentrations of 10 to 15%, as opposed to aqueous systems in which high enhancement was seen with 1% enhancer. As an example, a permeation increase of seven and ten times was obtained with 1.5 mg/ml 5-FU and IDU, respectively, from PG systems containing 15% decyl-MSO.

The data reported on the effect of two enhancers, oleic acid and decyl-MSO on THC, chosen as a model of a highly lipophilic molecule, shed more light on the selective enhancement effect by decyl-MSO.[28] In this work it was found that 1% decyl-MSO does not affect the skin permeation course of THC from unsaturated PG-ethanol (PG-EtOH) solutions (Figure 4). Moreover, in the presence of 1% decyl-MSO in a PG:EtOH:H_2O unsaturated THC system the skin permeation flux of THC was slightly decreased. In a similar system the permeation of 5-FU increased by 14-fold (Figure 5). Touitou and Fabin[28] also measured the effect of water on the permeability coefficients of THC and 5-FU, as a control, in systems without enhancer. It was found that while in the presence of 30% water, the permeation of THC was increased by almost 11 times, 5-FU skin permeation flux was not affected.

From the data reviewed[10,27,28] it is clear that the amplitude of drug permeation-enhancing effect of decyl-MSO is highly dependent on drug characteristics and carrier composition.

The observation that decyl-MSO has less enhancing effect on hydrophobic drugs[6,10,28] was further confirmed by the work of Goodman and Barry.[11,29] These authors find that decyl-MSO was more efficient in promoting the human skin permeation of 5-FU than that of estradiol.

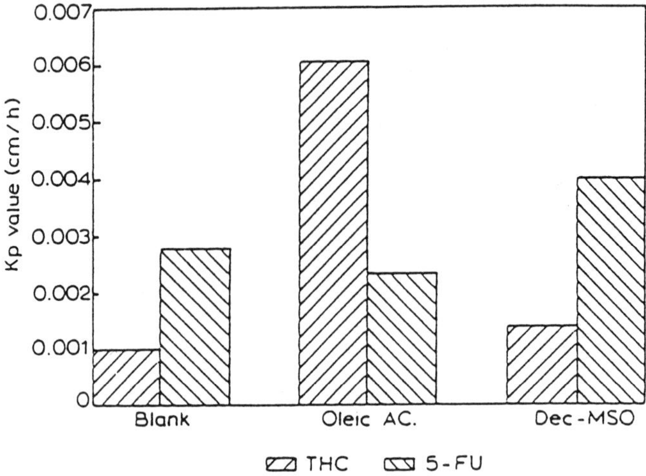

Figure 4 Effect of oleic acid and decyl-MSO on the skin permeability coefficient *(K_p)* of THC and 5-FU in PG:EtOH solutions.

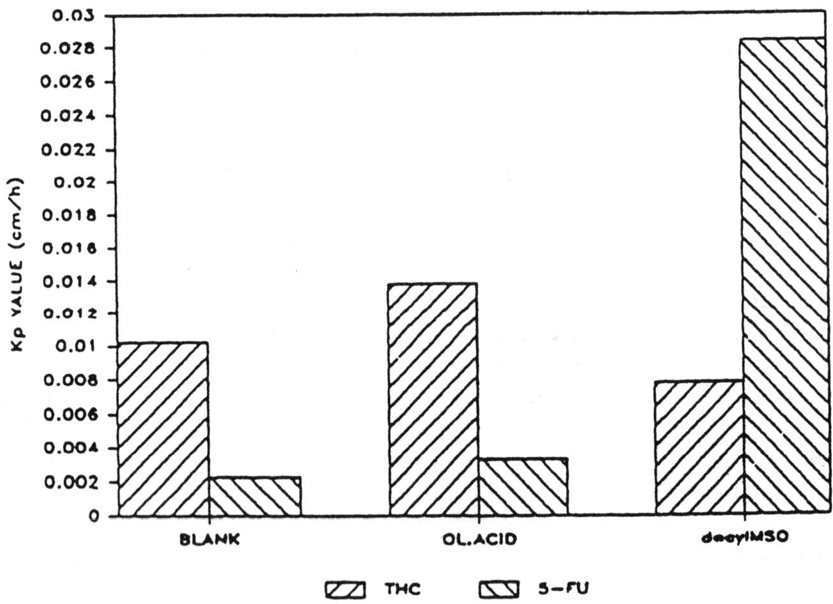

Figure 5 Effect of oleic acid and decyl-MSO on the skin permeability coefficient *(K_p)* of THC and 5-FU in PG:EtOH solutions containing 30% water.

Choi et al.[16] found that permeation through hairless mouse skin of phenyl propanolamine, propranolol, acyclovir, and hydrocortisone from buffer solutions increased with increasing concentrations of decyl-MSO up to a limiting permeability coefficient value of 0.1 cm/h; in those systems the permeation lag time values were drastically shortened relative to control systems with no enhancer. These authors discovered that propranolol and phenyl propanolamine solubilized decyl-MSO probably by forming mixed micelles. They concluded that the structural alterations, associated with decyl-MSO, were permanent. In the diffusion experiments carried out in this study no detectable recovery of barrier function of hairless mouse skin was seen.

Penetration enhancement of peptides obtained with decyl-MSO is of special interest. Pharmacologically potent peptides are important active agents, but their delivery through the noninvasive routes of administration is problematic. The skin is an effective barrier to the penetration of large ionic molecules such as peptides. One of the approaches tested for promoting peptide skin permeation is the use of chemical enhancers. Weber et al.[9] tested the effect of decyl-MSO on the transcutaneous absorption of the octapeptide SMS 201–995, a somatostatin analogue. Experiments were carried out *in vitro* on hairless mouse skin and human cadaver skin and *in vivo* in mice. The authors reported that the addition of 1% decyl-MSO resulted in rapid transdermal transport of peptide *in vitro;* the amount that permeated the hairless mouse skin in 24 h was 20 $\mu g/cm^2$. The application to mice of a transdermal patch containing 10 mg of SMS analogue and decyl-MSO gave plasma levels of peptide >8000 pg/ml in 2 h. It is noteworthy that in these studies the amount of peptide that permeated the skin both in *in vitro* and *in vivo* experiments was measured by using a radioimmunoassay specific for SMS.

Choi et al.[14] investigated the effect of decyl-MSO on the metabolism and transport through hairless mouse skin of amino acids, dipeptides, and the pentapeptide, enkephalin. These authors showed that complex metabolism of peptides in the skin can be partially overcome by the use of inhibitors and pH adjustment. Increased permeability of the amino acids and peptide tested was measured from systems in which enhancer, pH adjustment, and inhibitors were combined.

III. MECHANISM OF SKIN PERMEATION ENHANCEMENT BY DECYL-MSO

It is believed that decyl-MSO, as with many other penetration enhancers, may increase permeation by interfering with the barrier nature of the horny layer of the skin. Lipid and protein modifications induced in this layer appear to be related mainly to the amphiphilic nature of the enhancer. In an aqueous vehicle this molecule exhibits surface-active properties.

Figure 6 illustrates the surface tension vs. concentration dependence of aqueous solutions of decyl-MSO. The sharp break in the surface tension vs. concentration curve corresponds to a critical micelle concentration value of 5×10^{-3} *M* (0.12%).[10]

The following two observations can be related to the surface activity and micelle formation of an amphiphilic molecule:

1. Decyl-MSO is effective mainly in an aqueous medium.
2. The skin permeation enhancing effect in aqueous solutions drastically increases at decyl-MSO concentrations higher than 0.1%.

The prominent penetration enhancing activity of decyl-MSO occurs at concentrations above the threshold of micellization. This effect was clearly seen with a number of hydrophilic molecules.[6,8,10–12,29]

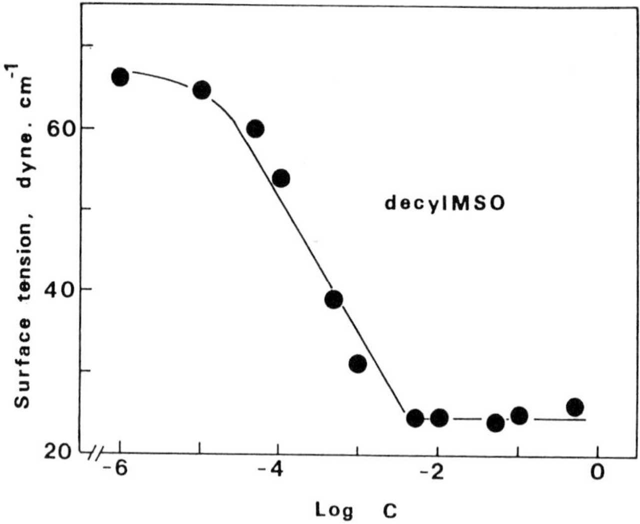

Figure 6 Surface tension vs. log concentrations of decyl-MSO in aqueous solutions tested at 23°C by means of a Fisher surface tensiometer.

Differential scanning calorimetry experiments could shed further light on how enhancers modify phase transitions within the stratum corneum (SC) and alter its structure. According to Barry,[30] the value of four main transition temperatures (T1 to T4), each representing a different kind of lipid–lipid or lipid–protein interaction were changed in skin treated with decyl-MSO. The values of T2 (lipid melting), T3 (lipid or lipid–protein association thermal events), and T4 (protein denaturation) have been lowered, with T1 (sebaceous lipid melting) having disappeared.

Figure 7 presents the thermal behavior of human callus treated with 1% decyl-MSO aqueous solution for 24 h at 20°C. The thermograms clearly show that the melting transitions have been accentuated and shifted by hydration and almost completely erased by treatment with decyl-MSO. These thermal changes indicate that the enhancer interacts with both the protein and lipids domains by changing protein conformation and by affecting lipid packing.

Figure 8 schematically shows the different effect of 1% decyl-MSO on the skin permeation of two model drugs, one hydrophilic (5FU), and one lipophilic (THC from PG-EtOH solutions with and without the addition of water).[28] Its effectiveness only in aqueous solutions at a 1% concentration suggests that this amphiphile is active as a penetration enhancer for a hydrophilic molecule which exists in a micellar form in water. The micelles may interact with both lipid and protein components of the horny layer, thus aiding permeation through the skin. On the other hand, the availability to the skin of lipophilic compounds such as THC may be reduced in a decyl-MSO micellar system, this step now becoming the rate-limiting step in the overall permeation process. The effect of the addition of water to a PG-EtOH system was explained by the authors[28] as an increase in the thermodynamic activity of THC rather than as a hydration effect because the permeation course of 5-FU from a similar aqueous system without enhancer was not changed.

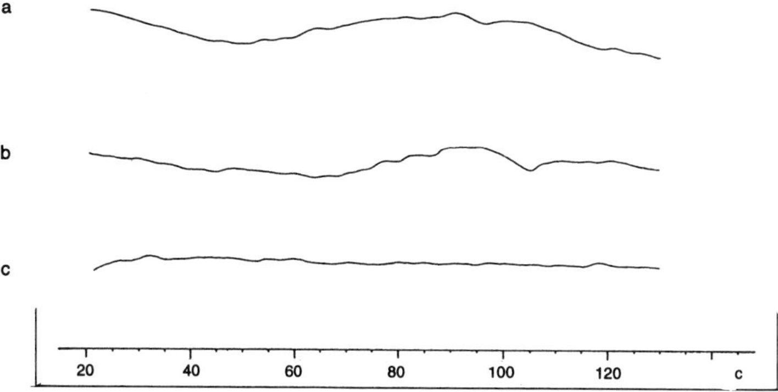

Figure 7 Differential scanning calorimetry of human callus: (a) dry; (b) hydrated; (c) treated with 1% w/v decyl-MSO aqueous solution.

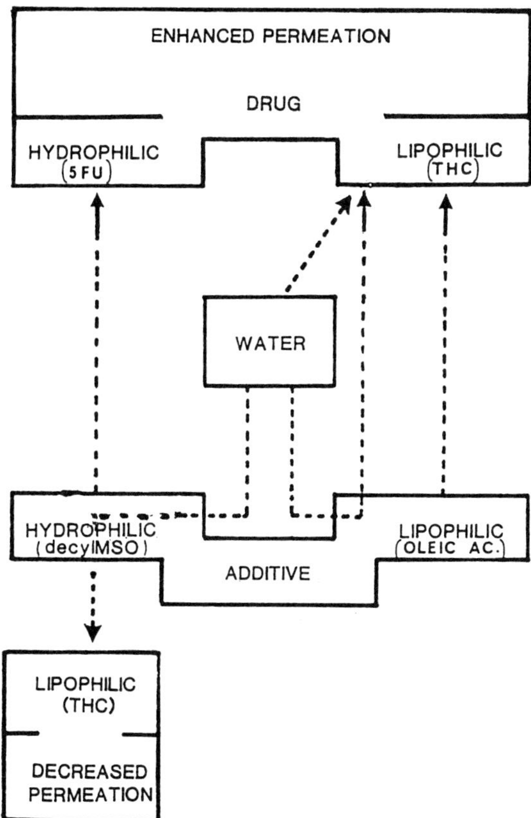

Figure 8 Selective effect of oleic acid and decyl-MSO on the skin permeation of the lipophilic THC and the hydrophilic 5-FU.

In conclusion, decyl-MSO may alter the skin permeation of other molecules by inducing modifications in the membrane structure and/or by interfering with the permeant thermodynamic activity.

REFERENCES

1. **Barry, B. W.,** *Dermatological Formulations,* Vol. 18, Marcel Dekker, New York, 1983, 162.
2. **Sekura, D. L. and Scala, J.,** The percutaneous absorption of alkyl methyl sulphoxides, *Adv. Biol. Skin,* 12, 257, 1972.
3. **Hucker, H. B., Ahmad, P. M., and Miller, E. A.,** Absorption, distribution, and metabolism of dimethylsulphoxide in the rat, rabbit, and guinea pig, *J. Pharmacol. Exp. Ther.,* 154, 176, 1966.
4. **McCullough, J. L., Snyder, D. S., Weinstein, G. D., Friedland, A., and Stein, B.,** Factors affecting human percutaneous penetration of methotrexate and its analogs *in vitro, J. Invest. Dermatol.,* 66, 103, 1976.
5. **Chowhan, Z. T. and Pritchard, R.,** Effect of surfactants on percutaneous absorption of naproxen. I. Comparisons of rabbit, rat and human excised skin, *J. Pharm. Sci.,* 67, 1272, 1978.
6. **Cooper, E. R.,** Effect of decyl methyl sulphoxide on skin penetration, in *Proc. Int. Symp. Solution Behavior of Surfactants: Theoretical and Applied Aspects,* Vol. 2, Mittal, K. L. and Fendler, E. J., Eds., Plenum Press, New York, 1982, 1505.
7. **Aungst, B. J., Rogers, N. J., and Shefter, E.,** Enhancement of naloxone penetration through human skin *in vitro* using fatty acids, fatty alcohols, surfactants, sulphoxides and amides, *Int. J. Pharm.,* 33, 225, 1986.
8. **Barry, B. W. and Bennett, S. L.,** Effect of penetration enhancers on the permeation of mannitol, hydrocortisone and progesterone through human skin, *J. Pharm. Pharmacol.,* 39, 535, 1987.
9. **Weber, C. J., Jicha, D., Matz, S., Siverly, J., O'Dorisio, T., Strausberg, L., Laurencot, J., McLarty, A., Norton, J., Kazim, M., and Reentsma, K.,** Passage of stomatostatin analogue across human and mouse skin, *Surgery (St. Louis),* 102, 974, 1987.
10. **Touitou, E.,** Skin permeation enhancement by n-decyl methyl sulphoxide: effect of solvent systems and insights on mechanism of action, *Int. J. Pharm.,* 43, 1, 1988.
11. **Goodman, M. and Barry, B. W.,** Action of penetration enhancers on human skin as assessed by the permeation of model drugs 5-fluorouracil and estradiol. I. Infinite dose technique, *J. Invest. Dermatol.,* 91, 323, 1988.
12. **Mitra, A. K. and Wirtanen, D. J.,** The effect of skin penetration enhancers on the transdermal delivery of pyridostigmine bromide, *Drug Dev. Ind. Pharm.,* 15, 1855, 1989.
13. **Aungst, B. J., Blake, J. A., Rogers, N. J., and Hussain, M. A.,** Transdermal oxymorphone formulation development and methods for evaluating flux and lag times for two skin permeation-enhancing vehicles, *J. Pharm. Sci.,* 79, 1072, 1990.
14. **Choi, H. K., Flynn, G. L., and Amidon, G. L.,** Transdermal delivery of bioactive peptides: the effect of n-decyl methyl sulphoxide, pH, and inhibitors on enkephalin metabolism and transport, *Pharm. Res.,* 7, 1099, 1990.
15. **Wearley, L. and Chien, Y. W.,** Enhancement of the *in vitro* skin permeability of azidothymidine (AZT) via iontophoresis and chemical enhancer, *Pharm. Res.,* 7, 34, 1990.
16. **Choi, H. K., Amidon, G. L., and Flynn, G. L.,** Some general influences of n-decylmethyl sulphoxide on the permeation of drugs across hairless mouse skin, *J. Invest. Dermatol.,* 96, 822, 1991.
17. **Valia, K. H.,** European Patent Appl. EP 492930, A2, 1992.
18. **MacMillan, F. S. K., Lyness, W. I.,** US Patent 3,839,566, 1974.
19. **Weber, C. J., Kazim, M., Reemtsma, K., and Nicholson, J. F.,** WO 8505036, 1985.
20. **Gale, R. M. and Enscore, D. J.,** Ger. Offen. DE 3614843, A1, 1986.
21. **Flora, L.,** Ger. Offen. DE 2731366, 1978.
22. **Griffiths, H. A. and Sanderson, F. D.,** Canadian Patent Appl. CA 2022632, AA, 1991.
23. **Smith, D. E.,** US Patent 4,046,886, 1977.
24. **Chowhan, Z. T., Pritchard, R., Rooks, W. H., and Tomolonis, A.,** Effect of surfactants on percutaneous absorption of naproxen. II. *In vitro* and *in vivo* correlation in rats, *J. Pharm. Sci.,* 67, 1645, 1978.

25. **Frank, S. B.,** Topical treatment of acne with a tetracycline preparation: results of a multi-group study, *Cutis,* 17, 539, 1976.
26. **Smith, J. G., Jr., Chalker, D. K., and Wehr, R. F.,** The effectiveness of topical and oral tetracycline for acne, *South. Med. J.,* 69, 695, 1976.
27. **Touitou, E. and Abed, L.,** Effect of propylene glycol, Azone® and n-decylmethyl sulphoxide on skin permeation kinetics of 5-fluorouracil, *Int. J. Pharm.,* 27, 89, 1985.
28. **Touitou, E. and Fabin, B.,** Altered skin permeation of a highly lipophilic molecule: tetrahydrocannabinol, *Int. J. Pharm.,* 43, 17, 1988.
29. **Goodman, M. and Barry, B. W.,** Lipid-protein-partitioning (LPP) theory of skin enhancer activity: finite dose technique, *Int. J. Pharm.,* 57, 29, 1989.
30. **Barry, B. W.,** Lipid-protein-partitioning theory of skin penetration enhancement, *J. Control. Rel.,* 15, 237, 1991.

Chapter 5.2

Dimethylsulfoxide

Thomas J. Franz, Paul A. Lehman, and Matthew K. Kagy

CONTENTS

I. BACKGROUND

The recorded history of dimethylsulfoxide (DMSO) began in 1867 following its synthesis from dimethylsulfide by a Russian chemist, Alexander Saytzeff.[1] Dimethylsulfoxide was found by chemists to have remarkable solvent properties which led to its widespread use both in the laboratory and for industrial processes. It is commercially produced in Europe from coal and petroleum and in the U.S. from lignin, a by-product of the paper industry.

Dimethylsulfoxide first burst onto the medical headlines in the 1960s and was the subject of much basic research, clinical investigation, and controversy. Following reports of its therapeutic potential in 1964,[2] it quickly became the subject of numerous clinical trials for a wide spectrum of unrelated disorders. Diseases as diverse as arthritis, scleroderma, musculoskeletal disorders, genitourinary conditions, headache, and others were said to respond to this "wonder drug";[3–5] its ability to facilitate drug movement through membranes was also noted. Clinical evaluation was halted by the U.S. Food and Drug Administration in 1965 when reports of ocular toxicity in animal studies began to surface. However, a year later some studies were allowed to continue for serious conditions for which no effective forms of therapy were available (scleroderma, herpes zoster, severe rheumatoid arthritis).

When no clear evidence of human ocular toxicity emerged from these limited studies, clinical evaluation of DMSO in less severe conditions was again allowed to proceed. Despite the fervor that enveloped the early investigative efforts on DMSO, little evidence of exceptional clinical efficacy emerged. Today, in the U.S. only one product is approved for human use and two for veterinary use. Rimso-50®, the only product approved for human use, is a 50% DMSO solution indicated for the treatment of interstitial cystitis by direct intravesicular instillation. Domoso® gel and solution, 90% DMSO in water, are recommended as topical treatment to reduce acute swelling due to trauma in dogs and horses. Synotic® otic solution, a combination of 0.01%

0-8493-2605-2/95/$0.00+$.50

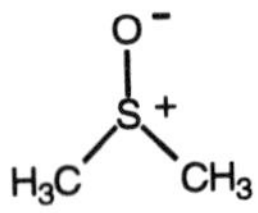

Figure 1 The polarized form of DMSO.

Table 1 Physical Properties Of DMSO

Property	Value
Freezing point, °C	18.55
Boiling point at atm, °C	189.0
Enthalpy of fusion, kcal/mol	3.43
Enthalpy of vaporization, kcal/mol at 25°C	12.64
Density, g/ml at 25°C	1.0958
Refractive index, *D* line at 25°C	1.4473
Dielectric constant, 25°C, 8 mc	46.7
Dipole moment, *D* at 20°C	4.3
pK_a	31.3
Conductivity, ohm/cm at 20°C	3×10^{-8}
Surface tension, dyne/cm at 25°C	42.86
Viscosity, c.p. at 25°C	1.99
Kf, °C/mol/1000 g	3.8

Note: mc = megacycles, c.p. = centipoise.

Data from MacGregor, W.S., *Biological Actions of Dimethyl Sulfoxide, Ann. N. Y. Acad. Sci.*, Leake, C.D., Ed., 141, 1967, p. 3.

fluocinolone acetonide and 60% DMSO, is indicated for the relief of pruritus and inflammation associated with acute and chronic otitis in the dog.

II. CHEMISTRY

The chemistry of DMSO was reviewed by MacGregor.[6] It is a clear, colorless liquid with unusual physical-chemical properties that make it a unique solvent. It is a dipolar, aprotic solvent with a high dielectric constant due to the polarity of the sulfur–oxygen bond (Figure 1). The combination of polarity and geometry favor considerable association into chains in the liquid state. This organization of the liquid structure by dipole attraction is reflected in a number of unusual physical constants, among them a relatively high freezing and boiling point (Table 1).

The dielectric constant of DMSO is sufficiently high, reported to be one third greater than that of methanol, to impart good solubility properties for ionic and polar substances. Many salts are completely ionized in this solvent at concentrations below 10^{-3} *M.* Dimethylsulfoxide is also capable of solvating cations because of the increased electron density of the oxygen atom. The dipolar nature of DMSO does not result in activation of the hydrogens of the methyl groups, and for this reason DMSO is only weakly acidic. Protons are removed only by strong bases such as sodium hydride. Although it cannot usually donate its own protons in chemical reactions, it can act as an acceptor for protons in hydrogen bonding and, thus, acts as a Lewis base.

Dimethylsulfoxide has strong affinity for water due to its propensity to form hydrogen bonds, the DMSO–water bond being 1.33 times stronger than the water–water bond. Like alcohol, DMSO mixes in all proportions with water. As a result of its hygroscopic nature, when exposed to room air, it will absorb water and be diluted to a concentration of only 66 to 67%. Hydration of DMSO is an exothermic reaction and this is readily appreciated when working with this compound. Highly concentrated solutions of DMSO will freeze in the refrigerator, but at lower concentrations (20% or less) it can act as an antifreeze due to its hydrogen bonding capacity that interferes with the tendency of water to form a crystalline structure.

III. EFFECT ON PERCUTANEOUS ABSORPTION

A. EARLY STUDIES

Although the first medical use of DMSO appeared to be as a cryopreservative,[7] the chance observation that this material could be tasted shortly after contacting the skin suggested that it rapidly penetrated the cutaneous barrier, and led some to examine its enhancer properties. Indeed, among the first experiments cited by Jacob et al.[2] enumerating the diverse activities of DMSO were those showing enhanced absorption of drugs through another epithelial structure, the urinary bladder of dogs. These findings — rapid absorption through human skin and increased absorption of drugs through the dog bladder — when coupled with the observations that it could prevent the damaging effects of freezing and thawing in cells, led quickly to the belief that DMSO could easily penetrate all cell membranes. Studies to investigate its potential enhancement effects in skin logically followed and the unique capacity of DMSO to enhance percutaneous absorption was quickly confirmed.[8–19]

The first to document the potent effects of DMSO on the skin were Stoughton and Fritsch.[8] Their studies, based largely on *in vivo* bioassays, showed that pharmacologic effects could be enhanced when DMSO was incorporated into the vehicle. Using hexopyrronium bromide (quaternary anticholinergic) to inhibit sweating, naphazoline hydrochloride (adrenergic agonist) to produce vasoconstriction, and fluocinolone acetonide (anti-inflammatory corticosteroid) to produce vasoconstriction, they found that the dose response curve for each drug was shifted toward lower drug concentrations when 10 to 50% DMSO was added to an alcohol vehicle. Limited *in vitro* studies were also conducted and demonstrated that DMSO promoted the absorption of both ^{14}C-hydrocortisone and ^{14}C-hexopyrronium chloride through human skin.

In a subsequent study Stoughton[10] demonstrated the rapidity with which DMSO exerted its effect. Two corticosteroids, ^{14}C-hydrocortisone and ^{14}C-fluocinolone acetonide, were applied to the forearm of human subjects from both an alcohol vehicle and an emulsion cream base into which DMSO had been incorporated at 40%. The corticosteroids were left in place for 30, 120, or 240 min, then washed off with soap and water or alcohol in a prescribed manner, and the amount of drug remaining in the stratum corneum (SC) was determined with a surface counter. In comparison to control vehicles the presence of DMSO resulted in a tenfold increase in drug content after only a 30-min application and much of the retained material was resistant to washoff (Table 2). Increasing the application time to 120 or 240 min led only to small additional increases in retained drug. It was subsequently found that the retained radioactivity persisted in the skin for approximately 2 weeks (Table 3).

Table 2 Establishment of SC Reservoir Following 30-Min Application (% of applied dose retained)

	Hydrocortisone[a]		
	1 SW	**3 SW**	**3 A**
40% DMSO/alcohol	35.1	24.2	16.1
40% DMSO/cream base	23.4	20.1	12.5
Alcohol control	2.1	0.7	0.2
Cream base control	2.4	0.5	0.2
	Fluocinolone Acetonide[a]		
	1 SW	**3 SW**	**3 A**
40% DMSO/alcohol	33.1	29.4	25.0
40% DMSO/cream base	24.2	18.5	15.2
Alcohol control	1.4	0.6	0.3
Cream base control	0.9	0.3	0.1

[a] (no. of washes) SW = soap and water wash, (no. of washes) A = alcohol wash.
Data from Stoughton, R. B., *Arch. Dermatol.*, 91, 657, 1965.

Table 3 Percent of Applied Dose Retained in SC

	Days After Application					
	0	**2**	**4**	**8**	**12**	**16**
Hydrocortisone						
40% DMSO/alcohol	36	16	6	3	1.5	1.1
Alcohol control	2.2	0	0	0	0	0
Fluocinolone acetonide						
40% DMSO/alcohol	34	15	7	3	0.8	0.1
Alcohol control	1.8	0.8	0	0	0	0

Data from Stoughton, R. B., *Arch. Dermatol.*, 91, 657, 1965.

However, because almost all of the retained material could be removed immediately by complete tape stripping (to glistening) of the SC, it was aptly said that DMSO had established a SC "reservoir".

One of the observations emerging from early studies was the marked concentration dependence of the enhancement effect, particularly when water was used as the cosolvent. This can be seen in the work of Kligman,[11] who conducted a series of novel *in vivo* and *in vitro* experiments with a diverse group of compounds ranging from steroids to fluorescent dyes. Using tape stripping to assess penetration into the SC *in vivo,* it was found that the fluorescent dye tetrachlorosalicylanilide could penetrate to the very base of the horny layer in only a few minutes when the DMSO concentration was 60% or above. The same endpoint took 2 h with an ethylene glycol monomethylether vehicle and 6 d with a petrolatum vehicle. A similar effect was noted with the fluorescent antibiotic demethylchlortetracycline. Penetration to the base of the horny layer took substantially less time when the vehicle was 50% DMSO or higher. From water alone, the time for complete penetration was >3 h. At 50, 70, and 90% DMSO the time was reduced to 120, 55, and 20 min, respectively.

Similar results were obtained by Sweeney et al.[12] Absorption of ^3H_2O through human cadaver skin *in vitro* was not enhanced until the DMSO concentration was above 60%. Likewise, Elfbaum and Laden[17] found that the absorption of picric acid *in vitro* through guinea pig skin increased markedly at DMSO concentrations above 60%.

In comparing the work of those who used water as a cosolvent to the previously cited work of Stoughton,[8,10] it appears that enhancement can be obtained at lower DMSO concentrations when ethyl alcohol is used as the cosolvent.

B. RECENT STUDIES

A study to more closely examine the mechanism of permeability enhancement by DMSO and separate kinetic from thermodynamic effects was conducted by Kurihara-Bergstrom et al.[20] The absorption of volatile alkanols of increasing hydrophobicity through hairless mouse skin and the effects induced by increasing concentrations of DMSO were measured. A unique feature of the study was the use of volatile probes because this permitted independent determination of activity coefficients through the measurement of vapor pressure and allowed for experimentally determined permeability coefficients to be normalized to unit activity in the vehicle.

In this study steady-state absorption of methanol, butanol, and octanol was measured and the permeability coefficients determined according to:

$$(dm/dt)_{ss} = AP(C) \tag{1}$$

where $(dm/dt)_{ss}$ is the quasi-steady-state rate of absorption across the skin, A is area, P is the permeability coefficient, and C is the concentration of one of the test permeants in the donor phase. Because it can be shown that:

$$P = \frac{D}{h}\frac{\gamma_v}{\gamma_m} \tag{2}$$

combining Equations 1 and 2 yields:

$$(dm/dt)_{ss} = A\frac{D}{h}\frac{\gamma_v}{\gamma_m}(C) \tag{3}$$

where γ_v and γ_m are activity coefficients of the permeant species in the donor solution (vehicle) and membrane, respectively, and h is the thickness of the membrane. Equation 3 shows that the rate of absorption is directly related to the activity coefficient in the vehicle and that attempts to elucidate the mechanism by which DMSO enhances flux must account for this variable. Equation 3 also shows that the flux is inversely related to the activity coefficient in the membrane and, because no independent measure of this factor exists, it is inseparable from D and h and the three appear in the permeability coefficient as a set. In fact, all three factors would be expected to be sensitive to significant transformations of barrier structure.

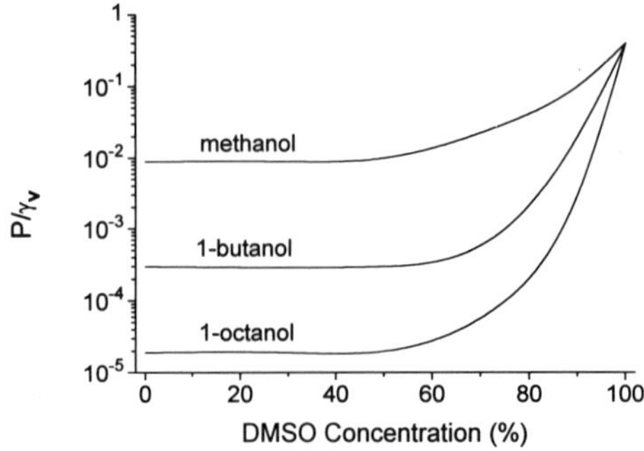

Figure 2 Normalized permeability coefficients for methanol, butanol, and octanol as a function of DMSO concentration in water.[20]

Of particular interest is the situation in which $D/h \cdot \gamma_m$ remains constant; i.e., barrier structure is unaltered. In this condition the product of $P \times \gamma_v$ is predicted to be constant:

$$P\frac{1}{\gamma_v} = \frac{D}{h}\frac{1}{\gamma_m} \tag{4}$$

Thus, if γ_v is independently known, one can rigorously determine whether a changing vehicle composition, i.e., increasing levels of DMSO, affects permeability strictly through the thermodynamics of solution or if it also induces a change in barrier properties.

Aqueous solutions of DMSO at 0, 30, 50, 75, 90, and 100% concentration were studied. When DMSO solutions were placed on both sides of the skin (balanced configuration) in a two-compartment diffusion cell, normalized (activity-adjusted) permeability coefficients of ethanol, butanol, and octanol did not change at DMSO concentrations of 0 to 50% (Figure 2). Thus, as predicted from Equation 4, the barrier was unaffected by these concentrations of DMSO. However, at 75% and above activity-adjusted permeability coefficients increased markedly in a systematic fashion. Application of neat DMSO to both sides of the skin resulted in permeability coefficients which were maximal and approximately equal for all three alcohols. Barrier function was impaired to such an extent that its discriminatory capacity was abolished.

The data of Figure 2 are particularly interesting in that a large increase appears to exist in octanol absorption at higher DMSO levels. In fact, this is not the case. The excellent solvent capacity of DMSO for octanol is such that the activity coefficient of octanol is reduced over three orders of magnitude in going from 0 to 100% DMSO (Figure 3). Thus, the rate of octanol absorption through hairless mouse skin is actually *reduced* at intermediate DMSO concentrations and does not increase until the barrier is effectively destroyed by application of neat solvent to both sides of the skin. It is clear from these data that the magnitude of permeability enhancement may be different for hydrophobic and hydrophilic compounds, and that simple measurement of net effects (i.e., changes in the rate of absorption) do not accurately reflect

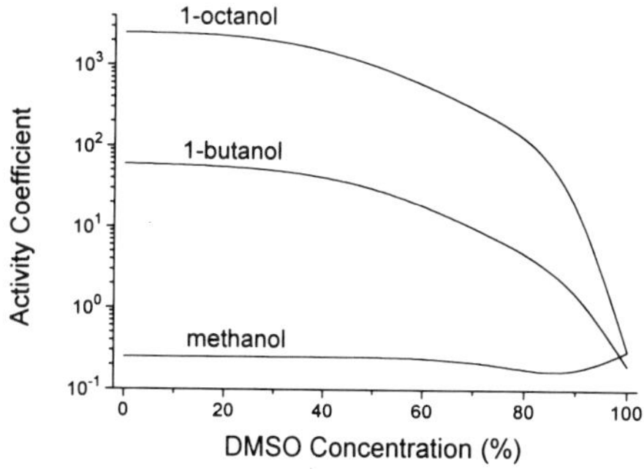

Figure 3 Activity coefficients of methanol, butanol, and octanol as function of DMSO concentration in water.[20]

significant changes in underlying events when competing factors are moving in opposite directions. Others have also found the DMSO enhancing effect to be dependent upon the water solubility of the compound studied.[21]

Further complicating the picture with respect to the mechanism of action of DMSO is the observation by Kurihara-Bergstrom et al.[20] that the effects on skin permeability could be quite different if the solvent was applied to only the outside of the skin (asymmetric application), duplicating clinical use conditions, rather than to both sides of the skin. This was most evident when neat solvent was applied and when the probe molecule was hydrophobic. The rate of absorption of methanol was little affected by the application regimen, but that of octanol differed by an order of magnitude (Figure 4). Octanol absorption was actually inhibited when neat DMSO was used as the donor solution and isotonic saline used as the receptor, but was enhanced when neat DMSO was used as both donor and receptor. It was postulated that competing solvent flows, DMSO moving inward and water outward, as in the first situation, may be introducing significant variables not accounted for in Equation 3.

One factor measured in the study of Kurihara-Bergstrom et al.[20] that correlated nicely with the permeability enhancing capacity of DMSO was the change in the amount of material extracted from the SC (Figure 5). Little change in the dry weight of the barrier layer was found following a 2-h exposure to 50% or less DMSO:H_2O. However, at higher concentrations weight loss increased significantly, to as high as 18% in neat solvent, and the abrupt change in the shape of the curve paralleled that seen with the permeability coefficient. Others also showed the ability of DMSO to extract significant amounts of material from the skin, although a detailed analysis of components extracted has not been done.[22]

In a companion study by Kurihara-Bergstrom et al.[23] the same experimental design was employed to determine the effect of DMSO on the percutaneous absorption of the antiviral agent vidarabine (ara-A). As before, the concentration dependence of the DMSO effect was observed and the results varied as the manner of application varied, balanced vs. asymmetric (Figure 6) At low DMSO concentrations absorption was inhibited, in keeping with enhanced drug solubility, and therefore reduced thermodynamic activity. At higher concentrations, however, the permeability coefficient increased systematically over an order of magnitude and was maximal in neat DMSO.

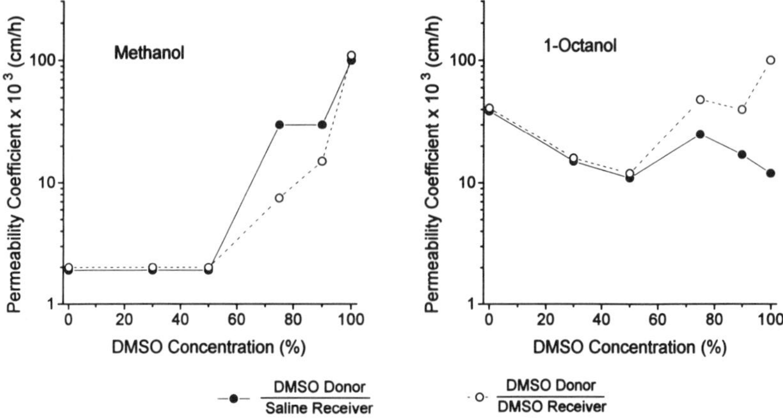

Figure 4 Change in permeability coefficient for methanol and octanol as function of DMSO concentration and method of application of DMSO, balanced or asymmetric.[20]

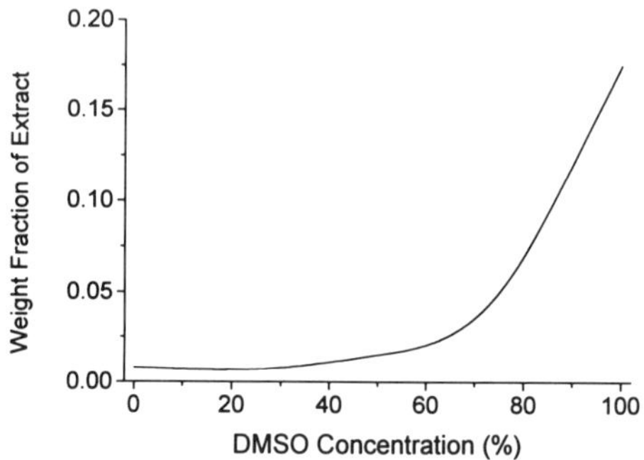

Figure 5 Dry weight of SC removed after 2-h exposure to various DMSO concentrations.[20]

Although a complete understanding of the basis for the differences in absorption observed depending upon the manner of DMSO application is lacking, the situation most relevant to the clinical use of this enhancer is that in which saline is used as the receptor phase (asymmetric application). The results cited show that it is vital for *in vitro* studies to appropriately mimic real-life situations when the intent is to develop drug formulations for animal or human use.

Other studies have been conducted to examine the ability of DMSO to increase skin permeability to active therapeutic agents, some of which have even progressed to clinical evaluation.[24–28] The results to date have been mixed. Although little doubt exists concerning the ability of DMSO to enhance absorption, clinical efficacy does not automatically follow.

One recent investigation, which combined both laboratory and clinical studies, is of particular interest because it not only supports the data of earlier workers, who noted the rapidity with which DMSO exerts its action, but also shows that large doses of DMSO are not required to enhance absorption.[28] Whereas many of the prior studies essentially used an infinite dose of drug-containing DMSO solutions to

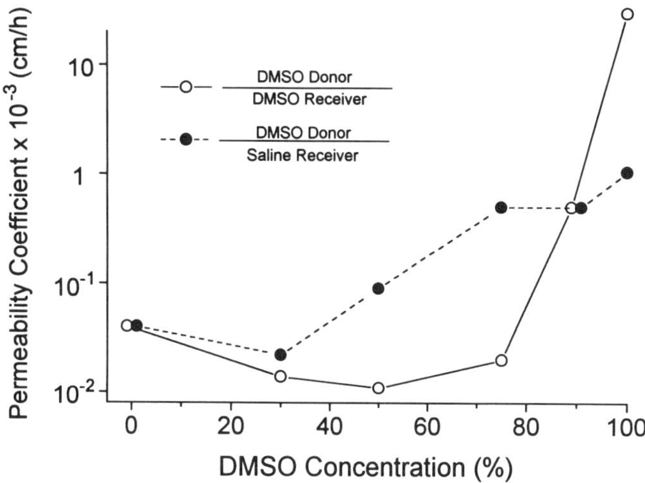

Figure 6 Change in permeability coefficient for ara-A as function of DMSO concentration and method of application of DMSO, balanced or asymmetric.[23]

achieve enhancement, the *in vitro* portion of this study used doses approximating those that were subsequently used clinically (i.e., 20 μl/cm²).

Various concentrations of lidocaine-free base ranging from 1 to 50% were incorporated into 70% DMSO in ethanol, and the rate and extent of absorption measured *in vitro* through human cadaver skin using the finite dose technique. Not only did the incorporation of DMSO lead to significantly increased lidocaine absorption over other commonly used topical anesthetic formulations (Figure 7), but examination of the rates of absorption found that enhancement occurred rapidly. The peak flux of lidocaine occurred at 1 to 2 h (Figure 8), which is in keeping with the observation of Stoughton[10] that it took approximately 30 min to establish a SC reservoir for corticosteroids. In this case, because lidocaine had to penetrate the full thickness of the epidermis as well as some dermis prior to its detection in the receptor solution, a somewhat longer transit time was expected. Clinical evaluation of 25% lidocaine in 70% DMSO, the formulation having maximum bioavailability, found it to have a high degree of efficacy in the prevention of pain associated with laser therapy of vascular malformations.

IV. CLINICAL AND HISTOPATHOLOGIC OBSERVATIONS

A number of investigations examined the cutaneous response to DMSO in animals and humans.[29–34] Topical application can elicit visible reactions, the extent of which are dependent upon three factors: DMSO concentration, total dose (finite vs. infinite application), and method of exposure (occluded vs. open).

Approximately 50% of human subjects will exhibit a local reaction to open application of a finite dose of 60% DMSO, and the percentage increases with increasing concentration.[29] Erythema and, in some subjects, weals (hives) will be noted. The latter begin around hair shafts as small papules, possibly a result of follicular diffusion, then coalesce to form a single weal. The reaction can begin

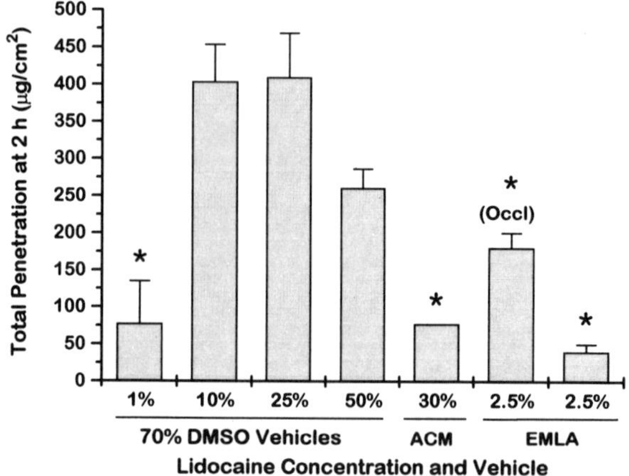

Figure 7 Total amount of drug absorbed *in vitro* 2 h after topical application. Data are the means ± SE from duplicate determinations on two donor skin samples (except acid mantle cream, 1 donor skin). ACM = acid mantle cream; EMLA data combine lidocaine and prilocaine; Occl = occluded dose (all others unoccluded). * Data significantly different from the 25% lidocaine in 70% DMSO-ethanol formulation ($p < 0.01$).[28]

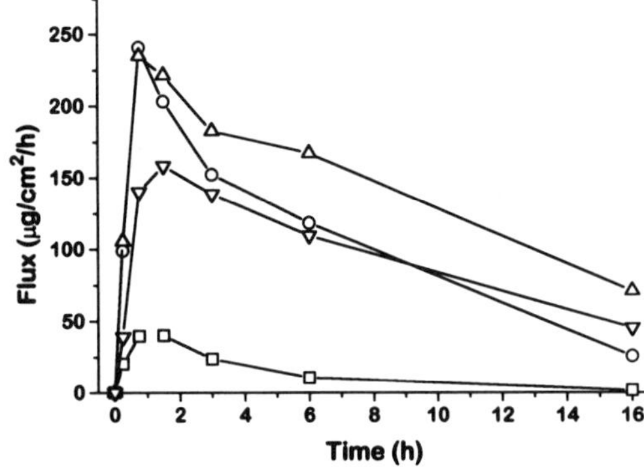

Figure 8 Rate of absorption of various concentrations of lidocaine from 70% DMSO-ethanol solution plotted as flux vs. the mid-time point of the sampling period. Data are the means of duplicate determinations on two donor skin samples. Lidocaine concentrations in 70% DMSO are □ 1% (w/v), ○ 10% (w/v), Δ 25% (w/v), ∇ 50% (w/v).[28]

within minutes, a consequence of histamine liberation, and take up to 40 to 50 min to develop fully. However, many variables impact on this reaction, including individual susceptibility, DMSO concentration, dose, and body site.[29,30] Examination of these reactions microscopically reveals the cells of the epidermis to be swollen with shrunken nuclei and, in some areas, ruptured to form open clefts or microvesicles.[29,31] Application of 80% DMSO under occlusion for 24 h can lead to frank necrosis of the skin and bullae formation.[32]

Kligman[31] pointed out that the skin can accommodate or "harden" following repeated exposure to DMSO. Daily applications of 90% DMSO under occlusion to the backs of human subjects resulted in the development of a dermatitis within 24 h, which increased in severity for 2 weeks, then regressed with continued application, so that by 35 d the skin had almost returned to normal.

Montes et al.[33] examined electron microscopic changes occurring in the SC of guinea pig skin following DMSO treatment and compared the results to those obtained from an untreated contralateral site. Application (50 to 200 μl/cm^2) of 90% DMSO led rapidly to the destruction of the normal morphology of the SC. As early as 30 min following dosing the cells in the deeper layers of the barrier appear to be enlarged and vacuolated. Islands of electron-dense material were present within the vacuoles, but only occasionally was this found to have the fibrillar pattern characteristic of keratin. In many locations separation of SC from the underlying granular layer occurred, giving rise to clefts. All of these changes could still be observed 48 h post-treatment.

Although the intermediate portion of the horny layer seemed to be somewhat less affected than the basal portion, significant morphologic changes were also observed in the most superficial layers. The normal keratin pattern was either lost, leaving the cytoplasm to appear "homogeneously amorphous", or in some cases complete loss of all intracellular contents occurred. The cell membranes, however, remained intact.

V. MECHANISM OF ACTION

Although the precise mechanism of action of DMSO remains a matter for speculation, key elements underlying its enhancer properties must be taken into account: (1) it acts quickly, e.g., a drug reservoir can be established in the SC in 30 min or less,[10] and (2) high concentrations (>60% in water) are essential.[11,12,17,20,23] Simple destruction of the barrier through extraction of critical components could be proposed and evidence for this hypothesis is abundant. Electron microscopic changes are found throughout the guinea pig SC 30 min following exposure to 90% DMSO.[33] Loss of barrier mass has been documented following DMSO exposure,[20,22] showing a concentration dependence that correlates with changes in absorption.[20]

It is also possible that more subtle changes underlie the enhancement effect of DMSO and that some observations cited above (e.g., extraction of barrier components) only reflect long-term effects not essential to its immediate action. Elfbaum and Laden[35] suggested that DMSO promotes swelling and unfolding of certain proteins within the cells of the SC and exerts its enhancer effect through this mechanism. Rammler and Zaffaroni[36] offer a similar view and suggest that enhancement could result from reversible changes in protein configuration secondary to replacement of bound water molecules by DMSO.

A more comprehensive view has been offered by Barry.[37] Enhancer activity may occur via two fundamental mechanisms: its superb solvent properties, which increase drug partitioning into the barrier, and its effects on barrier constituents, leading to greatly reduced diffusional resistance (this may occur via more than one mechanism). The first suggests that DMSO could act by its mere presence in the SC, independent of any destructive or protein/lipid altering activities, creating solvent-filled spaces with greater solubility for drugs than untreated SC. This would explain the need for high concentrations of DMSO. The second effect could occur through a number of mechanisms. Above 60% concentration DMSO appears to affect barrier lipids, as determined by differential scanning calorimetry, leading to greater fluidity and, hence, less resistance to diffusion. At lower DMSO concentrations, down to 20%, evidence of interaction with SC proteins was found. Thus, DMSO may preferentially move initially into the corneocytes, displacing bound water from proteins and leading to a more solvated (swollen) environment, then (at higher concentrations) displace water from polar head groups of intercellular lipids, leading to highly solvated channels between lipid bilayers. Interaction between DMSO and the polar head groups of intercellular lipids may also lead to less packing of the hydrocarbon tails that form the core of each bilayer because of the larger solvation shell created around the head group. The result would be increased fluidity within the core of the bilayer and a reduction in the resistance of this pathway to diffusion.

REFERENCES

1. **Brayton, C. F.,** Dimethyl sulfoxide (DMSO): a review, *Cornell Vet.,* 76, 61, 1986.
2. **Jacob, S. W., Bischel, M., and Herschler, R. J.,** Dimethyl sulfoxide (DMSO): a new concept in pharmacotherapy, *Curr. Ther. Res.,* 6, 134, 1964.
3. **Leake, C. D., Ed.,** *Biological Actions of Dimethyl Sulfoxide, Ann. N. Y. Acad. Sci.,* 141, 1967.
4. **Jacob, S. W. et al.,** *Dimethyl Sulfoxide. Basic Concepts of DMSO,* Marcel Dekker, New York, 1971.
5. **Jacob, S. W. and Herschler, R., Eds.,** *Biological Actions of Dimethyl Sulfoxide, Ann. N. Y. Acad. Sci.,* 243, 1975.
6. **MacGregor, W. S.,** The chemical and physical properties of DMSO, in *Biological Actions of Dimethyl Sulfoxide, Ann. N. Y. Acad. Sci.,* Leake, C. D., Ed., 141, 1967, p. 3.
7. **Lovelock, J. E. and Bishop, M. W. H.,** Prevention of freezing damage to living cells by dimethylsulphoxide, *Nature,* 183, 1394, 1959.
8. **Stoughton, R. B. and Fritsch, W.,** Influence of dimethyl sulfoxide on human percutaneous absorption, *Arch. Dermatol.,* 90, 512, 1964.
9. **Horitz, A. and Weber, K. J.,** Skin penetrating property of drugs dissolved in dimethyl sulfoxide (DMSO) and other vehicles, *Life Sci.,* 3, 1389, 1964.
10. **Stoughton, R. B.,** Dimethyl sulfoxide induction of a steroid reservoir in human skin, *Arch. Dermatol.,* 91, 657, 1965.
11. **Kligman, A. M.,** Topical pharmacology and toxicology of dimethyl sulfoxide. I., *JAMA,* 193, 796, 1965.
12. **Sweeney, T. M., Downes, A. M., and Matoltsy, A. G.,** The effect of dimethyl sulfoxide on the epidermal water barrier, *J. Invest. Dermatol.,* 46, 300, 1966.
13. **Kastin, A. J., Akire, A., and Schally, A. V.,** Topical absorption of polypeptides with dimethyl sulfoxide, *Arch. Dermatol.,* 93, 471, 1966.
14. **Djan, T. I. and Gunberg, D. L.,** Percutaneous absorption of two steroids dissolved in dimethyl sulfoxide in the immature female rat, in *Biological Actions of Dimethyl Sulfoxide, Annals of the New York Academy of Sci.,* Leake, C. D., Ed., 141, 406, 1967.
15. **Maibach, H. I. and Feldmann, R. J.,** The effect of DMSO on percutaneous penetration of hydrocortisone and testosterone in man, in *Biological Actions of Dimethyl Sulfoxide, Ann. N. Y. Acad. Sci.,* Leake, C. D., Ed., 141, 423, 1967.
16. **McDermot, H. L., Finkbeiner, A. J., Wills, W. J., and Heggie, R. M.,** The enhancement of penetration of an organophosphorous anti-cholinesterase through guinea pig skin by dimethyl sulphoxide, *Can. J. Physiol. Pharm.,* 45, 299, 1967.
17. **Elfbaum, S. G. and Laden, K.,** The effect of dimethyl sulfoxide on percutaneous absorption: a mechanistic study. I., *J. Soc. Cosmet. Chem.,* 19, 119, 1968.
18. **Elfbaum, S. G. and Laden, K.,** The effect of dimethyl sulfoxide on percutaneous absorption: a mechanistic study. II. *J. Soc. Cosmet. Chem.,* 19, 163, 1968.
19. **Dugard, P. H. and Embery, G.,** The influence of dimethyl sulphoxide on the percutaneous migration of potassium butyl (^{35}S) sulphate, potassium methyl (^{35}S) and sodium (^{35}S) sulphate, *Br. J. Dermatol.,* 81 (Suppl. 4), 69, 1969.

20. **Kurihara-Bergstrom, T., Flynn, G. L., and Higuchi, W. I.,** Physico-chemical study of percutaneous absorption enhancement by dimethyl sulfoxide: kinetic and thermodynamic determinants of dimethyl sulfoxide mediated mass transfer of alkanols, *J. Pharm. Sci.,* 75, 479, 1986.
21. **Boman, A.,** Percutaneous absorption of 3 organic solvents in the guinea pig. V. Effect of "accelerants", *Contact Dermatitis,* 21, 304, 1989.
22. **Embery, G. and Dugard, P. H.,** The isolation of dimethyl sulfoxide soluble components from human epidermal preparations: a possible mechanism of action of dimethyl sulfoxide in effecting percutaneous migration phenomena, *J. Invest. Dermatol.,* 57, 308, 1971.
23. **Kurihara-Bergstrom, T., Flynn, G. L., and Higuchi, W. I.,** Physico-chemical study of percutaneous absorption enhancement by dimethyl sulfoxide: dimethyl sulfoxide mediation of vidarabine (ara-A) permeation of hairless mouse skin, *J. Invest. Dermatol.,* 89, 274, 1987.
24. **Parker, J. D.,** A double-blind trial of idoxuridine in recurrent genital herpes, *J. Antimicrob. Chemother.,* 3(Suppl. A), 131, 1977.
25. **Silvestri, D. L., Corey, L., and Holmes, K. K.,** Ineffectiveness of topical idoxuridine in dimethyl sulfoxide for therapy for genital herpes, *JAMA,* 248, 953, 1982.
26. **Franz, T. J.,** On the bioavailability of topical formulations of clindamycin hydrochloride, *J. Am. Acad. Dermatol.,* 9, 66, 1983.
27. **Sidwell, R. W., Huffman, J. H., Call, E., Alaghamandan, H., and Dixon, G. J.,** Effect of vidarabine in dimethyl sulfoxide vehicle on type 1 herpes virus-induced cutaneous lesions in laboratory animals, *Chemotherapy,* 33, 141, 1987.
28. **Mallory, S. B., Lehman, P. A., Vanderpool, D. R., and Franz, T. J.,** Topical lidocaine for anesthesia in patients undergoing pulsed dye laser treatment for vascular malformations, *Pediatr. Dermatol.,* 10, 370, 1993.
29. **Sulzberger, M. B., Cortese, T. A., Fishman, L., Wiley, H. S., and Peyakovich, P. S.,** Some effects of DMSO on human skin *in vivo,* in *Biological Actions of Dimethyl Sulfoxide, Ann. N. Y. Acad. Sci.,* Leake, C. D., Ed., 141, 437, 1967.
30. **Frosch, P. J., Duncan, S., and Kligman, A. M.,** Cutaneous biometrics. I. The response of human skin to dimethyl sulphoxide, *Br. J. Dermatol.,* 102, 263, 1980.
31. **Kligman, A. M.,** Dimethyl sulfoxide. II., *JAMA,* 193, 932, 1965.
32. **Skog, E. and Wahlberg, J. E.,** Effect of dimethyl sulfoxide on skin, *Acta Derm. Venereol.,* 47, 426, 1967.
33. **Montes, L. F., Day, J. L., Wand, C. J., and Kennedy, L.,** Ultrastructural changes in the horny layer following local application of dimethyl sulfoxide, *J. Invest. Dermatol.,* 48, 184, 1967.
34. **Shackleford, J. M. and Yielding, K. L.,** Ultrastructural studies of barrier restoration in epidermis of hairless mice following dimethyl sulfoxide application, *J. Cutaneous Pathol.,* 11, 259, 1984.
35. **Elfbaum, S. G. and Laden, K.,** The effect of dimethyl sulphoxide on percutaneous absorption: a mechanistic study. III., *J. Soc. Cosmet. Chem.,* 19, 841, 1968.
36. **Rammler, D. H. and Zaffaroni, A.,** Biological implications of DMSO based on a review of its chemical properties, in *Biological Actions of Dimethyl Sulfoxide, Ann. N. Y. Acad. Sci.,* Leake, C. D., Ed., 141, 13, 1967.
37. **Barry, B. W.,** Mode of action of penetration enhancers in human skin, *J. Control. Rel.,* 6, 85, 1987.

Chapter 6.1

Azone®

Geoffrey Allan

CONTENTS

I. INTRODUCTION

Azone® is the registered trademark of the chemical substance laurocapram (1-dodecyl azacycloheptan-2-one). Azone® is a novel chemical skin penetration enhancer that was developed specifically as a pharmaceutical vehicle for incorporation into both topical and transdermal drug delivery systems to facilitate and control delivery of drugs across the stratum corneum (SC).[1]

This chapter is a review of studies related to the mechanism of action of this novel agent and an overview of the body of data generated with this material attesting to its safety, from a regulatory perspective, for use as a pharmaceutical excipient in novel drug delivery systems.

0-8493-2605-2/95/$0.00+$.50

II. MECHANISM OF ACTION

A. PHYSICOCHEMICAL PROPERTIES OF AZONE®

Azone® is a clear, amber-colored liquid with a relative molecular mass of 281.49 Da, a melting point of –7°C, and a boiling point of 160°C at 0.05 mmHg. The octanol-water partition coefficient estimated from Hansch Analysis is 6.21, demonstrating it to be an extremely lipophilic material.

Azone® is compatible with most organic solvents and is an excellent solubilizer of a wide variety of drugs. It can be readily incorporated into a variety of formulation systems, and shows a high degree of chemical stability and excipient compatibility.

B. INTERACTION WITH STRATUM CORNEUM LIPIDS

Although the mechanisms by which Azone® interacts with the SC lipids is still under investigation, it appears that a direct interaction with the intercellular lipids to increase the degree of fluidity of the hydrophobic regions of the intercellular lamellar structure explains its ability to decrease the diffusional resistance of the skin.

SC lipids are primarily composed of cholesterol derivatives and ceramides with smaller amounts of other materials such as fatty acids and triglycerides. The lipids are present in a distinct, structured bilayer lamellae, thereby providing a substantial hydrophobic barrier. It is believed that the stability of the lamellar structure is dependent upon electrostatic interactions between the polar head groups and hydrophobic interactions between the alkyl chains of the component lipids. It is clear from various structure activity studies that the C_{12} alkyl chain of Azone® corresponds to the dimensions of the cholesterol skeleton, leading to the hypothesis that disruption of ceramide–cholesterol or cholesterol–cholesterol interactions is an important factor in the penetration-enhancing activity of Azone®.

A molecular model describing the electrostatic interaction of Azone® with the SC lipids has been proposed by Brain and Walters,[2] and the reader is referred to this work for further discussion.

C. EFFECT ON SKIN PENETRATION

The effect of Azone® on the penetration of a wide variety of drugs has been extensively studied since the early 1980s. It is clear that Azone® is an effective enhancer for both a number of hydrophilic and hydrophobic drugs of varying molecular weight, including peptide molecules such as insulin and vasopressin.[3,4] Azone® is generally used at low concentrations, 1 to 5%, and its enhancement activity can be increased further by the use of cosolvents such as propylene glycol (PG).

Although Azone® may be considered to be a universal skin penetration enhancer, it is clear that skin penetration of drugs is dependent upon a number of other key factors such as the solubility and degree of ionization of the drug in the delivery vehicles. It is therefore important when designing a multicomponent delivery vehicle that the interplay between all of the controlling factors influencing skin penetration is understood.

III. PHARMACOLOGICAL AND TOXICOLOGICAL PROPERTIES OF AZONE®

A. PHARMACOLOGICAL ACTIONS

In addition to its principal biological activity as a dermal penetration enhancer, Azone® does exhibit a secondary pharmacological action, virucidal activity.[5] This discovery was made as a result of observations that Azone® enhanced the penetration and efficacy of the antiviral substance, trifluorothymidine. In this series of experiments Azone® reduced viral titers of cultures of herpes simplex viruses, HSV-1 and HSV-2, and inhibited the number and size of cutaneous HSV-1 lesions in guinea pigs.

B. TOXICOLOGICAL ACTIONS

Because Azone® is considered a new chemical entity, a thorough and very extensive toxicology program has been conducted in mice, rats, guinea pigs, rabbits, and monkeys to determine its toxicity potential. No adverse systemic or dermal toxicity has been observed in studies ranging from 1 month to lifetime dermal exposure.

In single-dose toxicity studies the oral LD_{50} of 100% Azone® is approximately 7.4 and 9.0 g/kg in mice and rats, respectively. When 100% Azone® is applied dermally to rats, a similar LD_{50} value of 7.3 g/kg is obtained.

Acute ocular irritation studies conducted in rabbits revealed that Azone® exhibited a slight irritating effect at high concentrations, with frequent applications producing a mild conjunctival hyperemia.

In multidose dermal toxicity studies, with up to 30 d of applications, concentrations of Azone® of 10 to 50% were slightly irritating to hairless mice, considerably to severely irritating to rats, and mildly to moderately irritating to rabbits and guinea pigs. With dermal applications for up to 6 months in mice, Azone® at concentrations up to 5% caused a mild to moderate irritation of the treated skin with no detectable systemic effects. Similarly, in rats and cynomolgus monkeys Azone® at the same concentrations for up to 6 months caused a mild, reversible dermal irritation with no systemic effects. The dermal changes noted following the application of Azone® were considered to be consistent with findings following long-term exposure to mild irritants.

The potential tumorigenic effects of Azone® by repeated daily dermal applications was evaluated in both mice and rats. No evidence of a dermal tumorigenic effect was found in either species at concentrations at least 30 times the anticipated human dose. In rats, although no evidence of carcinogenicity was found at the site of dermal application, a small, though not statistically significant increase was observed in the incidence of oral/nasal squamous cell tumors in rats treated with Azone®.

Azone® has been shown to be neither genotoxic nor mutagenic in appropriate mammalian and bacterial bioassays. Reproduction studies in rats with Azone® showed no interference with reproduction or adverse effect on offspring. Teratology studies in mice and rabbits with Azone® demonstrated no evidence of compound-related effects, no evidence of embryotoxicity or teratogenicity, and no effect on litter parameters, embryonic development, or fetal development.

C. EXCRETION PROFILE OF AZONE® FOLLOWING HUMAN DERMAL APPLICATION

A number of studies have been conducted to examine the dermal absorption and excretion of Azone® following dermal application. In two studies using radiotracer methodology with single-dose administration of 100% Azone®, either under unoccluded or occlusive conditions, minimal absorption of the material (<1%) was demonstrated.[6] Most of the applied radiotracer was recovered from the skin surface. Most of the radioactivity detected in skin strippings was found in tape strips that sampled the outermost layers of the SC. No radioactivity was detected in the blood and extremely small quantities were recovered in the feces (0.005%).

A recent study evaluated the absorption of Azone® following repetitive dermal application.[7] In this study Azone® (1.6%) was incorporated into a topical cream base containing PG and applied dermally to human subjects under conditions similar to that which would be used in clinical practice. Azone® was applied for 21 d and small tracer quantities of radiolabel were periodically applied for quantitative urinary recovery. The study demonstrated that Azone® was minimally absorbed, with <3% of the applied dose being recovered in the urine, which did not increase with repetitive application.

IV. CLINICAL STUDIES WITH AZONE®

Several clinical studies were conducted in normal adult volunteers to investigate the skin irritancy and sensitization potential of different concentrations of Azone®. In addition, as part of a number of drug development programs, several clinical trials were performed to evaluate the clinical efficacy of Azone®-containing formulations. The clinical efficacy of triamcinolone acetonide/Azone®- and methotrexate/Azone®-containing formulations are briefly reviewed.

A. CLINICAL SAFETY STUDIES

1. Twenty-One-Day Studies of Cumulative Irritation

Several clinical studies were conducted in normal adult volunteers to investigate the irritancy potential of different concentrations of Azone® with various delivery systems. In one study, each of the 11 subjects was treated with 2, 5, 25, 50, and 100% Azone® in a Neutrogena® vehicle and with three control preparations (Neutrogena, mineral oil, and Vaseline® Intensive Care lotion). The materials were delivered using a Webril patch with occlusion, applied to the same site, for 5 d/week over a 21-d period. Azone® in concentrations up through 50% was not irritating; at a concentration of 100%, Azone® was more irritating than a mineral oil control in one of the 11 subjects.

In another study, ten subjects received 100% Azone® in a poroplastic patch along with a control patch containing water only. Patches were applied 5 d/week for 21 d to the same sites. None of the subjects reacted to either treatment.

In a third study, 26 subjects were exposed to 46% Azone® incorporated into occluded Webril patches, applied 5 d/week for 21 d. Estimates of skin irritation on a five-point scale were made daily at the time of patch removal. Low irritancy potential was seen.

A study of 12 subjects was conducted to assess the correlation of two physiological measures of skin irritation, transepidermal water loss and cutaneous blood velocity, with traditional visual measures of irritation. Each subject had 12 test sites, six on each side of the back. One concentration of sodium lauryl sulfate (1%) and five concentrations of Azone® (0, 1, 3, 10, and 30%) were used; each concentration was applied to duplicate sites, one on each side of the back. The six sites on one side of the back were covered with a Webril patch, and the six sites on the other side were left uncovered. Measurements of irritation were conducted at baseline, 7, 14, and 21 d. The sites without patches were unaffected by all treatments, whereas the sites with patches containing sodium lauryl sulfate (1%) and 10 and 30% Azone® were irritated.

2. Modified Draize Skin Sensitization Study

To evaluate the potential for Azone® to induce irritation and sensitization, a repeated-insult patch test was performed on 200 subjects by using the modified Draize method. Test patches with 50% Azone® were applied with occlusion to the same site, three times, for a 3-week induction period. Two weeks later, the same kind of patch was applied to a site not previously exposed to Azone®. After 21 d, the challenge patch was removed, and the degree of inflammation was evaluated. No evidence of allergic contact sensitization was found.

3. Photoirritation Study

The photoirritation potential of 100% Azone® was investigated in ten normal subjects by using a modification of the Marzulli procedure. Test sites were prepared by tape stripping and then were moistened with 100% Azone®. One hour later, the sites were irradiated and were evaluated after 24 h. No evidence of photoirritation was observed.

The potential of 100% Azone® for irritation and photosensitization was assessed by using a repeated-insult patch test on 25 normal subjects; the modified Draize procedure was used. The test site was irradiated when each patch was removed. A challenge patch was applied for 24 h to a test site not previously exposed or irradiated, and the new site was irradiated. Four days later the challenge site was evaluated. No evidence for allergic or photoallergic contact sensitization was observed.

4. Summary

Clinical studies demonstrate that human skin can tolerate repeated applications of Azone® over an extended period. Irritation tends to be associated with the use of high concentrations of Azone® and with the use of occlusive patches on the application site.

B. CLINICAL STUDIES WITH AZONE® CONTAINING FORMULATIONS

1. Triamcinolone Acetonide

Triamcinolone acetonide is a synthetic corticosteroid with a variety of systemic and topical applicabilities. The efficacy of triamcinolone preparations with Azone® was assessed in clinical studies of two dermatological disorders, psoriasis vulgaris and atopic dermatitis.

In psoriasis studies, adults with psoriasis vulgaris were randomized into three treatment groups: triamcinolone acetonide 0.05% plus Azone® 1.6%, triamcinolone 0.05% alone, and Azone® 1.6% alone. Subjects applied test medication to all lesions twice daily for 6 weeks. Subjects were evaluated for severity of the disease at baseline, days 8, 15, 29, and 43 of treatment, and 2 weeks after treatment ended. Erythema, induration, and scaling were rated in addition to global change in disease status.

All treatments, including Azone® alone, were associated with improvement over baseline; however, a slight decline occurred after treatment ended. Patients treated with triamcinolone plus Azone® showed significantly greater improvement after 6 weeks of treatment than those treated with Azone® alone, whereas treatment with triamcinolone alone and with Azone® alone did not differ in effect after 6 weeks. No serious adverse events occurred, and reports of treatment-emergent adverse experiences did not differ among the three treatment groups.

In atopic dermatitis studies, adults with atopic dermatitis were randomized into three treatment groups: triamcinolone acetonide 0.05% plus Azone® 1.6%, triamcinolone 0.05% alone, and Azone® 1.6% alone. Subjects applied test medication to all lesions twice daily for 2 weeks. Subjects were evaluated for severity of the disease by rating erythema, induration, and pruritus and global evaluations.

Triamcinolone plus Azone® was generally associated with greater improvement than triamcinolone alone at days 3 and 7. At day 15, patients treated with triamcinolone plus Azone® showed greater improvement than those treated with triamcinolone alone, and the difference was statistically significant. Furthermore, triamcinolone plus Azone® was associated with significantly greater improvement than Azone® alone from day 3 through day 15. During the same period, patients treated with triamcinolone alone showed significantly greater in some, but not all, of the measures than patients treated with Azone® alone.

No serious adverse events were reported. The most common treatment-emergent adverse experience reported, exacerbation of symptoms, was believed by the investigators to represent disease progression, rather than an effect of treatment.

2. Methotrexate

Methotrexate is an antimetabolite that is used in the systemic treatment of certain neoplastic diseases, adult rheumatoid arthritis, and severe psoriasis. Because of the extreme toxicity of this drug, its use in the treatment of psoriasis is restricted to patients for whom the condition is both severe and insufficiently responsive to less extreme forms of therapy. As a water-soluble medication, methotrexate alone does not readily penetrate the SC. The use of Azone® as a vehicle for topically applied methotrexate has been investigated in a number of studies.

In one study[8] four treatments were used: 3% Azone® in a gel formulation with methotrexate concentrated at 0.1, 0.5, or 1.0%, or the 3% Azone® formulation alone. Each subject received two different, randomly assigned treatments on separate sites. Test medication was applied twice daily for 6 weeks.

All treatments, including Azone® alone, were associated with progressive improvement over the 6-week treatment period. In all groups improvement reached a maximum at 6 weeks, and declined during the week after treatment ended. All treatment sites were significantly improved over untreated sites during all 6 weeks of therapy. At 6 weeks, improvement in the sites treated with 1% methotrexate was significantly greater than improvement in the sites treated with Azone® alone.

No systemic side effects were observed from the hematological and biochemical profiles; furthermore, methotrexate was not detected in the serum, suggesting that most or all of the applied drug remained at the site of treatment. The lack of improvement at untreated sites provided further evidence that the observed therapeutic effects occurred locally in the skin. These preliminary results suggest that Azone® may facilitate the percutaneous penetration of methotrexate.

The pharmacokinetic characteristics of a topical 1% methotrexate-3% Azone® gel were assessed in nine patients with moderately severe psoriasis.[9] Methotrexate was applied every 12 h for 3.5 d to psoriatic lesions, drug was discontinued, and after at least a 5-d washout period, patients received three doses of 5 mg orally every 12 h.

Methotrexate concentrations in serum and urine were measured by a kinetic enzyme assay based on the competitive inhibition of dihydrofolate reductase. In this study percutaneous absorption of methotrexate ranged from 0.01 to 1.2% of the administered dose.

Adverse side effects of the topical preparation were primarily transient pruritus and burning and stinging in psoriatic lesions in six patients. Interestingly, after only 4 d of topical therapy, one patient showed no change, one patient had moderate improvement, and seven patients had slight improvement of their psoriasis.

In a more recent study, the effects of a 1% topical methotrexate formulation containing Azone® on psoriatic lesions in a double-blind paired, placebo-controlled randomed study were evaluated.[10] In this study involving 53 subjects topical application of a 1% methotrexate formulation resulted in a marked improvement in psoriatic status. Treatment significantly reduced the total psoriasis score over the 8-week treatment period when compared to placebo. At the end of the treatment period, the majority of subjects were characterized as having marked improvement in their psoriasis lesion. In contrast, none of the subjects receiving placebo demonstrated a marked improvement in their psoriasis lesion at any time throughout the treatment period. No serious adverse events were noted throughout the duration of the study, although skin discomfort caused the premature dropout of six subjects from the study.

V. CONCLUSIONS

Azone® has been subjected to an extensive series of toxicological tests in both rodents and primates. No adverse systemic or dermal toxicity was observed in studies ranging from 1 month to lifetime dermal exposure. Safety studies conducted with Azone® in human subjects show that this compound is not irritating or allergenic when applied to human skin. Dermal absorption studies in humans demonstrate that Azone® is readily absorbed into the SC, but is minimally absorbed into the systemic circulation even after prolonged application.

When Azone® is combined with topically applied medications indicated for the skin disorders of psoriasis and atopic dermatitis, the clinical efficacy of the Azone®-containing formulations is greater than formulations containing the primary drug alone. These observations demonstrate the importance of facilitated drug penetration in contributing to clinical efficacy.

REFERENCES

1. **Stoughton, R. B.,** Enhanced percutaneous penetration with 1-dodecyl acycloheptan-2-one, *Arch. Dermatol.,* 118, 474, 1982.
2. **Brain, K. R. and Walters, K. A.,** Molecular modeling of skin permeation enhancement by chemical agents, in *Pharmaceutical Skin Penetration Enhancement,* Walters, K. A. and Hadgraft, J., Eds., Marcel Dekker, New York, 1993, chap. 18.
3. **Wiecher, J. W. and De Zeeuw, R. A.,** Transdermal drug delivery: efficacy and potential applications of the penetration enhancer Azone®, in *Drug Design and Delivery,* Vol. 6, Honan, M., Ed., Harwood Academic Publishers, London, 1990, chap. 5.
4. **Hadgraft, J., Williams, D. G., and Allan, G.,** Azone®, Mechanisms of action and clinical effect, in *Pharmaceutical Skin Penetration Enhancement,* Walters, K. A. and Hadgraft, J., Eds., Marcel Dekker, New York, chap. 7, 1993.

5. **Spruance, S. L., McKeough, M., Sugibayashi, K., Robertson, F., Gaede, P., and Clark, D. S.,** Effect of Azone® and propylene glycol on penetration of trifluorothymidine through skin and efficacy of different topical formulations against cutaneous herpes simplex virus infections in guinea pigs, *Antimicrob. Agents Chemother.*, 26, 819, 1984.
6. **Wiechers, T. W., Drenth, B. F., Jonkman, J. H., and De Zeevw, R. A.,** Percutaneous absorption and elimination of the penetration enhancer Azone® in humans, *Pharm. Res.*, 4, 519, 1987.
7. **Wester, R. C., Melendres, J., Sedik, L., and Maibach, H. I.,** Percutaneous absorption of Azone® following single and multiple doses to human volunteers, *J. Pharm. Sci.*, 83, 124, 1994.
8. **Weinstein, G. D., McCullough, J. C., and Olsen, E.,** Topical methotrexate therapy for psoriasis, *Arch. Dermatol.*, 125, 227, 1989.
9. **Olsen, E., Cato, A., Meyer, C., Beughman, S., and Allan, G.,** A Pharmacokinetic Study of Topical Methotrexate/Azone® in Patients with Psoriasis, presented at 5th Int. Psoriasis Symp., San Francisco, July, 1991.
10. **Allan, G., Nolan, J. C., and Swinehart, J. M.,** Topical Methotrexate in the Treatment of Psoriasis, Proc. 3rd Int. Conf. Prediction of Percutaneous Penetration, La Grande Molte, France, April, 1993.

Chapter 6.2

Human SC Barrier Impairment by *N*-Alkyl-Azacycloheptanones: A Mechanistic Study of Drug Flux Enhancement, Azone® Mobility, and Protein and Lipid Perturbation

Joke A. Bouwstra and Harry E. Boddé

CONTENTS

I. INTRODUCTION

The main function of the outermost layer of the skin, the stratum corneum (SC), is to provide a barrier to evaporation of water from the underlying viable cell layers and

0-8493-2605-2/95/$0.00+$.50

to protect the organism against undesirable substances from the environment. The SC consists of dead, flattened cells embedded in lipid lamellar phases. The interior of the cells consists of keratin. For most substances the barrier resides mainly in the intercellular lipid domains. The major lipid classes found in the SC are ceramides, triglycerides, free fatty acids, and cholesterol.[1] These include a unique heterogeneous group of ceramides. No phospholipids are found in the SC. Successful percutaneous delivery of drugs relies strongly on adequate reduction of the barrier capacity of the SC, which can in principle be achieved via the use of penetration enhancers. It is expected that in order to be effective, penetration enhancers be capable of perturbing the SC barrier efficiently to increase its permeability for drugs. Successful development of skin penetration enhancers will depend greatly on a thorough understanding of the barrier function of SC and the mechanism of action of penetration enhancers. This implies that studies are required of the lipid organization in human SC, and of mechanisms, by which the lipid organization can be modified by skin penetration enhancers. In the past much effort was made to elucidate the mechanisms involved in increasing the absorption rate of drugs by penetration enhancers. Among the extensively studied penetration enhancers are oleic acid,[2–7] oleyl surfactants,[8,9] terpenes,[10–14] alcohols[15–21], dimethylsulfoxide,[22–25] Azone®,[26–40] and analogues of Azone®.[41–43]

This chapter deals with studies performed to elucidate the mechanisms leading to increased absorption with drugs after treatment of a series of *N*-alkyl-azocycloheptan-2-ones (*N*-alkyl azones) including Azone® solubilized in propylene glycol (PG). The structure of the *N*-alkyl azones is given in Figure 1. The series of *N*-alkylazacycloheptanones was designed in such a way that a systematic increase of the alkyl chain length occurred from hexyl to hexadecyl; this made it possible to systematically investigate the relationship between the molecular structure of the Azone® derivatives and their lipid barrier perturbation properties. In recent studies[44] the transport route of $HgCl_2$ across human skin was visualized at the ultrastructural level. These studies revealed that the intercellular route of $HgCl_2$ dominates and that only after longer transport times do the apical corneocytes tend to take up $HgCl_2$. In additional studies the influence on *N*-alkyl Azones® of the transport route of $HgCl_2$ was determined. These studies indicated that treatment with higher alkyl Azones® in PG tends to favor the intercellular route even further,[45] demonstrating the importance of lipid–enhancer interactions in understanding the mode of action of penetration enhancers on the skin barrier function.

II. MATERIAL AND METHODS

A. ISOLATION OF STRATUM CORNEUM AND TREATMENT WITH PROPYLENE GLYCOL AND ALKYL AZONES®

Abdomen or mammary skin obtained from the hospital was dermatomed to a thickness of 200 μm. The SC was separated from the epidermis by incubation in an 0.1% trypsin solution in a phosphate buffered saline solution (PBS, pH 7.4) on filter paper at 4°C overnight. Then the SC was incubated for 1 h at 37°C. The SC was mechanically separated from the epidermis and treated with an 0.1% trypsin inhibitor in PBS, pH 7.4. Finally, the SC was stored in a desiccator over silica gel. Before use the SC was hydrated over a 27% NaBr salt solution.

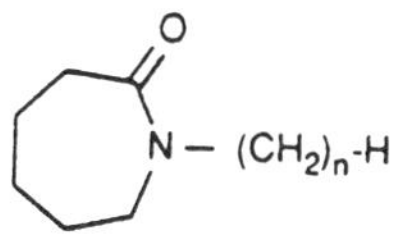

Figure 1 The molecular structure of the series of *N*-alkyl Azones®; *n* is the number of C atoms in the hydrocarbon chain.

Treatment with PG or 0.15 *M* *N*-alkyl Azones® in PG was carried out for a period of 24 h. The *N*-alkyl Azones® studied were hexyl Azone® (C_6), octyl Azone® (C_8), decyl Azone® (C_{10}), dodecyl Azone® (C_{12}), tetradecyl Azone® (C_{14}), and hexadecyl Azone® (C_{16}).

B. *IN VITRO* FLUX STUDIES

Skin penetration studies were carried out using a hydrophilic drug, a small peptide, 9-desglycinamide,8-arginine vasopressin (DGAVP) citrate and a lipophilic drug, nitroglycerin. SC was sandwiched between two silastic sheeting membranes and clamped in a diffusion cell.[46] To avoid stagnant water layers the donor compartment that contained 1 ml of a peptide or 1 ml of a nitroglycerin solution was stirred throughout the experiment. The area of diffusion was 0.79 cm^2. The acceptor phase was pumped through at a rate of 1 ml/h. The samples were collected at 1-h intervals with a fraction collector[46] and analyzed for the concentration of either DGAVP, using an radioimmunoassay[47] or nitroglycerin[48] using gas chromatography.

C. DIFFERENTIAL THERMAL ANALYSIS

The thermal behavior of the SC was studied with differential thermal analysis (DTA; Maple Instruments, The Netherlands). Approximately 20 mg of hydrated SC was used in each experiment. All measurements were carried out with hermetically sealed sample pans in order to avoid evaporation of water. The SC was scanned between 273 and 403 K at a heating rate of 2 K/min. In the case of PG-treated or *N*-alkyl Azones® in PG-treated SC, first the samples were heated to 55°C, equilibrated for 14 h, then cooled down to 273 K, after which a second run was started between 273 and 403 K. This was necessary because nonequilibrated treated SC had an exothermal peak at 55°C.[49] The maxima of the endothermal peaks were taken as transition temperatures.

D. SMALL-ANGLE X-RAY DIFFRACTION (SAXD)

Measurements were carried out at the synchrotron radiation station in Daresbury using station 8.2. A description of the experimental setup is given in Reference 50. The diffraction curves are all plotted as a function of Q, the scattering vector, which is defined as $Q = (4\pi \sin \theta/\lambda)$, where λ is the wavelength (0.154 nm) and θ is the scattering angle. In a lamellar phase the positions of the peaks are directly related to their spacings in the following way:[51] the position of the *n*th order diffraction peak (Q_n) is directly related to the periodicity (d) by $Q_n = 2\pi\, n/d$, in which n is the order of the peak.

E. WIDE-ANGLE X-RAY DIFFRACTION (WAXD)

Measurements were carried out at the synchrotron radiation source in Daresbury using station 7.2. A description of the experimental setup is given in Reference 52.

The diffraction patterns were recorded on a photographic film with two-dimensional detection. The positions of the reflections are indicated by their spacings.

F. FREEZE-FRACTURE ELECTRON MICROSCOPY (FFEM)

Enhancer-treated and -untreated SC were cut into small pieces and mounted in cylindrically shaped sample holders designed[53] to facilitate perpendicular cross-fractures. The samples were cryofixed in liquid propane, using the plunching method (KF80, Reichert Jung, Austria). The frozen samples were placed in a Balzers BAF400 D freeze-etching device (Balzers, Lichtenstein) on a table that was precooled to –150°C. After evacuation to 2×10^{-6} Pa, the specimens were fractured. The fracture plane was replicated by evaporation first of Pt/C at a 45° angle and subsequently of C at an angle of 90°. The replicas were cleaned using a procedure described elsewhere.[54]

G. FREEZE-SUBSTITUTION ELECTRON MICROSCOPY (FSEM) WITH RUO_4 POSTFIXATION

The SC was incubated first with 5% glutaraldehyde and then with 0.5% w/w RuO_4 in a cacodylate buffer, pH 6.8. Freeze substitution was carried out in a CS-Auto (Reichert-Jung, Austria) at a temperature of –90°C for 48 h. The substitution medium was pure methanol which contained 1% w/w osmium tetroxide (OsO_4), 0.5% uranyl acetate, and 3% glutaraldehyde. After freeze substitution, the temperature was raised to –45°C, and the methanol replaced gradually by lowicryl HM20. The polymerization was carried out by exposure of the monomer mixture to UV light. The samples were sectioned and visualized in a 201 Analytical Electron Microscope (AEM) or a 410 AEM (Phillips, The Netherlands).

H. NUCLEAR MAGNETIC RESONANCE SPECTROSCOPY (NMR)

The synthesis of the alkyl chain deuterated C_{12} Azone® is described in References 55 and 56. SC samples were treated as follows:

1. Untreated SC was used to verify whether SC provides a ^{2}H-NMR signal (so-called natural abundance)
2. Treatment of SC for 24 h with 0.15 *M* perdeuterated C_{12} Azone® followed by a PG wash
3. Treatment of SC for a few minutes followed by a wash with PG to verify the absence of chain deuterated C_{12} Azone® contamination after the PG wash procedure.

The 61.4 MHz ^{2}H-NMR data were collected on a Bruker MSL400 spectrometer using a standard wideline probe. For recording the spectra a quadrupole solid $\pi/2_x$-T-$\pi/2_y$-T pulse sequence with quadrupole detection and phase cycling was used with a $\pi/2$ pulse length of 2.7 μs and t = 20 μs. The SC was oriented with respect to the magnetic field.

III. RESULTS

A. FLUX STUDIES

Figure 2A displays the enhancement factor obtained for nitroglycerin without pretreatment of the series of *N*-alkyl Azones®.[48] No significant increase in the transport rate of nitroglycerin was observed between PG and C_6 Azone® in PG-treated skin. However, after pretreatment with C_8 Azone® in PG a significant increase in the

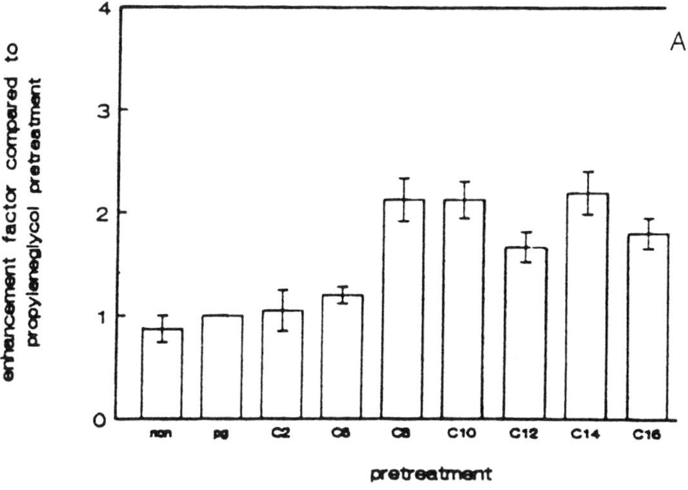

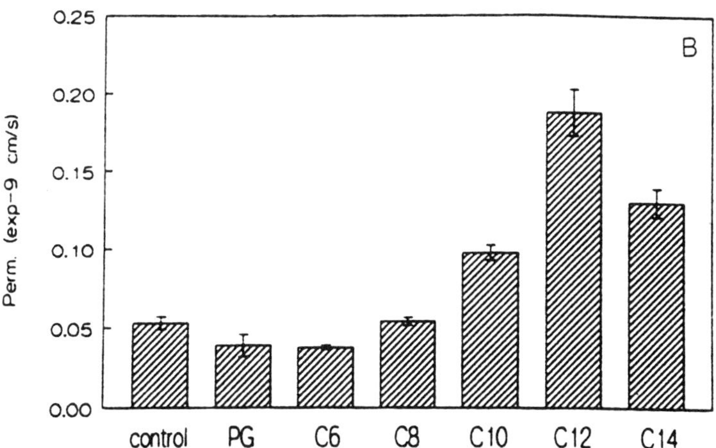

Figure 2 (A) Nitroglycerin flux enhancement ratios as a function of Azone® pretreatment. (B) DGAVP permeabilities as a function of Azone® pretreatments.

diffusion rate of nitroglycerin was observed. A further increase in alkyl chain length of the Azones® did not increase the absorption rate.

Figure 2B displays the permeability coefficients of DGAVP calculated from the fluxes.[46] Pretreatment with PG and C_6 Azone® in PG did not affect the penetration of DGAVP across human SC, but further elongation of the alkyl chain gradually increased the transport of DGAVP through the human SC. C_{12} Azone® in PG treatment resulted in the strongest effect on the DGAVP transport.

B. DIFFERENTIAL THERMAL ANALYSIS

In Figure 3 a typical example of the thermal behavior of the human SC between 0° and 120°C is shown. Four transitions were found in this temperature region, as indicated in the figure. The transition around 37°C (310 K), denoted by 1 in the

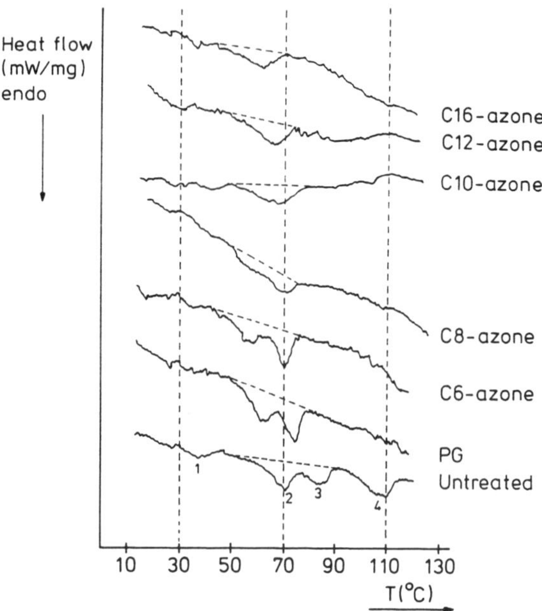

Figure 3 Influence of *N*-alkyl Azones® and PG on the thermal behavior of human SC.

figure, was ascribed to a change in the lateral packing of the lipids from an orthorhombic to a hexagonal lateral packing.[52,57] The transition around 68°C (341 K), denoted by 2 in the curve, was also thought to be based on a lipid transition due to the reversible character of the transition. However, it is not clear whether this transition is due only to a disordering of the lamellae observed between 60 and 75°C[50] or to a hexagonal to liquid transition of the lateral packing of the lipids. Recently it was found[58] that the hexagonal to liquid transition of the lipids takes place between 62 and 85°C. The third thermal transition, located at approximately 87°C, was partly irreversible, and therefore assigned to lipids bound to proteins.[59] The fourth thermal transition, at 107°C (380 K), was completely irreversible, and therefore assigned to proteins.

Figure 3 also shows the influence of PG and a series of alkyl Azones® solubilized in PG on the thermal behavior of human SC. After pretreatment with PG or alkyl Azones® in PG the protein peak disappeared. This is most likely due to extraction of water from the proteins by PG. Van Duzee[60] reported that the enthalpy involved in the protein denaturation at 107°C is very sensitive to the amount of water present in the SC; below a water content of 15% no thermal transition was observed at 107°C. Another change observed after treatment with PG was a reduction in the area under the peak at 37°C. This might indicate that part of the lipids in the orthorhombic lattice transformed to a hexagonal or liquid phase. The enthalpy involved in the two transitions present at 67° and 85°C, respectively, did not change, but the two peaks were shifted to a lower temperature region. The shift in temperature was about 10°C, which was rather large.

The experiments in which the effects of the various *N*-alkyl Azones® were studied[49,61] revealed that treatment with C_6 Azone® in PG did not change the thermal behavior of SC when compared to PG-treated SC, except for a minor shift in transition temperature of the second and third thermal transitions. Furthermore, the transition at 37°C could still be observed. The situation changed by prolonging the alkyl chains of the Azones®, and thus, after treatment with C_8 azone the second and third transition were no longer resolved. This trend was continued by further prolonging the alkyl chain length of the Azones®. The total enthalpy involved in the two transitions decreased gradually to half the value obtained in untreated SC. From these experiments one cannot deduce whether one of the two transitions disappeared and the other transition shifted to lower temperatures or whether both transitions gradually changed in temperature and enthalpy. However, most likely the second thermal transition disappeared because otherwise the addition of *N*-alkyl Azones® would lead to an increase in transition temperatures, which is unlikely. Although not always clearly observed, the curves indicate that the first thermal transition is still present, even after treatment with C_{16} Azone® in PG. It seems that lipids are partly packed in an orthorhombic lattice, even after treatment with C_{16} Azone®.

C. SMALL-ANGLE X-RAY DIFFRACTION

The diffraction curves of untreated SC are presented in Figure 4. The diffraction curve at room temperature exhibited two peaks, a strong and a weak diffraction peak, both consisting of a main position and a shoulder on the right-hand side. The positions of the main peaks and shoulders cannot be explained by one lamellar phase because the positions are not located at the same interpeak distances. However, after heating to 120°C and cooling to room temperature the diffraction pattern of the SC contained a series of diffraction peaks, which were located at equidistant positions. Comparison of the control curve with the diffraction curves obtained after recrystallization resulted in the conclusion that the diffraction curve of the control SC can be explained by two lamellar phases with periodicities of 13.4 and 6.4 nm, respectively.

After treatment with PG no change in the diffraction pattern was observed, as shown in Figure 5. It seems that no effect on the periodicity of the phases and the stacking of the lamellae was observed. After treatment with C_8, C_{10}, C_{12}, C_{14}, and C_{16} Azone® in PG the diffraction peaks disappeared. However from the curves it could not be concluded whether only the stacking of the lamellae disappeared or whether the lamellae disappeared completely.

D. WIDE-ANGLE X-RAY DIFFRACTION

The WAXD patterns are shown in Figure 6. The pattern of untreated SC displayed two very strong reflections at 0.415 and 0.375 nm, respectively, revealing an orthorhombic structure.[49] Sometimes weak reflections based on crystalline cholesterol were present in the diffraction pattern. Two very diffuse broad diffraction rings were present at 0.96 and 0.46 nm spacings, indicative of soft keratin, although α-keratin cannot be fully excluded because the 0.96 nm ring was slightly nonisotropic, when SC was oriented with respect to the primary beam.

After treatment with PG, a ring with high intensity at 0.46 nm spacing was observed in the WAXD pattern. The appearance of the ring and its high intensity was different than the 0.46 nm ring in the pattern of untreated SC. The diffuse diffraction ring was not present in the diffraction pattern of PG alone and therefore cannot be

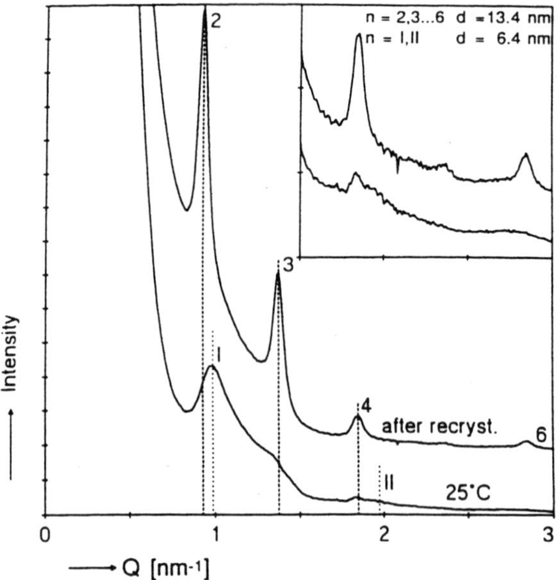

Figure 4 The diffraction curve of untreated SC and after heating to 120°C and cooling to room temperature.

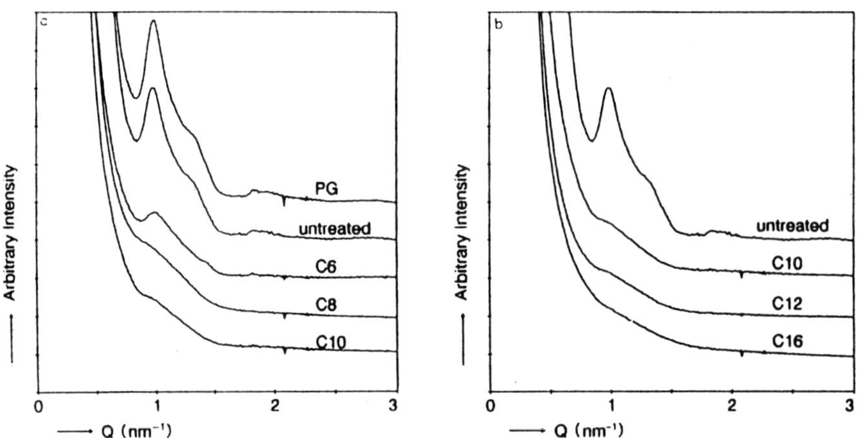

Figure 5 The influence of *N*-alkyl Azones® and PG on the lamellar ordering of the human SC.

ascribed to the solvent only. The origin of the broad diffuse diffraction ring is not yet understood, although at least three possibilities exist:

1. The diffraction ring may be due to a mixture of lipids and PG. Lipids in a liquid phase cause a broad 0.46-nm reflection in the WAXD pattern. For explaining the high intensity of the 0.46 nm diffraction ring a substantial part of the intercellular lipids must be solubilized in PG and form a separate phase. Because it is thought that ceramides, cholesterol, and free fatty acids are essential for the formation of lamellar phases[1] it is

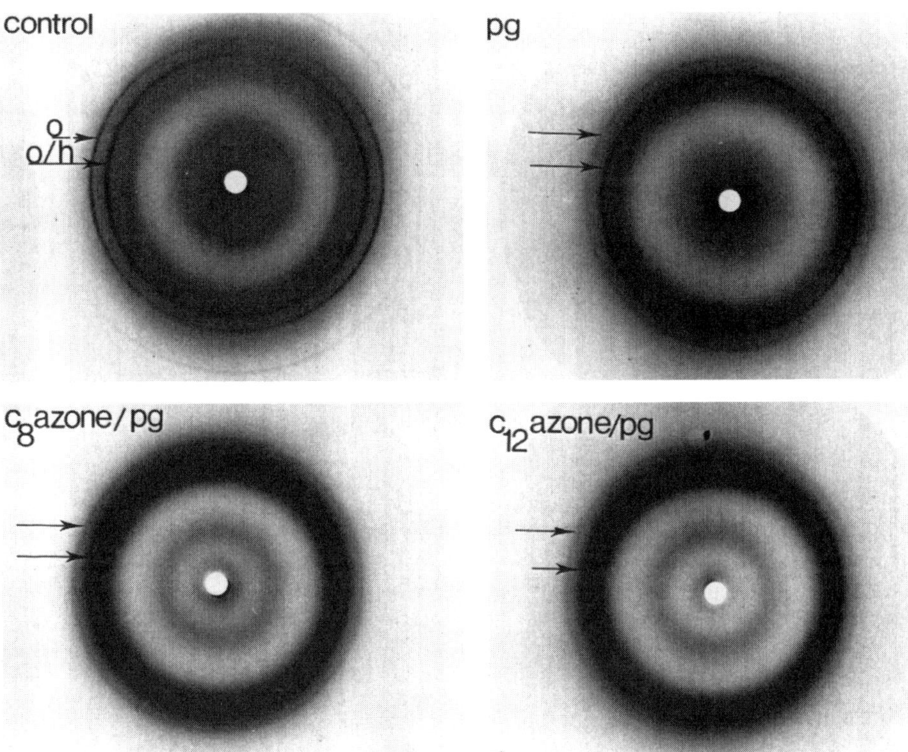

Figure 6 The WAXD pattern of human SC, control, PG treated, C_8 Azone® in PG, and C_{12} Azone® in PG.

not likely that these lipids form a mixture with PG without changing the lamellar periodicity.

2. A second possibility is intercalation of PG in the hydrocarbon regions of the lipid bilayers in the SC, leading to a swelling of the lateral packing of a part of the lipids, and thus a possible transition from a crystalline to a liquid phase. This transition would not lead to a change in the lamellar periodicity. Besides the absorption of PG in the lipid lamellae, a separate PG liquid phase may be present. No information can be deduced from the WAXD pattern about the presence of a liquid PG phase because pure PG does not induce a ring in the diffraction pattern.
3. A third possibility is that a substantial amount of PG penetrates into the corneocytes, after which PG forms a complex with the keratin that results in the additional diffuse strong diffraction ring at 0.46 nm, the same spacing at which one of the amorphous soft keratin reflections is located (see above). Propylene glycol changes the thermal behavior of proteins/keratin in the SC and thus that PG has an influence on the keratin (see above).

Apart from the additional ring no changes in the diffraction pattern were found after treatment with PG. The orthorhombic hydrocarbon packing was still present and the corresponding spacings did not change significantly. This is in agreement with the presence of the thermal transition at 37°C after treatment of *N*-alkyl Azones® which corresponds with the orthorhombic-hexagonal lateral packing (see above).

Although the reflections were weak as compared to untreated SC, no conclusion can be drawn about changes in the amount of lipids packed in the orthorhombic lattice because PG is an excellent X-ray absorber, and reduces the intensity of the reflections. In other words, part of the orthorhombic phase may have disappeared but this would only be detectable using quantitative measurements. This was not possible with available diffraction patterns.

After treatment with the series of *N*-alkyl Azones® no further changes in the lipid chain packing were observed, but the higher order reflections based on the lamellar phases disappeared. This is in agreement with the findings obtained by SAXD (see above).

E. FREEZE-FRACTURE ELECTRON MICROSCOPY

Electron micrographs of untreated hydrated SC are shown in Figure 7. The fracture planes are approximately perpendicular to the surface of the SC. Corneocytes could be recognized by rough fracture surfaces due to the keratin filaments. The lipid regions are characterized by smooth surfaces, occasionally interrupted by fractures across the lipid bilayers, showing up as sharp edges in the fracture plane. Desmosomes recognizable as groups of densely packed protein particles were frequently visualized on the surfaces of the corneocytes. After pretreatment with PG, the ultrastructure of the SC did not change significantly. Large regions of smooth surfaces occasionally showing steps could be visualized in the intercellular spaces. No fractures that might suggest the presence of a separate PG phase were visualized in the intercellular spaces. This, in fact, excludes the explanation that the presence of the isotropic broad diffraction ring in the WAXD pattern could be caused by the presence of a separate lipid-rich PG phase in the intercellular regions. Pretreatment with C_8 Azone® in PG changed the structure of the lipids in the intercellular regions. The lipid structure became less ordered. More specifically, the clear distinction between smooth fracture planes along the lamellae and the sharp steps produced by cross-fractures had disappeared, and a much rougher, less anisotropic fracturing behavior appeared. Disorder occurred most pronounced in the center of the intercellular spaces. Close to the corneocyte envelopes, much less perturbed lipid lamellae were still visible. C_{12} Azone® in PG induced a further aggravation in the disordering of the lamellae. However, even in strongly perturbed lipid regions, lamellae were still present in the direct vicinity of the corneocyte envelopes. It is obvious that *N*-alkyl Azones® induced perturbation of the lamellar structure mainly in the center of the intercellular spaces. Perturbation of the lamellar stacking is in agreement with the findings obtained by SAXD (see above).

F. FREEZE-SUBSTITUTION ELECTRON MICROSCOPY

Electron micrographs of untreated SC are shown in Figure 8. In large areas of the intercellular spaces the lipid lamellae (LL) repeating units were characterized by two broad translucent bands and one narrow translucent band between which electron dense bands were located. The pattern was similar to that found in mouse[62] and pig[63] SC. The periodicity was approximately 13 nm, which corresponded to the periodicity of one of the two lamellar phases found by SAXD (see above). The lamellae were mainly oriented parallel to the surface of the SC, which is in agreement with the findings by WAXD. The nonisotropic 0.415 and 0.375 nm reflections using WAXD

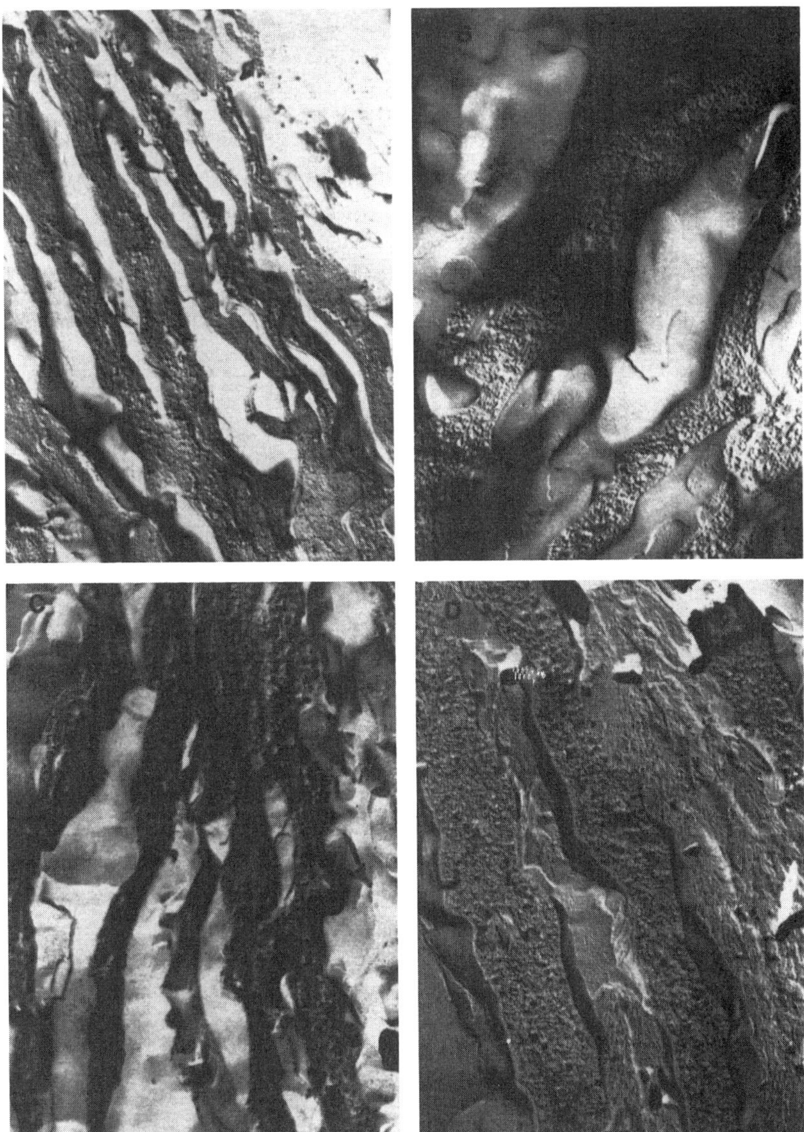

Figure 7 Electron micrographs of freeze-fracture replicas of untreated, PG treated, C_8 Azone® in PG, and C_{12} Azone® in treated human SC.

when the SC was oriented parallel with respect to the primary beam[49] obviously reflects the same preferred orientation of the lamellae. In some regions the broad–broad–narrow sequence was not present; this might be an artefact due to poor penetration of RuO_4 in the SC, a nonperpendicular sectioning direction to the lamellae, or another lipid lamellar phase may be present. However, the spacings in these regions did not correspond with the 6.4-nm phase found with X-ray diffraction (see above). Furthermore, intercellular grey regions were found. In these regions

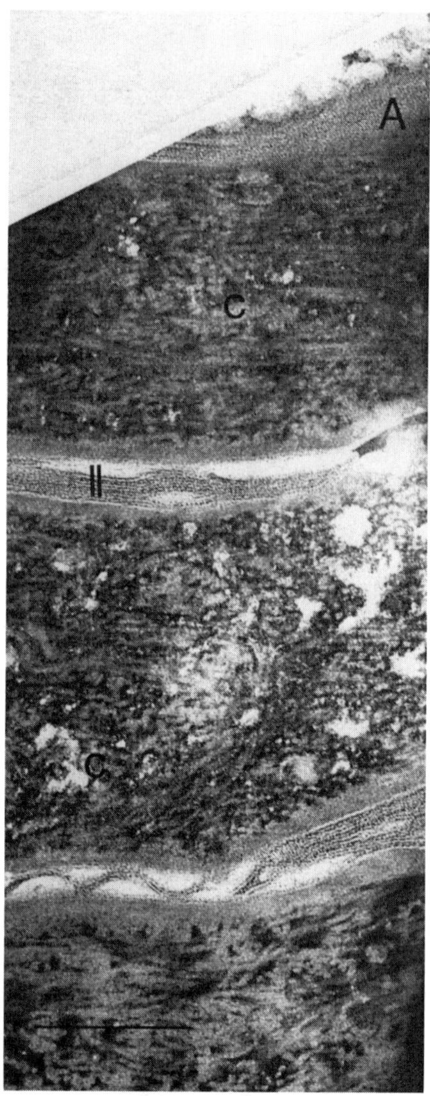

Figure 8 Electron micrographs of FSEM of (A) untreated, (B) PG treated, (C) C_8 Azone® in PG, and (D) C_{12} Azone® in PG-treated human SC. bar = 100 nm; C = corneocytes; LL = Lipid lamellae; SL = single lamellae; CE = corneocyte envelope; d = desmosome.

lipid bilayers could be visualized only along the cell boundaries, while toward the center of the domain one finds an amorphous pattern. Desmosomes interrupting the lipid bilayers were present in the intercellular spaces. The keratin filaments were visualized inside the corneocytes. It was shown that these filaments were aligned mainly parallel to the SC surface. After treatment with PG or hexyl Azone® in PG, no significant changes in the lipid lamellar stacking could be visualized (not shown). The broad–broad–narrow electronlucent bands were still present and their periodicity

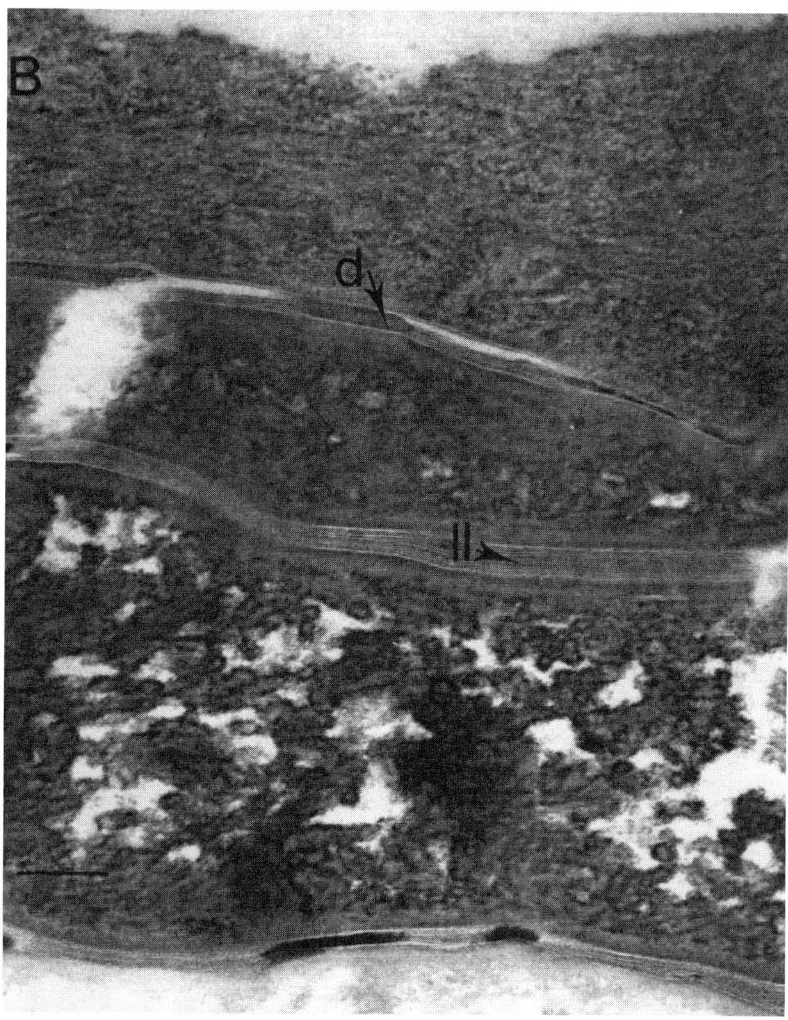

Figure 8 (continued)

did not change compared to the pattern observed in untreated SC. This is in agreement with the results obtained with FFEM and SAXD. However, treatment with C_8 Azone® and C_{12} Azone® in PG did result in a loss of the lamellar stacking in large regions in the SC (see Figure 8). In these regions the single lamellae (SL) consist of two broad electronlucent bands between which a narrow electron-dense band is located. This change in appearance may indicate a change in lipid organization inside the lamellae. A change in lipid lateral packing was not observed by WAXD, but the interpretations of the WAXD pattern were hampered for two reasons: (1) no conclusions can be drawn based on changes in intensities of the 0.415 and 0.375 nm rings and (2) new diffraction rings may be obscured by the dense, broad 0.46 nm ring.

Furthermore, close to cell boundaries intercellular lipid bilayers (L) were often still present. The decrease in lamellar ordering confirms the results obtained with

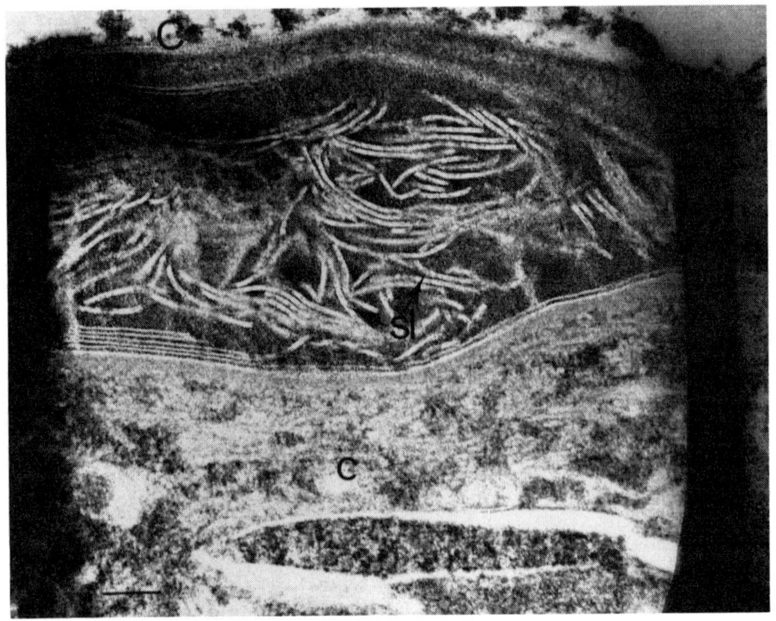

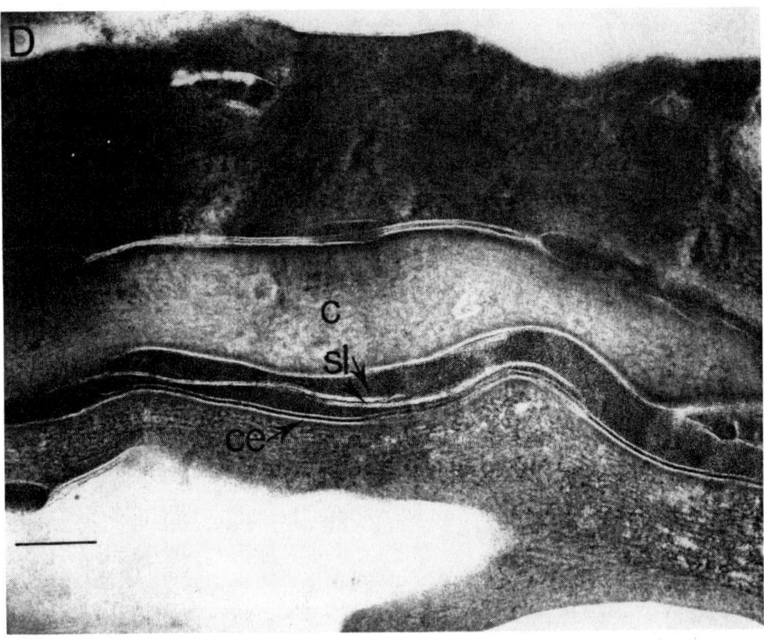

Figure 8 (continued)

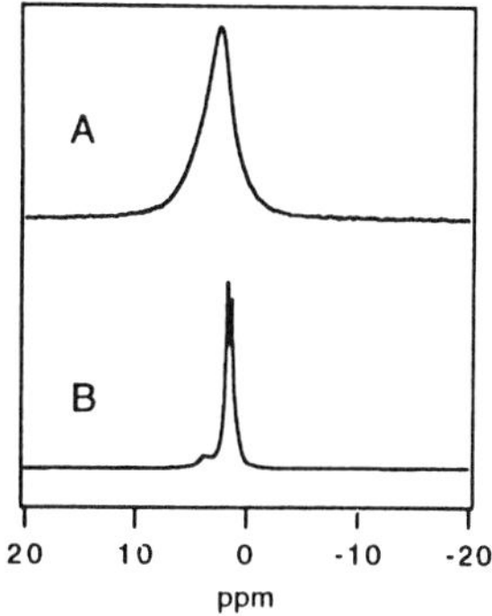

Figure 9 ^{2}H-NMR spectra at room temperature. (A) Human SC pretreated for 24 h with a 0.15 *M* solution of chain-deuterated C_{12} Azone®. (B) Solution of 0.15 *M* chain-deuterated Azone® in PG.

SAXD: the diffraction peaks disappeared after treatment with C_8 and C_{12} Azone® in PG. However, FSEM with RuO_4 postfixation revealed that lamellae were still present in the SC after treatment with C_8 and C_{12} Azone® in PG. This is in agreement with the FFEM results.

G. NUCLEAR MAGNETIC RESONANCE SPECTROSCOPY

The complete absence of excess chain deuterated C_{12} Azone® on the SC surface after the wiping procedure was verified successfully. In addition the ^{2}H signal in the ^{2}H-NMR spectrum of untreated SC could not be resolved from the noise. These two necessary validation tests revealed that in deuterated C_{12} Azone-treated, postwiped SC the ^{2}H signal derives only from the deuterated C_{12} Azone® that is located inside the SC.

By using ^{2}H-NMR it is possible to obtain insight into the mobility and orientation of ^{2}H-labeled molecules and their immediate surroundings. In this study perdeuterated C_{12} Azone® revealed a signal in the ^{2}H-NMR spectrum that is characteristic for a fast isotropic motion (see Figure 9) (fast with respect to the linewidth of the ^{2}H line width, which appeared to be $\tau c < 0.6$ μs. As stated above, the majority of the lipids in the SC are in a gel or crystalline state. If C_{12} Azone® could be intercalated in the lamellae without changing the local environment a powder pattern would be expected. However, the isotropic relaxation behavior indicated that a large part of C_{12} Azone® was present in an isotropic solution and thus that either C_{12} Azone® was not intercalated in the bilayers or that C_{12} Azone® locally changed the lipid phase behavior. In an additional experiment SC samples treated with chain-deuterated C_{12} Azone® in PG were measured at 150 K, oriented at three different angles with respect to the SC surface (90° and 54 to 44°, the so-called magic angle). The samples were deliberately frozen so as to "fix" any preferred orientation that might exist at room temperature. The resulting characteristic ^{2}H-NMR powder patterns turned out to be identical in all three cases, clearly demonstrating the absence of a preferred orientation of C_{12} Azone® in the SC samples. Each of these spectra consisted of a superposition of two powder patterns, with quadrupole splittings of 126 and 36 kHz, characteristic for static methylene and the end-methyl groups of the alkyl chain of C_{12} Azone®, respectively.

IV. DISCUSSION

A. FLUX STUDIES

The permeability coefficients of DGAVP did not change significantly after pretreatment with PG or C_6 Azone® in PG. An elongation of the *N*-alkyl Azones® increased the permeability coefficient of DGAVP gradually. A maximum value was derived with C_{12} Azone® in PG. The effect of *N*-alkyl Azones® on the permeability of nitroglycerin was different than that of DGAVP. The permeability of SC for nitroglycerin changed abruptly only after pretreatment with C_{12} Azone® and higher alkyl Azones® in PG. It seems that the alkyl chain length of *N*-alkyl Azones® needs to be longer to affect the transport of lipophilic drugs compared to that of hydrophilic drugs. This finding suggests a difference in pathways, in that nitroglycerin would travel in a more lipophilic domain than DGAVP in the intercellular lipid lamellae.

B. STRUCTURAL CHANGES OBSERVED IN HUMAN STRATUM CORNEUM

1. Propylene Glycol

Treatment of the SC with PG did not change the ordering and periodicity of the lamellae in human SC as determined with SAXD. Wide-angle X-ray diffraction revealed the presence of a strong reflection with a spacing of 0.46 nm, which was absent in untreated SC. One explanation of this reflection is the existence of a separate phase of PG mixed with lipids. However, neither FSEM nor FFEM studies revealed separate phases in the intercellular spaces. An alternative mechanism that explains the presence of the 0.46-nm reflection is intercalation of PG in the hydrocarbon regions of the lamellae without swelling the lamellae. A small amount of PG may be present in the lamellar phases because PG did influence the lipid transition temperatures (see Section III.B). However, it is unlikely that large amounts of PG were absorbed in these phases without changing the lamellar periodicity. Because no new intercellular phases were found in the intercellular regions, the excess PG was most likely absorbed in the corneocytes. The disappearance of the protein peak at 107°C after treatment with PG is a strong indication that PG interacts with proteins, possibly keratin, inside the corneocytes.

2. *N*-Alkyl Azones®

The mechanism by which *N*-alkyl Azones® interact with the SC and change the barrier properties of the SC is very complicated and depends on the alkyl chain length. The influence of hexyl Azone® in PG on the structure of human SC was similar to that of PG. However, when the SC was pretreated with octyl Azone® in PG, SAXD revealed a disordering of the lamellar stacking. Both FFEM and FSEM illustrated the nature of the disorder and confirmed the disordering of the lamellae. Furthermore, these techniques revealed that the disordering was more easily induced in the center of the intercellular spaces than close to cell boundaries, where lamellae were still present. In addition the micrographs obtained by FSEM revealed that the appearance of the lamellae after treatment with C_8 and C_{12} Azone® in PG differed from that of untreated SC. The Landmann units, consisting of a sequence of broad–broad–narrow electron translucent bands, were replaced by disordered lamellae that consist of only two broad electron translucent bands between which one narrow electron-dense band was located. Stacking of the latter would lead to a sequence of only broad electron translucent bands between which electron-dense bands would be located. It can be speculated that the C_8 and C_{12} Azone® treatments changed a part of the lateral packing of the lipids. That part of the lipid lateral packing remaining intact could be deduced from the WAXD pattern of *N*-alkyl Azone-treated human SC; reflections from an orthorhombic lateral packing were still present in the corresponding WAXD patterns. An incomplete change from orthorhombic/hexagonal to liquid packing also may explain the NMR results. If C_{12} Azone® induced a change in lateral packing in its local environment and simultaneously perturbed the lamellar ordering, isotropic relaxation behavior of C_{12} Azone® would indeed be expected. The difference in the effect of *N*-alkyl Azones® on nitroglycerin absorption vs. the DGAVP absorption rate is not yet understood. The difference may be due to a difference in hydrophilicity of the two drugs. As speculated previously,[64] it is possible that in following the likely intercellular pathway across the SC, DGAVP travels closer to the head group domain than does nitroglycerin, and that intercalating *N*-alkyl Azones® have a more pronounced local effect close to the head groups as compared to the center of the alkyl chain regions.

A study was performed recently[34] in which the extent of C_{12} Azone® accumulation in human SC was correlated with its effect on the diffusion coefficient of diazepam. These studies clearly demonstrated that the strongest increase in diffusion coefficient of diazepam was obtained at 12% w/w enhancer content of the SC. It is quite surprising that such large quantities of C_{12} Azone® can be absorbed in the SC. These quantities imply that on a molar basis the amount of enhancer in the SC exceeds that of the endogenous lipids. The same study also showed that an increase in enhancer uptake resulted in a stronger effect on the lipid thermal transitions around 70°C.

C. COMPARISON BETWEEN MODEL SYSTEMS AND SKIN

To further clarify the mode of action of Azones®, several studies were carried out using model systems. The reasons for using model systems is at least twofold. On the one hand, model systems minimize the technical difficulties often encountered when using intact SC, and on the other hand the composition of the model lipid systems can be varied to elucidate the role of individual classes of lipids in building the SC structure. In most of these studies on model systems carried out with either skin lipids[65] or phospholipids[66] it was shown that C_{12} Azone® has an effect on the lipid packing of the hydrocarbon chains inside the bilayers, and that this might correspond to that observed in intact SC. However, the addition of C_{12} Azone® to a lamellar phase, prepared from brain ceramides, free fatty acids and cholesterol,[67] or from hydrated phosphatidylcholine[68] did not reveal the disordering found in intact SC. This might be due to either lower concentrations of C_{12} Azone® in the model systems as compared to the SC or to a mismatch between the lipids in the SC and that used for the model systems (see Chapter 6.6).

In one of the studies Schuckler and Lee[65] studied the change in monolayer arrangement of free fatty acids, cholesterol, or brain ceramides and mixtures of three classes of lipids. It appeared that in the case of monolayers prepared only from free fatty acids the addition of C_{12} Azone® resulted in an almost ideal mixing behavior. The addition of cholesterol condensed the free fatty acid phase, but the addition of

C_{12} azone to this monolayer or to a monolayer prepared from ceramides, cholesterol, and free fatty acids favored the L_1-phase, which most closely resembles the liquid crystalline state. These results are in agreement with our observations on intact SC; ^{2}H-NMR experiments revealed that C_{12} Azone® induces a liquid microenvironment in human SC.

REFERENCES

1. **Schurer, N. J. and Elias, P. M., Eds.,** *The Biochemistry and Function of SC Lipids, Adv. Lipid Res.,* 24, 27, 1992.
2. **Yamada, M., Uda, Y., and Tanigawara, Y.,** Mechanism of enhancement of percutaneous absorption of molsidomine by oleic acid, *Chem. Pharm. Bull.,* 35(8), 3399, 1987.
3. **Francoeur, M. L., Golden, G. M., and Potts, R. O.,** Oleic acid: its effects on SC in relation to transdermal drug delivery, *Pharm. Res.,* 7, 621, 1990.
4. **Naik, A., Pechtold, L., Potts, R. O., and Guy, R. H.,** Mechanism of skin penetration enhancement, *in vivo,* in man, in *Prediction of Percutaneous Penetration,* Vol. 3, Brian, K. R., James, V. J., and Walters, K. A., Eds., STS Publishing, Cardiff, U.K., 1993, 161.
5. **Ongpipattanakul, B., Burnette, R., and Potts, R. O.,** Evidence that oleic acid exists as a separate phase within SC, *Pharm. Res.,* 8, 350, 1991.
6. **Tanojo, H., Junginger, H. E., and Boddé, H. E.,** Effects of oleic acid on human transepidermal water loss using ethanol or propylene glycol as vehicles, in *Prediction of Percutaneous Penetration,* Vol. 3, Brian, K. R., James, V. J., and Walters, K. A., Eds., STS Publishing, Cardiff, U.K., 1993, 319.
7. **Green, P. and Hadgraft, J.,** Facilitated transfer of cationic drugs across a lipoidal membrane by oleic acid and lauric acid, *Int. J. Pharm.,* 37, 251, 1987.
8. **Kadir, R., Tiemessen, H. L. G. M., Ponec, M., Junginger, H. E., and Boddé, H. E.,** Oleyl surfactants as skin penetration enhancers, in *Pharmaceutical Skin Penetration Enhancement,* Walters, K. A. and Hadgraft, J., Eds., Marcel Dekker, New York, 1993, 215.
9. **Walters, K. A., Walker, M., and Oleinik, O.,** Hydration and surfactant effects of methyl nicotinate penetration through hairless mouse skin, *J. Pharm. Pharmacol.,* 37, 76, 1985.
10. **Williams, A. C. and Barry, B. W.,** Terpenes and the lipid-protein partitioning theory of skin penetration enhancement, *Pharm. Res.,* 8, 17, 1991.
11. **Williams, A. C. and Barry, B. W.,** The enhancement index concept applied to terpene penetration enhancers for human skin and model lipophilic (oestradiol) and hydrophylic (5-fluorouacil) drugs, *Int. J. Pharm.,* 76, 157, 1991.
12. **Okamoto, H., Ohyabu, M., Hashida, M., and Sezaki, H.,** Enhanced penetration of mytomicin C through hairless mouse and rat skin by enhancers with terpene moieties, *J. Pharm. Pharmacol.,* 39, 531, 1987.
13. **Cornwell, P. A., Barry, B. W., Bouwstra, J. A., and Gooris, G. S.,** Small angle X-ray Diffraction investigations on the lipid barrier in human skin, in *Prediction of Percutaneous Penetration,* Vol. 3, Brian, K. R., James, V. J., and Walters, K. A., Eds., STS Publishing, Cardiff, U.K., 1993.
14. **Cornwell, P. A., Stoddart, C. P., Bouwstra, J. A., and Barry, B. W.,** *J. Pharm. Pharmacol.,* 46, 938-950, 1994.
15. **Kai, T., Mak, V. H. M., Potts, R. O., and Guy, R. H.,** Mechanism of skin penetration enhancement: effect of n-alcohols on the permeability barrier, *Proc. Int. Symp. Control. Bioact. Mater.,* 15, 211, 1988.
16. **Kurihara-Bergstrom, T., Knutson, K., De Noble, L. J., and Goates, C. Y.,** Percutaneous absorption of an ionic molecule by ethanol-water systems in human skin, *Pharm. Res.,* 7, 762, 1990.
17. **Bommannan, D., Potts, R. O., and Guy, R. H.,** Examination of the effect of ethanol on human SC *in vivo* using infrared spectroscopy, *J. Control. Rel.,* 16, 299, 1991.
18. **Liu, P., Kurihara-Bergstrom, T., and Good, W. R.,** Cotransport of estradiol and ethanol through human skin *in vitro*: understanding the permeant/enhancer flux relationship, *Pharm. Res.,* 8, 938, 1991.

19. **Cooper, E., Merritt, E., and Smith, R.,** Effect of fatty acids and alcohols on the penetration of acyclovir across human skin *in vitro*, *J. Pharm. Sci.*, 74, 688, 1985.
20. **Aungst, B. J., Rogers, N. J., and Shefter, E.,** Enhancement of naloxone penetration through human skin *in vitro* using fatty acids, fatty alcohols, surfactants, sulfoxides and amides, *Int. J. Pharm.*, 33, 225, 1986.
21. **Goldman, L., Igelman, J. M., and Kitzmiller, K.,** Investigative studies with DMSO in dermatology, *Ann. N.Y. Acad. Sci.*, 145, 435, 1986.
22. **Maibach, H. I. and Feldmann, R. J.,** The effect of DMSO on percutaneous penetration of hydrocortisone and testosterone in man, *Ann. N.Y. Acad. Sci.*, 141, 423, 1967.
23. **Goodman, M. and Barry, B. W.,** Differential scanning calorimetry of human SC: effect of penetration enhancers azone and DMSO, *Anal. Proc.*, 23, 397, 1986.
24. **Taylor, P. M. and Winfield, A. J.,** Studies of the mechanism of action of DMSO as penetration enhancer, *J. Pharm. Pharmacol.*, 39, 140P, 1987.
25. **Cramer, M. B. and Cates, L. A.,** Effect of dimethylsulfoxide and trimethylphosphine oxide on percutaneous absorption of corticosteroids in the rat, *J. Pharm. Sci.*, 63, 793, 1974.
26. **Stoughtton, R. and McClure, W.,** Azone® — a new non-toxic enhancer for cutaneous penetration, *Drug. Dev. Ind. Pharm.*, 9, 725, 1983.
27. **Morimoto, Y., Sugibayashi, K., Hosoya, K., and Higuchi, W. I.,** Penetration enhancing effect of Azone® on the transport of 5-fluorouracil across the hairless rat skin, *Int. J. Pharm.*, 32, 31, 1986.
28. **Lambert, W., Higuchi, W., Knutson, K., and Krill, S.,** Dose dependent enhancement effects of Azone® on skin permeability, *Pharm. Res.*, 6, 798, 1989.
29. **Chow, D., Kaka, I., and Wang, T.,** Concentration-dependent enhancement of 1-dodecyl-azacycloheptan-2-one on the percutaneous penetration kinetics of triamcinolone acetonide, *J. Pharm. Sci.*, 12, 1794, 1984.
30. **Sheth, N., Freeman, D., Higuchi, W., and Spruance, S.** The influence of azone, propylene glycol and polyethylene glycol on *in vitro* skin penetration of trifluorothymidine, *Int. J. Pharm.*, 28, 201, 1986.
31. **Sugibayashi, K., Hosaya, K., Moromoto, Y., and Higuchi, W.,** Effect of the absorption enhancer azone on the transport of 5-fluorouracil across hairless rat skin, *J. Pharm. Pharmacol.*, 37, 578, 1985.
32. **Wotton, P., Mollgaard, B., Hadgraft, J., and Hoelgaard, A.,** Vehicle effect on topical drug delivery. III. Effect of azone on the cutaneous permeation of metronidazole and propylene glycol, *Int. J. Pharm.*, 24, 19, 1985.
33. **Ruland, A. and Kreuter, J.,** Influence of various penetration enhancers on the *in vitro* permeation of amino acids across hairless mouse skin, *Int. J. Pharm.*, 85, 7, 1992.
34. **Schuckler, F. and Lee, G.,** Relating the concentration-dependent action of azone and dodecyl-l-pyroglutamate on the structure of excised human SC to changes in drug diffusivity, partition coefficient and flux, *Int. J. Pharm.*, 80, 81, 1992.
35. **Swart, P. W., Toulouse, F. A. M., and De Zeeuw, R. A.,** The influence of azone on the transdermal penetration of the dopamine D_2 agonist MN-0923 in freely moving rats, *Int. J. Pharm.*, 88, 165, 1992.
36. **Wiechers, J. W., Drenth, B. F. H., Adolfsen, F. A. W., Groothuis, G. M. M., and de Zeeuw, R. A.,** Disposition and metabolic profiling of the penetration enhancer Azone®. I. *In vivo* studies urinary profiles of hamster, rat and monkey, and man, *Pharm. Res.*, 5, 496, 1990.
37. **Wiechers, J. W., Drenth, B. F. H., Adolfsen, F. A. W., Gerding, T. K., Groothuis, G. M. M., and de Zeeuw, R. A.,** Disposition and metabolic profiling of the penetration enhancer Azone®. II. *In vitro* studies: liver perfusion, hepatocytes and liver microsomes using rat and human material, *Pharm. Res.*, 5, 1992.
38. **Bannerjee, P. S.,** Transdermal penetration of vasopressin. II. The influence of Azone® in *in vitro* and *in vivo* penetration, *Int. J. Pharm.*, 49, 199, 1989.
39. **Stoughton, R. B.,** Enhanced percutaneous penetration with 1-dodecylazocycloheptan-2-one, *Arch. Dermatol.*, 118, 474, 1982.
40. **Stoughton, R. B.,** Azone® (dodecylazocycloheptan-2-one) enhances percutaneous penetration, in *Psoriasis*, Farben, E. M., Ed., Grune & Stratton, Orlando, FL, 1982, 474.
41. **Hadgraft, J.,** Skin penetration enhancement, in *Prediction of Percutaneous Penetration*, Vol. 3, Brian, K. R., James, V. J., and Walters, K. A. Eds., STS Publishing, Cardiff, U.K., 1993, 138.

42. **Michniak, B. B., Player, M. R., Chapman, J. M., Jr., and Sowell, J. W., Sr.,** *In vitro* evaluation of a series of Azone® analogs as dermal penetration enhancers. I., *Int. J. Pharm.,* 91, 85, 1993.
43. **Michniak, B. B., Player, M. R., Fuhrman, L. C., Christensen, J. M., Chapman, J. M., and Sowell, J. W.,** *In vitro* evaluation of a series of Azone® analogs as dermal penetration enhancers. II. (Thio)amides, *Int. J. Pharm.,* 91, 1993.
44. **Boddé, H. E., van den Brink, I., Koerten, H. K., and de Haan, F. H. N.,** Visualization of *in vitro* percutaneous penetration of $HgCl_2$; transport through intercellular space versus cellular uptake through desmosomes, *J. Control. Rel.,* 15, 227, 1991.
45. **Boddé, H. E., Kruithof, M. A. M., Brussee, J., and Koerten, H. K.,** Visualisation of normal and enhanced $HgCl_2$ transport through human skin, *Int. J. Pharm.,* 53, 12, 1989.
46. **Hoogstraate, A. J., Verhoef, J., IJzerman, A. P., Spies, F., and Boddé, H. E.,** Kinetics, ultrastructural aspects and molecular modelling of transdermal peptide flux enhancement by N-alkylazaclycloheptanones, *Int. J. Pharm.,* 76, 37, 1991.
47. **Bree, J. B. M. M., de Boer, A. G., Danhof, M., Verhoef, J. C., van Wimersma Greidanus, T. B., and Breimer, D. D.,** Radioimmunoassay, of desglycinamide-arginine vasopressin and its application in a pharmacokinetic study in the rat, *Peptides,* 9, 555, 1988.
48. **Tiemessen, H. L. G. M., Boddé, H. E., Van Koppen, M., Bauer, W. C., and Junginger, H. E.,** A two-chambered diffusion cell with improved flow through characteristics for studying the drug permeation of biological membranes, *Acta Pharm. Tech.,* 34, 99, 1988.
49. **Bouwstra, J. A., Peschier, L., Brussee, J., and Boddé, H.,** Effect of N-alkyl-azocycloheptan-2-ones including azone on the thermal behaviour of human SC, *Int. J. Pharm.,* 52, 249, 1989.
50. **Bouwstra, J. A., Gooris, G. S., van der Spek, J. A., and Bras, W.,** The structure of human SC as determined with small-angle x-ray scattering, *J. Invest. Dermatol.,* 97, 1005, 1991.
51. **Franks, N. P. and Levine, Y. K.,** in *Membrane Spectroscopy,* Vol. 31, Grell, E., Ed., Springer-Verlag, New York, 1983, 437.
52. **Bouwstra, J. A., Gooris, G. S., and Bras, W.,** Structure of human SC as function of temperature and hydration: a wide-angle x-ray diffraction study, *Int. J. Pharm.,* 84, 205, 1992.
53. **Holman, B. P., Spies, F., and Boddé, H. E.,** An optimized freeze fracture replication procedure for human skin, *J. Invest. Dermatol.,* 94, 336, 1990.
54. **Hofland, H. E. J., Bouwstra, J. A., Boddé, H. E., Spies, F., and Junginger, H. E.,** Interactions between liposomes and human skin *in vitro*: freeze fracture electron microscopical visualization and small-angle x-ray studies, *Br. J. Dermatol.,* in press.
55. **Doorenbos, N. J. and Wu, M. T.,** Synthesis of some aza-A-homocholestanes by the Beckmann and Schmidt rearrangements in polyphosphoric acid, *J. Org. Chem.,* 26, 2548, 1961.
56. **Bezema, F. R., Marttin, E., Roemele, P. E. H., Salomons, M. A., Brussee, J., de Groot, H. J. M., Spies, F., and Boddé, H. E.,** ^{2}H NMR and freeze fracture electron microscopy reveal rapid isotropic motion and lipid perturbation by azone in human SC in, *Prediction of Percutaneous Penetration,* Vol. 3, Brian, K. R., James, V. J., and Walters, K. A., Eds., STS Publishing, Cardiff, U.K., 1993, 8.
57. **Wilkes, G. L., Nguyen, A.-L., and Wildhauer, R.,** Structure properties relations of human and neonatal rat SC, *Biochim. Biophys. Acta,* 304, 267, 1973.
58. **Bauwstra, J. A. and Cornwell, P.,** unpublished results.
59. **Knudsen, K., Potts, R. O., Guzek, D. B., Golden, G. M., McKie, J. E., Lambert, W. J., and Higuchi, W. I.,** Macro and molecular physical-chemical considerations in understanding drug transport in the SC, *J. Control. Rel.,* 2, 67, 1985.
60. **van Duzee, B. F.,** Thermal analysis of human SC, *J. Invest. Dermatol.,* 65, 404, 1975.
61. **Bouwstra, J. A., de Vries, M. A., Gooris, G. S., Bras, W., Brussee, W., and Ponec, M.,** Thermodynamic and structural aspects of the skin barrier, *J. Control. Rel.,* 15, 209, 1991.
62. **Hou, S. Y. E., Mitra, A. K., White, S., Menom, G. P., Ghadially, R., and Elias, P. M.,** *J. Invest. Dermatol.,* 96, 215, 1991.
63. **Swartzendruber, D. C.,** *Semin. Dermatol.,* 11, 157, 1992.
64. **Boddé, H. E., Ponec, M., IJzerman, A. P., Hoogstraate, A. J., Salomons, M. A., and Bouwstra, J. A.,** *In vitro* Analysis of QSAR in Wanted and Unwanted Effects of Azacycloheptanones as Transdermal Penetration Enhancers, in *Pharmaceutical Skin Penetration Enhancement,* Walters, K. A., and Hadgraft, J., Eds., Marcel Dekker, New York, 1993, 199.

65. **Schuckler, F. and Lee, G.,** The influence of Azone® on monolayer films of some SC lipids, *Int. J. Pharm.,* 70, 173, 1991.
66. **Lewis, D., Hadgraft, J., and Boddé, H. E.,** Mixed monolayer studies of DPPC with N-alkyl-aza-cycloheptanones at the air-water interface, in *Prediction of percutaneous Penetration/Methods Measurements, Modelling,* Scot, R. C., Guy, R. H., Boddé, H. E., Eds., ICB Technical Services, London, 1989, 355.
67. **Schuckler, F., Bouwstra, J. A., Gooris, G. S., and Lee, G.,** An X-ray diffraction study of some model SC lipids containing Azone® and dodecyl-L-pyroglutamate, *J. Control. Rel.,* 23, 27, 1993.
68. **Engblom, J. and Engstrom, S.,** Azone® and the formation of reversed mono- and bicontinuous lipid-water phases, *Int. J. Pharm.,* 98, 173, 1993.

Chapter 6.3

Enhanced Percutaneous Absorption of Azone® Following Single and Multiple Doses to Human Volunteers

Ronald C. Wester and Howard I. Maibach

CONTENTS

I. INTRODUCTION

Azone® (1-dodecylazacycloheptan-2-one) is an agent that has been shown to enhance the percutaneous absorption of drugs.[1,2] Azone® is believed to act on the stratum corneum (SC) by increasing fluidity of the lipid bilayers.[3,4] Because Azone® is nonpolar, it is thought to act by partitioning into the lipid bilayers, thereby disrupting the structure, and potentially allowing drug penetration to increase.[5] Previous clinical studies with single-dose administration show neat Azone® percutaneous absorption to be <1%.[6,7] A short-term, 4-d dosing sequence gave absorption of 3.5 ± 0.3%.[8] However, the effect of long-term multiple dosing of Azone® on the percutaneous absorption of Azone® has never been assessed. A study such as this is important because the mechanism of Azone®, disruption of the lipid bilayer structure, suggests a potential for enhanced percutaneous absorption with chronic administration.

II. EXPERIMENTAL

The study was an open-label study with nine normal volunteer outpatients (two males, seven females; ages 51 to 75 years) from whom informed consent had been obtained. Each day the subjects received a single application of Azone® cream (1.6%, 100 mg) to a 5 cm × 10 cm area of the ventral forearm. The dosing sequence was continual for 21 d. On days 1, 8, and 15, the subjects received a single application of the Azone® cream containing [^{14}C]-Azone® (47 μCi) to the same 5 cm × 10 cm skin area of the ventral forearm. The site was not occluded, and the volunteers could wear the clothing of their choice. The skin application site was washed with soap (50% Ivory® liquid) and water 24 h following application of all dosing material. Subjects collected all urine voided into plastic bags (used clinically for 24-h urine collection) for the 21-d duration of the study. A new bag was provided for each day. The subjects were told to collect every drop of their urine.

0-8493-2605-2/95/$0.00+$.50

Percutaneous absorption was determined from the urinary excretion of radioactivity following topical application of the [^{14}C]-Azone®. Excretion following day 1 application determines skin absorption of a single dose. Excretion following days 8 and 15 topical application determines skin absorption following chronic Azone® application.[9,10] Of the Azone® absorbed through skin, >94% is excreted in the urine.[6]

Urine samples were analyzed in duplicate for ^{14}C. A 5-ml aliquot of each urine sample was assayed in 10 ml of scintillation cocktail (Universol-ES, ICN, Costa Mesa, California) with a Packard 1500 liquid scintillation spectrophotometer. The cotton balls used in washing the site of application were individually counted in 10 ml of scintillation cocktail with the liquid scintillation spectrophotometer.

III. RESULTS

Table 1 gives the percent dose radioactivity excreted following daily topical exposure to Azone®. Excretion from days 1 to 7 topical application gave a single-dose percutaneous absorption of 1.84 ± 1.56% dose. Percutaneous absorption from days 8 to 15 skin application was 2.76 ± 1.91%, and the absorption from days 15 to 21 skin application was 2.72 ± 1.21%. Statistical analysis showed a significant difference for day 1 dosing vs. day 8 dosing ($p < 0.001$) and for day 1 dosing vs. day 15 dosing ($p < 0.008$). No difference was observed in percutaneous absorption for day 8 vs. day 15 dosing (Figure 1). The daily excretion patterns show that peak excretion occurred at 24 or 48 h following topical application (Figure 2). The data in Table 2 show that recovery of [^{14}C]-Azone® with soap and water wash at 24 h was only 1 or 2% applied dose for all three radioactive doses.

IV. DISCUSSION

The results show that an increase occurs in the absorption of Azone® with long-term multiple application, but that this enhanced self-absorption occurs early in use, and a steady-state absorption amount is established after the initial enhancement. Wiechers et al.[8] applied [^{14}C]-Azone® in cream containing triamcinolone acetonide for 12 h/d for four consecutive days. The site was occluded and washed each day with ethanol. The flux of Azone® increased during the study period, reaching a plateau in 2 to 3 d. Both occlusion and ethanol can enhance absorption. The present study confirms the initial enhanced absorption and establishes the steady-state absorption over the long term. This is done in a study design without occlusion, and with soap and water wash instead of ethanol, a procedure more natural to common use.

Changes in percutaneous absorption following repeated application have been shown not to occur in humans with malathion[10] and the steroids hydrocortisone, estradiol, and testosterone.[11] The results seen with Azone® may be due to initial changes in bilayer structure caused by the Azone®. After initial structural changes, a steady-state process in absorption is established. Multiple-dose application results in changes in absorption in animals. This has been shown for hydrocortisone in the rhesus monkey[9] and for malathion and benzoyl peroxide in the guinea pig.[11] The increased absorption in animals may be related in part to the washing process between repeated doses.[11] It is doubtful that skin washing affected the enhanced self-absorption seen with Azone®.

Table 1 Azone® Urinary Excretion Following Daily Topical Exposure for 21 Consecutive Days to Human Subjects

Subject	Percent Dose Excreted		
	Day 1	Day 8	Day 15
1	0.77	2.54	2.28
2	1.68	2.80	3.65
3	2.18	3.42	3.52
4	0.92	1.59	1.90
5	5.64	7.26	5.27
6	1.58	1.90	2.06
7	2.39	3.29	2.40
8	0.68	1.34	1.99
9	0.70	0.68	1.41
Mean	1.84	2.76	2.72
S.D.	1.56	1.91	1.21

Statistical Analysis

Comparison	*p*-value	Significance
Day 1 vs. day 8	0.001	Significant difference
Day 1 vs. day 15	0.008	Significant difference
Day 8 vs. day 15	0.904	Nonsignificant

Paired *t*-test (PRIMER, McGraw-Hill, Inc., 1988)

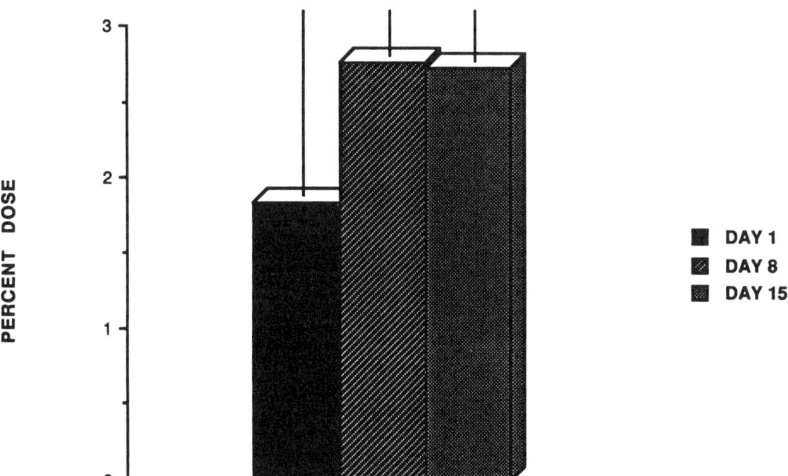

Figure 1 *In vivo* percutaneous absorption of Azone® in humans with repeated Azone® skin application (mean ± S. D.).

Previous reports on the percutaneous absorption of Azone® in humans show 0.13% absorbed after 4 h skin exposure[6] and 0.42% absorbed after 12 h skin exposure.[7] These absorption amounts give rates of 0.03%/h, assuming a steady-state rate of absorption. In the present study the first single-dose absorption of 1.84% over 24 h gives a higher absorption rate of 0.08%/h, assuming a steady-state rate of

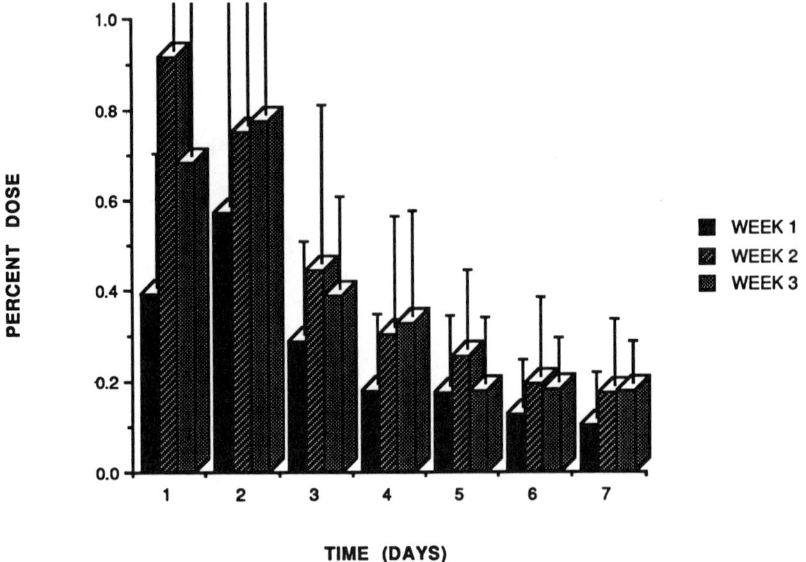

Figure 2 Daily radioactivity excretion following repeated skin application of [^{14}C]-Azone® to human subjects (mean ± S. D.).

Table 2 Soap And Water Wash Recovery Of Azone® From Human Subjects[a]

	Percent Dose Excreted		
Subject	**Day 1**	**Day 8**	**Day 15**
1	2.23	2.74	1.21
2	0.79	1.19	1.48
3	0.72	0.49	0.40
4	4.80	3.15	1.52
5	0.60	0.37	0.73
6	0.45	0.54	0.63
7	0.41	0.16	0.24
8	7.26	1.49	1.23
9	0.17	0.21	3.09
Mean	1.94	1.15	1.17
S.D.	2.47	1.11	0.85

[a] Wash sequence = 1 soap, 1 water rinse, 1 soap, 2 water rinses.

absorption. This may be due to differences in study design. Another possibility is that the initial effect of absorption enhancement is occurring, and the rate of absorption steadily increases.

The soap and water wash process failed to recover >1 or 2% of the applied topical dose. This is probably due to lack of solubility of Azone® in the soap and water wash. Previous studies in humans recovered >90% of Azone® from skin using repeated ethanol washes.[6,8]

Thus, Azone® can enhance its own absorption as well as that of other compounds. Washing the skin site of application with soap and water only recovered 1 to 2% of applied radioactivity. Previous published studies recovered the Azone® dose with ethanol washes. Thus, a potential accumulation of Azone® in skin could occur. This should be considered relevant for any pharmacological or toxicological evaluation of formulations containing Azone®.

V. SUMMARY

Azone® is an agent that has been shown to enhance percutaneous absorption of drugs. Azone® is thought to act by partitioning into skin lipid bilayers, thereby disrupting the structure. An open-label study was done with nine volunteers (two males, seven females; ages 51 to 75 years) in which Azone® cream (1.6%; 100 mg) was topically dosed to a 5 cm × 10 cm area of the ventral forearm for 21 consecutive days. On days 1, 8, and 15, the Azone® cream contained 47 μCi [^{14}C]-Azone®. The skin application site was washed with soap and water after each 24-h dosing. Percutaneous absorption was determined by urinary radioactivity excretion. The [^{14}C]-Azone® was ring labeled [^{14}C-2-cycloheptan]. Radiochemical purity was >98.6% and cold azone purity was 99%.

Percutaneous absorption of the first dose (day 1) was 1.84 ± 1.56% (SD) of applied dose for 24-h skin application time. Day 8 percutaneous absorption, after repeated application, increased significantly ($p < 0.002$) to 2.76 ± 1.91%. Day 15 percutaneous absorption, after continued repeated application, stayed the same at 2.72 ± 1.21%. In humans repeated application of Azone® results in an initial self-absorption enhancement, probably due to its mechanism of action. However, steady-state percutaneous absorption of Azone® is established after this initial change. Thus, Azone® can enhance its own absorption as well as that of other compounds. This should be considered relevant for any pharmacological or toxicological evaluation.

Washing the skin site of application with soap and water only recovered 1 or 2% of applied radioactivity. Previous published studies recovered the Azone® dose with ethanol washes. Thus, a potential accumulation of Azone® in skin could occur.

REFERENCES

1. **Stoughton, R. B.,** Enhanced percutaneous penetration with 1-dodecylazacycloheptan-2-one, *Arch. Dermatol.,* 118, 474, 1982.
2. **Stoughton, R. B. and McClure, W. O.,** Azone®: a new non-toxic enhancer of cutaneous penetration, *Drug Dev. Ind. Pharm.,* 9, 725, 1983.
3. **Stoughton, R. B. and Barry, B. W.,** Differential scanning calorimetry (DSC) of human SC; effect of Azone®, *J. Pharm. Pharmacol.,* 37 (Suppl.), 80, 1985.
4. **Beastall, J. C., Hadgraft, J., and Washington, C.,** Mechanism of action of Azone® as a percutaneous penetration enhancer: lipid bilayer fluidity and transition temperature effects, *Int. J. Pharm.,* 43, 207, 1988.
5. **Landmann, L.,** The epidermal permeability barrier. Comparison between *in vivo* and *in vitro* lipid structures, *Eur. J. Cell Biol.* 33, 258, 1984.
6. **Wiechers, J. W., Drenth, B. F. H., Jonkman, J. H. G., and De Zeeuw, R. A.,** Percutaneous absorption and elimination of the penetration enhancer Azone® in humans, *Pharm. Res.,* 519, 1987.
7. **Wiechers, J. W., Drenth, B. F. H., Jonkman, J. H. G., and De Zeeuw, R. A.,** Percutaneous absorption, metabolism and elimination of the penetration enhancer Azone® in humans after prolonged application under occlusion, *Int. J. Pharm.,* 47, 43, 1988.

8. **Wiechers, J. W., Drenth, B. F. H., Jonkman, J. H. G., and De Zeeuw, R. A.,** Percutaneous absorption, metabolic profiling, and excretion of the penetration enhancer Azone® after multiple dosing of an Azone-containing triamcinolone acetonide cream in humans, *J. Pharm. Sci.,* 79, 1111, 1990.
9. **Wester, R. C., Noonan, P. K., and Maibach, H. I.,** Percutaneous absorption of hydrocortisone increases with long-term administration: *in vivo* studies in the Rhesus monkey, *Arch. Dermatol.,* 116, 186, 1980.
10. **Wester, R. C., Maibach, H. I., Bucks, D. A. W., and Guy, R. H.,** Malathion percutaneous absorption after repeated administration to man, *Toxicol. Appl. Pharmacol.,* 68, 116, 1983.
11. **Bucks, D. A. W., Maibach, H. I., and Guy, R. H.,** *In vivo* percutaneous absorption: effect of repeated application versus single dose, in *Percutaneous Absorption,* 2nd ed., Bronaugh, R. and Maibach, H., Eds., Marcel Dekker, New York, 1989, 633.

Chapter 6.4

Metabolism of the Penetration Enhancer Azone®: *In Vivo* and *In Vitro* Studies in the Hamster, Rat, Monkey, and Human*

Johann W. Wiechers

CONTENTS

I. INTRODUCTION

The need for penetration enhancers in transdermal drug delivery is discussed elsewhere in this book. They may facilitate skin penetration by interacting with the skin or by increasing the release of drug from its vehicle.[1,2] The most widely used penetration enhancers in the past were aprotic solvents, such as sulfoxides (dimethylsulfoxide, decylmethylsulfoxide), amides (dimethylformamide, dimethylacetamide), and cyclic amides (2-pyrrolidone, *N*-methyl-2-pyrrolidone). However, these compounds showed a considerable extent of irritancy, toxicity, and/or odor.[3]

* The studies described in this chapter were performed in the Departments of Analytical Chemistry and Toxicology, Pharmacology and Therapeutics of the University Centre for Pharmacy, Groningen, The Netherlands.

0-8493-2605-2/95/$0.00+$.50

Stoughton demonstrated the potentials of 1-dodecylazacycloheptan-2-one or laurocapram (Azone) as a penetration enhancer for a wide variety of drugs, such as antibiotics and steroids,[4,5] and its wider potential as a penetration enhancer has been reviewed.[6] This chapter focuses on the metabolism of Azone® as observed in the hamster, rat, monkey, and human in *in vivo* and *in vitro* studies. With the ultimate aim of structure elucidation of the human metabolites, the percutaneous absorption of Azone® itself through human skin, rather than its effect on skin absorption of other penetrants, was studied either when applied as a single dose to human skin as a neat liquid[7,8] or as a constituent of a cream in a multiple-dosing regimen.[9,10] Unfortunately for structure elucidation, the absorption of Azone® through human skin was low. While over 97% of the administered dose was recovered from the skin, <0.5% could be detected in the excreta, predominantly in the urine.[7,8] Subsequent *in vivo* studies were set up in species other than human in which Azone® was expected to be more readily absorbed, in order to generate larger quantities of metabolites.[11] For the same reason *in vitro* studies were undertaken using the metabolizing organs and organelles of humans and rats.

II. *IN VIVO* STUDIES[11]

A. METABOLISM OF AZONE® IN THE HAMSTER *IN VIVO*

1-[1-^{14}C]Dodecylazacycloheptan-2-one (Atomlight, North Billerica, MA) was given as a bolus injection to male Syrian hamsters *(Mesocricetus auratus)* as described previously.[11] Bile and urine were collected for a period of 24 h. Recovery of radioactivity in this study was 71.5%, 91.4% of which was found in the urine and 8.6% in the bile. The metabolic profile of the radioactivity retrieved in the urine was assessed by fractionating and analyzing the column effluent for radioactivity after separation by reversed-phase high-performance liquid chromatography (RP-HPLC).[11] A linear gradient from 100% 0.01 *M* phosphate buffer pH 6.8 to 100% methanol in 60 min, followed by a 15-min 100% methanol flush, was used to separate the Azone® metabolites in hamster urine, followed by offline scintillation counting. The metabolic profile in the urine of the hamster is depicted in Figure 1A. Some radioactivity was found to elute at the retention time of Azone® itself at 60 to 63 min, at a relative concentration of 8.8% of the total amount of eluted radioactivity. It seems likely that this peak corresponds to unchanged Azone®, also because this compound continued to have the same retention time as Azone® in other elution profiles. However, the majority of the metabolites were more polar in nature than Azone®.

B. METABOLISM OF AZONE® IN THE MONKEY *IN VIVO*

1-[1-^{14}C]Dodecylazacycloheptan-2-one was dosed intravenously to male cynomolgus monkeys *(Macaca fasicularis).* Urine and feces were collected separately for a period of 5 d. Further experimental detail can be found in Reference 11. Recovery of radioactivity in this study was 88.1%, 94.6% of which was found in the urine and 5.4% in the feces. A concave rather than a linear gradient elution profile was used in the same RP-HPLC setup described above for the separation of the hamster metabolites. This resulted in a shift toward longer retention times for the medium polar compounds, whereas the retention times of the nonpolar compounds, eluting during the methanol flush (60 to 75 min), remained virtually unaffected. The

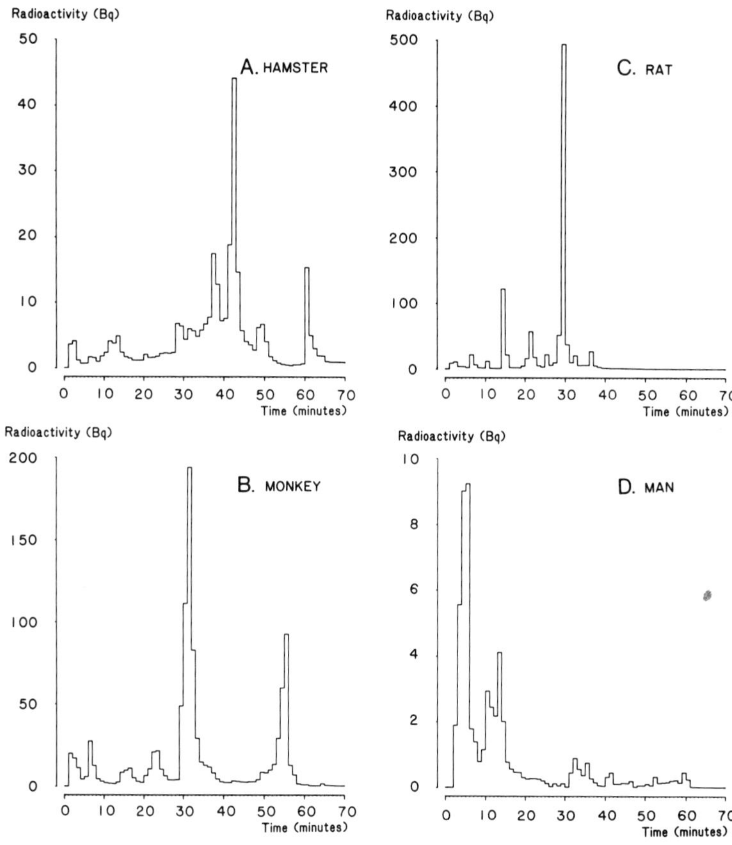

Figure 1 Urinary metabolic profile of chain-labeled ^{14}C-Azone®-derived radioactivity after intravenous administration to hamsters (0 to 24 h; A), monkeys (4 to 12 h; B), and rats (60 to 90 min; C), and after dermal application to humans (12 to 24 h; D). Volume injected: 100 (A), 20 (B), 50 (C), and 2000 µl (D). (From Wiechers, J. W., Drenth, B. F. H., Adolfsen, F. A. W., Prins, L., and De Zeeuw, R. A., *Pharm. Res.,* 7, 496, 1990. With permission.)

chromatogram of the urinary metabolites in the 4 to 12 h fraction is given in Figure 1B. A similar profile was obtained for the 0 to 4 h urine fraction. During the first 12 h after dosing 89% of the total urinary radioactivity was excreted. In contrast to the hamster urine no unchanged Azone® could be detected in the monkey urine, while the cluster seen at around 56 min in the monkey urine using the concave gradient coincided with the 40 min cluster in the hamster urine (linear gradient).

C. METABOLISM OF AZONE® IN THE RAT *IN VIVO*

1-[1-^{14}C]Dodecylazacycloheptan-2-one was dosed intravenously to male Wistar rats and bile and urine were collected over a period of 3 h.[11] Recovery of radioactivity in this study in urine and bile was 38.5%, 77.4% of which was retrieved in the urine and 22.6% in the bile. Another 9.9% of the applied dose could be retrieved in the organs and the blood. Low amounts of radioactivity in the lungs make expiration unlikely as a possible route of elimination of Azone®-derived radioactivity. The concave

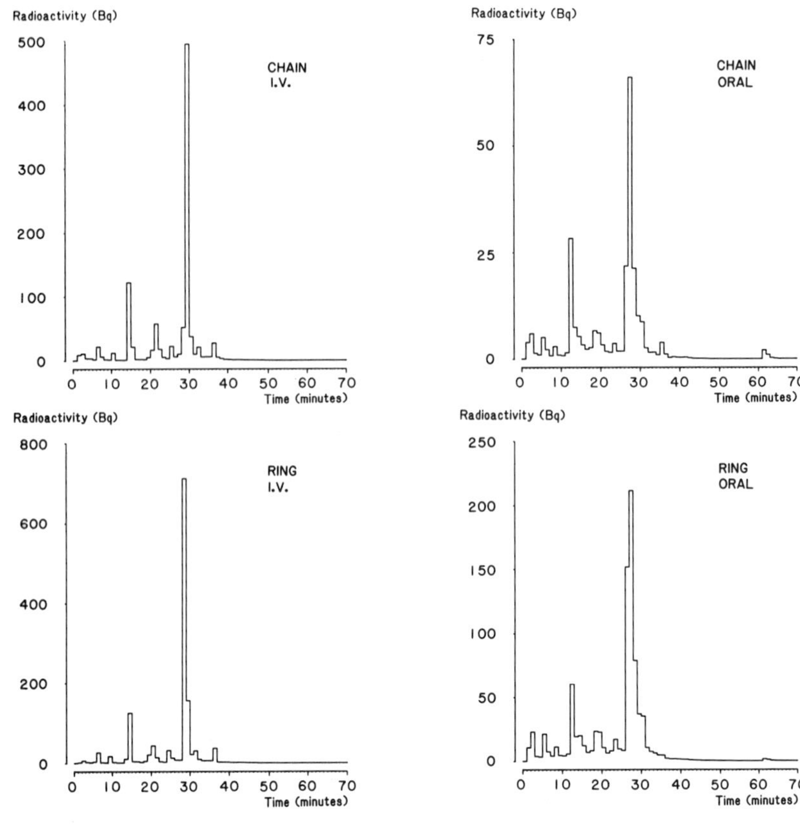

Figure 2 Urinary metabolic profiles of ^{14}C-Azone®-derived radioactivity after intravenous (left; 60 to 90 min) and oral administration (right; 90 to 120 min) of chain- (top) and ring-labeled Azone® (bottom) to rats. Volume injected: 50 μl. (From Wiechers, J. W., Drenth, B. F. H., Adolfsen, F. A. W., Prins, L., and De Zeeuw, R. A., *Pharm. Res.*, 7, 496, 1990. With permission.)

elution gradient was used to separate the metabolites of Azone® in the rat urine. The urinary profile of the 60 to 90 min postdose fraction is given in Figure 1C.

Azone® labeled in the ring (1-dodecylazacycloheptan-2-[^{14}C]one) as well as the previously used Azone® labeled in the chain (1-[1-^{14}C]dodecylazacycloheptan-2-one) were intravenously and orally dosed to male Wistar rats to study the influence of the position of the ^{14}C label in the Azone® molecule, as well as the route of administration on the metabolic profile. Results are shown in Figure 2. Independent of the position of the label, some radioactivity was found to elute at the Azone® position in the chromatograms after oral administration, whereas no unchanged Azone® was detectable in the urinary metabolic profile after intravenous administration. Apart from this observation and minor differences in the relative abundance of the individual peaks, the urinary metabolic profiles after intravenous and oral administration were essentially the same. Likewise, no differences could be seen between the radiochromatograms using two different positions of the radioisotope within the Azone® molecule. It was therefore concluded that gastrointestinal metabolism of Azone® in the rat did not occur or was similar to systemic metabolism, and complete removal of the dodecyl side chain or cleavage of the ring followed by removal of the carboxyl group did not occur. Topical administration was not tested as skin metabolism of Azone® during skin passage in humans had already been shown not to occur.[12]

D. METABOLISM OF AZONE® IN HUMAN *IN VIVO*

1-[1-^{14}C]Dodecylazacycloheptan-2-one was applied to the volar aspect of the forearm of volunteers for 12 h under occlusion as described previously.[8] Urine, feces, and plasma samples were collected throughout the 5.5 d following the application of the dose. Percutaneously absorbed Azone®-derived radioactivity was predominantly excreted in the urine (97.2%) after extensive metabolism to polar metabolites. Figure 1D shows a urinary profile, 12 to 24 h after application of the dose, obtained after concentrating the urine sample by lyophilization and extraction with methanol. The same concave elution pattern was used to separate the urinary metabolites, making the profile directly comparable to those of the monkey and the rat. Although some peaks appear to be present in the same positions in the radiochromatograms as compared to rats and monkeys, it is clear that the bulk of the metabolites is more polar than those in the rat urine and much more polar than those in the monkey urine. The metabolites found in the hamster urine were even that lipophilic that another elution profile had to be used. Human and hamster metabolites are therefore certainly not similar.

In another study Azone® was applied to the volar aspect of the forearm in a cream at a concentration of 1.6% for 12 h under occlusion on four consecutive days.[9] Different parts of the application areas were stripped 28 times at 1, 20, and 44 h after removal of the last dose, using commercial cellophane translucent tape (3M, Leiden, The Netherlands). All 28 strips from one point in time were combined and Azone-derived radioactivity extracted as described previously.[12] The metabolic profile of the ^{14}C-Azone® derived radioactivity in the tape strip extract obtained from the stripping procedure at 1 h after removal of the last dose showed only the parent compound, except for a minor amount of radioactivity in the front (see Figure 3). This small peak most likely originated from the tritiated drug triamcinolone acetonide that was coadministered in the cream. The radiochromatograms at 20 and 44 h showed similar profiles, yet at much lower concentrations due to the rapid disappearance of Azone® from the stratum corneum (SC).[12] It could therefore be concluded that only unchanged Azone® was present in the SC.

Urine from this multiple dosing study was also analyzed using the previously mentioned concave gradient elution in RP-HPLC. Like the profile in human urine in Figure 1D most of the radioactivity was excreted as very polar metabolites eluting within 20 min. A nonpolar compound was observed at 65 min, suspected to be unchanged Azone® that would elute at 63 to 64 minutes under these conditions.[9] Only once before was a lipophilic metabolite of Azone® seen in human urine: a peak eluting at around 58 min, positively identified not to be Azone® by spiking the urine.[8]

E. CONCLUSIONS OF *IN VIVO* METABOLISM STUDIES USING AZONE®

Topical administration of Azone® to humans resulted in absorption of the penetration enhancer by the SC, where it could only be found as the parent compound. Subsequent absorption and metabolism resulted in a mixture of at least three mainly polar

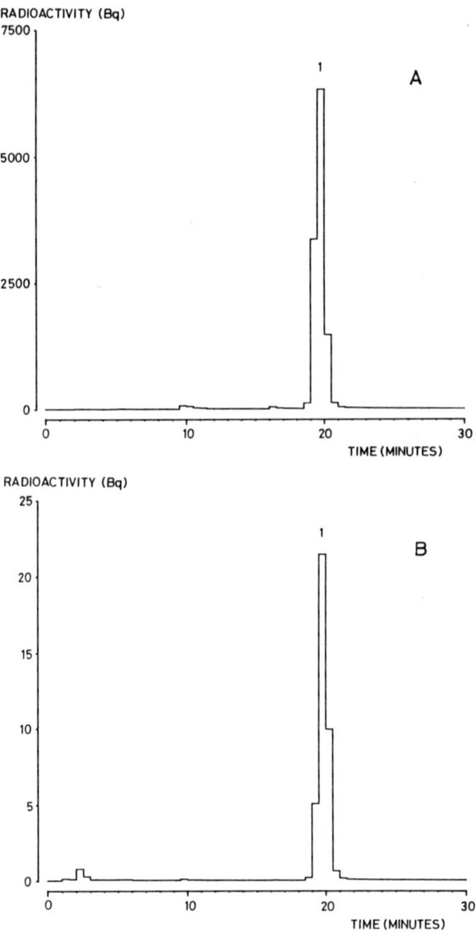

Figure 3 Radiochromatograms of ^{14}C-Azone-derived radioactivity in the dosage (A) and the tape extracts at 1 h after removal of the dose (B). (From Wiechers, J. W., Herder, R. E., Drenth, B. F. H., and De Zeeuw, R. A., *J. Soc. Cosmet. Chem.*, 40, 367, 1989. With permission.)

metabolites (0 to 18 min) and a possible fourth metabolite of a polarity closely similar to Azone®. At least four other metabolites, present in minute quantities, could be observed. Regardless of the way in which Azone® was dosed (single dose of neat Azone® with or without occlusion, multiple application from a cream), its percutaneous absorption was low and did not yield sufficient quantities of metabolites for structure elucidation. Hamster, monkey, and rat were therefore investigated to see whether they could act as a source of metabolites of Azone®. Therefore, the compound was injected intravenously, thereby avoiding the problem of limited absorption. Extensive systemic metabolism occurred in all species, but both qualitative and quantitative differences were observed. The polarity of the bulk of the metabolites increased from hamster to monkey to rat to human. Only the hamster consistently excreted minor amounts of unchanged Azone®. Some of the polar major human metabolites could be detected in rat urine, while minor metabolites of moderate polarity were retrieved in monkey urine as well. Finally, total cleavage of the dodecyl side chain could be excluded in rats and gastrointestinal metabolism in rats did not occur or was similar to systemic metabolism.

The above suggests at least the initial metabolic pathways of Azone® to be similar, and the observed metabolic differences between the animal species and humans could be the result of prolonged residence time in the human body as well as the availability and/or utilization of different enzyme systems by humans. Therefore, using the metabolizing organs or organelles of rat and humans *in vitro* may help to unravel the bioconversion of Azone®.

III. *IN VITRO* STUDIES

This section describes the results of *in vitro* studies performed to regenerate the human urinary metabolic profile, using human hepatocytes and microsomes. In order to explain the observed differences in the metabolic profiles of the various animal species, rat liver material was also used in the perfused liver technique, and in hepatocyte and microsome experiments.

A. METABOLISM OF AZONE® IN THE RAT *IN VITRO*

1. Rat Liver Perfusion

Isolated rat liver perfusions were carried out according to the method of Meijer et al.[13] The liver of a male Wistar rat (ca. 230 g), anesthetized with urethane (1.28 g/kg body weight), was isolated and the portal and hepatic veins and the bile duct were cannulated. Subsequently, the liver was placed in a thermostatically controlled cabinet at 37°C, and was recirculatingly perfused by a Krebs-bicarbonate-glucose buffer solution (pH 7.4) containing 1% bovine serum albumin as a physiological drug carrier. The perfusate was introduced via the portal vein and drained via the hepatic veins. It was circulated by a peristaltic roller pump acting on silicon rubber tubing at a rate of 28 ml/min, i.e., 3.5 ml/g of liver per minute, which is higher than normal liver blood flow to attain adequate oxygenation. The perfusate, the temperature of which was maintained at 37°C, was oxygenated by carbogen (O_2/CO_2 95/5 v/v). The pH was kept at 7.40 ± 0.05 and carefully controlled by mixing O_2 to the O_2/CO_2 gas flow. Bile flow was maintained by replacing the excreted bile salts. This was done by a constant infusion of 15 μmol/h of sodium taurocholate in physiological saline. The infusion rate was 0.9 ml/h. The experiment began with the addition of 9.3 μl of methanolic solution of 1-dodecylazacycloheptan-2-[^{14}C]one to the main perfusion medium reservoir that contained a total volume of 100 ml. In this way 0.51 μmol of Azone® was dosed containing 4.65 μCi. Bile was continuously collected via the cannula in ice-cooled counting vials in 15- or 30-min fractions. Samples of 1 ml were taken from the perfusate at 5, 10, 20, 30, 45, 60, 90, and 105 min after dosing. At 105 min, the perfusion was terminated and the liver was homogenized in a threefold volume of ice-cold KCl buffer (0.154 *M*).

Figure 4 shows the radiochromatograms of the isolated liver perfusate at 10, 30, and 105 min, eluted with the same concave gradient and solvents as described for the monkey, rat, and human urine in the *in vivo* experiments. Peak 11, therefore, is unchanged Azone®. It can be seen that Azone® is metabolized to more polar metabolites as time goes by. The bile also contained metabolites, and only minor amounts of radioactivity at 63 min elution time could be seen, suggesting that Azone® is almost completely metabolized before being excreted (profiles not shown). Peaks 4,

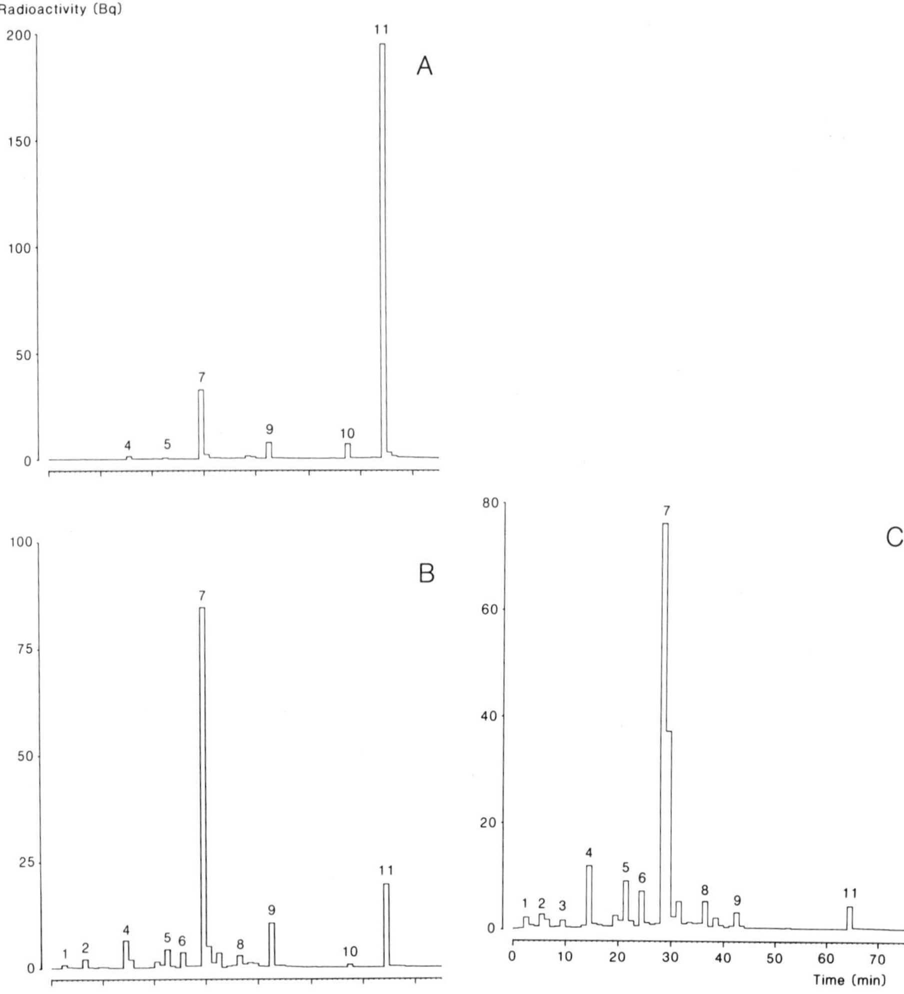

Figure 4 Rat liver perfusion: radiochromatograms of the perfusate at 10 (A), 30 (B), and 105 min (C) following concave gradient elution. Volume injected: 200 µl.

7, and 8 of the perfusate profile (Figure 4) were also present in relatively large amounts in the bile.

A good correlation exists between the metabolic profiles of the *in vitro* and the *in vivo* biofluids. The perfusate at 105 min (Figure 4C) resembles the rat *in vivo* urinary profile (Figure 1C) remarkably well, as do the rat perfusion biliary profile (60 to 105 min fraction) and the *in vivo* biliary profile (radiochromatograms not shown). This indicates that the liver is indeed the primary organ in the metabolism of Azone® in the rat. The perfusate at 10 min (Figure 4A) contains predominantly unchanged Azone®. Its metabolism resulted essentially in one major compound (peak 7), the relative concentration of which remained almost constant after 30 min (around 55%). This peak was shown to be susceptible to pH changes of the eluent, and moved toward longer retention times (40 min) at pH 5.1. Increasing the pH to 7.6, however, had no influence on the retention time of peak 7, which indicates that this compound is ionized to a higher extent at pH 6.8 than at pH 5.1. At longer perfusion times, the more polar peaks with retention times of <30 min are formed. Whether these are formed by a second transformation (e.g., a phase II conjugation reaction) out of metabolites such as compounds 7, 9, and 10, or directly out of Azone® (peak 11) cannot be concluded from these radiochromatograms.

2. Rat Hepatocyte Experiments

Isolated rat hepatocytes were obtained by digestion of the liver through collagenase perfusion of the organ and subsequent differential centrifugation. A modification of the procedure of Berry and Friend,[14] as described by Braakman, et al.,[15] was performed. Rat hepatocytes were suspended in Krebs-Henseleit bicarbonate buffer, pH 7.40, containing 1% bovine serum albumin to a concentration of 3.1×10^6 cells per milliliter and kept on ice until use. The viability of the cells was tested with trypan blue (0.2% final concentration). Viability was >95%. Three milliliters of this hepatocyte suspension were preincubated for 30 min in a shaking water bath at 37°C under carbogen. The experiment was initiated by the addition of 30 μl of a 317 μ*M* 1-dodecylazacycloheptan-2-[^{14}C]one emulsion in water, containing 0.1% dimethylsulfoxide (DMSO) as the emulsifier, resulting in a final concentration of 3.1 μ*M* Azone®, and a radioactive concentration of 0.0277 μCi/ml. After 1, 5, and 30 min 1 ml aliquots were taken which were immediately placed on ice to terminate the reaction. The aliquots were centrifuged for 10 min at 13,000 RPM, and the supernatants stored at –20°C until analysis. The pellet was washed with 1 ml of cold saline and the wash water was stored at –20°C. Subsequently the hepatocytes were lysed by adding 1 ml of a methanol/water mixture (50/50 v/v) to the pellet. The remainder of the hepatocytes were centrifuged and the supernatant was stored at –20°C until analysis.

The radiochromatograms of the supernatant and the hepatocyte content are shown in Figures 5 and 6, respectively. The radiochromatogram of the hepatocyte wash at 30 min (not shown) closely resembles that of the supernatant at 30 min. As with the perfusate in the rat liver perfusion, the rat hepatocyte incubation medium has a dual function. At the same time it serves as the dosing solution and the excretion medium, but now for both the "urinary" and "biliary" metabolites. The radiochromatograms in Figures 5 and 6 indicate a fast, yet time-dependent metabolism of Azone® in the rat hepatocyte. After just 1 min, the relative concentration of Azone® in the hepatocyte is only 20.7% and the majority of the Azone-derived radioactivity is present in nonpolar metabolites eluting between 50 and 60 min, although small quantities of polar compounds can already be seen (Figure 6A). After an incubation period of 30 min, however, these nonpolar compounds have almost completely disappeared (Figure 6C), but not into the incubation medium (see Figure 5). This suggest that these nonpolar compounds are biotransformation products of transient character.

The similarity of the radiochromatograms of the supernatant at the end of the experiment (Figure 5C) and that of the rat *in vivo* urine (Figure 1C) is striking, and demonstrates the excellent correlation between the *in vitro* rat hepatocyte experiment and *in vivo* metabolism in the rat. This resemblance suggests that the "urinary" metabolites are emitted by the hepatocyte into the incubation medium, whereas the "biliary" metabolites remain in the hepatocyte itself as the resemblance between the rat hepatocyte content and the rat *in vivo* biliary profiles (not shown) is very good.

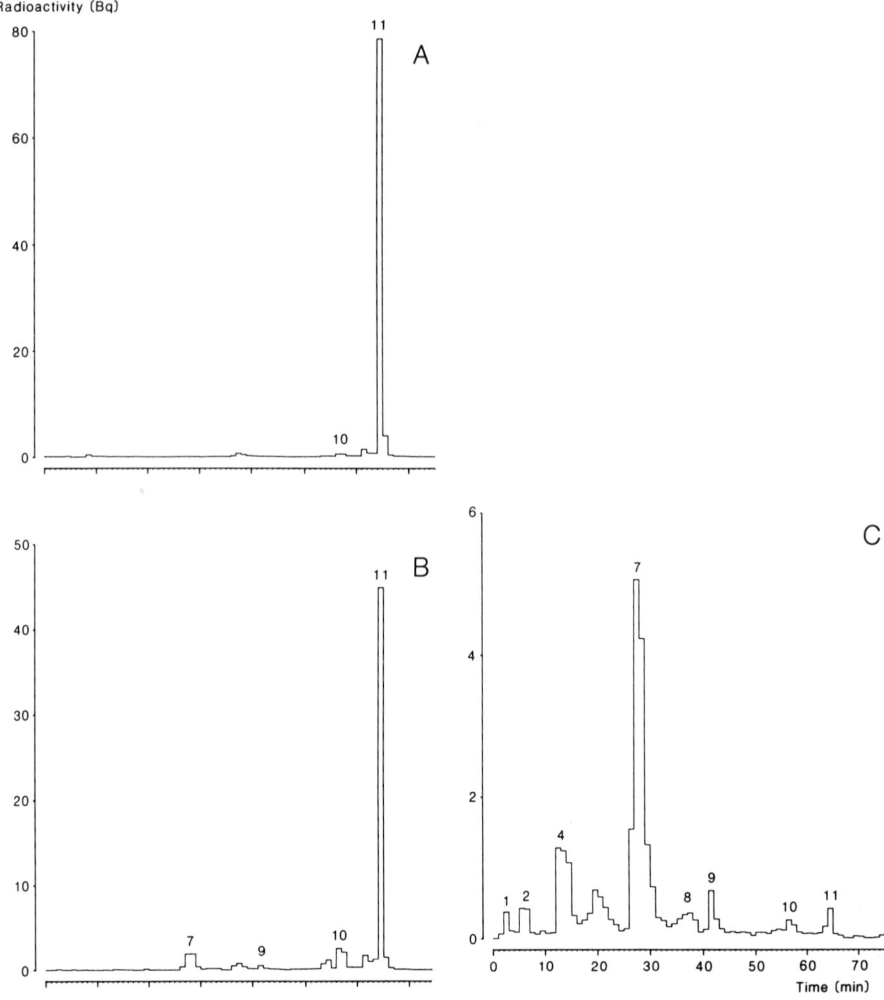

Figure 5 Rat hepatocytes: radiochromatograms of the supernatant at 1 (A), 5 (B), and 30 min (C) following concave gradient elution. Volume injected: 100 (A, B) and 20 μl (C). Peak numbers refer to peaks in Figure 4 that elute with the same retention time and are given for the purpose of comparison.

3. Rat Microsome Experiments

Fasted male Wistar rats (ca. 200 g) were killed by cervical dislocation and the livers were rapidly removed. Microsomes were obtained by fractional centrifugation of the liver homogenate according to Chowdhury and Arias,[16] with slight modifications as described by Gerding et al.[17] The incubation medium consisted of 50 m*M* Tris-HCl buffer, pH 7.4, 5 m*M* $MgCl_2$, 10 m*M* nicotinamide, 2 m*M* NADPH, 73 μ*M* ^{14}C-Azone® (0.672 μCi), and 4.14 mg rat microsomal protein in a final incubation volume of 1 ml. In order to activate the cofactor for oxidative drug metabolism, NADPH, all constituents except the microsomes were preincubated for a period of 5 min in a shaking water bath at 37°C. The reactions were initiated by the addition of the microsomal suspension, and the mixture was incubated at 37°C for 60 min. Metabolic

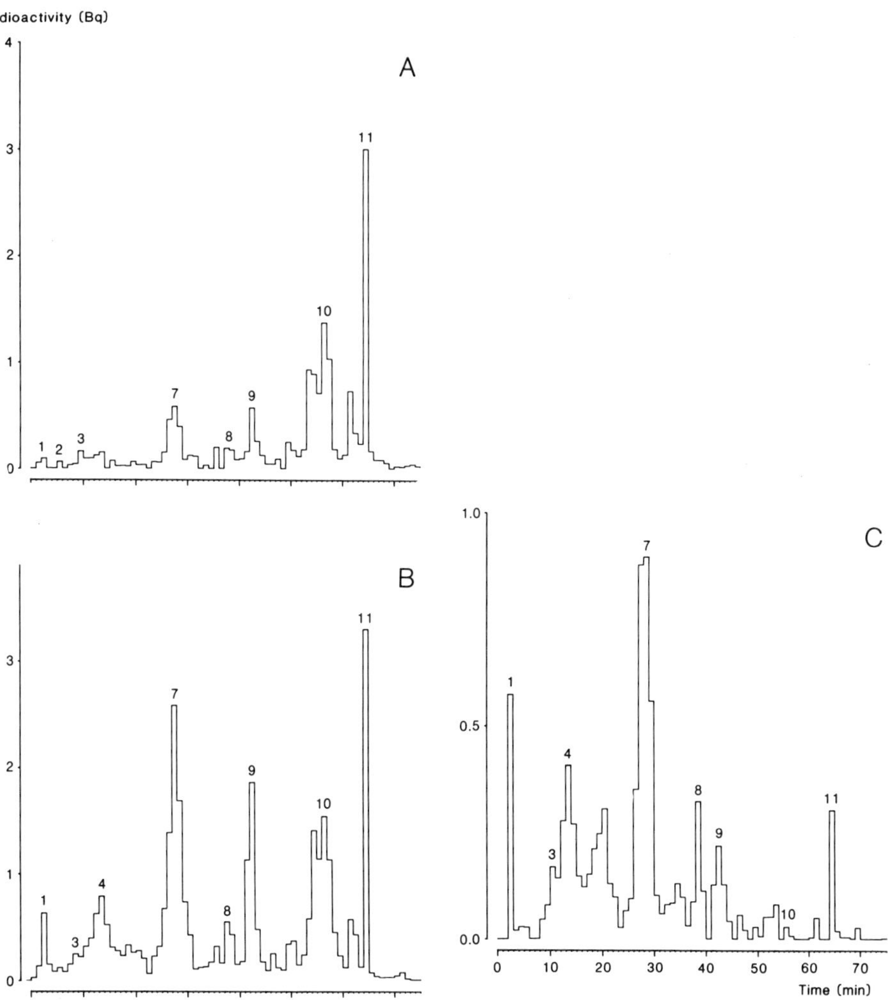

Figure 6 Rat hepatocytes: radiochromatograms of the hepatocyte content at 1 (A), 5 (B), and 30 min (C) following concave gradient elution. Volume injected: 100 µl. Peak numbers refer to peaks in Figure 4 that elute with the same retention time and are given for the purpose of comparison.

reactions were terminated by placing the vials on ice. After centrifugation of the incubation mixtures, the clear supernatant was decanted and stored at –20°C until analysis.

The recovery of Azone®-derived radioactivity in these experiments was low, 51.5%. The remainder of the radioactivity could be shown to have adhered to the walls of the centrifugation tubes. Metabolic profiling of the incubation media using concave gradient elution as described above resulted in a cluster of peaks eluting at retention times between 56 and 65 min. Isocratic elution (methanol/phosphate buffer 0.01 *M,* pH 6.8 (85/15 v/v)) was therefore regarded to be more suitable to separate these peaks, and the resulting chromatogram is shown in Figure 7A. Azone® eluted at 15 min under these conditions. The parent compound (peak 11) was hardly present in the medium following the 60-min incubation (<1%). The broad peak in the "polar

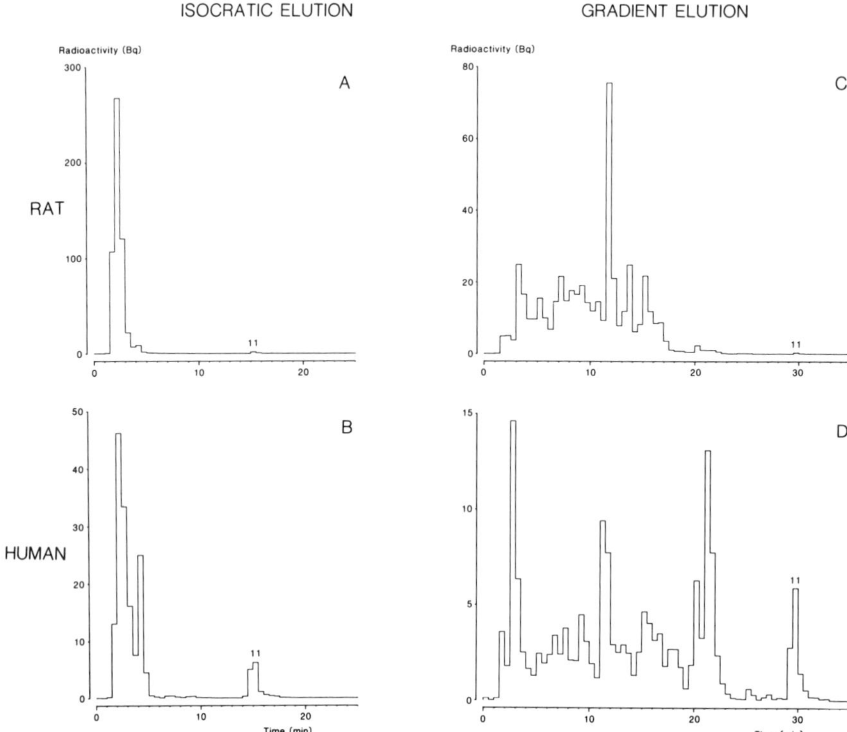

Figure 7 Microsomes: radiochromatograms of the supernatant using rat (A and C) and human microsomes (B and D), following isocratic (A and B) and linear gradient elution (C and D). Volume injected: 50 μl. Peak numbers refer to peaks in Figure 4 that elute with the same retention time and are given for the purpose of comparison.

part" of the profile, however, suggested the existence of more than one compound. Therefore, another linear gradient from methanol/phosphate buffer 0.01 *M,* pH 6.8 (50/50 v/v), to methanol in 30 min followed by a methanol flush was used, and the resulting radiochromatogram is shown in Figure 7B. Unchanged Azone® now eluted at 30 min, while the largest peak eluted at 12 min.

The experiments indicate that rat microsomes are not capable of bioconverting Azone® to the more polar metabolites encountered in the *in vivo* profile (Figure 1C). Nevertheless, they seem to be capable of generating the transient metabolites as observed in the hepatocyte experiments. It is very possible, then, that Azone® undergoes phase I metabolism in the microsomes (endoplasmic reticulum), which is a well-known phenomenon.[18] However, it cannot be further metabolized in phase II conjugation reactions in the microsomes. Despite the presence of the microsomal enzyme UDP-glucuronyltransferase, glucuronidation is impossible because the cofactor UDP-glucuronic acid has not been added to the incubation medium. All other phase II conjugation reactions are impossible because the necessary enzymes are present in the cytosol, which is discarded during preparation of the microsomes. Such a sequence of reactions would explain the poor *in vivo/in vitro* metabolism correlation.

B. METABOLISM OF AZONE® IN HUMANS *IN VITRO*

1. Human Hepatocyte Experiments

Human hepatocytes were prepared by collagenase digestion of human liver tissue according to a modification of the method of isolation of rat hepatocytes in cooperation with the Human Liver Group Gröningen.[19] The concentration of human hepatocytes was 0.8×10^6 cells per milliliter and the viability as determined by trypan blue exclusion was 65%. Five milliliters of this hepatocyte suspension were preincubated for 40 min in a shaking water bath at 37°C under carbogen. The experiment began with the addition of 50 μl of a 317 μ*M* ^{14}C-Azone® emulsion in water, containing 0.02% Triton® X-100 as the emulsifier, resulting in a final concentration of 3.1 μ*M* Azone®, corresponding to 0.0277 μCi/ml. After 30, 60, and 120 min, aliquots of 1.5, 1.5, and 2 ml were taken which were immediately placed on ice to terminate metabolic reactions. Supernatant, hepatocyte wash, and hepatocyte content were obtained as described above for rat hepatocytes. Wash volumes were adapted for the smaller amount of hepatocytes. This time, the hepatocytes were lysed using 100% methanol.

Recovery of radioactivity in the various samples was 42.6%. The better part of the remainder of the radioactivity could be detected in the pellet of the lysed hepatocytes. Of the radioactivity in the samples, 84.1% was retrieved in the supernatant, 7.5% in the hepatocyte content, 7.4% in the hepatocyte wash, and only 1.0% in the vial wash. The same time dependency observed in the supernatant of rat hepatocytes was seen in the radiochromatograms of the supernatant of the human hepatocytes (Figure 8). Unfortunately, due to the low amounts of radioactivity in the hepatocyte content samples, proper chromatographic analysis of these samples was impossible.

Uptake of substances by human hepatocytes is often much slower as compared to those of rats.[19] The time span of the human incubation experiment was therefore expanded to compensate this effect. Nevertheless, radioactivity in the supernatant was still predominantly present as unchanged Azone® at all three time points (Figure 8). This decreased rate of uptake by the human hepatocyte[19] as well as the observed slower metabolic rate of the human hepatocytes[20] may be reasons for the apparent discrepancy between the *in vitro* hepatocyte supernatant profile at 120 min (Figure 8C) and the human *in vivo* urinary profile (Figure 1D). Yet, apparently a fair resemblance exists with the rat *in vitro* profiles (Figures 4, 5, and 6) and rat urinary *in vivo* profile (Figure 1C), especially with regard to peaks 4 and 7.

Of special interest is the cluster of nonpolar metabolites eluting at 50 to 60 min. These metabolites were only found in the rat hepatocyte and not in their *in vivo* profiles, suggesting them to be of transient character. When using human hepatocytes, they were found outside the hepatocyte in the supernatant (Figure 8B) and therefore must have been excreted. Compounds having these retention times have sometimes been found in the human *in vivo* urinary metabolic profile which might be in accordance with the excretion by the human hepatocyte. Another explanation for the occurrence of the transient metabolites in the supernatant of the human hepatocyte experiment may be a higher susceptibility of the human hepatocyte membrane to Azone® as compared to that of the rat. Azone®, a penetration enhancer, is known to make membranes more permeable.

Although human hepatocytes experiments have demonstrated excellent correlation with human metabolites *in vivo* with other drugs,[20] the human hepatocytes metabolized Azone® to compounds only slightly more polar than Azone® itself,

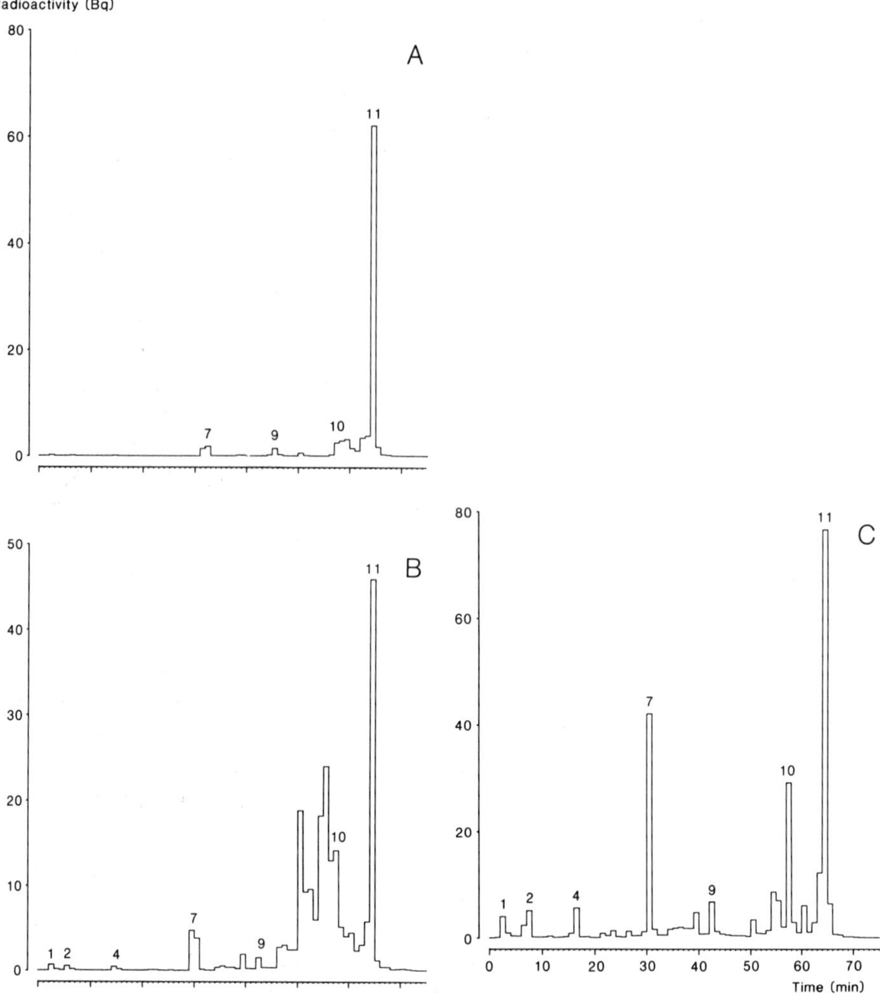

Figure 8 Human hepatocytes: radiochromatograms of the supernatant at 30 (A), 60 (B), and 120 min (C) following concave gradient elution. Volume injected: 200 (A, B) and 500 μl (C). Peak numbers refer to peaks in Figure 4 that elute with the same retention time and are given for the purpose of comparison.

which showed a closer resemblance to the rat *in vivo* urinary profile rather than to the human *in vivo* urinary profile. This may be due to the relatively short duration of the human hepatocyte experiment, or to the involvement of extrahepatic metabolizing organs in the bioconversion of Azone® in humans *in vivo.*

2. Human Microsome Experiments

A small part of a frozen human liver that was previously perfused with a mixture of DMSO, fetal calf serum, and Krebs buffer (1:2:7) to remove blood traces was treated as described above for the preparation of rat microsomes. The incubation procedure with human microsomes was similar to that using rat microsomes, the only difference being that the incubation medium now contained 1.92 mg of human microsomal protein.

Recovery of Azone®-derived radioactivity was low, 47.1%, the remainder again having adhered to the walls of the centrifugation tubes. As with the rat microsome experiments, the concave gradient elution resulted in a cluster of peaks eluting at retention times between 56 and 65 min. Therefore, the other elution profiles (isocratic and shallow linear gradient elution; see rat microsome experiments for details) were used to separate the metabolites. The radiochromatograms are depicted in Figures 7B and D. Higher levels of the unchanged Azone® could be detected in the human microsomal incubation medium (8.5%), relative to the rat microsomal incubation medium (<1%). The two profiles in Figures 7C (rat) and 7D (human) show substantial differences, both qualitatively and quantitatively. The largest peak in the rat elutes at 12 min, whereas the human material shows three major peaks, at 3, 11, and 21 min.

Using these chromatographic systems, differences in the initial steps in metabolism between the two species could be demonstrated. This could very well explain the observed differences in the *in vivo* rat and human urinary profiles. On the other hand, the occurrence of some peaks in both the rat and human microsomal profiles may explain the partial overlap of the urinary *in vivo* metabolic profiles of rat and humans.

C. CONCLUSIONS OF *IN VITRO* METABOLISM STUDIES USING AZONE®

Although the metabolites encountered in human urine *in vivo* were not observed in the described *in vitro* experiments, these studies suggest that the use of rat and human liver material may produce valuable information on the initial breakdown of Azone® in these two species. Moreover, as some of the main metabolites produced by human hepatocytes also appeared to be produced by *in vitro* experiments with rat material, the latter may provide a suitable approach to obtain larger quantities for metabolite identification. Hence, careful utilization of the various *in vitro* techniques discussed above appears to provide promising avenues to unravel the initial metabolic pathways of Azone® in humans as well as rats. Once these initial pathways have been established, it may be possible to further clarify the pathways leading to the very polar metabolites that are found in human urine.

IV. SPECULATIONS ON THE METABOLIZING ORGAN AND THE STRUCTURE OF THE METABOLITES OF AZONE®

During its passage through the body, the Azone® molecule penetrates through the skin, is taken up by the blood, transported to all organs, including the liver, and excreted into urine and feces. Based on the discussed experimental findings, it can be speculated that Azone® is predominantly metabolized by the liver. First, metabolism in the SC could be excluded.[12] Subsequently, it was shown that gastrointestinal metabolism of Azone® did not occur or was similar to systemic metabolism.[11] Of the two possibilities, only the liver was studied in more detail. The isolated rat liver clearly demonstrated its ability to metabolize Azone® in accordance with the *in vivo* profiles. These findings clearly indicate that the liver is the primary organ in the metabolism of Azone®, at least in the rat.

No intact human liver was available to conclusively demonstrate the same for the metabolism of Azone® in humans. The rat hepatocyte experiments demonstrated a good correlation between the supernatant at the end of the experiment (Figure 5C) and the rat *in vivo* urine (Figure 1C). Were the liver also the primary organ in the metabolism of Azone® in humans, a good correlation between the human hepatocyte supernatant (Figure 8C) and the human *in vivo* urinary profiles (Figure 1D) would be anticipated. Unfortunately, this correlation was not as good as that for the rat. As explained above, this is likely to be due to the slower uptake of Azone® by the human hepatocyte relative to the rat hepatocyte is sound. The lower viability and concentration of the human hepatocytes slow down the metabolic rate even further. In humans, therefore, Azone® may be primarily metabolized by the liver, although the involvement of other organs cannot be excluded.

None of the methodologies used during these metabolism studies resulted in the generation of sufficient quantities of metabolites of Azone® to allow structure elucidation. Human percutaneous absorption of Azone® was too low, while intravenously administered Azone® in animals resulted in different metabolic profiles. Only the intermediary human metabolite 7 was found to be ionizable. Complete removal of the dodecyl side chain from the Azone® molecule did not occur, which would have resulted in the generation of ε-caprolactam. The metabolism of this compound has been studied in rats.[21] As with Azone®, ε-caprolactam is metabolized to a number of compounds which are excreted in the urine. One of these metabolites is 6-aminohexanoic acid, the hydrolysis product of ε-caprolactam. Two other metabolites have been identified as 6-amino-4-hydroxyhexanoic acid and the corresponding 6-amino-1,4-caprolactone.[21] If the metabolism of Azone® would follow similar metabolic pathways, then *N*-dodecyl-6-aminohexanoic acid, *N*-dodecyl-6-amino-4-hydroxyhexanoic acid, and *N*-dodecyl-6-amino-1,4-caprolactone could be possible metabolites. All these structures do still contain the originally ^{14}C-labeled carbonyl and α-carbon atoms. However, taking the lipophilicity of these structures into account, it seems more likely that these structures are the transient metabolites rather than the final metabolites encountered in human urine. Larger quantities of human metabolites of Azone® will be necessary before proper structure identification by techniques such as mass spectroscopy and nuclear magnetic resonance can be done.

ACKNOWLEDGMENT

The author would like to thank his colleagues in the Department of Analytical Chemistry and Toxicology (Prof. Dr. R. A. de Zeeuw) and the Department of Pharmacology and Therapeutics (Prof. Dr. D. K. F. Meijer) of the University Centre of Pharmacy, Gröningen, The Netherlands. The help and practical advice of Drs. G. M. M. Groothuis and G. W. Sandker during the human hepatocyte experiments is very much appreciated. These studies were supported in part by Whitby Research, Inc., Richmond, VA.

REFERENCES

1. **Wiechers, J. W.,** The barrier function of the skin in relation to percutaneous absorption of drugs, *Pharm. Wkbl. Sci. Ed.,* 11, 185, 1989.
2. **Woodford, R. and Barry, B. W.,** Penetration enhancers and the percutaneous absorption of drugs: an update, *J. Toxicol. Cut. Ocul. Toxicol.,* 5, 165, 1986.

3. **Barry, B. W.,** Optimizing percutaneous absorption, in *Percutaneous Absorption. Mechanisms, Methodology, Drug Delivery,* Bronaugh, R. L. and Maibach, H. I., Eds., Marcel Dekker, New York, 1985, 489.
4. **Stoughton, R. B.,** Enhanced percutaneous penetration with 1-dodecylazacycloheptan-2-one, *Arch. Dermatol.,* 118, 474, 1982.
5. **Stoughton, R. B. and McClure, W. O.,** Azone®: A new non-toxic enhancer of cutaneous penetration, *Drug Dev. Ind. Pharm.,* 9, 725, 1983.
6. **Wiechers, J. W. and De Zeeuw, R. A.,** Transdermal drug delivery: efficacy and potential applications of the penetration enhancer Azone®, *Drug Des. Deliv.,* 6, 87, 1990.
7. **Wiechers, J. W., Drenth, B. F. H., Jonkman, J. H. G., and De Zeeuw, R. A.,** Percutaneous absorption and elimination of the penetration enhancer Azone® in humans, *Pharm. Res.,* 4, 519, 1987.
8. **Wiechers, J. W., Drenth, B. F. H., Jonkman, J. H. G., and De Zeeuw, R. A.,** Percutaneous absorption, metabolism, and elimination of the penetration enhancer Azone® in humans after prolonged application under occlusion, *Int. J. Pharm.,* 47, 43, 1988.
9. **Wiechers, J. W., Drenth, B. F. H., Jonkman, J. H. G., and De Zeeuw, R. A.,** Percutaneous absorption, metabolic profiling, and excretion of the penetration enhancer Azone® after multiple dosing of an Azone-containing triamcinolone acetonide cream in humans, *J. Pharm. Sci.,* 79, 111, 1990.
10. **Wester, R. C., Melendres, J., Sedik, L., and Maibach, H. I.,** Percutaneous absorption of Azone® following single and multiple doses to human volunteers, *J. Pharm. Sci.,* 83, 124, 1994.
11. **Wiechers, J. W., Drenth, B. F. H., Adolfsen, F. A. W., Prins, L., and De Zeeuw, R. A.,** Disposition and metabolic profiling of the penetration enhancer Azone®. I. *In vivo* studies: urinary profiles of hamster, rat, monkey and man, *Pharm. Res.,* 7, 496, 1990.
12. **Wiechers, J. W., Herder, R. E., Drenth, B. F. H., and De Zeeuw, R. A.,** Skin stripping as a potential method to determine *in vivo* cutaneous metabolism of topically applied drugs, *J. Soc. Cosmet. Chem.,* 40, 367, 1989.
13. **Meijer, D. K. F., Keulemans, K., and Mulder, G. J.,** Isolated perfused rat liver technique, in *Methods in Enzymology, Vol. 77: Detoxification and Drug Metabolism: Conjugation and Related Systems,* Jacoby, W. B., Ed., Academic Press, New York, 1981, 81.
14. **Berry, M. N. and Friend, D. S.,** High yield preparation of isolated rat liver parenchymal cells. A biochemical and fine structural study, *J. Cell Biol.,* 43, 506, 1969.
15. **Braakman, L. J., Pijning, T., Verest, O., Weert, B., Meijer, D. F. K., and Groothuis, G. M. M.,** Vesicular uptake systems for the cation lucigenin in the rat hepatocyte, *Mol. Pharmacol.,* 36, 537, 1989.
16. **Chowdhury, J. R. and Arias, I. M.,** Dismutation of bilirubin monoglucuronide, in *Methods in Enzymology, Vol. 77: Detoxification and Drug Metabolism: Conjugation and Related Systems,* Jacoby, W. B., Ed., Academic Press, New York, 1981, 192.
17. **Gerding, T. K., Drenth, B. F. H., and De Zeeuw, R. A.,** Isotopic separation of the drug N-0437 and its diastereomeric glucuronides by high-performance liquid chromatography, *Anal. Biochem.,* 171, 382, 1988.
18. **Gibson, G. G. and Skett, P.,** *Introduction to Drug Metabolism,* Chapman & Hall, London, 1986, chap. 1.
19. **Sandker, G. W., Weert, B., Olinga, P., Wolters, H., Slooff, M. J. H., Meijer, D. K. F., and Groothuis, G. M. M.,** Characterization of transport in isolated human hepatocytes. A study with the bile acid taurocholic acid, the uncharged ouabain and the organic cations vecuronium and recuronium, *Biochem. Pharmacol.,* 47, 2193, 1994.
20. **Sandker, G. W., Vos, R. M. E., Delbressine, L. P. C., Slooff, M. J. H., Meijer, D. K. F., and Groothuis, G. M. M.,** Metabolism of three pharmacologically active drugs in isolated human and rat hepatocytes — analysis of interspecies variability and comparison with metabolism *in vivo, Xenobiotica,* 24, 143, 1994.
21. **Kerschner, L. E.,** Studies on Pectic Substances from Dietary Fiber Sources. I. Identification of Caprolactam Metabolites. II, Ph.D. thesis, Cornell University, Ithaca, NY, 1983.

Chapter 6.5

Azone® Analogues as Penetration Enhancers

Bozena B. Michniak

CONTENTS

I. INTRODUCTION

Azone®, laurocapram, 1-dodecylhexahydro-2*H*-azepine-2-one (Figure 1), is one of a series of *N*-alkylated cyclic amides and was patented in 1976 as a penetration enhancer.[1–11] Several other compounds are known to enhance drug penetration through the stratum corneum (SC) such as dimethylsulfoxide, dimethylacetamide, selected terpenes, 2-pyrrolidinone, phosphine oxides, and surfactants.[12–15] Many, however, have not been used clinically because of suspected pharmacological activity or potential toxicity problems.

Azone® has been shown to be an effective enhancer in relatively low concentrations (1 to 10%) for a variety of hydrophilic and lipophilic drugs.[16] Two pharmacokinetic studies indicate that pure Azone® is poorly absorbed into the human body, and although it rapidly penetrates into the upper levels of the skin, it does not accumulate there. The small quantity that is absorbed is readily metabolized and excreted in the urine.[17–20] A modified Draize test on 200 subjects suggested that Azone® did not induce any allergic contact sensitization, although some mild irritation was initially observed.[21] Skin irritation occurred when Azone® was applied in conjunction with other formulation excipients, particularly propylene glycol (PG). This effect was significant with high concentrations of PG.[22]

It must be stressed that the final degree of enhancement produced by these compounds depends upon the vehicle, additional formulation excipients, solubility parameters, level of skin hydration (occluded/nonoccluded), enhancer concentration, skin model chosen *(in vivo/in vitro),* skin thickness, species chosen (hairless mouse, human), application site, age, sex, skin condition (presence or absence of a functioning barrier), etc.

Most studies utilize a variety of techniques, which can pose problems when comparisons need to be made. A continual effort has been made over the years to identify compounds with activity similar to or surpassing that of Azone®. Many of these investigations have the additional objective of relating enhancer chemical

0-8493-2605-2/95/$0.00+$.50

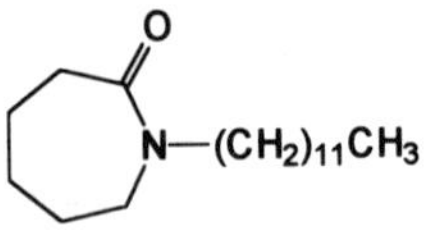

O
N—$(CH_2)_{11}CH_3$

Figure 1 Chemical structure of Azone®.

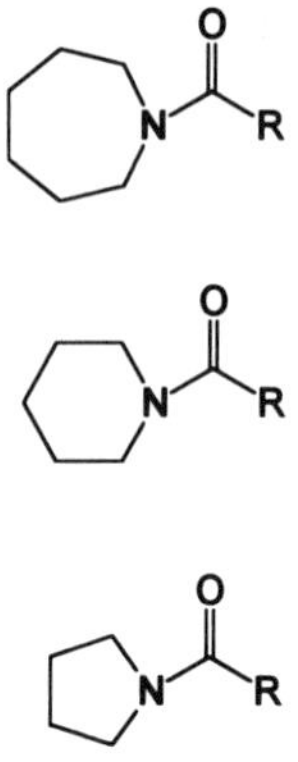

R	Compound
$-(CH_2)_6CH_3$	**1**
$-(CH_2)_{10}CH_3$	**2**
$-(CH_2)_{14}CH_3$	**3**
$-(CH_2)_6CH_3$	**4**
$-(CH_2)_{10}CH_3$	**5**
$-(CH_2)_{14}CH_3$	**6**
$-(CH_2)_6CH_3$	**7**
$-(CH_2)_{10}CH_3$	**8**
$-(CH_2)_{14}CH_3$	**9**

Figure 2 Hexamethylene lauramide **(2)** and its derivatives.

structures to their activity and possible mechanisms of action. One approach has been to examine agents with modified Azone® structures — the Azone® analogue approach.

II. HEXAMETHYLENE LAURAMIDE DERIVATIVES

Hexamethylene lauramide (hexahydro-1-lauroyl-1*H*-azepine) was evaluated together with several amides of cyclic amines (pyrrolidine, piperidine, and hexahydro-1*H*-azepine) (Figure 2).[23] These were tested using hairless mouse skin both *in vitro* and *in vivo.* For the *in vitro* study, the enhancers were applied at 5% (w/w) in 20% (w/w) PG, and this was adjusted to 100% (w/w) with alcohol. Model drugs tested were hydrocortisone 1%, griseofulvin 1%, and erythromycin 2%. Hexamethylene lauramide (**2**) was found to be the most effective broad spectrum compound. For hydrocortisone, percent of diffusion ± S.D. was 70 ± 8 with **3;** 67 ± 6 with **2;** 46 ± 8 with **1;** and 64 ± 6 with Azone® (Table 1). The *in vitro* diffusion of hydrocortisone was also determined following pretreatment with enhancers *in vivo.* The data suggested that the longer the pretreatment, the lower the amount of hydrocortisone penetrated, and also that penetration through dead skin was slower than that through living skin.

All amides showed penetration enhancement to variable degrees, depending on the model drug used. In general, larger rings and longer chains seemed to have a higher enhancing ability. It must be noted, however, that all compounds exhibited relatively high enhancement *in vitro,* and major differences between the enhancers were observed only in the *in vivo* studies.

Table 1 Diffusion of Model Drugs Through Hairless Mouse Skin

	% Diffusion ± S.D.[a]		
Enhancer	**Hydrocortisone (1%)**	**Griseofulvin (1%)**	**Erythromycin (2%)**
Control	1.4 ± 1	<1	1.6 ± 0.5
1	46 ± 8	6 ± 2	21 ± 10
2	67 ± 6	31 ± 17	20 ± 10
3	70 ± 8	14 ± 7	22 ± 12
4	41 ± 17	17[b]	19 ± 7
5	67 ± 7	33 ± 15	18 ± 5
6	64 ± 10	33[b]	23 ± 7
7	15 ± 2	ND[c]	2 ± 1
8	83 ± 11	26 ± 5	18 ± 3
9	60 ± 9	ND	35 ± 10
Azone®	64 ± 6	36 ± 19	24 ± 10

[a] $n = 5$ to 12.
[b] $n = 2$.
[c] Not determined.

From Mirejovsky, D. and Takruri, H., *J. Pharm. Sci.*, 75, 1089, 1986. Reproduced with permission of the American Pharmaceutical Association.

These investigations were continued by Tang-Liu et al.[24] using hexamethylene lauramide as enhancer and hydrocortisone as the model drug. This study utilized the rat isolated sandwich skin flap model, which allowed direct measurement of drug levels in the skin blood supply as well as in the systemic circulation. The skin penetration of 1% w/w hydrocortisone into the systemic circulation increased 3.5-fold following topical application of a formulation containing the steroid and 21% hexamethylene lauramide. The authors found high concentrations (3000-fold) of enhancer in the epidermis as compared to that in cutaneous blood. The enhancer was recovered in urine (85%) and feces (13%). Hexamethylene lauramide was metabolized extensively to a polar species, but no attempt was made to identify the metabolites.

III. AZACYCLOALKANONE DERIVATIVES

Okamoto et al.[25] screened nine azacycloalkanone analogues with 5-, 6-, and 7-membered rings using guinea pig skin *in vitro* and model drug 6-mercaptopurine. The enhancers included: 1-geranylazacycloheptan-2-one **(10),** 1-farnesylazacycloheptan-2-one **(11),** 1-geranylgeranylazacycloheptan-2-one **(12),** 1-(3,7-dimethyloctyl)azacycloheptan-2-one **(13),** 1-(3,7,11-trimethyldodecyl)azacycloheptan-2-one **(14),** 1-geranylazacyclohexan-2-one **(15),** 1-geranylgeranylazacyclohexan-2-one **(16),** 1-geranylazacyclopentan-2,5-dione **(17),** 1-farnesylazacyclopentan-2-one **(18),** and Azone® (Figures 1 and 3). Skin retention and percutaneous penetration of 6-mercaptopurine was significantly enhanced by pretreatment of the skin with **10, 11,** and **18.** These compounds were also found to be the least irritating to the skin. Compounds **13, 16,** and Azone® showed the largest daily primary irritation indices for erythema and edema following 24-h application of enhancer (100%). Longer carbon chain lengths, e.g., C_{20}, produced less enhancement. No correlation was noted between enhancer activity and ring size.

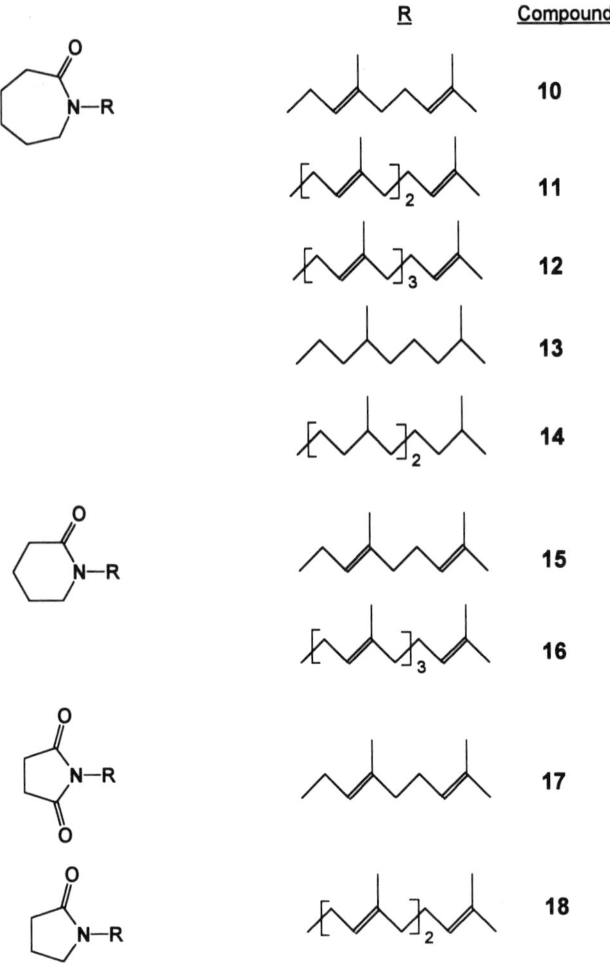

Figure 3 1-alkyl- and 1-alkenylazacycloalkanone derivatives.

An increase in the number of carbonyl groupings in the ring also caused a reduction in activity. Enhancers **11** and **15** were the most active for both 6-mercaptopurine and mitomycin C.[26,27] In a later study the penetration of indomethacin, triamcinolone acetonide, 5-fluorouracil, sulfanilic acid, butylparaben, and acyclovir, in addition to 6-mercaptopurine, was investigated using Azone®, **10,** and **11** in aqueous and ethanolic systems.[28] Drugs possessing *n*-octanol/water partition coefficients close to 1.0 e.g., 5-fluorouracil and 6-mercaptopurine, exhibited higher penetration rates following pretreatment with these enhancers. The enhancement was highest using the aqueous system.

Several studies dealt with the correlation of enhancer activity and the effects on the SC lipids, with reference to *N*-alkylazacycloheptanones[29–32] (see also Chapter 6.2 of this book). Several Azones® were synthesized by Hoogstraate et al.,[29] including C_6, C_8, C_{10}, C_{12}, and C_{14}. Permeation studies were conducted using human SC *in vitro* pretreated with 0.15 *M* enhancer in PG, and two model drugs, nitroglycerin and desglycinamide-8-arginine vasopressin (5 m*M*).[29,30] Control peptide flux was 1 pmol/h/cm^2 (donor drug concentration: 5 m*M*). The permeability coefficient was 5.3 ± 0.6 × 10^{-11} cm/s. Enhancement ratios (E.R.) were highest for C_{14} (E.R. = 2.5) and C_{12} Azone® (E.R. = 3.5). Enhancement ratios with nitroglycerin (0.05% in 5% ethanol) were highest with C_8, C_{10}, and C_{14} Azones®.

Thermal analysis of the SC following treatment with *N*-alkylazones with C_6 chains or longer showed the highest mobility of lipids.[31,32] Small-angle X-ray studies showed that larger chain lengths (C_{10} or more) significantly affected the order of the lamellar lipid structure.[31,33] It was also concluded from IC_{50} cytotoxicity values that a correlation existed between membrane-mediated toxic effects and increasing enhancement effects.[30]

Schückler and Lee[34] studied the transport of diazepam through human SC following treatment with 0 to 30% w/w Azone® and dodecyl-L-pyroglutamate (DLP). Azone® was found to have a significant influence on diffusivity as compared to DLP at concentrations of 0 to 12%. Permeation rates were higher or relatively the same for both enhancers up to this concentration. At loading concentrations of 10 to 24% DLP showed a sudden increase as compared to Azone® permeation, which plateaued at this range.

Differential scanning calorimetry (DSC) data indicated that less DLP was taken up by the SC as compared to Azone®; hence, higher concentrations of DLP were required to cause lipid disruption patterns similar to those produced by Azone®.

Several azocycloalkanone derivatives were tested in hairless mouse skin *in vitro* using a saturated suspension of hydrocortisone 21-acetate in PG.[35,36] All enhancers were applied at 0.4 *M* in the same vehicle 1 h prior to the model drug. Chemical structures of the seven enhancers tested are given in Figure 4.

Enhancers **24** and **25** gave similar 24-h receptor concentrations (Q_{24}) to Azone®; however, skin contents of the steroid were higher with **20, 21, 22, 23,** and **24** than with Azone®. However, all enhancers showed some degree of enhancement as compared to the control (no enhancer) (Table 2).

IV. CYCLOHEXANONE DERIVATIVES

Akitoshi et al.[37] investigated several cyclohexanone derivatives on the percutaneous penetration of indomethacin and ketoprofen from gel ointments through shaved rat skin *in vivo* (Figure 5). The drugs were incorporated in carboxyvinyl polymer/sodium polyacrylate gels and 1.5 g was applied in a glass cell to the skin of the rat. The absorption of both drugs was significantly enhanced by 2-*t*-butylcyclohexanone **(29),** then by 2,6-dimethylcyclohexanone **(28)** and 4-*t*-butylcyclohexanone **(30),** and little if any effect was seen with cyclohexanone and its 2-methyl and 3-methyl analogues (**26** and **27**). In general, dimethyl derivatives were more effective than monomethyl derivatives.

2-*n*-Octylcyclohexanone was the most effective enhancer and parabolic behavior was observed for the series; i.e., enhancement increased initially with increasing carbon chain length, reached a maximum, and then decreased. Such behavior was reported for other series of enhancers, e.g., alkanols and alkanoic acids[38] and saturated fatty acids.[39] Quan et al.[40] concluded that the cyclohexanone derivatives exert

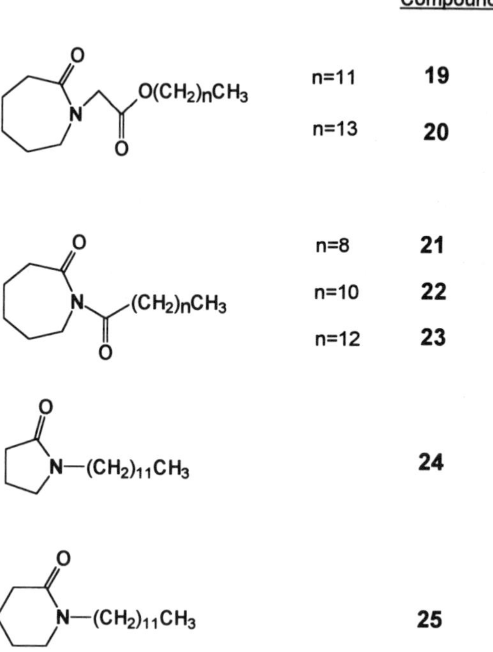

Figure 4 Azacycloalkanone derivatives.

Table 2 Effect of Enhancers **19** to **25** on 24-h Diffusion Cell Receptor Concentrations (Q_{24}) and Skin Contents of Hydrocortisone 21-Acetate (HCA) of Hairless Mouse Skin

Enhancer in PG[a]	Q_{24} (μM)	E.R.[b] $_{Q_{24}}$	Skin HCA Content (μg/g)	Skin HC[c] Content (μg/g)	E.R.[b] (HC + HCA)
Control (n = 8)	0.751 ± 0.250	1.00	285.2 ± 21.6	ND[e]	1.0
Azone® (n = 5)	28.760 ± 4.624	38.30	410.6 ± 34.4	9.9 ± 2.5	1.5
19	2.905 ± 1.092	3.87	435.7 ± 37.9	13.5 ± 1.9	1.6
20[d]	2.411 ± 1.046	3.25	2167.4 ± 85.9	ND	7.6
21	11.231 ± 3.065	14.96	508.4 ± 18.3	7.3 ± 2.1	1.8
22	13.780 ± 3.595	18.35	650.3 ± 28.4	6.1 ± 0.9	2.3
23	16.059 ± 3.989	21.38	675.3 ± 29.6	9.8 ± 0.8	2.4
24	25.371 ± 2.179	33.78	624.5 ± 16.9	9.5 ± 1.2	2.2
25	26.564 ± 3.199	35.37	431.0 ± 20.4	12.1 ± 2.4	1.6

[a] Propylene glycol.
[b] Enhancement ratio.
[c] Hydrocortisone.
[d] Applied at 0.136 M (saturation solubility).
[e] Not detected.

From Michniak, B.B., Player, M.R., Chapman, M.J., Jr., and Sowell, J.W., Sr., *Int. J. Pharm.*, 91, 85, 1993 and Michniak, B.B., Player, M.R., Fuhrman, L.C., Christensen, C.A., Chapman, J.M., Jr., and Sowell, J.W., Sr., *Int. J. Pharm.*, 94, 203, 1993. With permission.

	Compound
2-methyl	**26**
3-methyl	**27**
2,6-dimethyl	**28**
2-*t*-butyl	**29**
4-*t*-butyl	**30**
m=3; 2-n-butyl	**31**
m=5; 2-n-hexyl	**32**
m=7; 2-n-octyl	**33**
m=9; 2-n-decyl	**34**
m=11; 2-n-lauryl	**35**
m=15; 2-n-cetyl	**36**

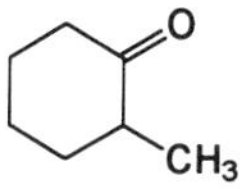

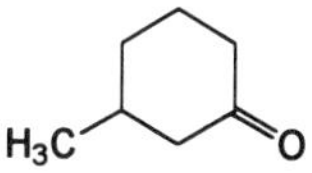

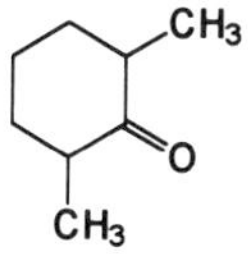

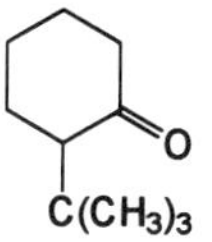

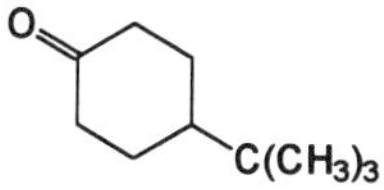

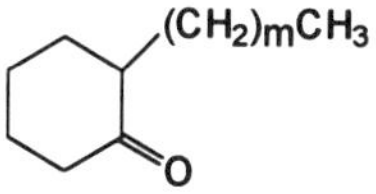

Figure 5 Cyclohexanone and 2-*n*-alkyl cyclohexanone derivatives tested as potential enhancers.

their enhancement by fluidizing and modifying the hydrophobic barrier of the SC. These studies were performed using differential scanning calorimetry and pig SC.

V. MISCELLANEOUS DERIVATIVES

Michniak et al.[35,36] synthesized and screened 14 Azone® analogues using hairless mouse skin *in vitro* and the model drug hydrocortisone 21-acetate (Figure 6). Compound **37** exhibited the highest enhancement ratio for model drug amounts delivered across the skin as well as into the skin (Table 3). Most of the derivatives were not as effective as Azone® in delivering steroid transdermally, but **37, 39, 43, 44, 45,** and **46** all delivered more drug than Azone® into full-thickness hairless mouse skin. Thioamide enhancers were less effective than their oxygen-containing counterparts (**44, 45, 46**). The difference between drug delivery transdermally and skin retention

		Compound
$O(CH_2)_2N(CH_2)_nCH_3$ cyclic	n=9	**37**
	n=11	**38**
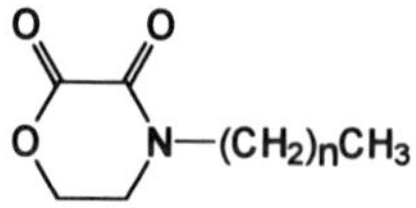	n=11	**39**
	n=13	**40**
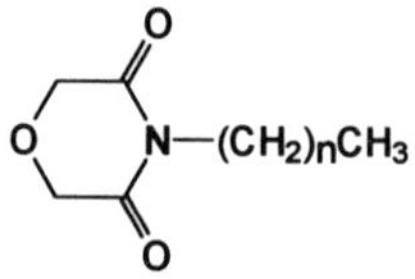	n=11	**41**
	n=13	**42**
$N-(CH_2)_{11}CH_3$		**43**
$N-(CH_2)_{11}CH_3$		**44**
$N-(CH_2)_{11}CH_3$		**45**
$N-(CH_2)_{11}CH_3$		**46**
$(CH_2)_{10}CH_3$		**47**
$(CH_2)_{10}CH_3$		**48**
$(CH_2)_{10}CH_3$		**49**
$(CH_2)_{10}CH_3$		**50**

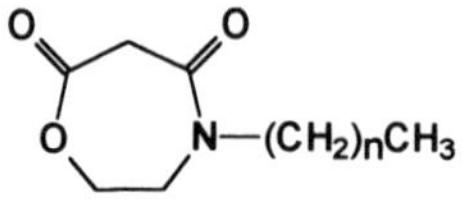

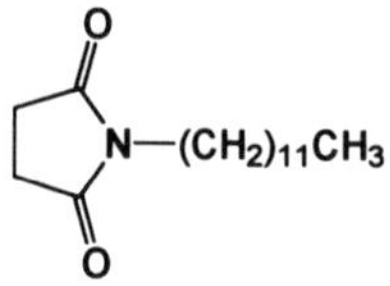

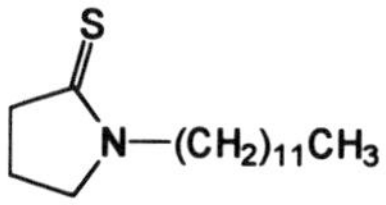

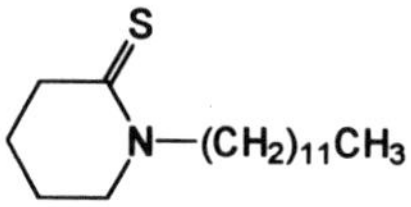

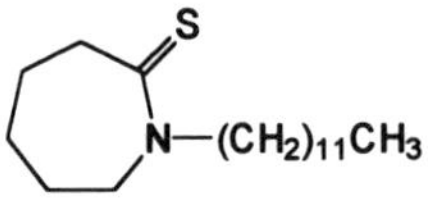

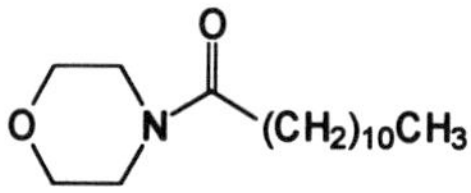

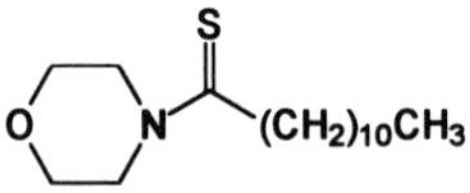

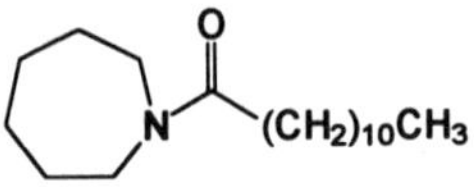

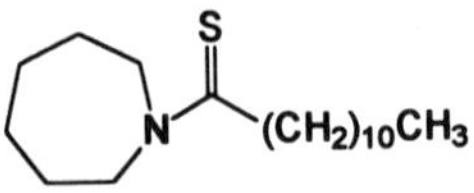

Figure 6 Azone® analogues tested as enhancers in hairless mouse skin using hydrocortisone 21-acetate.

Table 3 Effect Of Enhancers **37** To **50** On 24-h Diffusion Cell Receptor Concentrations (Q_{24}) And Skin Contents Of Hydrocortisone 21-Acetate (HCA) Of Hairless Mouse Skin

Enhancer in PG[a]	Q_{24} (μ*M*)	E.R.$^{b}_{Q_{24}}$	Skin HCA Content (μg/g)	Skin HC[c] Content (μg/g)	E.R.[b] Skin (HC + HCA)
Control (*n* = 8)	0.751 ± 0.250	1.00	285.2 ± 21.6	ND[e]	1.0
Azone® (*n* = 5)	28.760 ± 4.624	38.30	410.6 ± 34.4	9.9 ± 2.5	1.5
37 (*n* = 5)	57.471 ± 6.425	76.89	1467.9 ± 95.0	27.6 ± 3.4	5.2
38 (*n* = 5)	22.475 ± 4.299	29.93	324.2 ± 23.9	20.1 ± 2.3	1.2
39[d] (*n* = 5)	14.782 ± 1.995	19.68	729.4 ± 25.7	3.7 ± 0.7	2.6
40[d] (*n* = 5)	4.362 ± 1.486	5.81	296.1 ± 21.3	2.1 ± 0.6	1.1
41 (*n* = 5)	9.635 ± 1.626	12.83	337.7 ± 18.2	6.6 ± 1.2	1.2
42 (*n* = 5)	10.874 ± 2.091	14.48	360.8 ± 19.5	8.6 ± 2.1	1.3
43 (*n* = 5)	11.150 ± 3.152	14.85	874.4 ± 29.2	11.3 ± 3.6	3.1
44[d] (*n* = 5)	8.640 ± 1.399	11.50	598.7 ± 19.9	6.7 ± 1.1	2.1
45[d] (*n* = 5)	6.529 ± 1.986	8.69	571.8 ± 20.7	2.0 ± 0.9	2.0
46[d] (*n* = 5)	2.259 ± 0.564	3.00	541.3 ± 15.6	ND	1.9
47 (*n* = 5)	22.039 ± 2.066	29.35	274.5 ± 17.5	6.9 ± 1.1	1.0
48[d] (*n* = 5)	4.391 ± 0.099	5.85	245.2 ± 21.9	ND	0.9
49 (*n* = 5)	14.307 ± 1.708	19.05	412.3 ± 20.6	9.9 ± 2.2	1.5
50[d] (*n* = 5)	5.091 ± 1.151	6.78	272.8 ± 10.2	ND	1.0

[a] Propylene glycol.
[b] Enhancement ratio.
[c] Hydrocortisone.
[d] Applied at saturation solubility: **39** at 0.113 *M;* **40** at 0.051 *M;* **44** at 0.179 *M;* **45** at 0.187 *M;* **46** at 0.163 *M;* **48** at 0.069 *M;* and **50** at 0.090 *M.*
[e] Not detected.

From Michniak, B.B., Player, M.R., Chapman, J.M., Jr., and Sowell, J.W., Sr., *Int. J. Pharm.,* 91, 85, 1993 and Michniak, B.B., Player, M.R., Fuhrman, L.C., Christensen, C.A., Chapman, J.M., Jr., and Sowell, J.W., Sr., *Int. J. Pharm.,* 94, 203, 1993. With permission.

may be useful when enhancer selection is made for either transdermal patches or topical formulations.

Several azacycloalkenes were patented in 1992 by Minaskanian and Peck[41] as transdermal enhancers: 1-*n*-dodecylazacyclohept-3-ene-2-one; 1-*n*-dodecylazacyclohept-4-ene-2-one; 1-*n*-dodecyl-3-methylazacyclohept-3-ene-2-one; 1-*n*-dodecyl-3-methylazacyclohept-4-ene-2-one; 1-*n*-dodecanoylazacyclohept-3-ene-2-one; 1-*n*-dodecanoylazacyclohept-4-ene-2-one; 1-*n*-dodecanoylazacylohept-3-ene; 1-*n*-dodecanoylazacyclohept-4-ene; 1-*n*-dodecanoylazacyclopent-3-ene; 1-*n*-dodecylazacyclohept-3-ene-2-thione; and 1-*n*-dodecylazacyclohept-4-ene-2-thione. All were recommended for use in several dosage forms at a concentration between 1 and 10%.

Bonina et al.[42] reported a novel prodrug approach using 1-alkylazacycloalkan-2-one esters of indomethacin (Figure 7). 1-Methylazacycloalkan-2-one esters were unstable in aqueous media, but 1-ethyl derivatives were more stable. The latter also exhibited greater percutaneous penetration through human skin *in vitro.* When flux was plotted against the lipophilic index of esters **51** to **58,** a parabolic relationship was observed, the maximum being reported with ester **56.** Control indomethacin flux μg/cm²/h ± S.D. was 0.083 ± 0.016; for **55:** 0.287 ± 0.013; **56:** 0.343 ± 0.007; **57:** 0.275 ± 0.011, and **58:** 0.068 ± 0.028.

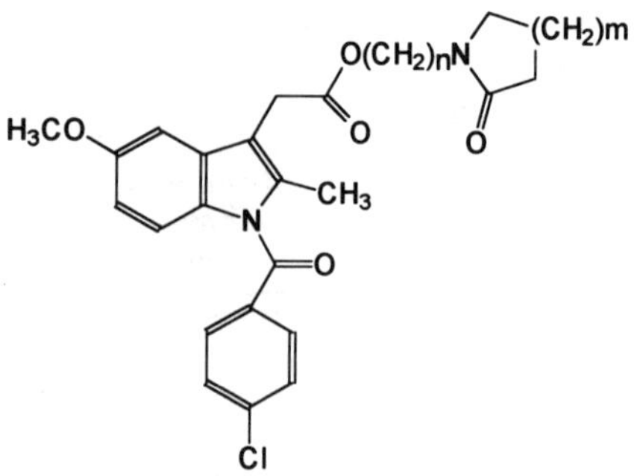

n=1; m=1	**51**
n=1; m=2	**52**
n=1; m=3	**53**
n=1; m=4	**54**
n=2; m=1	**55**
n=2; m=2	**56**
n=2; m=3	**57**
n=2; m=4	**58**

Figure 7 Chemical structures of 1-alkylazacycloalkan-2-one esters of indomethacin.

ACKNOWLEDGMENT

The author wishes to thank Mark Player, M.D. for helpful discussions and for the preparation of figures, and Emily Willingham for typing the manuscript.

REFERENCES

1. **Rajadhyaksha, V. J.,** U.S. Patent 3,989,815, 1976.
2. **Rajadhyaksha, V. J.,** U.S. Patent 3,991,203, 1976.
3. **Rajadhyaksha, V. J.,** U.S. Patent 4,122,170, 1978.
4. **Rajadhyaksha, V. J.,** U.S. Patent 4,405,616, 1983.
5. **Rajadhyaksha, V. J.,** U.S. Patent 4,415,563, 1983.
6. **Rajadhyaksha, V. J.,** U.S. Patent 4,423,040, 1983.
7. **Rajadhyaksha, V. J.,** U.S. Patent 4,424,210, 1984.
8. **Rajadhyaksha, V. J.,** U.S. Patent 4,444,762, 1984.
9. **Rajadhyaksha, V. J.,** U.S. Patent 3,989,816, 1976.
10. **Rajadhyaksha, V. J.,** U.S. Patent 4,316,893, 1982.
11. **Rajadhyaksha, V. J., Peck, J. V., and Miniskanian, G.,** U.S. Patent 4,422,970, 1983.
12. **Stoughton, R. B. and Fritsch, W. E.,** Influence of dimethylsulfoxide (DMSO) on human percutaneous absorption, *Arch. Dermatol.*, 90, 512, 1964.
13. **Barry, B. W.,** *Dermatological Formulations: Percutaneous Absorption,* Marcel Dekker, New York, 1983, 160.
14. **Munro, D. D. and Stoughton, R. B.,** Dimethylacetamide (DMAC) and dimethylformamide (DMFA) effect on percutaneous absorption, *Arch. Dermatol.*, 92, 585, 1965.
15. **Williams, A. C. and Barry, B. W.,** Terpenes and the lipid-protein-partitioning theory of skin penetration enhancement, *Pharm. Res.*, 8, 17, 1991.

16. **Hadgraft, J., Williams, D. G., and Allan, G.,** Azone®. Mechanisms of action and clinical effect, in *Pharmaceutical Skin Penetration Enhancement,* Walters, K. A. and Hadgraft, J., Eds., Marcel Dekker, New York, 1993, 182.
17. **Wiechers, J. W., Jonkman, J. H. G., and de Zeeuw, R. A.,** Percutaneous absorption and elimination of the penetration enhancer Azone® in humans, *Pharm. Res.,* 4, 519, 1987.
18. **Wiechers, J. W., Drenth, B. F. H., Jonkman, J. H. G., and de Zeeuw, R. A.,** Percutaneous absorption, metabolic profiling, and excretion of the penetration enhancer Azone® after multiple dosing of an Azone-containing triaminolone acetonide cream in humans, *J. Pharm. Sci.,* 79, 111, 1990.
19. **Wiechers, J. W., Drenth, B. F. H., Adolfson, F. A., Prins, L., and de Zeeuw, R. A.,** Disposition and metabolic profiling of the penetration enhancer Azone®. I. *In vivo* studies: urinary profiles of hamster, rat, monkey, and man, *Pharm. Res.,* 7, 496, 1990.
20. **Wiechers, J. W., Drenth, B., Jonkman, J., and de Zeeuw, R. A.,** Percutaneous absorption of triaminolone acetonide from creams with and without Azone® in humans *in vivo, Int. J. Pharm.,* 66, 53, 1990.
21. Data on file, Whitby Research, Inc., Richmond, VA.
22. **Vaidyanathan, R., Rajdhyaksha, V. J., Kim, B. K., and Anisko, J. J.,** Azone®, in *Transdermal Delivery of Drugs,* Vol. 2, Kydonieus, A. F. and Berner, B., Eds., CRC Press, Boca Raton, FL, 1987, 68.
23. **Mirejovsky, D. and Takruri, H.,** Dermal penetration enhancement profile of hexamethylene lauramide and its homologues: *in vitro* versus *in vivo* behavior of enhancers in the penetration of hydrocortisone, *J. Pharm. Sci.,* 75, 1089, 1986.
24. **Tang-Liu, D., Neff, J., Zolezio, H., and Sandri, R.,** Percutaneous and systemic disposition of hexamethylene lauramide and its penetration enhancement effect on hydrocortisone in a rat sandwich skin-flap model, *Pharm. Res.,* 5, 477, 1988.
25. **Okamoto, H., Hashida, M., and Sezaki, H.,** Structure-activity relationship of 1-alkyl- or 1-alkenylazacycloalkanone derivatives as percutaneous penetration enhancers, *J. Pharm. Sci.,* 77, 418, 1988.
26. **Okamoto, H., Ohyabu, M., Hashida, M., and Sezaki, H.,** Enhanced penetration of mitomycin C through hairless mouse and rat skin by enhancers with terpene moieties, *J. Pharm. Pharmacol.,* 39, 531, 1987.
27. **Okamoto, H., Tsukahara, H., Hashida, M., and Sezaki, H.,** Effect of 1-alkyl- or 1-alkenylazacycloalkanone derivatives on penetration of mitomycin C through rat skin, *Chem. Pharm. Bull.,* 35, 4605, 1987.
28. **Okamoto, H., Hashida, M., and Sezaki, H.,** Effect of 1-alkyl- or 1-alkenylazacycloalkanone derivatives on the penetration of drugs with different lipophilicities through guinea pig skin, *J. Pharm. Sci.,* 80, 39, 1991.
29. **Hoogstraate, A. J., Verhoef, J., Brussee, J., IJzerman, A. P., Spies, F., and Boddé, H. E.,** Kinetics, ultrastructural aspects and molecular modeling of transdermal peptide flux enhancement by *N*-alkylazacycloheptanones, *Int. J. Pharm.,* 76, 37, 1991.
30. **Boddé, H. H., Ponec, M., IJzerman, A. P., Hoogstraate, A. J., Salomons, M. A., and Bouwstra, J.,** *In vitro* analysis of QSAR in wanted and unwanted effects of azacycloheptanones as transdermal penetration enhancers, in *Pharmaceutical Skin Penetration Enhancement,* Walters, K. A. and Hadgraft, J., Eds., Marcel Dekker, New York, 1993, 199.
31. **Bouwstra, J. A., Gooris, G. S., Brussee, J., Salomons-de Vries, M. A., and Bras, W.,** The influence of alkyl-azones on the ordering of the lamellae in human SC, *Int. J. Pharm.,* 79, 141, 1992.
32. **Bouwstra, J. A., Peschier, L. J. C., Brussee, J., and Boddé, H. E.,** Effect of *N*-azacyclohepan-2-ones including Azone® on the thermal behavior of human SC, *Int. J. Pharm.,* 52, 47, 1989.
33. **Bouwstra, J. A., DeVries, M. A., Bras, W., Brussee, J., and Gooris, G. S.,** The influence of C_n azones on the structure and thermal behavior of human SC, *Proc. Int. Symp. Control. Rel. Bioact. Mater.,* 17, 33, 1990.
34. **Schückler, F. and Lee, G.,** Relating the concentration-dependent action of Azone® and dodecyl-L-pyroglutamate on the structure of excised human SC to changes in drug diffusivity, partition coefficient, and flux, *Int. J. Pharm.,* 80, 81, 1992.
35. **Michniak, B. B., Player, M. R., Chapman, J. M., Jr., and Sowell, J. W., Sr.,** *In vitro* evaluation of a series of Azone® analogs as dermal penetration enhancers. I., *Int. J. Pharm.,* 91, 85, 1993.

36. **Michniak, B. B., Player, M. R., Fuhrman, L. C., Christensen, C. A., Chapman, J. M., Jr., and Sowell, J. W., Sr.,** *In vitro* evaluation of a series of Azone® analogs as dermal penetration enhancers. II. (Thio)amides, *Int. J. Pharm.,* 94, 203, 1993.
37. **Akitoshi, Y., Takayama, K., Machida, Y., and Nagai, T.,** Effect of cyclohexanone derivatives on percutaneous absorption of ketoprofen and indomethacin, *Drug Des. Deliv.,* 2, 239, 1988.
38. **Liron, Z. and Cohen, S.,** Percutaneous absorption of alkanoic acids. II. Application of regular solution theory, *J. Pharm. Sci.,* 73, 538, 1984.
39. **Chien, Y. W.,** Development concepts and practice in transdermal therapeutic systems, in *Transdermal Controlled Systemic Medications,* Chien, Y. W., Ed., Marcel Dekker, New York, 1987, 73.
40. **Quan, D., Takayama, K., and Nagai, T.,** Effect of cyclohexanone derivatives on *in vitro* percutaneous absorption of indomethacin, *Drug Des. Deliv.,* 4, 323, 1989.
41. **Minaskanian, G. and Peck, J. V.,** U.S. Patent 5,142,044, 1992.
42. **Bonina, F. P., Montenegro, L., De Capraris, P., Bousquet, E., and Tirendi, S.,** 1-Alkylazacycloalkan-2-one esters as prodrugs of indomethacin for improved delivery through human skin, *Int. J. Pharm.,* 77, 21, 1991.

Chapter 6.6

Interaction of Azone® with Model Lipid Systems

Geoffrey Lee

CONTENTS

I. INTRODUCTION

Goodman and Barry's work in the mid 1980s using differential scanning calorimetry (DSC) showed that Azone® (1-dodecylazacycloheptan-2-one) interacts strongly with the lipid fraction of intact human stratum corneum (SC).[1–3] Based on this evidence, Barry[4] postulated the molecular locations for the action of Azone® within the intercellular lipid structure. His intuitive suggestion was that the Azone® molecule inserts within the hydrocarbon region of the extended bilayer structure formed by the SC lipids. The geometric packing is disturbed and the fluidity is increased, resulting in a substantial decrease in the barrier property of the intercellular lipid structure.

Although Barry could provide no structural evidence to support his hypothysis, he had at least attempted to explain the enhancing action of Azone® on the molecular level. The molecular interactions between Azone® and the SC lipid structure are, however, difficult to examine because of the relative inaccessibility of the latter to direct experiment; the lipid structure exists only in small amounts between compressed layers of corneocytes. The DSC technique provides no direct structural information and is notoriously liable to overinterpretation. X-ray scattering provides direct evidence of the structural changes induced by Azone® in the intercellular lipid fraction of intact SC,[5] but requires a high-power X-ray source to obtain satisfactory resolution for the tiny amounts of lipid present. Fourier transform infrared spectroscopy (FTIR) is a readily available method for identifying molecular interactions in lipid systems,[6] but again, the resolution is poor with intact SC.[7] Additionally, the unknown lipid composition of the particular SC membrane under examination complicates spectral interpretation.

Because of these technical difficulties with intact SC membranes, some researchers have used artificial lipid systems to serve as models for the lipid fraction of the SC. Their composition is known precisely and can be varied at will to examine the importance of individual components.[8,9] The influence of a foreign substance such as Azone® on their structure can be readily determined using standard techniques. The selection of suitable model lipids is clearly a critical question. Table 1 shows us the

0-8493-2605-2/95/$0.00+$.50

Table 1 Lipid Composition Of Abdominal Human SC[10,11]

Substance	mol%
Polar lipids	
Phosphatidylethanolamine	Trace
Cholesterol sulfate	2
Neutral lipids	
Cholesterol	22
Fatty acids	42
C14:0 3.8%	
C16:0 36.8%	
C16:1 3.6%	
C18:0 9.9%	
C18:1 33.1%	
C18:2 12.5%	
C20:0 0.3%	
C20:1 trace	
C22:0 trace	
Triglycerides	Trace
Hydrocarbons, sterol wax esters	10
Sphingolipids	
Ceramides	24

lipid composition determined for abdominal SC and discussed by Elias.[10] The free fatty acids, sphingolipids and cholesterol together make up >85 mol% of the total lipids. The ratio of saturated:unsaturated fatty acids present is approximately 1:1.[11] Of note is the virtual absence of phospholipids. This complex mixture forms the extended intercellular bilayer structure which can be seen within intact SC using RuO_4 staining.[12] The action of Azone® has been examined using either phospholipids, acknowledged SC lipids, or other amphiphiles. Three different types of lipid structure have been investigated:

1. Aqueous dispersions of liposomes
2. Monomolecular lipid films at the water–air interface
3. Extended bilayer structures prepared from mixtures of lipid and water

This chapter considers critically the results obtained with each of these studies.

II. STUDIES ON LIPOSOMAL DISPERSIONS

Evidence that Azone® can influence the fluidity of lipid acyl chains was first obtained using aqueous dispersions of multilamellar vesicles (MLVs). Beastall et al.[13] selected L-α-dipalmitoyl phosphatidylcholine (DPPC) as a model lipid. A questionable choice, perhaps, as its $L_{\beta'}$-L_α transition temperature (T_m) of 41.4°C is much lower than the endothermic lipid transition found at 68° to 75°C with intact human SC.[14] The effect of Azone® on this T_m was determined by measuring the decrease in turbidity of an MLV dispersion, which occurs as the temperature increases through T_m. This technique was sufficiently sensitive to detect the L_β-$L_{\beta'}$ pretransition of the DPPC at 30°C (see Figure 1). The presence of Azone® within the MLVs reduces T_m linearly (Figure 2) as well as broadening the transition and abolishing the pretransition. The inclusion of approximately 50 mol% Azone® reduces T_m sufficiently to produce a

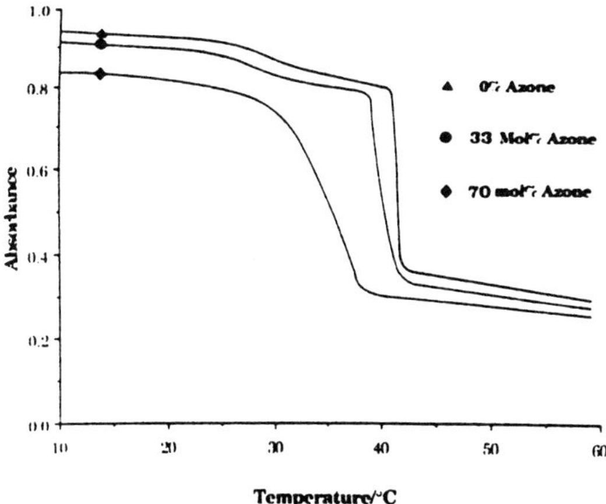

Figure 1 Absorbance-temperature profiles for DPPC MLVs containing Azone®. (From Beastall, J. et al., *Int. J. Pharm.*, 43, 207, 1988. With permission.)

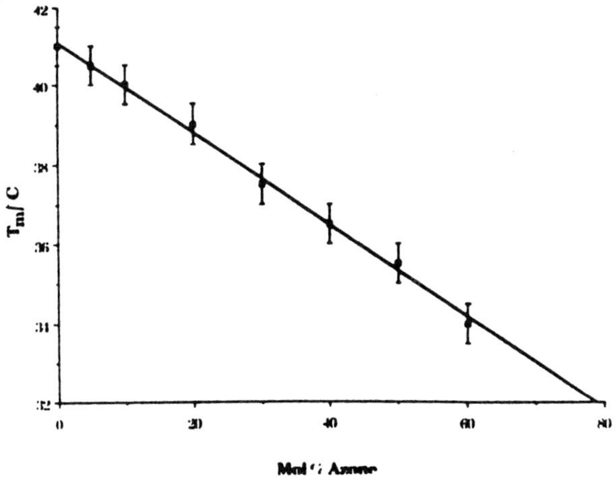

Figure 2 Transition temperature of DPPC MLVs as a function of Azone® concentration. (From Beastall, J. et al., *Int. J. Pharm.*, 43, 207, 1988. With permission.)

liquid crystalline structure at SC temperature (approximately 35°C). The authors' conclusion that topically applied Azone® could induce the same effect within intact SC is, however, flawed because of the much higher transition temperature of the SC lipids. Much more convincing is their finding, using the lipophilic fluorescent probe, pyrene, that Azone® alters the lipid fluidity of DPPC in small unilamellar vesicles (SUVs). The ratio of pyrene excimer:monomer emission at 35°C, I_e:I_m, a direct measure of lipid fluidity[15] at SC temperature, increases on addition of Azone® (Figure 3). This result indicates unequivocally that the presence of Azone® within the SUVs increases fluidity of the acyl chain region of the DPPC bilayers at SC temperature.

Beastall's finding concerning T_m was verified by Rolland et al.[16,17] with MLVs examined using DSC. Azone® had a strong influence on the endothermic transitions

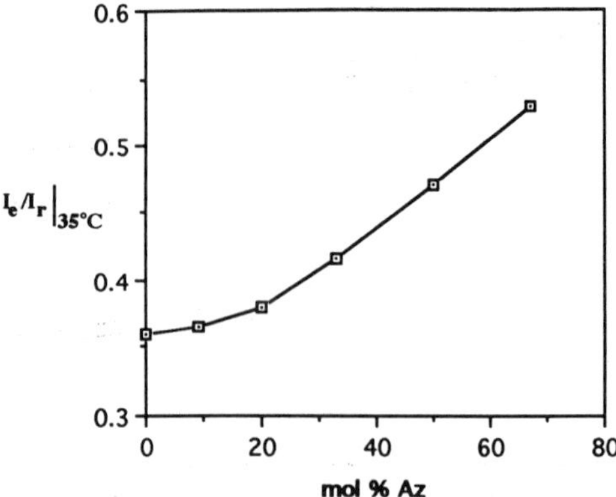

Figure 3 Pyrene excimer:monomer emission ratio at 35°C (I_e:I_m) as a function of Azone® concentration in DPPC MLVs. (Data taken from Beastall, J. et al., *Int. J. Pharm.*, 43, 207, 1988.)

of the DPPC MLVs. The L_β-$L_{\beta'}$ pretransition at 35°C vanishes at Azone® concentrations above 5 mol% (Figure 4), while the $L_{\beta'}$-L_α transition peak is broadened and shifted to lower temperatures (Figure 5). This is essentially the same result as Beastall's (see above), except that the values for T_m in the presence of Azone® are consistently approximately 1°C lower. The relevance of these changes in an endothermic transition that all lie above SC temperature, for lipid fluidity at 35°C is unclear. The authors' suggestion that DPPC MLVs would be a suitable model for the intercellular lipids of the SC is clearly not justified by the results given.

The questionable choice of DPPC is readily avoided by using acknowledged SC lipids. It has been known for some time that SUVs can be prepared from model SC lipids. A mixture of only cholesterol and ceramides did not form liposomes.[19] However, the addition of fatty acids to give the composition in Table 1 led to the successful production of SUVs. Salomons-de Vries et al.[19] prepared MLVs from cholesterol:ceramides:stearic acid (30:48:22 w/w), which showed a single endothermic transition at 73°C. This is within the range of 68 to 75°C seen with SC which is attributed to disordering of the lamellar phase of the intercellular lipids.[15] The incorporation of Azone® reduced the temperature of the endothermic transition and caused a second endothermic peak of unknown origin to appear at 50°C.[19] Again, no conclusion about the effect on lipid fluidity at SC temperature can be drawn, although Azone® clearly caused disruption of the bilayers. This was confirmed by measuring the release rate of carboxyl fluorescein from the liposomes, which was substantially increased by the incorporation of Azone®. This effect was not evident for a shorter chain (C_6) Azone®, indicating the importance for transport enhancement of its position within the bilayer.

The curvature of spherical liposomes is not an important factor when using them as a model for linear bilayer structures. Azone® has a large head group as compared with its alkyl chain volume, giving a small critical packing parameter (e.g., its "spoon" conformation[20]). Assuming an average bilayer hydrocarbon thickness *(a)* of 4.0 nm, the outside:inside lipid ratio ($R^2/(R-a)^2$) for SUVs of radius *(R)* 100 nm is only 1.085. The curvature experienced by each molecule in the vesicle wall is, therefore, only slightly different from the linear geometry ($\lim_{R\to\infty} R^2/(R-a)^2 = 1.0$) in a bilayer.

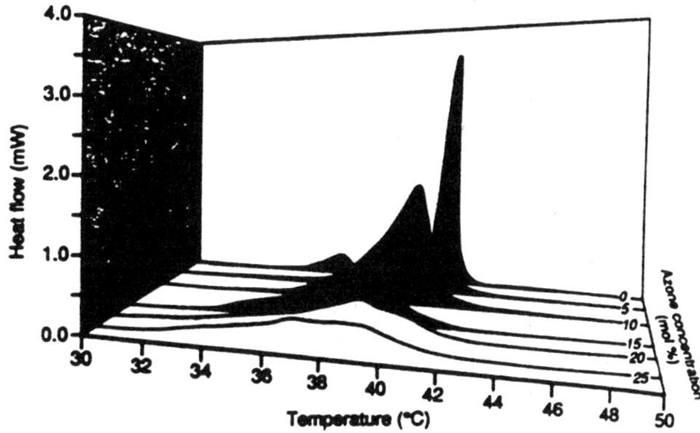

Figure 4 DSC scans of DPPC MLVs containing increasing concentrations of Azone®. (From Rolland, A. et al., *Int. J. Pharm.*, 76, 217, 1991. With permission.)

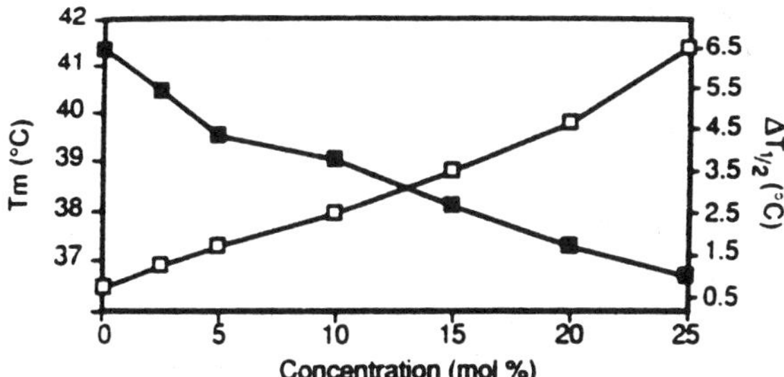

Figure 5 Effect of Azone® concentration on transition temperature of DPPC MLVs. (From Rolland, A. et al., *Int. J. Pharm.*, 76, 217, 1991. With permission.)

The use of DSC in these studies shows only that endothermic lipid transitions are altered by Azone®. It cannot provide a picture at the molecular level. The conclusion often drawn from DSC results, that Azone® intercolates between the acyl chains of the lipids, perturbs bilayer organization, and thus increases fluidity,[16] is clearly axiomatic, but strictly speaking cannot be proven by DSC alone.

III. STUDIES ON MONOMOLECULAR FILMS

The way Azone® increases the fluidity of lipid acyl chains was examined on the molecular level using a Langmuir trough. We recall that the behavior of film pressure, π *(A, T),* as a function of area per molecule, *A,* is classified as either solid (S), liquid condensed (L2), liquid expanded (L1), or gaseous (G).[21] Convincing FTIR evidence[22] shows that L2 and L1 monolayers are realistic models for the gel and liquid crystalline states, respectively, of lipid acyl chains. The influence of Azone® on the compression behavior of such films was first examined using DPPC as a model lipid.[20] The characteristic L1–L2 transition in the compression isotherm of DPPC was progressively attenuated by increasing the mole fraction of Azone® (X_{Az}) within the monolayer (Figure 6). Above $X_{Az} = 0.3$ only an expanded L1 film could be formed. Azone® thus severely reduced the ability of DPPC to form a gel-like L2

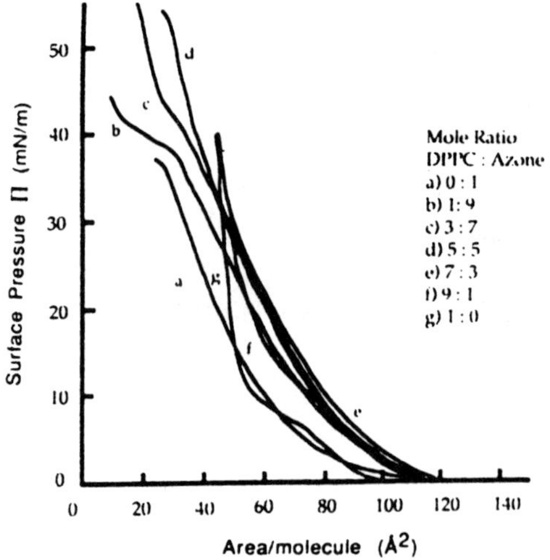

Figure 6 Compression isotherms of DPPC and Azone® mixed monolayers at 25°C. (From Lewis, D. and Hadgraft, J., *Int. J. Pharm.*, 65, 211, 1990. With permission.)

state at high film pressures. Of particular relevance is the positive deviation (up to 30%) from ideal mixing of the Azone® with DPPC (Figure 7a). This film expansion even occurs at the high film pressures corresponding to an initial gel-like state (e.g., π = 25 mN/m). Here, then, is direct evidence that Azone® promotes acyl chain disorder, resulting in the expansion of a gel phase monolayer. The authors suggested that the polar amide linkage of the cycloheptanone head group is oriented toward the underlying water surface, giving a large, effective head group surface area (the preferred "spoon" configuration). The C_{12} chain cannot adequately fill the resulting space available between the acyl chains of the DPPC, thereby causing free-volume defects within the monolayer. Greater dynamic freedom is now available to the acyl chains of the DPPC, promoting disorder. In a subsequent study Azones® having longer alkyl chains were found less effective in expanding the DPPC monolayers.[23] A C_{14} chain shows only slight positive deviation from ideal mixing (Figure 7b), whereas with a C_{16} chain the effect is negligible (Figure 7c). Again, this suggests that its position within the monolayer is important. The longer chains locate deep within the hydrophobic region, where a linear configuration is preferred that does not induce free-volume defects.

Schückler and Lee[24] examined monolayers of the three major SC lipids, fatty acids, cholesterol and ceramides. The fatty acids comprise almost half of the total SC lipids (molar ratio), and form an expanded L1 film (Figure 8). Its weak condensation results from the high proportion of unsaturated acyl chains present, which hinders the close packing necessary for an L2 film. With increasing mole fraction of Azone® the π-A curve remains of the L1 type with no change in compressibility, $c_s = 1/A \cdot 2A/2\pi$. No film expansion is observed (Figure 9a) and ideal mixing occurs at the highest film pressure. The Azone® molecule is, therefore, accommodated between the free-volume-forming unsaturated acyl chains. The highly condensed S-type film seen with cholesterol is transformed to an L1 state above $X_{Az} = 0.2$ (Figure 10). Here, the negative deviation from ideality at all film pressures is substantial (Figure 9b). Azone® is forced into a condensed state by the cholesterol, reducing its effective head

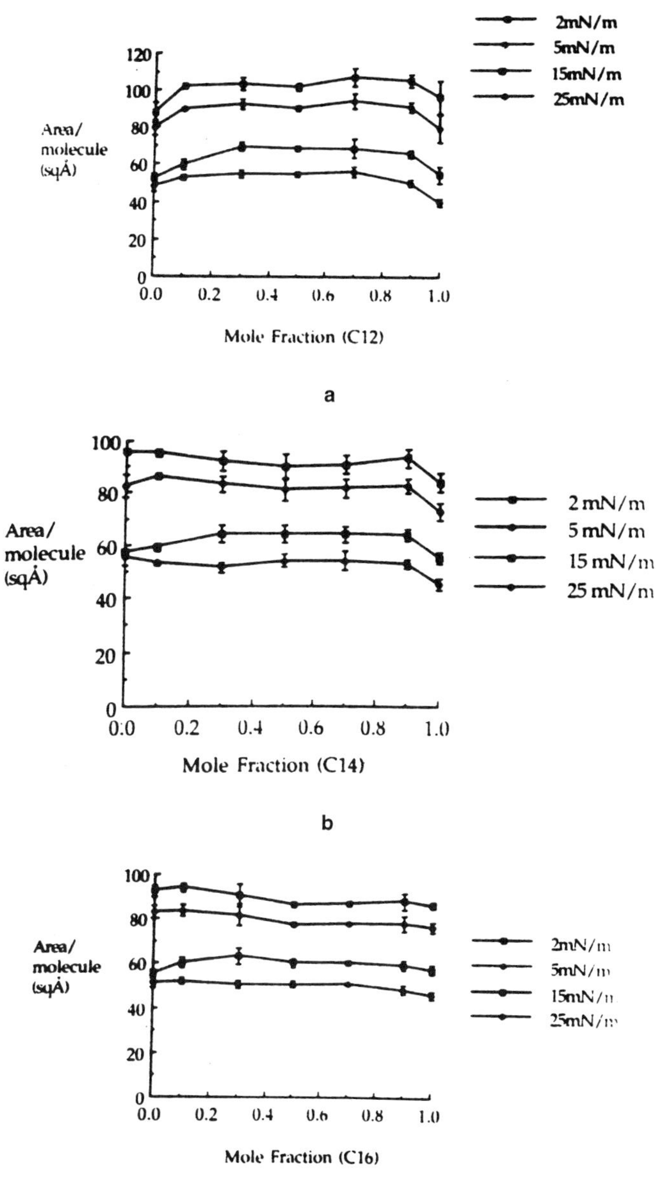

Figure 7 Average area per molecule as a function of mole fraction Azone® in mixed monolayers with DPPC at various film pressures. (a) C_{12}; (b) C_{14}; (c) C_{16}. (From Lewis, D. et al. *Prediction of Percutaneous Penetration,* IBC Technical Services, London, 1991. With permission.)

group surface area. It cannot adopt its "spoon" configuration at low X_{Az}. The L2-type monolayer of type IV ceramides (Figure 11) is similarly transformed to an L1 state, and the area per molecule initially drops (Figure 9c), indicating that Azone® induces the same conformational change in the ceramide packing of its L1 state. At low film pressure, ideal mixing occurs up to 100% Azone®, indicating that Azone® exists in

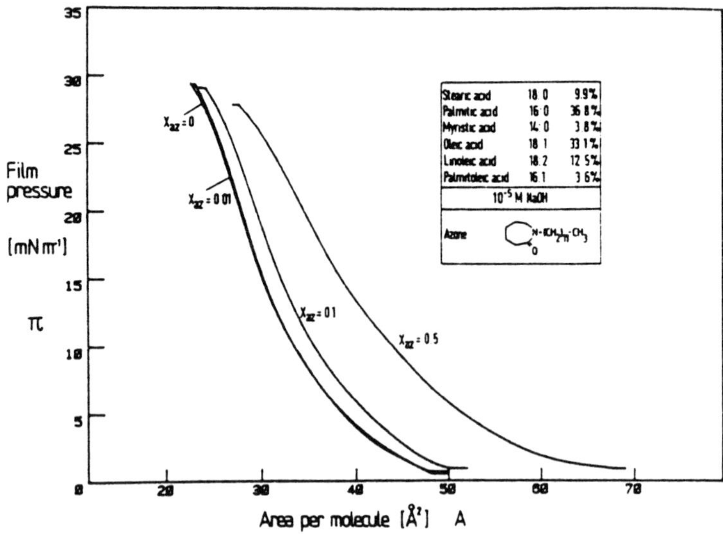

Figure 8 π–A diagram for mixed fatty acids containing increasing mole fraction of Azone®. (From Schückler, F. and Lee, G., *Int. J. Pharm.*, 70, 173, 1991. With permission.)

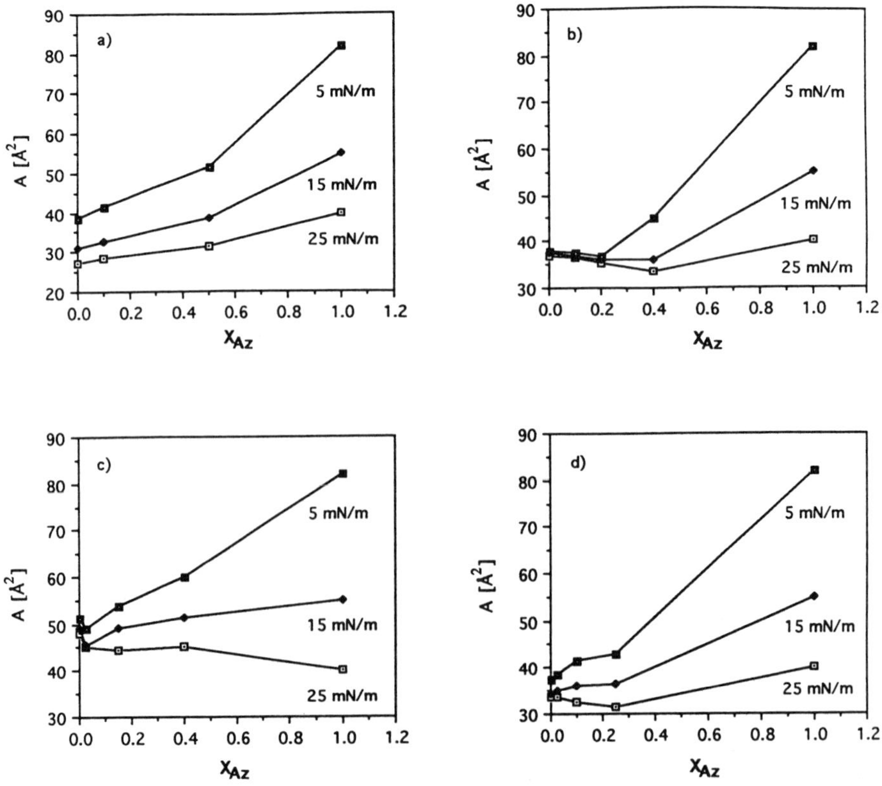

Figure 9 Average area per molecule as a function of mole fraction Azone® in mixed monolayers at various film pressures. (a) Fatty acids, (b) cholesterol, (c) ceramides, (d) model SC lipid mixture.

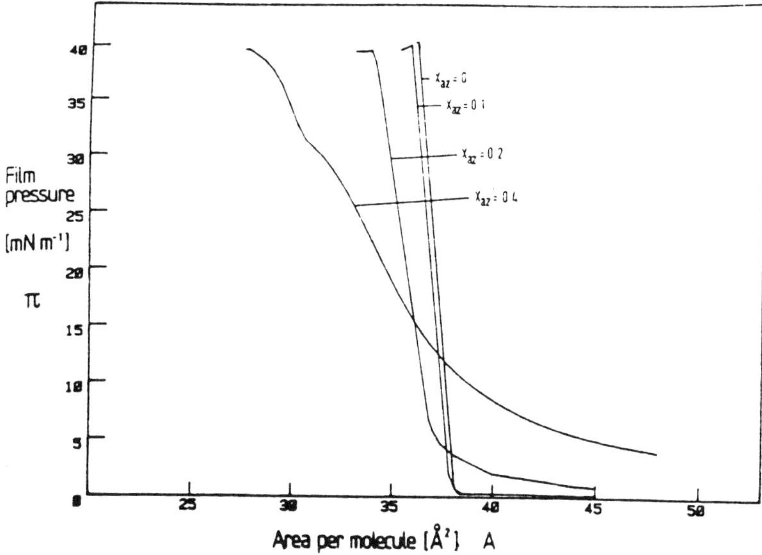

Figure 10 π–A diagram for cholesterol containing increasing mole fractions of Azone®. (From Schückler, F. and Lee, G., *Int. J. Pharm.,* 70, 173, 1991. With permission.)

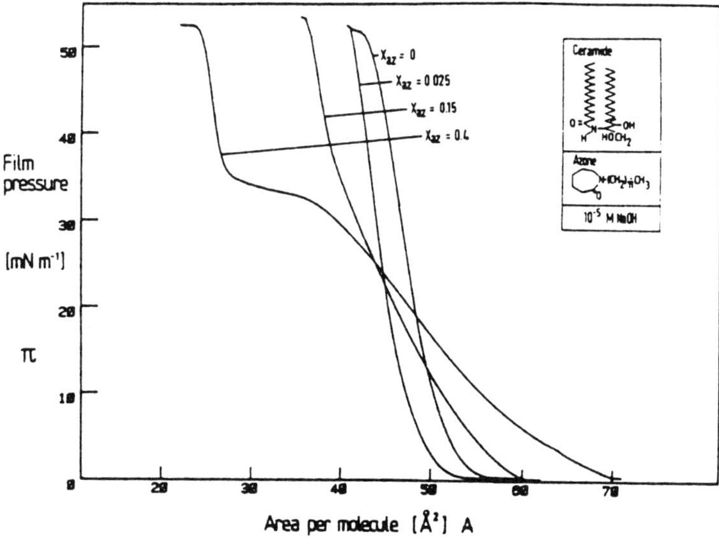

Figure 11 π–A diagram for ceramides containing increasing mole fractions of Azone®. (From Schückler, F. and Lee, G., *Int. J. Pharm.,* 70, 173, 1991. With permission.)

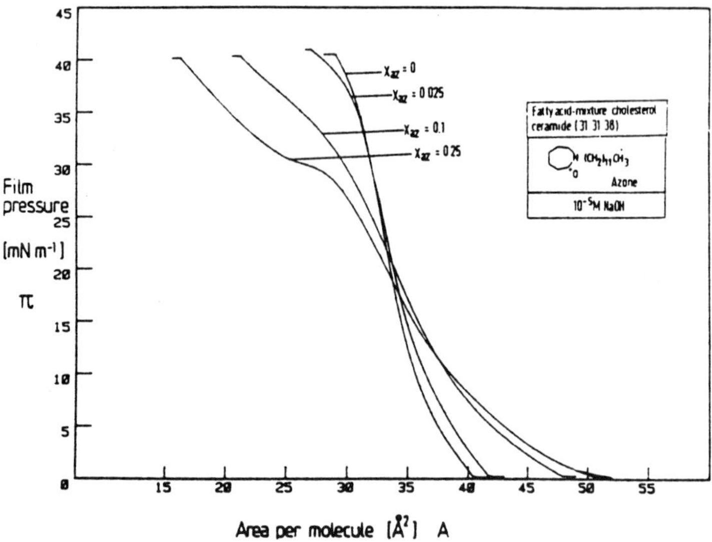

Figure 12 π–A diagram for model SC lipid mixture containing increasing mole fractions of Azone®. (From Schückler, F. and Lee, G., *Int. J. Pharm.*, 70, 173, 1991. With permission.)

its "spoon" conformation. This would explain why at higher film pressures slight indications of film expansion are seen, although they are much weaker than that seen with DPPC.[20]

A combination of the fatty acids, cholesterol, and ceramide (31:31:38 by weight) produced an L2 film (Figure 12). It was shown[24] that the condensed nature of this film is caused by the cholesterol and not the ceramides, and the cholesterol molecule fills the spaces between the unsaturated acyl chains of the fatty acids more effectively. With increasing mole fraction of Azone® the π-A curve is transformed to an L1 state, and a slight negative deviation from ideal mixing occurs at all film pressures (Figure 9d). This film contraction, despite the change from L2 to L1 behavior, can occur only if Azone® is incorporated within the monolayer of SC model lipids in a linear configuration, as already seen with cholesterol monolayers. It has been suggested that Azone's amide group loses direct contact with the water when under compression.[25] The area per molecule for this conformation is 36 Å² at $\pi = 25$ mN/m. Inserting this value at $X_{Az} = 1.0$ in Figure 9d gives ideal mixing at the highest film pressure corresponding to a gel phase. Azone® is, therefore, intercolated in this configuration within the mixed model SC lipid monolayer. These experiments were repeated by Harrison et al.,[23] with the same results.

From the monolayer studies we conclude that in the case of the phospholipid DPPC 7 fluidization is a result of lateral expansion of the lipid layers. This may be caused by intercolation of the Azone® molecule in its "spoon" configuration, which results in an increase in free volume within the acyl chain region of the lipids, giving increased acyl chain mobility. Azone® causes no lateral expansion of monolayers of mixed SC lipids (fatty acids, cholesterol and ceramides), indicating it is intercolated in a linear configuration. Even so, its effective head group area is larger than that of the mixed SC lipids, causing free-volume defects and promoting acyl chain disorder.

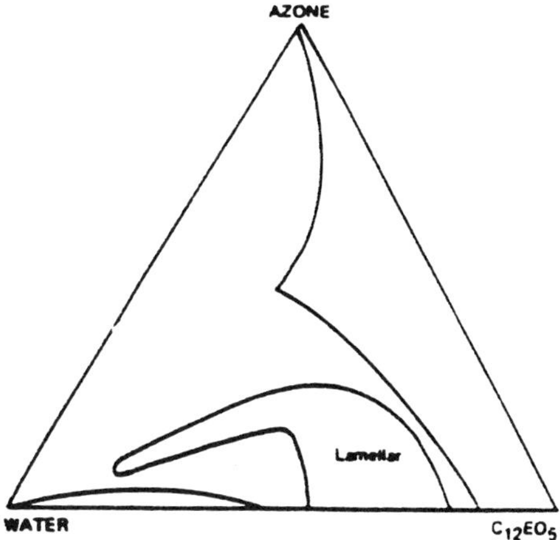

Figure 13 Phase diagram at 298 K for the system *n*-dodecyl pentaoxyethylene glycol ether/water/Azone®. (From Ward, A. and Tallon, R., *Topical Drug Delivery Formulation,* Marcel Dekker, New York, 1990. With permission.)

Although it appears that Azone® interacts differently with DPPC than with the model SC lipids, the result, decreased acyl chain condensation, is the same in both cases.

IV. STUDIES ON EXTENDED BILAYER STRUCTURES

The use of liposomes and monomolecular films to investigate the fluidization of model lipids by Azone®, as described in the previous sections, can be criticized on three grounds. First, it is not known if all of the components are incorporated into the liposomes. Second, the conformation and position of the Azone® molecule within a monolayer may differ from that within a bilayer. Third, it is not possible to investigate possible changes in lipid phase behavior with the Langmuir trough. All of these limitations can be avoided by using three-dimensional lipid bilayer structures.

Ward and Tallon's[26] choice of a lamellar phase composed of hydrated *n*-dodecyl pentaoxyethylene glycol ether resulted in an L_α state at the test temperature. The results are, nevertheless, of great interest, as the authors considered Azone's distribution within the bilayer. The phase diagram presented for the system surfactant/water/Azone® shows convincingly that the surfactant–water bilayer can incorporate up to 35% (w/w) Azone® without undergoing a phase change (Figure 13). Increasing the Azone® concentration within this range produces greater lamellar repeat distance (Figure 14). A comparison of the ^{13}C shifts in the lamellar phase with those in polar and nonpolar solvents indicated that the Azone's cycloheptanone ring is located in the polar environment of the bilayer–water interface.[27] The resulting enhanced hydrogen-bonding interactions cause an increase in the quadrupolar splitting (Figure 15) from greater order of the water molecules bound to the ethylene oxide groups. The continuous nature of this increase indicates that the degree of penetration of the Azone® molecule is concentration dependent. At low Azone® concentrations one finds only partial penetration, the Azone® being localized within the hydrophobic layer. This increases to 100% at the point of maximum repeat distance and maximum quadrupole water splitting. A clue to the subsequent decrease in repeat distance

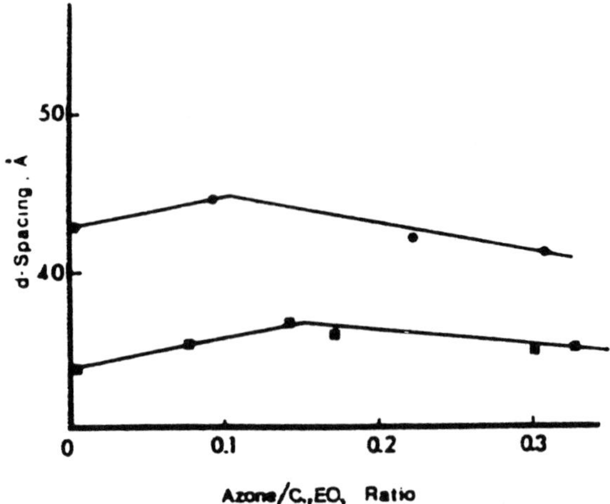

Figure 14 Lamellar repeat distance of the system *n*-dodecyl pentaoxyethylene glycol ether/water as a function of Azone® content ■ 30% w/w water; • 45% w/w water. (From Ward, A. and Tallon, R., *Topical Drug Delivery Formulation,* Marcel Dekker, New York, 1990. With permission.)

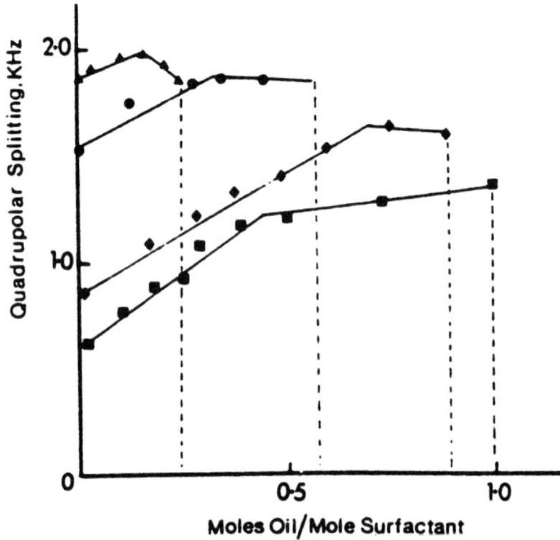

Figure 15 Effect of Azone® on quadrupolar water splitting in lamellar phase of *n*-dodecyl pentaoxyethylene glycol ether/water ▲ 22% water; • 30% water; ◆ 40% water; ■ 44% water. (From Ward, A. and Tallon, R., *Drug. Dev. Ind. Pharm.,* 14, 1155, 1988. With permission.)

(Figure 14) is obtained from the phase diagram (Figure 13). The addition of more than approximately 15% Azone® to the L_α phase increases the water capacity of the latter from 50 to about 85% (w/w). The authors propose that at this Azone® concentration, increased penetration of water into the bilayer is favored, causing decreased repeat distance. As a result, a simultaneous halt to the increase in quadru-

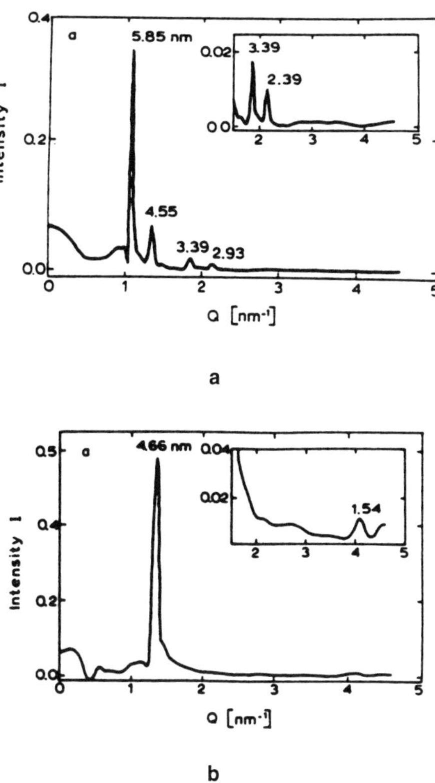

Figure 16 X-ray diffraction patterns of mixture of six major SC fatty acids: (a) 0% Azone®; (b) 30% Azone®. (From Schückler, F. et al., *J. Control. Rel.,* 23, 27, 1993. With permission.)

pole water splitting (Figure 15) takes place at this point. Thus, the incorporation of Azone® into the surfactant bilayer leads to an increased ability of fluid bilayers to take up water.

Schückler et al.[28] examined the influence of Azone® on a liquid crystal composed of the six major fatty acids of the SC (cf. Table 1). The X-ray diffraction pattern of this system, seen in Figure 16a, is that of mixed hexagonal [5.85 nm, 3.39 nm ($1/\sqrt{3}$), and 2.93 nm (1/2)] and lamellar (4.55 nm) periodicity. Increasing concentration of Azone® progressively attenuated the H_{II} structure and simultaneously promoted the lamellar structure without altering the repeat distances of either. With >30% w/w Azone®, only an anisotropic, pure L_α phase remained (Figure 16b). The authors explained these changes by considering that Azone® has a large head group surface area as compared with its alkyl chain volume, implying a small critical packing parameter. This must be true for both linear and "spoon" conformations. Interpolation of the Azone® molecules between the acyl chains of the H_{II} structure would, therefore, increase the average interfacial area per lipid/Azone® molecule and induce the observed H_{II}-L_α transition. Engblom and Engström[25] found, however, exactly the contrary effect for the action of Azone® on an $L\alpha$ phase composed of hydrated phosphatidylcholine. The addition of more than approximately 20% w/w Azone®

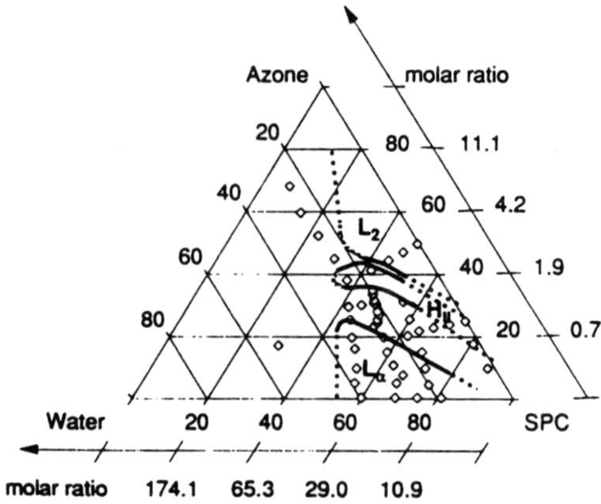

Figure 17 Phase diagram for system phosphatidylcholine/water/Azone®. (From Engblom, J. and Engström, S., *Int. J. Pharm.*, 98, 173, 1993. With permission.)

caused an L_α-H_{II} transition, as illustrated by the phase diagram for the system (Figure 17). On structural grounds this would, however, necessitate a large critical packing parameter which increases the inside-to-outside curvature of the bilayers. The authors mention that diffraction patterns (unfortunately not given in the paper) show that Azone® is not only anchored in the interfacial region, but also distributed within the hydrocarbon core.[25] Although this agrees with Ward and Tallon's[26] results, described above, such positioning would not necessarily favor an L_α-H_{II} transition.

Schückler et al.[28] also examined the action of Azone® on a system composed of the fatty acids, cholesterol and ceramides. These build a pure gel-phase bilayer structure *in vitro* at SC temperature (Figure 18a), probably L_β.[9] The addition of up to 30% w/w Azone® caused only a slight increase in repeat distance, but no attenuation of the lamellar periodicity (cf. Figure 18b). The authors note substantial discrepancies in the repeat distances with intermediate Azone® concentrations as well as the existence of crystalline cholesterol (reflections at approximately 3.40 and 1.70 nm). They concluded that the L_β structure can accommodate up to 30% Azone®, intercolated between the hydrocarbon chains with only lateral swelling of the bilayers. Again, this can be attributed to the geometry of the Azone® molecule, whose head group ring is large compared with its alkyl-chain volume. Unfortunately, this study did not encompass higher Azone® concentrations, where a phase change must occur at some point. The great utility of such model SC lipids was, however, clearly demonstrated. A combination of diffusion studies with X-ray diffraction and FTIR offers great possibilities. Carpe diem!

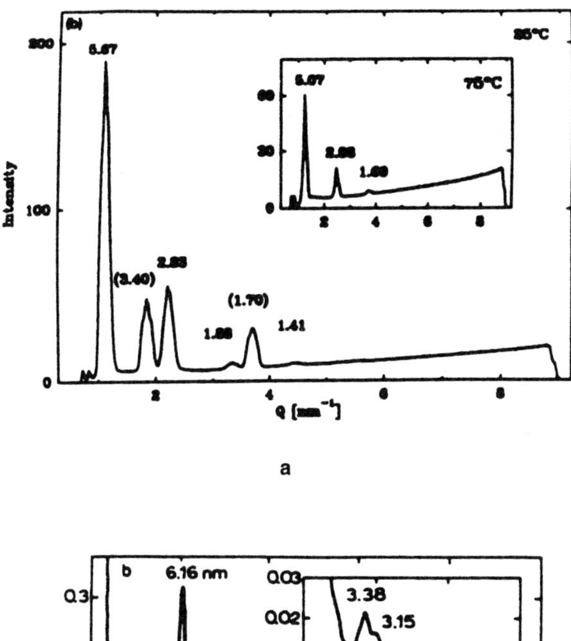

a

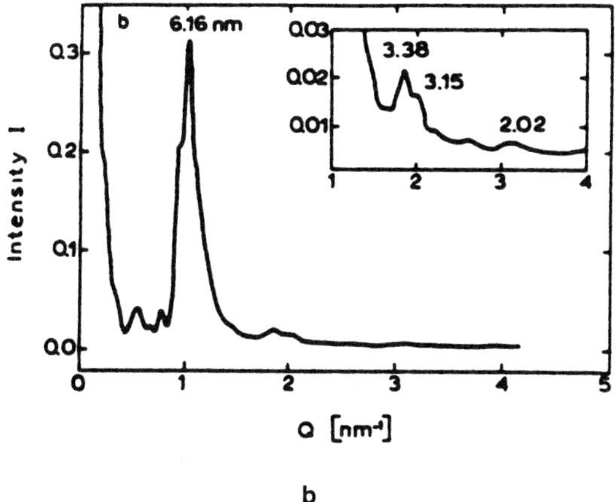

b

Figure 18 X-ray diffraction patterns of model SC lipid mixture: (a) 0% Azone®. (From Lieckfeldt, R. et al., *Biochim. Biophys. Acta,* 1151, 182, 1993. With permission.) (b) 30% Azone®. (From Schückler, F. et al., *J. Control. Rel.,* 23, 27, 1993. With permission.)

REFERENCES

1. **Goodman, M. and Barry, B. W.,** Differential scanning calorimetry (DSC) of human SC: effect of Azone®, *J. Pharm. Pharmacol.,* 37 (Suppl.), 80P, 1985.
2. **Goodman, M. and Barry, B. W.,** Differential scanning calorimetry of human SC: effect of penetration enhancers Azone® and DMSO, *Anal. Proc.,* 26, 397, 1986.
3. **Goodman, M. and Barry, B. W.,** Action of skin penetration enhancers Azone®, oleic acid and decylmethylsulphoxide; permeation and differential scanning calorimetry (DSC) studies, *J. Pharm. Pharmacol.,* 38 (Suppl.), 71P, 1986.
4. **Barry, B. W.,** Lipid-protein-partitioning theory of skin penetration enhancement, *J. Control. Rel.,* 15, 237, 1991.
5. **Bouwstra, J., de Vries, M., Gooris, G., Bras, J., and Porree, M.,** Thermodynamic and structural aspects of the skin barrier, *J. Control. Rel.,* 15, 209, 1991.

6. **Casal, H. and Mantsch, H.,** Polymorphic phase behaviour of phospholipid membranes studied by infrared spectroscopy, *Biochim. Biophys. Acta,* 779, 381, 1984.
7. **Ongpipattanakul, B., Burnette, R., Potts, R., and Francoer, M.,** Evidence that oleic acid exists in a separate phase within SC lipids, *Pharm. Res.,* 8, 350, 1991.
8. **Abraham, W. and Downing, D.,** Deuterium NMR investigation of polymorphism in SC lipids, *Biochim. Biophys. Acta,* 1068, 189, 1991.
9. **Lieckfeldt, R., Villalain, J., Gomez-Fernandez, J., and Lee, G.,** Diffusivity and structural polymorphism in some model SC lipid systems, *Biochim. Biophys. Acta,* 1151, 182, 1993.
10. **Elias, P.,** The importance of epidermal lipids for the SC barrier, in *Topical Drug Delivery Formulations,* Osbourne, D. and Amann, A., Eds., Marcel Dekker, New York, 1990, chap. 2.
11. **Lampe, M., Burlingame, A., Whitney, J., Williams, M., Brown, B., Roitman, E., and Elias, P.,** Human SC lipids: characterisation and regional variations, *J. Lipids Res.,* 24, 120, 1983.
12. **Elias, P.,** Epidermal barrier function: intercellular lamellar lipid structures, origin, composition and metabolism, *J. Control. Rel.,* 15, 199, 1991.
13. **Beastall, J., Hadgraft, J., and Washington, C.,** Mechanism of action of Azone® as a percutaneous penetration enhancer: lipid bilayer fluidity and transition temperature effects, *Int. J. Pharm.,* 43, 207, 1988.
14. **Potts, R.,** Physical characterisation of the SC: the relationship of mechanical and barrier properties to lipid and protein structure, in *Transdermal Drug Delivery,* Hadgraft, J. and Guy, R., Eds, Marcel Dekker, New York, 1989, chap. 2.
15. **Galla, H. and Sackmann, E.,** Lateral pyrene diffusion in the hydrophobic region of membranes: use of pyrene excimers as optical probes, *Biochim. Biophys. Acta,* 339, 103, 1974.
16. **Rolland, A., Brzokewicz, A., Shroot, B., and Jamoulle, J.,** Effect of penetration enhancers on the phase transition of multilamellar liposomes of dipalmitoylphosphatidyl choline. A study by differential scanning calorimetry, *Int. J. Pharm.,* 76, 217, 1991.
17. **Rolland, A., Brzokewicz, A., Shroot, B., and Jamoulle, J.,** A differential scanning calorimetric study of the effect of penetration enhancers on the thermal behaviour of dipalmitoylphosphatidyl choline multilamellar liposomes, in *Prediction of Percutaneous Penetration,* Scott, R., Guy, R., Hadgraft, J., and Boddé, H., Eds., IBC Technical Services, London, 1991, 365.
18. **Abraham, W. and Downing, D.,** Factors affecting the formation, morphology and permeability of SC lipid bilayers *in vitro,* in *Prediction of Percutaneous Penetration,* Scott, R., Guy, R., and Hadgraft, J., Eds., IBC Technical Services, London, 1990, 110.
19. **Salomons-de Vries, M., Gooris, G., Holl, C., Ponec, M., and Bouwstra, J.,** Liposomes as model system for lipid bilayers in SC, in *Proc. Int. Symp. Control. Rel. Bioact. Mater.,* 18, 515, 1991.
20. **Lewis, D. and Hadgraft, I.,** Mixed monolayers of diplamitoylphosphatidyl choline with Azone® or oleic acid at the air-water interface, *Int. J. Pharm.,* 65, 211, 1990.
21. **Adamson, A.,** *Physical Chemistry of Surfaces,* Wiley-Interscience, New York, 1982, 124.
22. **Mitchell, M. and Dluhy, R.,** In-situ FT-IR investigations of phospholipid monolayer phase transitions at the air-water interface, *J. Am. Chem. Soc.,* 110, 712, 1988.
23. **Lewis, D., Hadgraft, J., and Boddé, H.,** Mixed monolayer studies of DPPC with N-alkyl-azacycloheptanones at the air-water interface, in *Prediction of Percutaneous Penetration,* Scott, R., Guy, R., Hadgraft, J., and Boddé, H., Eds., IBC Technical Services, London, 1991, 355.
24. **Schückler, F. and Lee, G.,** The influence of Azone® on monomolecular films of some SC lipids, *Int. J. Pharm.,* 70, 173, 1991.
25. **Engblom, J. and Engström, S.,** Azone® and the formation of reversed mono- and bicontinuous lipid-water phases, *Int. J. Pharm.,* 98, 173, 1993.
26. **Ward, A. and Tallon, R.,** Penetration enhancer incorporation in bilayers, *Drug Dev. Ind. Pharm.,* 14, 1155, 1988.
27. **Ward, A. and Tallon, R.,** Penetration enhancer incorporation in bilayer, in *Topical Drug Delivery Formulation,* Osborne, D. and Amann, A., Eds., Marcel Dekker, New York, 1990, chap. 4.
28. **Schückler, F., Bouwstra, J., Gooris, G., and Lee, G.,** An X-ray diffraction study of some model SC lipids containing Azone® and dodecyl-L-pyroglutamate, *J. Control. Rel.,* 23, 27, 1993.
29. **Harrison, K., Brain, K., and Hadgraft, J.,** The effects of penetration modifiers on stratum corneum lipid monolayers, *Proceed. Int. Symp. Contr. Rel. Bioact. Mater.,* 27, 477, 1994.

Chapter 7.1

Pyrrolidones as Penetration Enhancers

Hitoshi Sasaki, Koyo Nishida, and Junzo Nakamura

CONTENTS

I. INTRODUCTION

2-Pyrrolidone (2-P) and *N*-methyl-2-pyrrolidone (NMP) are versatile solvents that are widely established in the petrochemical industry. Recently they became of great interest to the pharmaceutical industry as a transdermal penetration enhancer. Both 2-P and NMP can be used with a variety of drugs to promote penetration and to establish a reservoir of drug in the stratum corneum (SC).[1–3] Another pyrrolidone, pyroglutamic acid (PGA; 2-pyrrolidone-5-carboxylic acid), is a component of the natural moisturizing factor in skin, which is responsible for hydration of SC.[4]

Recently, *N*-dodecylazacycloheptan-2-one (Azone®) was developed as a potential enhancer without severe side effect. Azone® and NMP have a similar ring structure but different alkyl chains. Development of various pyrrolidone derivatives is progressing to improve the enhancing effect and to investigate the enhancing mechanism.

II. CHARACTERISTICS AND ENHANCING EFFECT

Table 1 shows structures of typical pyrrolidone derivatives reported as a penetration enhancer. Their lipophilicities were widely varied according to the substituted functions. The percutaneous absorption behavior and localization in the SC of the enhancer itself, according to its physicochemical property, can be considered as the most important factors controlling the enhancing activity and side effects.

0-8493-2605-2/95/$0.00+$.50

Table 1 Structure of 2-Pyrrolidone Derivatives as Penetration Enhancer

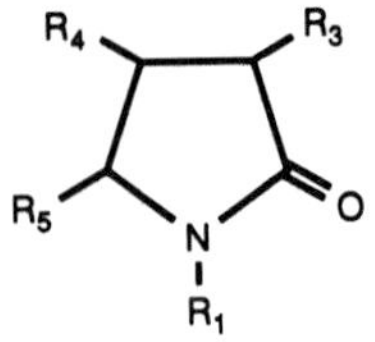

Name or Abbreviation	Substitution	Lipophilicity[a]
2-Pyrrolidone and lower alkylated pyrrolidones		
2-Pyrrolidone (2-P)	No substitution	H
N-Methyl-2-pyrrolidone (NMP)	R_1 = $-CH_3$	H
5-Methyl-2-pyrrolidone	R_5 = $-CH_3$	H
N-Ethyl-2-pyrrolidone	R_1 = $-C_2H_5$	H
1,5-Dimethyl-2-pyrrolidone	R_1 = $-CH_3$; R_5 = $-CH$	H
Lower alkylated *N*-substituted-2-pyrrolidones		
R_1 = alkyl (C_1–C_{18}), phenyl, benzyl; R_3, R_4, R_5 = lower alkyl		H-VL
N-Alkyl-2-pyrrolidones and its 4-substituted derivatives		
N-Hexyl-2-pyrrolidone (NHP)	R_1 = $-(CH_2)_4CH_3$	L
N-Lauryl-2-pyrrolidone (NLP)	R_1 = $-(CH_2)_{11}CH_3$	VL
4-Carboxy-NMP	R_1 = $-CH_3$; R_4 = $-COOH$	VH
4-Carboxy-NHP	R_1 = $-(CH_2)_4CH_3$; R_4 = $-COOH$	L
4-Carboxy-NLP	R_1 = $-(CH_2)_{11}CH_3$; R_4 = $-COOH$	VL
4-Methoxycarbonyl-NMP	R_1 = $-CH_3$; R_4 = $-COOCH_3$	H
4-Methoxycarbonyl-NHP	R_1 = $-(CH_2)_4CH_3$; R_4 = $-COOCH_3$	HL
4-Methoxycarbonyl-NLP	R_1 = $-(CH_2)_{11}CH_3$; R_4 = $-COOCH_3$	VL
Pyroglutamic acid (PGA) derivatives		
PGA (2-pyrrolidone-5-carboxylic acid)	R_5 = $-COOH$	VH
PGA decyl ester	R_5 = $-COO(CH_2)_9CH_3$	VL
PGA oleyl ester	R_5 = $-COO(CH_2)_8CHCH(CH_2)_7CH_3$	VL
PGA dodecyl ester	R_5 = $-COO(CH_2)_{11}CH_3$	VL
Other pyrrolidone derivatives		
HPE-101	R_1 = $-(CH_2)_2$-S-$(CH_2)_9CH_3$	VL
N-Farnesyl-2-pyrrolidone	R_1 = $-(CH_2CHC(CH_3)CH_2)_2CH_2CHCH(CH_3)_2$	VL
3-Hydroxy-NMP	R_1 = $-CH_3$; R_3= $-OH$	VH
HEP-Dec	R_1 = $-(CH_2)_2$-OCO-$(CH_2)_8CH_3$	VL

[a] VH: very hydrophilic, H: hydrophilic, L: lipophilic, VL: very lipophilic.

A. 2-PYRROLIDONE AND ALKYLATED DERIVATIVES

2-Pyrrolidone and NMP are hygroscopic and aprotic solvents for pesticides, agricultural chemicals, and polymers, similar to dimethylsulfoxide. These are miscible with aqueous and organic solvent. Resh and Stoughton[5] reported the usefulness of NMP as a penetration enhancer for topical antibiotic treatment of acne vulgaris. 2-Pyrrolidone or *N*-lower alkyl-2-pyrrolidone was reported to have enhanced a penetration of a number of agents such as griseofulvin, theophylline, and oxytetracycline.[6] Under *in vitro* conditions, using the same solvent in donor and receptor, 2-P is not a strong penetration enhancer for methanol, caffeine, and octanol.[7] However, Southwell and Barry[1] demonstrated the high enhancing effect of 2-P on caffeine and aspirin penetrations by the *in vitro* finite dose technique ("*in vivo* mimic" method). Using the same technique, NMP greatly enhanced the penetration of ibuprofen, flurbiprofen, mannitol, hydrocortisone, and progesterone.

The effects of enhancers on the percutaneous absorption of betamethasone 17-benzoate were investigated by vasoconstrictor assay in human subjects.[2] *N*-Methyl-2-pyrrolidone with occlusion was the best enhancer of a group that included acetone, dimethylformamide, 2-P, *N*-ethyl-2-pyrrolidone, dimethylisosorbide, propylene glycol (PG), and *N*-*N*-diethyl-*m*-toluamide. The enhancing effect of 2-P on the penetration of hexyl nicotinate was also confirmed by measuring vasodilation with laser Doppler velocimetry.[3] Nelson Research owns many patents on enhancing vehicles, including lower alkylated *N*-substituted-2-pyrrolidones for anticancer agents, antibiotics, steroids, fungicidal agents, and hormones.[6]

A combining vehicle of NMP with lipophilic alkane or lipophilic alcohol was reported to exert a superior enhancing effect on drug percutaneous penetration.[8] Recent reports demonstrated the ability of penetration enhancers to increase the skin permeation of large polar molecules such as vasopressin or insulin. Bonina and Montenegro[9] reported that NMP, Azone®, and PG promoted heparin (average molecular weight 17,000) flux.

B. *N*-ALKYL-2-PYRROLIDONE AND ITS 4-SUBSTITUTED DERIVATIVES

Sasaki et al.[10] prepared eight pyrrolidone derivatives as penetration enhancers and compared them to NMP for their physicochemical characteristics, transdermal absorbabilities, and promoting actions on transdermal delivery of phenol red. The preparing pyrrolidones included *N*-methyl- (NMP), *N*-hexyl- (NHP), and *N*-lauryl-2-pyrrolidone (NLP), and their 4-carboxy or 4-methoxycarbonyl substituted derivatives. The structure of NLP is very similar to Azone®. The derivatives showed various lipophilicities due to introduction of the functional groups. *N*-Methyl-2-pyrrolidone significantly increased the penetration of phenol red through an isolated rat skin, although the dye applied alone could not transfer. The pyrrolidones NHP and NLP largely promoted a penetration of phenol red, with a lag time for dye appearance in the receptor. Pyrrolidones NMP and NHP showed high permeation of the enhancer itself, although NLP was hardly detected in the receptor. Introduction of the 4-carboxy or the 4-methoxycarbonyl group into *N*-alkyl-2-pyrrolidone reduced the enhancer permeability and decreased the promoting effect. The hydrolysis of 4-methoxycarbonyl derivatives to 4-carboxy derivatives in the skin was observed.

The relationship between the partition coefficient (PC) of derivatives and the penetration flux of phenol red is shown in Figure 1A. High lipophilicity of the enhancer is important for promoting a penetration of the hydrophilic compound. Figure 1B shows the relationship between the reciprocal value of lag time for phenol red appearance and concentration of pyrrolidones in the receptor at 3 and 10 h. An increase of flux of penetration enhancer resulted in a decrease of lag time, suggesting that the lag time includes the time for penetration of the enhancer into the skin. These derivatives also increased a retention of phenol red in skin. The skin accumulation of phenol red at 10 h has a linear relationship with the penetration flux of phenol red. It was also reported that *N*-alkyl-2-pyrrolidones promoted the penetration and skin accumulation of 5-fluorouracil, aminopyrine, flurbiprofen, triamcinolone acetonide, indomethacin, and sulfaguanidine.[11,12] The promoting action of *N*-alkyl-2-pyrrolidones was supported by an *in vivo* absorption experiment in rats.[10]

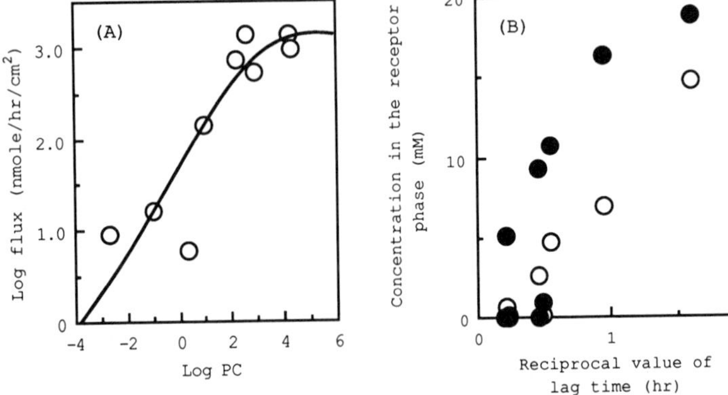

Figure 1 Relationship between log partition coefficient and flux of penetrants (A) and relationship between reciprocal value of lag time and concentration of pyrrolidones in the receptor phase (B). (B) Key: (○) concentration at 3 h, (•) concentration at 10 h. Each point is the mean of at least three experiments.

C. PYROGLUTAMIC ACID DERIVATIVES

Pyroglutamic acid and its derivatives are used as moisturizers in therapeutics and cosmetics. The enhancing effect of PGA is not clear. Lippold and Hackemüller[4] reported that the biological activity of benzyl nicotinate did not increase after treatment with PGA. However, the effectiveness of oleyl, decyl, and dodecyl ester of PGA was reported in enhancing the permeation of enalapril and clonidine across shed snake skin.[13]

D. 3-HYDROXY-*N*-METHYL-2-PYRROLIDONE

N-Methyl-2-pyrrolidone is biotransformed in the rat to a hydroxylated species such as 3-hydroxy- and 5-hydroxy-2-pyrrolidones, which upon acid hydrolysis under laboratory conditions yields the unsaturated product 4-(methylamino)-2-butenoic acid. The 3-hydroxy derivative of NMP is reported to have enhancement properties in the *in vitro* experiment using Franz cells.[13] Clioquinol penetration using the 3-hydroxy derivative was greater than in the controls by a factor of 1.8, and greater than NMP by a factor of 1.3. The NMP metabolite should be less toxic than that of NMP.

E. OTHER PYRROLIDONE DERIVATIVES

Okamoto et al.[14] investigated nine azacycloalkanone derivatives with an alkyl or terpene chain for their effects on the percutaneous penetration of 6-mercaptopurine through excised guinea pig skin. The number of carbonyl groups in chain affected the enhancing activity more effectively rather than the ring size. *N*-Farnesyl-2-pyrrolidone was one of the favorable enhancers. Yano et al.[15] reported that *N*-[2-(decylthio)ethyl]-2-pyrrolidone (HPE-101) significantly enhanced the excretion of nicotinic acid, 5-fluorouracil, estradiol, and triamcinolone acetonide, but not that of testosterone. Lambert et al.[16] demonstrated the usefulness of a biodegradable transdermal penetration enhancer, decanoic acid ester of *N*-(2-hydroxyethyl)-2-pyrrolidone (HEP-Dec). The ester linkage was readily cleaved by hydrolytic enzymes in plasma and skin. This enhancer increased the permeability of hydrocortisone through mouse skin by two orders of magnitude and showed much less irritation potential than traditional penetration enhancers.

Indomethacin prodrug having *N*-alkyl-2-pyrrolidone as a promoiety was designed from the basis of good skin penetration and an enhancing effect of pyrrolidones.[17] Some were able to penetrate through excised human skin better than the parent drug, although the mechanism was not clear.

III. ENHANCING MECHANISM

A. INFLUENCE OF FORMULATION AND CONDITION

The concentration of absorption enhancer in a formulation markedly influences the promotion of transdermal drug delivery. A decrease in the concentration of *N*-alkyl-2-pyrrolidones in a formulation was found to decrease the flux and skin accumulation, and to prolong the lag time for a steady-state penetration of phenol red.[18] This decreased enhancing effect can be explained by a decrease in penetration and skin accumulation of the enhancer.

Pretreatment of NMP, NHP, and NLP for 5 h shortened the lag time for a phenol red penetration.[18] The difference between the apparent lag times for coapplication (LT1) and pretreatment (LT2) was calculated as ELT. Phenol red flux, LT1, LT2, and ELT are listed in Table 2. LT2 is considered to be related to the process of diffusion of dye through the skin modified by the enhancer. The meaning of ELT is complicated, however, it reflects mainly the time during which the enhancer penetrates into the skin and shows a constant enhancing effect. A decrease in the concentration of the enhancer resulted in prolonging not only LT2, but also ELT. Removal of NHP from the donor side resulted in a decrease in the enhancing effect because rapid leakage of NHP from the skin into the receptor phase was observed.[18] *N*-Lauryl-2-pyrrolidone retained the enhancing effect after removal because of its high localization in lipophilic parts of the SC.

The vehicle in topical formulation is an important factor which controls the penetrations of not only the drug but also the enhancer itself. In an aqueous vehicle NMP showed little enhancing effect on transdermal penetration of phenol red and indomethacin as compared to that in isopropyl myristate vehicle.[19] Both NHP and NLP showed high enhancing effect in an aqueous vehicle. This inactivity of NMP can be explained by the poor penetration of NMP from the aqueous vehicle. Hoelgaard et al.[20] also reported that isopropyl myristate containing NMP showed higher percutaneous penetration of metronidazole associated with the release rate of NMP than PG.

Some vehicles can penetrate the SC and play the role of enhancer. Wotton et al.[21] demonstrated that Azone® enhanced the penetration of PG, and the enhanced PG penetration resulted in the enhanced transport of metronidazole. On the other hand, Sasaki et al.[22] found another mechanism in combining vehicles of NMP and NLP. *N*-Methyl-2-pyrrolidone promoted the rapid penetration of NLP into the skin, potentiated the enhancing effect of NLP on penetration of phenol red and 5-fluorouracil, and shortened the lag time. The enhancers increase each other's penetration into the skin and improve each other's enhancing activity. Therefore, the combining vehicle acts synergistically rather than additively.

Table 2 Flux and Apparent Lag Time for Phenol Red Penetration after Application with Pyrrolidone Derivatives (0.5 and 2 mmol/ml)

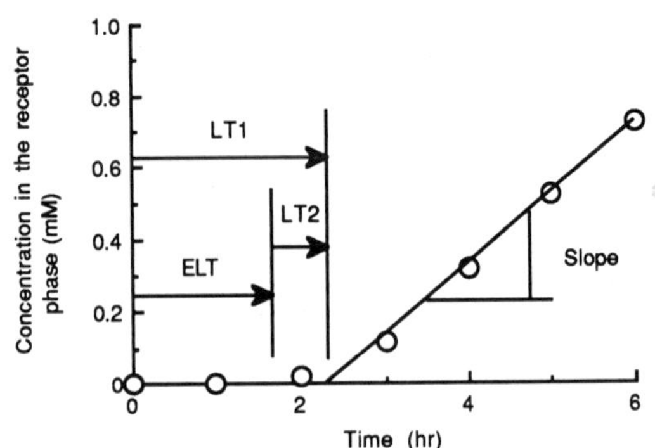

Enhancer	Conc. (mmol/ml)	Flux[a] (nmol/h/cm²)	LT1[b] (h)	LT2[c] (h)	ELT[d] (h)
NMP	2	16	0.62	0.87	−0.25
	0.5	4	2.12	0.51	1.61
NHP	2	1346	1.05	0.23	0.82
	0.5	38	2.68	1.21	1.47
NLP	2	1342	2.14	0.38	1.76
	0.5	418	4.70	1.24	3.46

[a] Flux = slope × receptor volume/available area.
[b] Lag time for phenol red penetration after coapplication with enhancer.
[c] Lag time for phenol red penetration after pretreatment with enhancer.
[d] ELT = LT1 − LT2.

B. INFLUENCE OF PENETRANTS

The SC is an ultradense membrane including hydrophilic and lipophilic domains. Many reports submitted polar route and nonpolar route for drug permeation according to drug lipophilicity. Southwell and Barry[7] investigated steady-state fluxes of polar methanol, nonpolar octanol, and intermediate compound caffeine in the *in vitro* experiment. They concluded that 2-P enhances drug permeation through the polar route of the skin by increasing the diffusivity, and reduces passage through the nonpolar route by decreasing diffusivity and partitioning.

Lipophilic enhancers such as Azone® predominantly enhanced hydrophilic drugs that penetrate through a polar route. The enhancing effects of NMP, NHP, and NLP on various penetrants were examined in the *in vitro* experiments.[11] Drug suspension was used as a formulation to determine the maximal flux. The enhancing effect (E_{pen}) and solubilizing effect (E_{sol}) were calculated as ratios of penetrant fluxes and penetrant solubilities in isopropyl myristate vehicle with and without enhancer, respectively. Figure 2 shows the relationship between partition coefficient of penetrant and E_{pen} (A) or E_{sol} (B).

If vehicle does not change the skin, the penetrant flux from the suspension is constant and E_{pen} is unity because the thermodynamic activities of penetrants are maximum in vehicle and in skin surface. However, in NHP and NLP an increase in

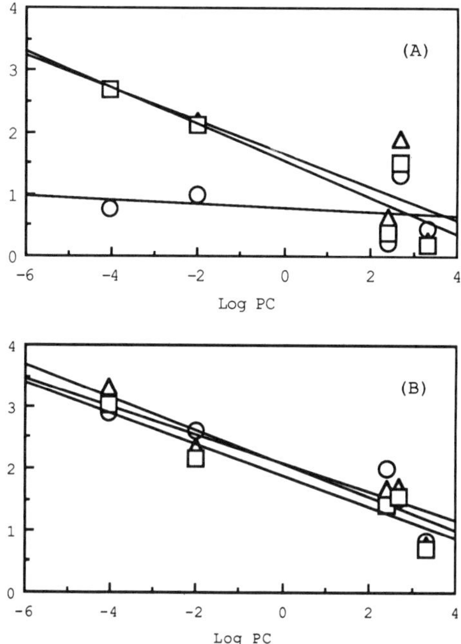

Figure 2 Relationships between log partition coefficient and log E_{pen} (A), or log E_{sol} (B). The lines through the data in (A) and (B) were obtained from a linear regression fit. Key: (○) NMP, (A) $y = -0.0308X + 0.769$, $r = 0.239$, (B) $y = -0.229X + 2.083$, $r = 0.911$; (Δ) NHP, (A) $y = -0.263X + 1.654$, $r = 0.834$, (B) $y = -0.266X + 2.089$, $r = 0.933$; (□) NLP, (A) $y = -0.296X + 1.517$, $r = 0.894$, (B) $y = -0.251X + 1.889$, $r = 0.943$. Each point is the mean of at least three experiments.

the hydrophilicity of penetrants showed an increase of E_{pen}. The slope for E_{pen} is almost equal to that for log E_{sol} in NHP and NLP. In fact, log E_{pen} showed a linear relationship with log E_{sol}. Lipophilic enhancer must be localized in lipophilic parts of the SC and must improve the solubility parameter of the SC by vehicle effect. The E_{pen} value of hydrophilic penetrant is especially increased by the enhancers because of its poor solubility in skin surfaces. The data analysis in this study can be simplified by using isopropyl myristate as a vehicle because of its similar solubility parameter to SC. On the other hand, NMP showed a high solubilizing effect but a low enhancing effect. It may be explained by a low localization of hydrophilic NMP in lipophilic parts of the SC at low concentrations.

A lipophilic ion pair of amide enhancer with anionic penetrant might cause the strong solubilizing capacity of pyrrolidones. However, *N*-alkyl-2-pyrrolidones showed a great enhancing effect on the penetration of even nonionic drugs.[12] El-Hinnawi and Najib[23] reported that the nitrogen of the pyrrolidone ring interacted with drug through hydrogen bonding. Hydrogen bonding may contribute to the solubilizing capacity.

C. INTERACTION WITH SKIN COMPONENTS

Elias[24] demonstrated the importance of lipid, qualitatively and quantitatively, in regulating the barrier properties of the SC. These lipids construct lamellar structures in the intercellular spaces of the SC and are closely associated with the keratin filaments. Sasaki et al.[25] demonstrated the effects of pyrrolidone derivatives on a release of 6-carboxyfluorescein from liposome. The lipophilic derivatives enhanced a release of hydrophilic dye and the enhancing effect showed a concentration dependency. Kim et al.[26] also reported that pyrrolidone derivatives disorder the liposomal membrane made with SC lipid. Barry[27] suggested, in a differential scanning calorimetry (DSC) work, that lipophilic enhancers appear to enter the lipid regions only where they disrupt the structure. The high enhancing effects of lipophilic pyrrolidones must be predominantly due to their interactions with structured lipids of the SC. More hydrophobic pyrrolidones penetrate more easily into the lipid and reduce the barrier function more effectively. Ogiso et al.[28] showed another mechanism in relation to lipids that Azone® interacts with structured lipids in the intercellular channels and releases them, thereby enhancing the penetration of drugs through the channels.

Oertel[29] reported that dimethylsulfoxide, which is an aprotic solvent as is NMP, induced a conformational change in the keratin filaments. Urea acts on skin protein as a keratolytic agent after prolonged contact with skin at high concentrations. The pyrrolidone derivatives slightly liberated the SH group of keratin, but did not change the electrophoresis pattern of keratin.[25] As the results of a DSC study show, NMP partitioned preferentially at low concentrations into the protein region rather than lipid of the SC and denatured α-keratin.[27] At high concentrations, NMP was able to interact with the SC lipid, increasing its fluidity. Also, NMP was reported to increase water content in the SC by determining skin conductance with an impedance meter.[25] Both NHP and NLP showed little influence on skin conductance. Hydration will become more important as an indirect enhancing effect in an aqueous vehicle.

IV. TOXICITY

A median lethal dose (LD_{50}) is 6.5 ml/kg for 2-P and 7.0 ml/kg for NMP in rat and guinea pig. *N*-Methyl-2-pyrrolidone is safe on nerve and blood at a dose of 0.25 mg/kg in rat and rabbit. After intravenous administration of double radiolabeled NMP, the half-lives of radioactivities in plasma were 7 and 9.9 h.[30] The major route of excretion was via the urine and accounted for 70% of the dose within 12 h. Topical application of NMP on skin also showed low toxicity. At high concentration, 2-P and NMP induced erythema in some human subjects, although this was usually short-lived.[2]

The acute toxicities of *N*-alkyl-2-pyrrolidones and its 4-substituted derivatives were observed at a dose of 500 mg/kg after intraperitoneal administration in mice.[31] These were comparable to those of observed with Azone® (LD_{50}, 232 mg/kg in mice) and nutritional compounds. The lipophilic enhancers such as NLP and Azone® may be more safe because of their poor skin penetration.

The primary skin irritations of *N*-alkyl-2-pyrrolidones and its 4-substituted derivatives were examined with rabbit dorsal skin.[31] Among the derivatives, NLP induced the most severe irritation similar to Azone®. The primary irritation indices of pyrrolidone derivatives were not relative to their accumulations in the skin but to their enhancing effects. Ponec et al.[32] also showed the parallel relationship between cytotoxicity in cultured human skin cells and penetration-enhancing capacity with *N*-alkylazacycloheptan-2-one derivatives. One approach to improve a balance between skin toxicity and enhancing effect is to develop a biodegradable enhancer. Some additives such as vitamin E and squalene in formulation were reported to reduce the erythema caused by lauroylsarcosine of a surfactant enhancer.[33]

REFERENCES

1. **Southwell, D. and Barry, B. W.,** Penetration enhancement in human skin; effect of 2-pyrrolidone, dimethylformamide and increased hydration on finite dose permeation of aspirin and caffeine, *Int. J. Pharm.,* 22, 291, 1984.
2. **Barry, B. W., Southwell, D., and Woodford, R.,** Optimization of bioavailability of topical steroids: penetration enhancers under occlusion, *J. Invest. Dermatol.,* 82, 49, 1984.
3. **Ryatt, K. S., Stevenson, J. M., Maibach, H. I., and Guy, R. H.,** Pharmacodynamic measurement of percutaneous penetration enhancement *in vivo, J. Pharm. Sci.,* 75, 374, 1986.
4. **Lippold, B. C. and Hackemüller, D.,** The influence of skin moisturizers on drug penetration *in vivo, Int. J. Pharm.,* 61, 205, 1990.
5. **Resh, W. and Stoughton, R. B.,** Topically applied antibiotics in acne vulgaris, *Arch. Dermatol.,* 112, 182, 1976.
6. **Barry, B. W.,** Properties that influence percutaneous absorption, in *Dermatological Formulations. Percutaneous Absorption,* Marcel Dekker, New York, 1983, 127.
7. **Southwell, D. and Barry, B. W.,** Penetration enhancers for human skin: mode of action of 2-pyrrolidone and dimethylformamide on partition and diffusion of model compounds water, n-alcohols, and caffeine, *J. Invest. Dermatol.,* 80, 507, 1983.
8. **Melendres, J. L., Nangia, A., Sedik, L., Hori, M., and Maibach, H. I.,** Nonane enhances propranolol hydrochloride penetration in human skin, *Int. J. Pharm.,* 92, 243, 1993.
9. **Bonina, F. P. and Montenegro, L.,** Penetration enhancer effects on *in vitro* percutaneous absorption of heparin sodium salt, *Int. J. Pharm.,* 82, 171, 1992.
10. **Sasaki, H., Kojima, M., Mori, Y., Nakamura, J., and Shibasaki, J.,** Enhancing effect of pyrrolidone derivatives on transdermal drug delivery. I., *Int. J. Pharm.,* 44, 15, 1988.
11. **Sasaki, H., Kojima, M., Mori, Y., Nakamura, J., and Shibasaki, J.,** Enhancing effect of pyrrolidone derivatives on transdermal penetration of 5-fluorouracil, triamcinolone acetonide, indomethacin, and flurbiprofen, *J. Pharm. Sci.,* 80, 533, 1991.
12. **Sasaki, H., Kojima, M., Nakamura, J., and Shibasaki, J.,** Enhancing effect of pyrrolidone derivatives on the transdermal penetration of sulfaguanidine, aminopyrine and sudan III, *J. Pharmacobio-Dyn.,* 13, 200, 1990.
13. **Santus, G. C. and Baker, R. W.,** Transdermal enhancer patent literature, *J. Control. Rel.,* 25, 1, 1993.
14. **Okamoto, H., Hashida, M., and Sezaki, H.,** Structure-activity relationship of 1-alkyl- or 1-alkenylazacycloalkanone derivatives as percutaneous penetration enhancers, *J. Pharm. Sci.,* 77, 418, 1988.
15. **Yano, T., Higo, N., Fukuda, K., Tsuji, M., Noda, K., and Otagiri, M.,** Further evaluation of a new penetration enhancer, HPE-101, *J. Pharm. Pharmacol.,* 45, 775, 1993.
16. **Lambert, W. J., Kudla, R. J., Holland, J. M., and Curry, J. T.,** A biodegradable transdermal penetration enhancer based on *N*-(2-hydroxyethyl)-2-pyrrolidone. I. Synthesis and characterization, *Int. J. Pharm.,* 95, 181, 1993.
17. **Bonina, F. P., Montenegro, L., De Capraris, P., Bousquet, E., and Tirendi, S.,** 1-Alkylazacycloalkan-2-one esters as prodrugs of indomethacin for improved delivery through human skin, *Int. J. Pharm.,* 77, 21, 1991.
18. **Sasaki, H., Kojima, M., Mori, Y., Nakamura, J., and Shibasaki, J.,** Enhancing effect of pyrrolidone derivatives on transdermal drug delivery. II. Effect of application concentration and pretreatment of enhancer, *Int. J. Pharm.,* 60, 177, 1990.
19. **Sasaki, H., Kojima, M., Nakamura, J., and Shibasaki, J.,** Enhancing effect of pyrrolidone derivatives on transdermal penetration of phenolsulfonphthalein and indomethacin from aqueous vehicle, *Chem. Pharm. Bull.,* 38, 797, 1990.
20. **Hoelgaard, A., Møllgaard, B., and Baker, E.,** Vehicle effect on topical drug delivery. IV. Effect of *N*-methylpyrrolidone and polar lipids on percutaneous drug transport, *Int. J. Pharm.,* 43, 233, 1988.

21. **Wotton, P. K., Møllgaard, B., Hadgraft, J., and Hoelgaard, A.,** Vehicle effect on topical drug delivery. III. Effect of Azone® on the cutaneous permeation of metronidazole and propylene glycol, *Int. J. Pharm.,* 24, 19, 1985.
22. **Sasaki, H., Kojima, M., Nakamura, J., and Shibasaki, J.,** Enhancing effect of combining two pyrrolidone vehicles on transdermal drug delivery, *J. Pharm. Pharmacol.,* 42, 196, 1990.
23. **El-Hinnawi, M. A. and Najib, N. M.,** Ibuprofen-polyvinylpyrrolidone dispersions. Proton nuclear magnetic resonance and infrared studies, *Int. J. Pharm.,* 37, 175, 1987.
24. **Elias, P. M.,** Epidermal barrier function: intercellular lamellar lipid structures, origin, composition and metabolism, *J. Control. Rel.,* 15, 199, 1991.
25. **Sasaki, H., Kishikawa, M., Nakamura, J., and Shibasaki, J.,** Effect of pyrrolidone derivatives on lipid membrane and protein conformation as transdermal penetration enhancer, *J. Pharmacobio-Dyn.,* 13, 468, 1990.
26. **Kim, C.-K., Hong, M.-S., Kim, Y.-B., and Han, S.-K.,** Effect of penetration enhancers (pyrrolidone derivatives) on multilamellar liposomes of SC lipid: a study by UV spectroscopy and differential scanning calorimetry, *Int. J. Pharm.,* 95, 43, 1993.
27. **Barry, B. W.,** Mode of action of penetration enhancers in human skin, *J. Control. Rel.,* 6, 85, 1987.
28. **Ogiso, T., Iwaki, M., Bechako, K., and Tsutsumi, Y.,** Enhancement of percutaneous absorption by laurocapram, *J. Pharm. Sci.,* 81, 762, 1992.
29. **Oertel, R. P.,** Protein conformational changes induced in human SC by organic sulfoxides: an infrared spectroscopic investigation, *Biopolymers,* 16, 2329, 1977.
30. **Wells, D. A. and Digenis, G. A.,** Disposition and metabolism of double-labeled [^{3}H and ^{14}C] *N*-methyl-2-pyrrolidinone in the rat, *Drug Metab. Dispos.,* 16, 243, 1988.
31. **Sasaki, H., Kojima, M., Nakamura, J., and Shibasaki, J.,** Acute toxicity and skin irritation of pyrrolidone derivatives as transdermal penetration enhancer, *Chem. Pharm. Bull.,* 38, 2308, 1990.
32. **Ponec, M., Haverkort, M., Soei, Y. L., Kempenaar, J., Brussee, J., and Boddé, H.,** Toxicity screening of *N*-alkylazacycloheptan-2-one derivatives in cultured human skin cells: structure-toxicity relationships, *J. Pharm. Sci.,* 78, 738, 1989.
33. **Aioi, A., Kuriyama, K., Shimizu, T., Yoshioka, M., and Uenoyama, S.,** Effects of vitamin E and squalene on skin irritation of a transdermal absorption enhancer, lauroylsarcosine, *Int. J. Pharm.,* 93, 1, 1993.

Chapter 7.2

Drug-Polyvinylpyrrolidone Coprecipitates

Owen I. Corrigan

CONTENTS

I. INTRODUCTION

The use of drug-polymer coprecipitates to improve the bioavailability of drugs of low solubility following oral administration has been advocated ever since the discovery of their remarkable dissolution-enhancing properties.[1–3] The polymers used are water soluble and the most commonly employed material is polyvinylpyrrolidone (PVP). In the original process the drug and the PVP were dissolved in a common solvent. The resulting solution was then evaporated to dryness, yielding a solid product known as a coprecipitate. The technique was first reported in 1965 as a method for preparing aqueous colloidal dispersions of β-carotene.[4] Enhanced dissolution rates of griseofulvin-PVP coprecipitates were next reported.[5] Then, enhanced *in vivo* absorption of rapidly dissolving reserpine-PVP coprecipitate in rats was obtained.[6] Similar findings were reported for other drugs of low aqueous solubility.[3] The increased dissolution rate of a drug-PVP coprecipitate, arising from an increased apparent solubility and decreased drug particle size, is highly likely to increase the absorption, i.e., bioavailability of a hydrophobic drug, because for such compounds dissolution is very often the rate-determining step governing absorption. However, drug dissolution is unlikely to be the rate-controlling element in the transdermal passage of a drug from a transdermal drug delivery system. The objective of this chapter is to consider the potential use of drug-PVP coprecipitates for enhancing the transdermal absorption of drugs.

0-8493-2605-2/95/$0.00+$.50

II. PROPERTIES OF POLYVINYLPYRROLIDONE

Polyvinylpyrrolidone has been used extensively for over 25 years as an excipient in a wide variety of pharmaceutical formulations, including products for oral, parenteral, and topical use. The versatility of PVP arises from its extremely low toxicity and its unique range of functional characteristics. Polyvinylpyrrolidone is a synthetic, water-soluble polymer consisting of linear chains of 1-vinyl-2 pyrrolidinone groups.[7] The molecular weight of the repeating unit is 111.16. A range of PVP products are commercially available for pharmaceutical use, with average molecular weights in the range 10,000 to 2.8 million.[7,8] Products are graded with reference to K-values determined by viscometry. The molecular weight affects not just viscosity, but also such properties as adhesiveness, glass transition and rate of solution. Polyvinylpyrrolidone has been shown to function as an anti-irritant when used as a component of topical and ophthalmic drug-containing products.[9,10] Among the physicochemical attributes of PVP that are likely to have biopharmaceutical consequences are a high solubility in a range of solvents, including water, the ability to form complexes with a wide range of drugs,[11,12] and the ability to prevent and/or retard crystal growth.[13–16] The latter two properties were linked to the ability of the polymer to promote the formation of high-energy drug phases in coprecipitates and also to its ability to stabilize these high-energy drug phases. Polyvinylpyrrolidone was linked to alterations in the absorption of a range of drug substances. Little, if any, data have been published relating specifically to transdermal drug delivery. However, a considerable amount of data relates to the effects of drug-PVP coprecipitates on membrane transport, which should provide strong guidelines as to their bioavailability-enhancing potential in transdermal systems.

III. THEORETICAL CONSIDERATIONS

The diffusion-controlled rate of transport, per unit surface area, of a drug across any barrier *(dQ/dt),* irrespective of its complexity, will be proportional to the drug concentration gradient and the overall permeability coefficient (P_e):

$$\frac{dQ}{dt} = P_e\left(C_d - C_r\right) \tag{1}$$

where C_d and C_r are the drug concentrations in the donor and receptor compartments, respectively. P_e may be defined as $K_S \cdot D/X$, where K_S is the partition coefficient for the interfacial partitioning of the drug from the vehicle onto the barrier phase, D is the apparent diffusivity of the drug in the barrier, and X is the thickness of the barrier.[17–19] In situations in which binding of the drug is occurring due to the presence of a nonabsorbable polymeric excipient, Equation 1 may be modified to take account of the effective decrease in drug concentration due to binding:[19]

$$\frac{dQ}{dt} = P_e\left(C_d - C_r\right)/\left(1 + k \cdot C_p\right) \tag{2}$$

where k is the equilibrium distribution constant of drug to polymer and C_p is the polymer concentration. At early times (i.e., when $C_r \sim 0$) the initial transport rate (G_i) is given by:

$$G_i = A \cdot P_e \cdot C_d \tag{3}$$

or when polymer binding occurs:

$$G_i = A \cdot P_e \cdot C_{td} / \left(1 + k \cdot C_p\right) \tag{4}$$

where A is the surface area and C_{td} is the total bulk drug concentration in the donor compartment, i.e., free plus bound. The above analysis shows that drug binding to a nonabsorbable polymeric excipient will decrease drug transport. However, by using a high-energy phase of the drug, such as those formed in drug-PVP coprecipitates, the flux of drug across the skin should be increased because C_d is effectively increased without altering P_e. This is in contrast to other solubility-enhancing strategies such as surfactant solubilization or cosolvent addition, which generally also decrease P_e.

IV. DRUG-POLYVINYLPYRROLIDONE INTERACTIONS

Polyvinylpyrrolidone is known to interact with a wide range of drugs forming complexes,[11,12] both in solution and in the solid state, and many of the novel functional properties of the polymer are thought to be related to these interactions. Investigations of complex formation between PVP and a number of phenolic compounds demonstrated the precipitation of an amorphous complex with phenol; the stoichiometry of the interaction was approximately one phenol molecule bound to every vinylpyrrolidone repeating unit. Molyneux and Frank[20] used an equilibrium dialysis technique to investigate the binding affinity of PVP for dissolved aromatic compounds. They found that the binding constants and hence the free energies of binding increased as the size of the aromatic system increased. An increase in the number of polar groups in the phenol–phloroglucinol series also led to an increase in the binding constant. Further studies[21] examined the effect of the interaction on the molecular size of the PVP polymer. With anionic compounds, viscometric results indicated that in general, the polymer expands. Light scattering data supported the viscometry findings. Plaizier-Vercammen obtained correlations among solubility,[22] octanol-water partition coefficient,[23] and binding of ligands to PVP. It was concluded that no highly specific orientation of the ligand with PVP occurred.

Binding also seems to play a part in the inhibition and retardation effects of PVP on crystal growth. Simonelli et al.[16] investigated the inhibition of sulfathiazole crystal growth by PVP from aqueous supersaturated solutions.[16] The minimum concentration of PVP required for complete inhibition of crystal growth was a function of the molecular weight of PVP used. The results suggested that the PVP concentration required to cause inhibition of crystal growth depended on the relative rates of transport of PVP and sulfathiazole to the crystal surface from the bulk solution. Polyvinylpyrrolidone not only retarded the rate of crystal growth, but also changed the growth pattern, leading to the development of roughened crystal surfaces. The rate of PVP transport to the crystal surface was insufficient to form a tightly packed film. It also appeared that the PVP was strongly bound to the sulfathiazole surface forming a polymer net on the surface, the mesh size of which dictated the supersaturation level necessary before growth could continue.[16] Sekikawa et al.[13] studied the effect of PVP on both the inhibition and retardation of crystallization of a range of compounds dissolved in ethanol solutions. The values of the binding constants at 50°C were in the same rank order as the inhibiting effect of PVP on drug crystallization.

V. THE NATURE OF THE DRUG PHASE IN POLYVINYLPYRROLIDONE COPRECIPITATES

In their classical study of sulfathiazole-PVP coprecipitates, Simonelli et al.[24] proposed the formation of a high-energy amorphous phase of drug in PVP-coprecipitate systems. The existence of such a phase was based on the results of X-ray diffraction and dissolution studies. The absence of characteristic diffraction peaks in the powder X-ray diffraction pattern of the drug when coprecipitates were compared to corresponding physical mixtures, was consistent with an amorphous form of drug. They also found that whereas the dissolution rates of sulfathiazole-PVP coprecipitates were qualitatively in agreement with the soluble complex model,[25] in the weight fraction range in which drug is expected to be the surface layer controlling dissolution, the observed rates were consistently higher (by a factor of 4) than those predicted from theory. Simonelli and co-workers postulated that this increased dissolution reflected the higher solubility of the amorphous high-energy phase. Thus, dissolution data could be used to factor out the contribution of increased solubility due to complex formation from that attributable to the high-energy drug phase. Subsequent detailed solubility studies of sulfathiazole-PVP coprecipitates confirmed the dissolution findings.[26] Other workers confirmed the amorphous nature of PVP-drug coprecipitates.[5,6,27] The inhibiting effect of PVP on crystallization, crystal growth, and phase transformation was demonstrated for many drugs in both organic and aqueous media.[12–16] The magnitude of this effect for a given drug was linked with the ability to form an amorphous coprecipitate. The molecular weight of the polymer and the structure of the drug are also determinants. Although the formation of high-energy drug phases in PVP-drug processed systems occurs with many drugs, the physicochemical requirements necessary to form such phases have not been elucidated.[27–29] The physicochemical nature of the high-energy drug phase present in coprecipitates is the subject of some debate. It has been possible to separate the relative contributions of free drug and soluble complex formation using dissolution,[24] solubility,[26] and membrane transport methodologies[19] (see below); all three methods yielded similar estimates of the activity increases for a given drug. Shefter and Cheng[30] measured drug solubility in PVP by differential scanning calorimetry DSC and related molecular dispersibility in the polymer to hydrogen bonding with the pyrrolidone moiety. They suggested that molecularly dispersed drug in the polymer probably accounts for the observed higher intrinsic dissolution rate of dispersions over physical mixtures. Evidence for the formation of different amorphous drug phases as well as molecularly bound drug in coprecipitate systems was reported.[31] Although most drugs exist at room temperature as crystalline solids, higher energy phases may be produced by appropriate processing. These range from crystalline polymorphs or pseudopolymorphs to amorphous forms.[32–34,37] It also appears that a range of amorphous states is possible for a given drug. Thus, Matsuda et al.[32] prepared two amorphous forms of frusemide using different spray drying conditions, each having different activation energies for the glass transition and crystallization processes. Furthermore, amorphous hydroflumethiazide produced by spray drying had an apparent solubility 1.6 times that of the pure crystalline drug phase, whereas the high-energy amorphous hydroflumethiazide present in hydroflumethiazide-PVP coprecipitates was approximately four times more soluble than that of the crystalline drug phase.[31] A better understanding of the nature of these high-energy drug forms is necessary to enable prediction of their activity and stability.

VI. ENHANCED MEMBRANE TRANSPORT WITH DRUG-POLYVINYLPYRROLIDONE COPRECIPITATES

Although not employing skin, a number of studies of drug transport across artificial membranes have been reported using drug-PVP coprecipitates.

A. SULFATHIAZOLE-POLYVINYLPYRROLIDONE COPRECIPITATES

The physicochemical studies outlined in the previous section indicated that the high-energy amorphous drug phase present in sulfathiazole-PVP (Povidone 10,000) coprecipitates exhibited thermodynamic activities approximately fourfold greater than that of the conventional crystalline form. The sulfathiazole flux across a cellophane membrane from a 5% PVP solution saturated with a sulfathiazole–PVP (1:3) coprecipitate was significantly greater than that obtained from solutions saturated with crystalline drug.[19] The ratio of the slopes was 3.5:1, comparable to the higher activity of the coprecipitate determined from dissolution data. Transport data obtained using solutions saturated with crystalline drug and containing 5% PVP gave fluxes slightly higher than those obtained in the absence of PVP. This effect was attributed to contributions from polymer-bound drug[17] and some polymer transport through the membrane. However, the results indicate that this "carrier" effect arising from drug-PVP complexation is almost an order of magnitude smaller than the thermodynamic effect.

B. HYDROCORTISONE-POLYVINYLPYRROLIDONE COPRECIPITATES

X-ray diffraction and dissolution data suggested that an amorphous high-energy form of hydrocortisone, with an activity 14 to 15 times that of the pure drug is present in these PVP coprecipitates. However, at the lower PVP weight fractions, even in the presence of up to 10% PVP, reconversion to the more stable form occurred during dissolution. In order to minimize this potential for nucleation and crystal growth, during membrane transport experiments, a 10:1 (PVP-drug) coprecipitate system was employed.[19] As was the case with sulfathiazole the flux from the PVP-containing solution, saturated with crystalline hydrocortisone, was about 15% higher than from the aqueous solution. Fluxes obtained from coprecipitate-containing systems were, however, considerably higher, the flux increasing with increasing hydrocortisone content. A comparison of the initial slopes indicates that the highest flux was about ten times that of unit activity. When the concentration of hydrocortisone was increased above 4.6 mg/ml, nucleation was observed in the donor solution and data deviated from the model predictions.[19]

Because attaining higher transport rates seemed to be limited by recrystallization, the nucleation and crystal growth inhibitors, Clayton yellow and dodecylamine

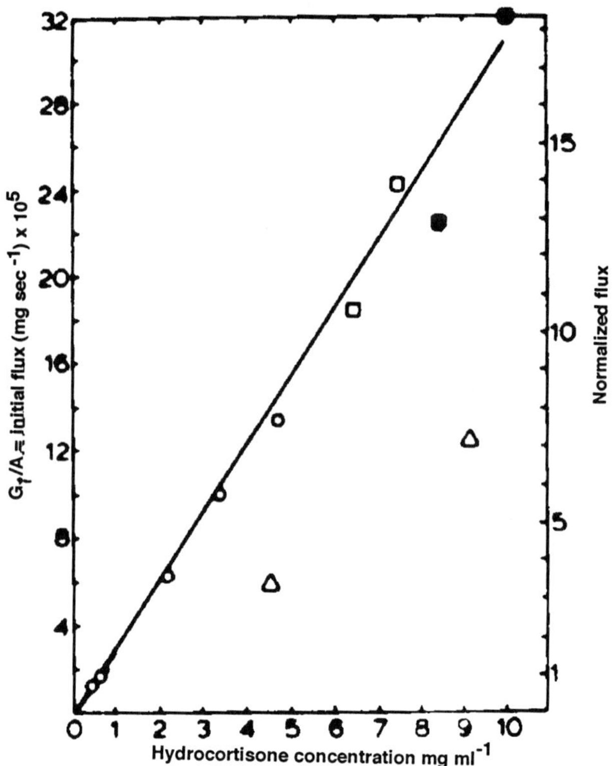

Figure 1 Initial hydrocortisone transport rate vs. drug concentration in 9.5% povidone prepared from 10:1 (PVP-drug) coprecipitate. Also included is the normalized flux (flux with coprecipitate/ flux with saturated solution of crystalline drug in 9.5% povidone). Key: ○, povidone 9.5%; □, povidone 9.5% plus Clayton yellow 0.05%; Δ, povidone 9.5% plus dodecylamine HCl 1%; ■, systems in which visible nucleation occurred during the experiment; —— theoretical assuming only membrane control. (Modified from Corrigan, O. I., Farvar, M. A., and Higuchi, W. I., *Int. J. Pharm.*, 5, 229, 1980. With permission.)

hydrochloride, were used in the membrane flux experiments and estimates made of the initial transport rates of hydrocortisone.[19] The actual and normalized values obtained are plotted, together with those estimated in the absence of Clayton yellow, vs. hydrocortisone total concentration in Figure 1. The good linear relationship, which includes the data from solutions which became cloudy, is evident, thus supporting the presence of a high-energy phase in coprecipitate systems. The relative maximum enhancement in membrane transport brought about by coprecipitate was 18- to 19-fold and in systems in which no nucleation was observed, 14- to 15-fold. These values are similar in magnitude to the relative enhancements observed in the intrinsic dissolution rate experiments.

Merkle[35] also investigated the hydrocortisone-PVP system using the Kollidon® 17 (molecular weight of 11,500) form of the polymer. Results of transport studies across cellophane dialysis membranes indicated a sixfold activity increase for the coprecipitates, containing drug fractions in the range 0.1 to 0.2, when compared to the crystalline phase. Up to a drug concentration of about 2 mg/ml the data were found to closely fit a linear relationship. Higher concentrations led to a rapid recrystallization of drug and deviations from linearity. Deviations from the optimum expected flux were attributed to complex binding and/or self-association, particularly the latter. Studies of higher molecular weight polymer fractions (i.e., 25,000 and 40,000) demonstrated the same basic principles, however, Merkle concluded that extent of self-association was higher in these systems. Merkle[35] also suggested that coprecipitation stabilizes nucleation embryos, thus preventing spontaneous recrystallization. The lower hydrocortisone activities reported for coprecipitates in the latter study[35] may have arisen from the different media employed (i.e., 5% PVP, which will inhibit/retard nucleation),[19] differences in the processes used to manufacture the coprecipitates, e.g., rate of evaporation/drying, cooling, etc., or characteristics of the PVP employed.

Aged samples were also studied and were found to have somewhat lower activities than fresh coprecipitates.[35] In essence, the aging of coprecipitated hydrocortisone was considered to be an association process in the solid state leading to aggregates in the colloidal range. From the differences in the relative activities of low and medium molecular weight PVP systems it can be concluded that the rate of the solid-state association depends on the molecular weight of the carrier. Because the hydrocortisone-PVP coprecipitate was the only example of such aging the author concluded that these results cannot be generalized to other drugs.[35]

C. NITRAZEPAM-POLYVINYLPYRROLIDONE COPRECIPITATES

Merkle also investigated the dynamic dialysis of nitrazepam-PVP coprecipitates using drug contents of 0.05 and 0.1 and the 11,500 and 25,000 mol wt polymer fractions. The results are shown in Figure 2. The maximum activity, as reflected by the enhanced flux, was found to be more than ten times higher than unit activity at saturation. The experimental data were close to the theoretical, assuming zero complex binding and association. Independent estimation of the binding constant gave a much lower value than that observed with hydrocortisone. Furthermore, no significant differences were observed on changing the molecular weight of the PVP used.[35]

D. DIGOXIN-POLYVINYLPYRROLIDONE COPRECIPITATES

Higuchi and Farvar[36] also investigated the digoxin-PVP system. While dissolution rate data yielded maximum rate enhancements of around 350-fold, the plateau region in the rate vs. composition diagram suggested that the high-energy phase had an activity 22 to 24 times that of crystalline digoxin. Figure 3 summarizes the membrane transport data for digoxin-povidone systems (1:10) as well as those for a saturated crystalline digoxin solution. The flux obtained was about 7.5 times that of the saturated solution when the total drug concentration in the donor chamber was about 8.3 times that of the saturated solution. Thus, most of the drug appears to be "free" under these conditions. The supersaturated solution remained clear for an indefinite period. When a 12.4-fold supersaturated solution was used, it became cloudy after about 6 h or more and the profile deviated from linearity. However, the addition of 1.0% Tween® 80 to this solution delayed the development of turbidity up to around 24 h. When the donor chamber drug concentration was increased to around 18 times saturation and Tween® 80 was included to inhibit nucleation a flux 20 times that for the saturated solution was obtained. Thus, the apparent supersaturations obtained under these conditions did in fact largely represent free drug, and indicated that the PVP levels used in these experiments and the 1.0% Tween® 80 had little or no

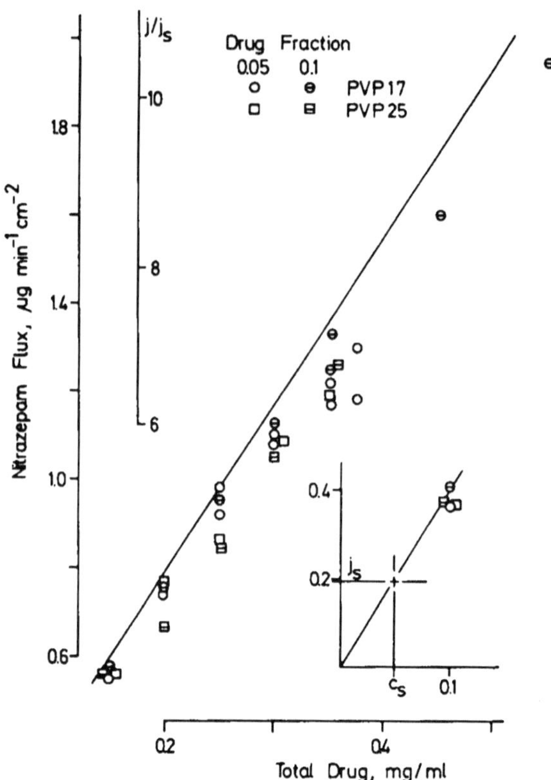

Figure 2 Nitrazepam flux resulting from dynamic dialysis of supersaturated solutions as a function of total drug concentration. Solid line indicates theoretical flux assuming zero complex binding and self-association. (From Merkle, H. P., *Proc. Int. Symp. Povidone,* Digenis, G. A. and Ansell, J., Eds., University of Kentucky, Lexington, 1983, 202. With permission.)

transport-retarding effect. The authors concluded that the enhanced fluxes found in these experiments were due mainly to increased thermodynamic activities rather than either intrinsic membrane effects or the transport of complexes. The maximum digoxin flux observed was close to the 22- to 24-fold enhancement found in the dissolution rate at the "plateau" region.[36]

E. OTHER DRUG-POLYVINYLPYRROLIDONE COPRECIPITATE SYSTEMS

Studies with the two other benzodiazepines, clonazepam and flunitrazepam, demonstrated supersaturation patterns similar to those observed with nitrazepam. Clonazepam showed a 14-fold increase in activity, while that observed with flunitrazepam was more than fivefold. Studies with prednisone were the least successful as rapid recrystallization of the drug to its low-energy form occurred. Maximum fluxes of only three and two times that of a normal saturated solution were achieved with the 11,500 and 25,000 mol wt PVP polymers, respectively. Merkle concluded that "although most drugs could be successfully coprecipitated to give solutions of highly elevated drug activities, the prednisone study shows that high drug activities do not

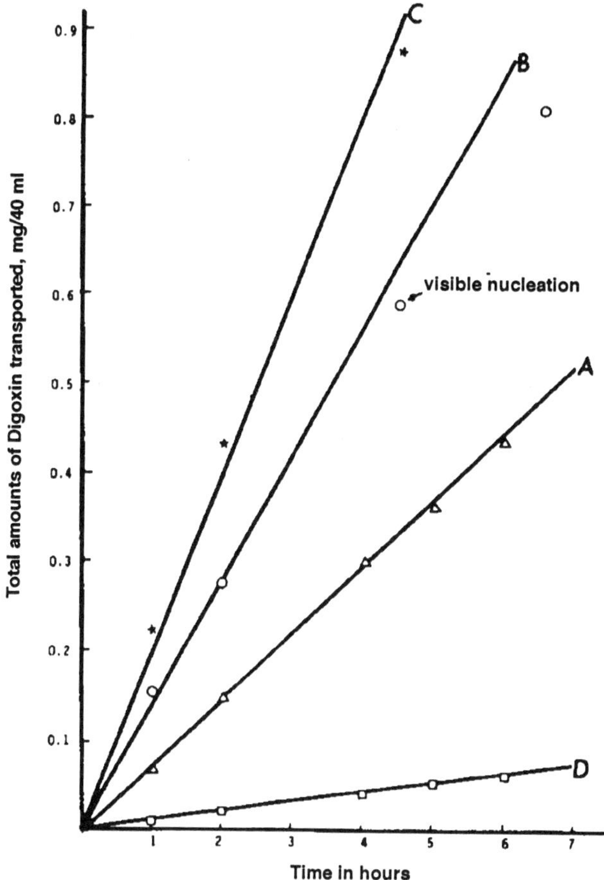

Figure 3 Fluxes of digoxin through a cellophane membrane from supersaturated solutions prepared by dissolving the 1:10 digoxin-PVP coprecipitate in aqueous media. Key: Δ, 0.283 mg/ml digoxin and 0.25% PVP; ○, 0.42 mg/ml digoxin and 0.55% PVP; ★, 0.61 mg/ml digoxin, 0.55% povidone, and 1.0% Tween® 80; □, digoxin (0.034 mg/ml). (From Higuchi, W. I. and Farrar, M. A., Proc. Int. Symp. Povidone, Digenis, G. A. and Ansell, J., Eds., University of Kentucky, Lexington, 1982, 71. With permission.)

solely depend on the use of PVP but also on the suitability of the drug itself. For a full understanding of the underlying mechanism, however, more work is needed on the dynamics and kinetics of supersaturated solutions."[35]

These results indicate that PVP-drug coprecipitates can generate stabilized supersaturated solutions with enhancements in drug transport across an artificial membrane, which may in some cases be as high as 10 to 25 times those obtained from saturated solutions prepared from the crystalline drug. As pointed out in the theory section, similar enhancements in rate should be obtained across biological membranes because the effect is on C_d and not P_e, irrespective of the complexity of P_e. To the author's knowledge no studies demonstrating enhanced transport with drug-PVP coprecipitates using skin samples as the membrane phase has been reported. However, enhanced transport from supersaturated systems across biological membranes, including skin and involving PVP as a stabilizer, has been reported.

VII. ENHANCED MEMBRANE TRANSPORT FROM RELATED SUPERSATURATED SYSTEMS

The induction of supersaturation through the use of volatile components in the vehicle was used by Coldman et al.[37] to enhance steroid penetration through human skin. Enhancements of eight- to tenfold were achieved and greater increases were limited by precipitation of the steroid. Kondo et al.[38] measured the bioavailability of nifedipine in rats following the application of supersaturated solutions. The vehicles employed included ternary solvent systems containing propyleneglycol:isopropyl myristate:acetone(25:2.5:89.5) with 3% drug. Evaporation of the acetone resulted in supersaturation, which in turn led to enhanced bioavailability. However, precipitation of drug occurred at the dosing site. The inclusion of polymeric additives such as 15% PVP (K-30) in this nonaqueous vehicle retarded precipitation and further enhanced transdermal bioavailability. This system gave a bioavailability enhancement, when compared to the saturated vehicles, of approximately 40-fold while the use of cellulose acetate phthalate as a crystal growth inhibitor resulted in an enhancement on the order of 75-fold as measured by the area under the concentration vs. time curve (AVC).

The use of aqueous-based supersaturated solutions stabilized by PVP to enhance membrane transport using the everted rat gut preparation has also been reported.[39] The drug employed was chlorothiazide and the maximum relative enhancement in membrane transport rate was fivefold. This relative enhancement was achieved with a system with a 5.8-fold supersaturation ratio stabilized with 10 mg/ml PVP. Increasing the PVP concentration to 50 mg/ml reduced the relative enhancement; however, it was still 2.4 times greater than that observed with the saturated solution. Systems with PVP concentrations below 10.0 mg/ml readily became cloudy on preparation, those containing 10.0 mg/ml PVP were metastable, while systems containing 50 mg/ml PVP remained clear. When the supersaturation ratio was increased to approximately 12-fold the 50 mg/ml PVP system also became cloudy and gave a membrane transport rate of 3.48 times that of the saturated solution. The results suggest that the enhanced transport rates from PVP-containing systems are due to the ability of PVP to retard and/or inhibit crystal growth. In addition the degree of supersaturation which can be sustained by PVP may be related to the solubility of the stabilized amorphous drug form.

VIII. CONCLUSIONS

The published research on drug-PVP coprecipitates reviewed in this chapter indicates that these systems contain high-energy amorphous drug phases which can increase membrane transport, in some cases by more than an order of magnitude. While these studies have not to date involved the use of skin as the membrane system no reason exists to doubt, from the published data, that similar enhancements are attainable through skin. However, our current understanding of the physicochemical properties of amorphous drug forms, either alone or when formed on processing with polymers such as PVP, is insufficient to allow prediction of their enhanced activity and hence to assess *a priori* their potential biopharmaceutical benefit for use in transdermal drug delivery systems. A further problem is their inherent physical instability. Many of the drug-PVP systems using artificial membranes studied to date have proved to be metastable, and whereas limited success has been achieved in their stabilization during the course of the membrane transport experiment using crystal growth inhibitors, much more research on stability issues, including that of long-term storage, is needed. Furthermore, no studies appear to have addressed the stability of drug-PVP coprecipitates on incorporation into vehicles for application to the skin. The latter is probably the major technical problem to be overcome before products of this nature can be marketed.

REFERENCES

1. **Chiou, W. L. and Riegelman, S.,** Pharmaceutical applications of solid dispersion systems, *J. Pharm. Sci.,* 60, 1281, 1971.
2. **Corrigan, O. I.,** Mechanisms of dissolution of fast release solid dispersions, *Drug Dev. Ind. Pharm.,* 11, 697, 1985.
3. **Ford, J. M.,** The current status of solid dispersions, *Pharm. Acta Helv.,* 61, 69, 1986.
4. **Tachibana, T. and Nakamura, A.,** Kolloide und naturliche makromolekule, *Kolloid-Z. Polym.,* 203, 130, 1965.
5. **Mayersohn, M. and Gibaldi, M.,** New method of solid-state dispersion for increasing dissolution rates, *J. Pharm. Sci.,* 55, 1323, 1966.
6. **Stupak, E. I. and Bates, T. R.,** Enhanced absorption and dissolution of reserpine from reserpine-polyvinylpyrrolidone coprecipitates, *J. Pharm. Sci.,* 61, 400, 1972.
7. **Patel, D. M.,** Povidone, in *Handbook of Pharmaceutical Excipients,* A Joint Publication of the American Pharmaceutical Association and the Pharmaceutical Society of Great Britain, The Pharmaceutical Press, London, 1986, 234.
8. **Jaiswal, D. K., Haldar, R. K., and Chaudhuri, R. K.,** Povidone K-120 as a superior binder and a dissolution enhancer for solid dosage forms, in *Proc. 11th Pharm. Technol. Conf.,* 2, 403, 1992.
9. **Goldemberg, R. L. and Safrin, L.,** Reduction of topical irritation, *J. Soc. Cosmet. Chem.,* 28, 667, 1977.
10. **Goldemberg, R. L.,** Anti-irritants, *J. Soc. Cosmet. Chem.,* 30, 415, 1979.
11. **Higuchi, T. and Kuramoto, R.,** Study of possible complex formation between macromolecules and certain pharmaceuticals. Polyvinylpyrrolidone with *p*-aminobenzoic acid, aminopyrine, benzoic acid, salicylic acid, *p*-hydroxybenzoic acid, *m*-hydroxybenzoic acid, citric acid and phenobarbital, *J. Am. Pharm. Assoc. (Sci. Ed.),* 43, 398, 1954.
12. **Guttman, D. and Higuchi, T.,** Study of possible complex formation between macromolecules and certain pharmaceuticals. The interaction of some phenolic compounds with polyethylene glycols, polypropylene glycols and polyvinylpyrrolidone, *J. Am. Pharm. Assoc. (Sci. Ed.),* 45, 659, 1956.
13. **Sekikawa, H., Nakano, M., and Arita, T.,** Inhibitory effect of polyvinylpyrrolidone on the crystallization of drugs, *Chem. Pharm. Bull.,* 26, 118, 1978.
14. **Sekikawa, H., Hori, R., Arita, T., Ito, K., and Nakano, M.,** Application of the cloud point method to the study of the interaction of PVP with some organic compounds in aqueous solution, *Chem. Pharm. Bull.,* 26, 2489, 1978.
15. **Ebian, A. R., Moustafa, M. A., Khalil, S. A., and Motawi, M. M.,** Effect of additives on the kinetics of interconversion of sulphamethoxydiazole crystal forms, *J. Pharm. Pharmacol.,* 25, 13, 1973.
16. **Simonelli, A. P., Mehta, S. C., and Higuchi, W. I.,** Inhibition of sulfathizole crystal growth by polyvinylpyrrolidone, *J. Pharm. Sci.,* 59, 633, 1970.
17. **Higuchi, T.,** Physical chemical analysis of percutaneous absorption process from creams and ointments, *J. Soc. Cosmet. Sci.,* 11, 86, 1960.
18. **Higuchi, W. I. and Higuchi, T.,** Theoretical analysis of diffusional movement through heterogeneous barriers, *J. Am. Pharm. Assoc. (Sci Ed.),* 49, 598, 1960.
19. **Corrigan, O. I., Farvar, M. A., and Higuchi, W. I.,** Drug membrane transport enhancement using high energy drug polyvinylpyrrolidone (PVP) coprecipitates, *Int. J. Pharm.,* 5, 229, 1980.

20. **Molyneux, P. and Frank, H. P.,** The interaction of polyvinylpyrrolidone with aromatic compounds in aqueous solutions. I. Thermodynamics of the binding equilibria and interaction forces, *J. Am. Chem. Soc.*, 85, 3169, 1961.
21. **Molyneux, P. and Frank, H. P.,** The interaction of polyvinylpyrrolidone with aromatic compounds in aqueous solutions. II. The effect of the interaction on the molecular size of the polymer, *J. Am. Chem. Soc.*, 85, 3175, 1961.
22. **Plaizier-Vercammen, J. A.,** Interaction of povidone with aromatic compounds. IV. Effect of macromolecular weight, solvent dielectric constant and ligand solubility on complex formation, *J. Pharm. Sci.*, 72, 1042, 1983.
23. **Plaizier-Vercammen, J. A.,** Interaction of povidone with aromatic compounds. VI. Use of partition coefficients (log Kd) to correlate with log P values and apparent Kd values to express the binding as a function of pH and pK_a, *J. Pharm. Sci.*, 76, 817, 1987.
24. **Simonelli, A. P., Mehta, S. C., and Higuchi, W. I.,** Dissolution rates of high energy sulfathiazole-povidone coprecipitates. I., *J. Pharm. Sci.*, 58, 538, 1969.
25. **Higuchi, W. I., Mir, N. A., and Desai, S. J.,** Dissolution rates of polyphase mixtures, *J. Pharm. Sci.*, 54, 1405, 1965.
26. **Simonelli, A. P., Mehta, S. C., and Higuchi, W. I.,** Dissolution rates of high energy sulfathiazole-povidone coprecipitates. II. Characterization of form of drug controlling its dissolution rate via solubility studies, *J. Pharm. Sci.*, 65, 355, 1976.
27. **Corrigan, O. I., and Timoney, R. F.,** The influence of polyvinylpyrrolidone (PVP) on the dissolution properties of hydroflumethiazide, *J. Pharm. Pharmacol.*, 27, 759, 1975.
28. **Junginger, H.,** Untersuchungen uber Spruheinbettungen von schwer wasserloslichen Arzneistoffen in Polymere, *Pharm. Ind.*, 39, 498, 1977.
29. **Mehta, S. C., Simonelli, A. P., and Higuchi, W. I.,** The effect of steroidal structure on the activity of its polyvinylpyrrolidone(PVP) coprecipitates, *Am. Ph.A. Meet. Abstr.*, 67, 1971.
30. **Shefter, E. and Cheng, K. C.,** Drug-polyvinylpyrrolidone (PVP) dispersions. A differential scanning calorimetric study, *Int. J. Pharm.*, 6, 179, 1980.
31. **Corrigan, O. I. and Holohan, E. M.,** Amorphous spray dried hydroflumethiazide-polyvinylpyrrolidone systems: physicochemical properties, *J. Pharm. Pharmacol.*, 36, 217, 1984.
32. **Matsuda, M., Otsuka, M., Onoe, M., and Talsumi, E.,** Amorphism and physicochemical stability of spray-dried frusemide, *J. Pharm. Pharmacol.*, 44, 627, 1992.
33. **Corrigan, O. I., Holohan, E. M., and Sabra, K.,** Amorphous forms of thiazide diuretics prepared by spray drying, *Int. J. Pharm.*, 18, 195, 1984.
34. **Shefter, E.,** Solubilization by solid state manipulation, in *Techniques of Solubilization of Drugs*, Yalkowsky, S. H., Eds., Marcel Dekker, New York, 1981, chap. 5.
35. **Merkle, H. P.,** Drug polyvinylpyrrolidone coprecipitates: kinetics of drug release and formation of supersaturated solutions, in *Proc. Int. Symp. Povidone,* Digenis, G. A. and Ansell, J., Eds., University of Kentucky, Lexington, 1983, 202.
36. **Higuchi, W. I. and Farvar, M. A.,** Drug membrane transport enhancement using high energy drug-povidone coprecipitates, in *Proc. Int. Symp. Povidone,* Digenis, G. A. and Ansell, J., Eds., University of Kentucky, Lexington, 1983, 71.
37. **Coldman, M. F., Poulsen, B. J., and Higuchi, T.,** Enhancement of percutaneous absorption by the use of volatile:nonvolatile systems as vehicles, *J. Pharm. Sci.*, 58, 1098, 1969.
38. **Kondo, S., Yamanaka, C., and Sugimoto, I.,** Enhancement of transdermal delivery by superfluous thermodynamic potential. III. Percutaneous absorption of nifedipine in rats, *J. Pharmacobio-Dyn.*, 10, 743, 1987.
39. **O'Driscoll, K. M. and Corrigan, O. I.,** Chlorthiazide-polyvinylpyrrolidone (PVP) interactions: influence on membrane permeation (everted rat intestine) and dissolution, *Drug. Dev. Ind. Pharm.*, 8, 547, 1982.

Chapter 7.3

Profile of Pirotiodecane (HPE-101): A New Potential Penetration Enhancer

Tadanori Yano, Yuji Shimozono, Takafumi Manako, Kazuya Fukuda, Shigenori Yahiro, and Kanji Noda

CONTENTS

I. INTRODUCTION

The development of the transdermal and transmucosal preparations in recent years has been marked, and the locally acting preparations as represented by the nonsteroidal agents and steroids, as well as by agents with systemic actions (e.g., nitroglycerin and protein preparations) have been developed. In general, the transdermal or transmucosal preparations present several advantages: capability of avoiding "the first pass effect" in the liver, acquisition of the steady state at the effective blood level, and easy regulation of doses (e.g., by discontinuation) and capability of alleviating adverse reactions. Conversely, they also possess some disadvantages, e.g., slow rate of drug absorption, slowness in action, and low amount of absorption which makes it difficult to reach the effective concentration. Therefore, it is indispensable to improve skin permeability for the development of better transdermal

0-8493-2605-2/95/$0.00+$.50

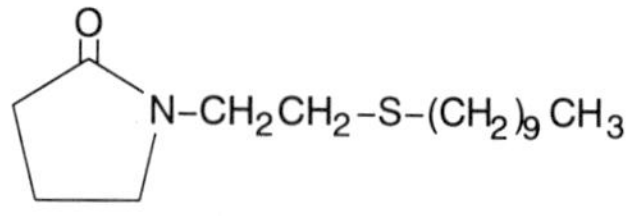

$$\text{(pyrrolidin-2-one)}\ N{-}CH_2CH_2{-}S{-}(CH_2)_9CH_3$$

Figure 1 Structure of pirotiodecane.

absorption preparations, and the needs for a safer penetration enhancer have increased.

From the aspects of physiology and safety of the skin, we first focused on a pyrrolidone derivative, a humectant ingredient of the skin, and cysteine, an amino acid constituting the keratin in the stratum corneum (SC). From the aspect of pharmaceutics, we initiated a study to create a transdermal penetration enhancer with excellent solubility and safety. Consequently, we discovered 1-[2-(decylthio)ethyl]azacyclopentan-2-one (pirotiodecane or HPE-101) (Figure 1). Subsequent studies have revealed that pirotiodecane is effective not only as a transdermal penetration enhancer, but also as a transmucosal penetration enhancer.

Following are summaries of pirotiodecane in terms of the physicochemical properties, penetration-enhancing action, pharmacokinetics, and safety.

II. PHYSICOCHEMICAL PROPERTIES

The physicochemical properties of pirotiodecane are shown in Table 1.

III. PENETRATION-ENHANCING ACTIONS

A. SCREENING

We synthesized methylthioethyl pyrrolidone (MTP), in which cysteine is ringed in consideration of the structure of 1-methyl-2-pyrrolidone, a compound conventionally known for its transdermal penetration-enhancing action, and the mercapto group is alkylated in consideration of the safety. This compound was used as a leading substance to synthesize several derivatives before examining them as penetration enhancers.

The following *in vivo* experiment was employed as the screening method for penetration-enhancing effects: a solution of ^{14}C-indomethacin in propylene glycol-ethanol (PG-EtOH) (9:1 v/v) was transdermally administered to hairless mouse back skin, and the cumulative urinary excretion rate of the radioactivity at a given time after administration was used as an index.

Results of the screening in terms of the penetration-enhancing effects of the candidate compounds listed in Figure 2 are shown in Figure 3. Especially potent actions were indicated for pirotiodecane and HN-2553, whose strengths were about 9.0-fold and about 8.7-fold greater than the control, respectively.[1]

B. DOSE RESPONSE

In the experiment conducted according to the diffusion cell method using the hairless mouse back skin, pirotiodecane, when administered at concentrations below 1%, significantly increased the permeation of pindolol in both the hydrophilic [ethanol-pH 6.0 phosphate buffer, (EtOH-PB), 1:1 v/v] and lipophilic (silicone) solvents,

Table 1 Physicochemical Properties of Pirotiodecane

Chemical structure	See Figure 1
Generic name	Pirotiodecane
Molecular formula	$C_{16}H_{31}NOS$
Molecular weight	285.49
Chemical name	1-[2-(decylthio)ethyl]azacyclopentan-2-one
Appearance	Clear liquid
Color	Colorless or pale yellow
Odor	Plactically odorless or slightly characteristic odor
Solubility	Miscible with methanol, acetonitrile, ethanol, acetone, ether, chloroform, and *n*-hexane Practically insoluble in water (<0.01 mg/ml)
Compatibility with vehicles	Compatible with white petrolatum, cetanol, stearyl alcohol, propylene glycol, PEG-400, PEG-4000, purified lanolin, white beeswax, isopropyl myristate, Witepsol H-5, Witepsol E-75, Span (40 and 80), Tween® (40, 60, 80, and 85), HCO-60, etc.
Specific gravity	d^{20}_{20}: 0.970
Refractive index	n^{20}_{20}: 1.493
Viscosity	28 centistokes (20°C)
Congealing point	16°C
Boiling point	180°–184°C (0.085 mmHg)
Partition coefficient	log P = 5.0 (*n*-octanol/water)
Stability	Stable for 3 years in amber-colored glass bottle at room temperature

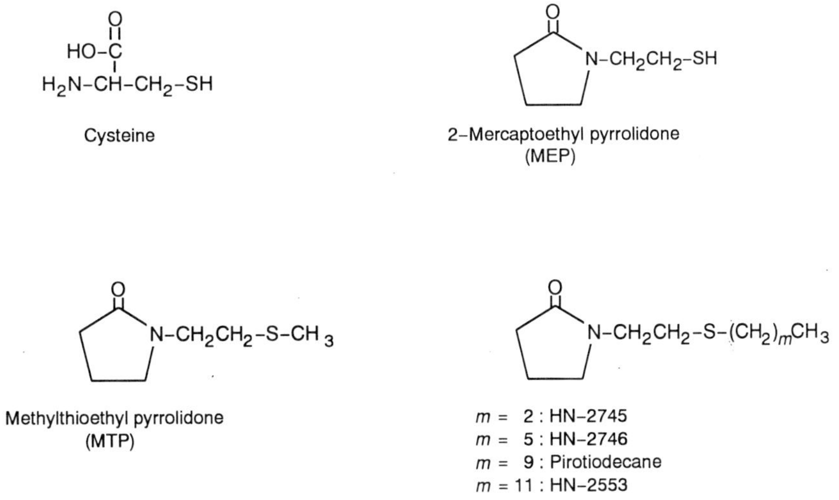

Figure 2 Structure of candidate penetration enhancer.

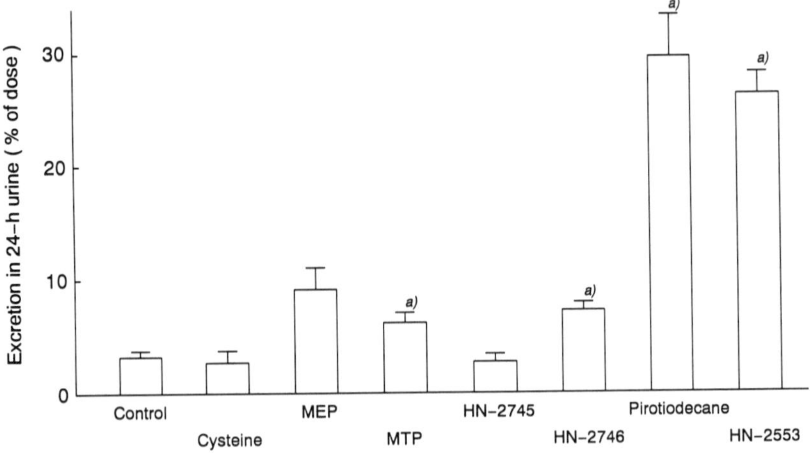

Figure 3 Excretion of radioactivity (% of dose) in 24-h urine after application to hairless mouse skin of ^{14}C-indomethacin alone or in combination with 3% solutions of various penetration enhancers in PG-EtOH. *(a)* Significant differences from the control: p <0.01.

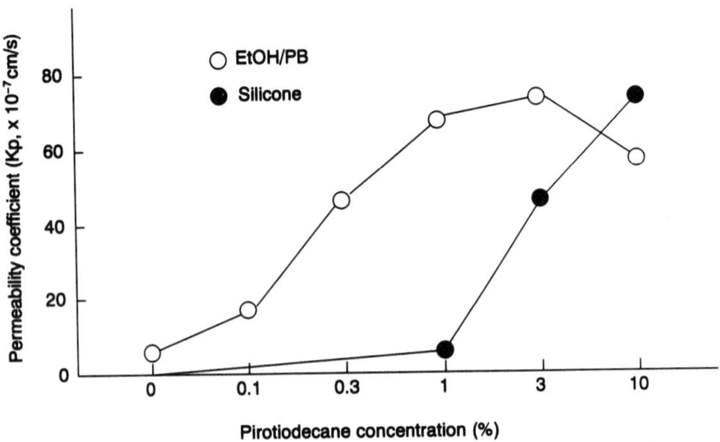

Figure 4 Effect of pirotiodecane concentration on the permeation of pindolol through hairless mouse skin in diffusion cells. Dosage of each drug: 10 m*M*/0.5 ml/0.785 cm². EtOH/PB: 50% ethanol-phosphate buffer (pH 6.0).

suggesting that the dose response of pirotiodecane may be different according to the solvent to be used (Figure 4).[2]

C. ACTIONS OF PIROTIODECANE ON DRUGS

Hydrophilic and lipophilic solvents were used to investigate the effects of pirotiodecane on several drugs according to the diffusion cell method using the hairless mouse back skin. Consequently, pirotiodecane enhanced skin permeability of all drugs; in all solvents examined, however, such action appeared to be relatively strong in the hydrophilic drugs (Figure 5).[3]

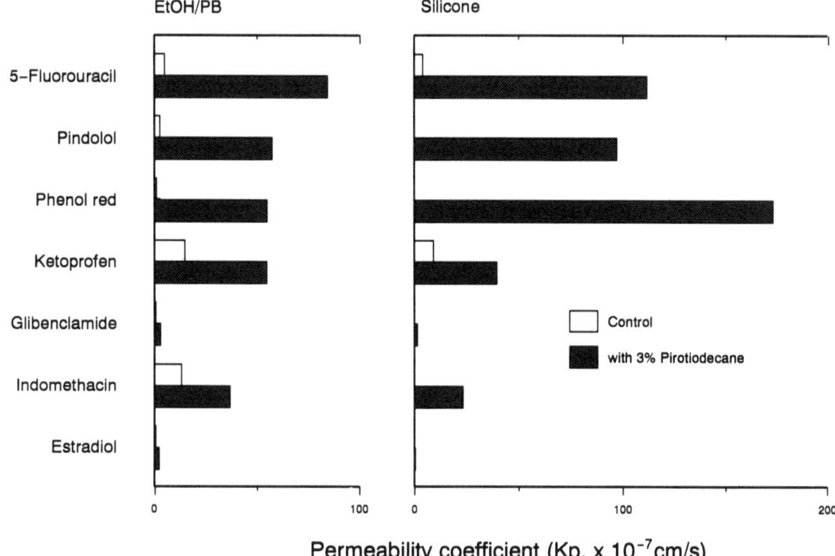

Figure 5 Enhancing effect of pirotiodecane on the permeation of various drugs through hairless mouse skin in diffusion cells. Dosage of each drug: 10 m*M*/0.5 ml/0.785 cm^2. EtOH/PB: 50% ethanol-phosphate buffer (pH 6.0).

D. PENETRATION-ENHANCING ACTIONS OF PIROTIODECANE IN SEVERAL PREPARATIONS

Pilot manufacture of five classes of indomethacin ointment and two classes of pindolol tape was conducted, and the penetration-enhancing action of pirotiodecane was assessed according to the diffusion cell method using the hairless mouse back skin. Pirotiodecane enhanced the skin permeability of the drug in all preparations examined.[4]

E. COMPARISON OF PIROTIODECANE TO SEVERAL PENETRATION ENHANCERS

Two classes of solvents were used to compare pirotiodecane to other penetration enhancers in terms of their strength of action according to the diffusion cell method using the hairless mouse back skin. Consequently, the following compounds potently enhanced skin permeability of pindolol (Figure 6): pirotiodecane, Azone®, and 1-menthol in the hydrophilic solvent (ethanol/phosphate buffer); and pirotiodecane and sodium lauryl sulfate in the lipophilic solvent (silicone). Thus, the penetration-enhancing action of pirotiodecane belongs to a category of relative potent strength in both solvent systems.[2]

F. MECHANISM OF ACTION

In the skin permeation test conducted according to the diffusion cell method using the hairless mouse back skin the skin permeation-enhancing action of pirotiodecane on indomethacin and pindolol almost disappeared due to detachment of the SC (Figure 7).[5] Furthermore, the enhancing action was more potent on the dissociated form than on molecular form of both drugs.[3] Thus, one of the mechanisms of action

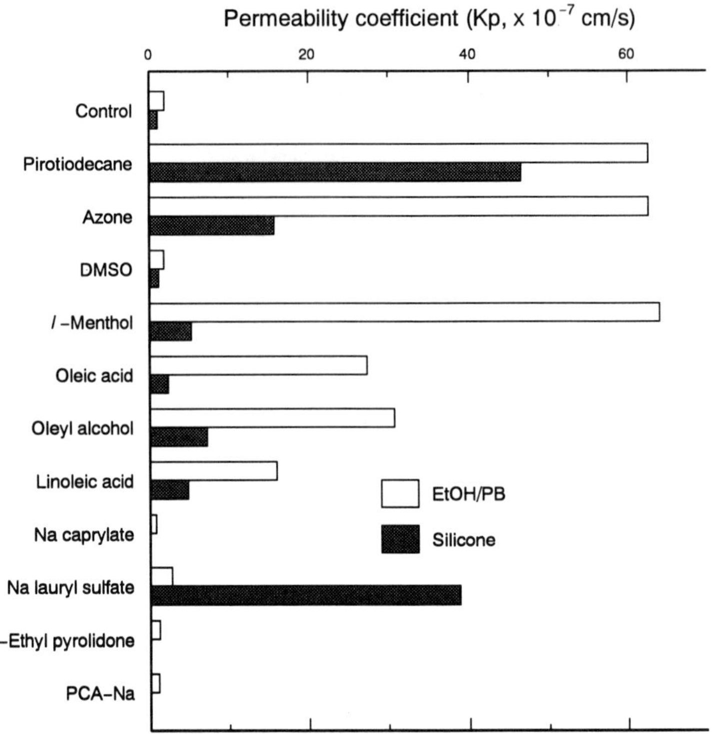

Figure 6 Enhancing effect of pirotiodecane on the permeation of pindolol through hairless mouse skin in diffusion cells. Dosage: 10 m*M*/0.5 ml/0.785 cm². EtOH/PB: 50% ethanol-phosphate buffer (pH 6.0).

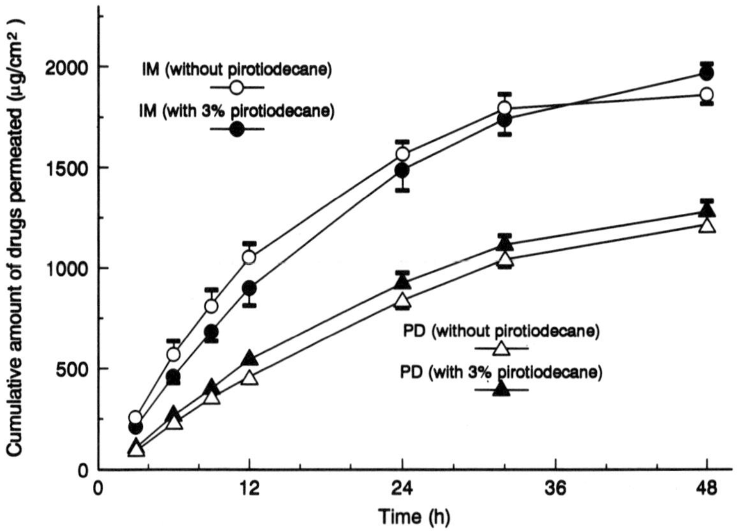

Figure 7 Effect of pirotiodecane on the permeation of indomethacin (IM) and pindolol (PD) through the stripped skin of hairless mice.

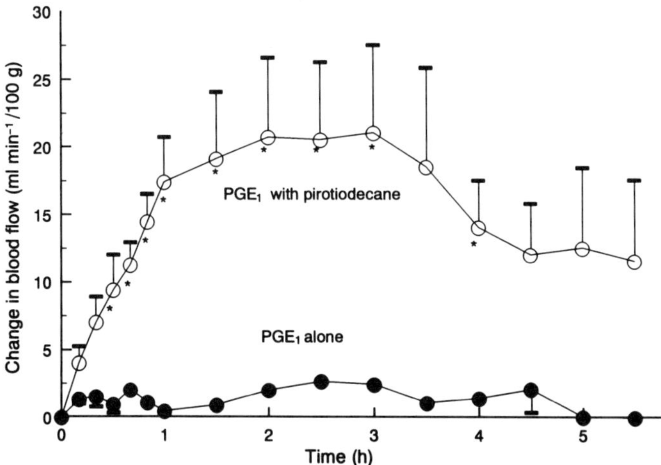

Figure 8 Changes in blood flow in the ear of rabbits after topical application of PGE_1 in FAPG ointment (500 mg, 0.01% w/w for PGE_1) supplemented with pirotiodecane (3% w/w). *, $p > 0.05$ vs. PGE_1 alone.

of pirotiodecane may be explained by hyperpermeability of the hydrophilic route in the SC.

G. FURTHER STUDIES

1. Effect on Transdermal Delivery of Prostaglandin E_1

Pirotiodecane was added to a fatty alcohol/propylene glycol (FAPG) ointment containing prostaglandin E_1 (PGE_1), and the ointment was applied onto the auricle of rabbits before measuring the skin blood flow; a marked increase in the blood flow as compared to the single preparation of PGE_1 was noted (Figure 8).[6] In the peripheral vascular occlusive sequelae model prepared by a bolus injection of sodium laurylate into the arterial auricularis caudalis in rabbits, the 3% pirotiodecane-added ointment containing PGE_1 markedly inhibited the progress of the lesion.[6]

2. Transmucosal Penetration-Enhancing Action

Rabbits with alloxan monohydrate-provoked diabetes mellitus were used to assess the insulin nasal penetration-enhancing action of pirotiodecane, employing the glucose level-decreasing action as an index; a significant decrease in glucose level was noted after the addition of 1% pirotiodecane (Figure 9).[7] Furthermore, pirotiodecane enhanced nasal absorption of inulin in rats, and such action has been reported to increase when combined with 2-hydroxypropyl-β-cyclodextrin (HP-β-CyD) (Figure 10).[8]

IV. PHARMACOKINETICS

A. ABSORPTION

Single intravenous administration (5 mg/kg) of pirotiodecane was performed in rats to investigate the pharmacokinetics. Consequently, blood concentrations of the radioactivity disappeared in a biphasic pattern. The half-lives were 0.40 and 6.06 h in

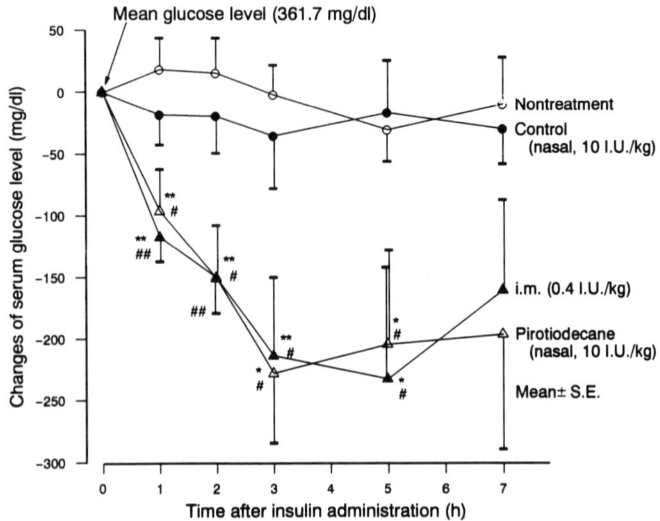

Figure 9 Changes in serum concentration of glucose in aloxan-induced diabetic rabbits nasally administered insulin with or without pirotiodecane (1% v/v). #, p <0.05; ##, p <0.01 vs. control; *, p <0.05; **, p <0.01 vs. nontreatment.

the α and β phases, respectively, while the AUC up to infinite time was 4.26 μg equiv. h/ml.

In the topical application (10 mg/kg) of pirotiodecane in rats, plasma concentrations of the radioactivity, despite continued application, reached maximum at 4 h postapplication and decreased thereafter (Figure 11). Thus, topically applied pirotiodecane is absorbed in relatively large amounts in the early stages after application. In addition, the half-lives of plasma concentrations postapplication were considerably shortened as compared to those during the application, suggesting that the absorption, although in trace amounts, may continue during the application.

B. DISTRIBUTION

Except for the skin at the site of application at the time of topical application, the organs which indicate specially high distribution at the time of single intravenous administration or single topical application of pirotiodecane in rats are the excretory organs, the liver and kidney; the organs showing especially high affinity have not been recognized. In the consecutive topical application study the organs showing accumulability were not recognized.

C. METABOLISM

Rabbits and rats were used to investigate the metabolism of pirotiodecane. The metabolism of pirotiodecane consists mainly in shortening the side chain due to the process in which the side chain undergoes ω-oxidation and subsequently suffers β-oxidation. Additionally, the metabolites, whose production is considered attributable to the oxidation of the atom S, *S*-dealkylation, or *S*-methylation, were identified. The conjugates with glucuronic acid and the conjugates with sulfuric acid were not identified.[9,10]

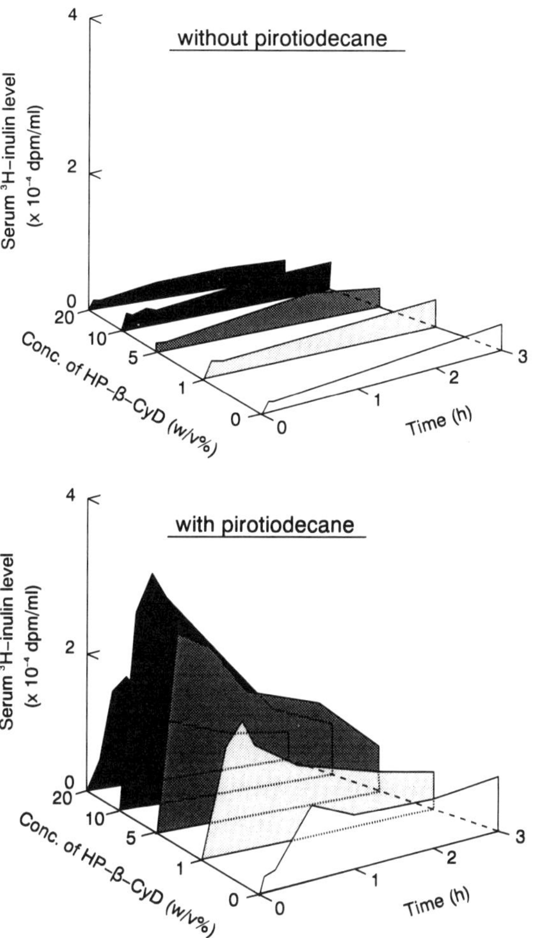

Figure 10 Effect of HP-β-CyD on the nasal absorption of inulin (2.5 μCi per body) with or without pirotiodecane (1% w/v) in rats.

D. EXCRETION

When administered intravenously or applied topically in rats, pirotiodecane is rapidly excreted, mainly to the urine. The urinary and fecal excretion rates to the dose by 72 h after intravenous administration (5 mg/kg) are 97.15 and 2.98%, respectively. The urinary and fecal excretion rates to the dose by 72 h after topical application (10 mg/ kg, 24 h) are 10.44 and 0.51%, respectively; these are equivalent to 95.5% of the amount of absorption (Figure 12). Moreover, 90.5% of the total amounts of urinary and fecal excretions by 72 h after application of pirotiodecane was already excreted by 24 h after application, suggesting that the excretion of pirotiodecane may be very rapid.

V. SAFETY

The LD_{50} values in single dose toxicity studies of pirotiodecane in rats, mice, and dogs are shown in Table 2.; the toxicity of pirotiodecane was found to be weak.

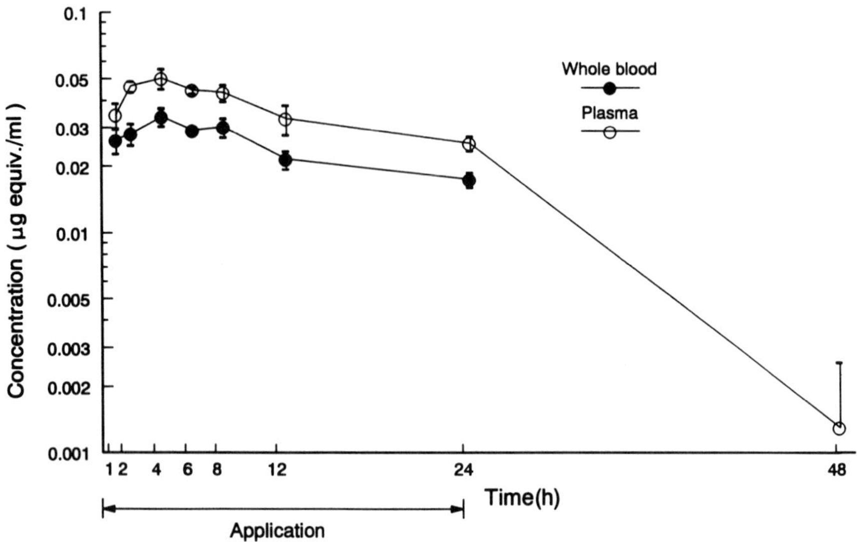

Figure 11 Whole blood and plasma concentration of radioactivity after a topical application of ^{14}C-pirotiodecane (10 mg/kg) to rats. Each point represents the mean ± S.E. of four rats.

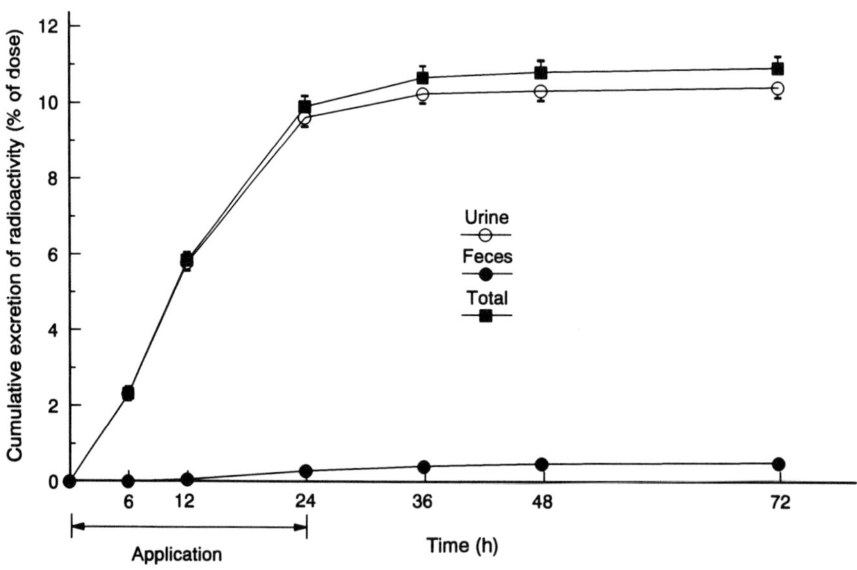

Figure 12 Cumulative excretion of radioactivity in urine and feces after a topical application of ^{14}C-pirotiodecane (10 mg/kg) to rats. Each point represents the mean ± S.E. of four rats.

Reversible changes in the skin at the site of application were noted at high doses in the 13-week repeated subcutaneous toxicity studies in rats and dogs; however, any other changes were not noted. The maximum nonaffecting dose was 16 mg/kg in rats and 15 mg/kg in dogs.

Table 2 Acute Toxicity of Pirotiodecane

Route of Administration	LD_{50} (mg/kg)				
	Rat		Mouse		Dog
	Male	Female	Male	Female	Male/Female
Oral	>5000	>5000	>5000	>5000	
Intraperitoneal	2041	2202	1607	1752	
Subcutaneous	>5000	>5000	>5000	>5000	>2000

In the study on administration prior to and in the early stages of pregnancy, the study on administration during the period of organogenesis, and the study on administration during the perinatal and lactation periods in rats, pirotiodecane had no effect on reproductive and developmental toxicity.

In the antigenicity studies using mice and guinea pigs pirotiodecane was negative in all of the passive cutaneous anaphylaxis reaction, active systemic anaphylaxis reaction, skin sensitization, and photosensitization. Furthermore, pirotiodecane was negative in the teratogenicity study.

In the primary skin irritation study, cumulative skin irritation study, and eye mucosa irritation study in rabbits conducted according to the Draize method, pirotiodecane, when administered at concentrations below 3%, presented mild irritation.

In addition, the 3% pirotiodecane-containing ointment of white petrolatum was applied to healthy male volunteers for 48 h; consequently, the ointment scarcely presented skin irritation. The intensity of the ointment was as strong as that of the commercialized ingredients, e.g., crotamiton and benzyl alcohol.

Thus, pirotiodecane is considered to present no problems in safety when used at concentrations below 3%.

VI. CONCLUSIONS

In general, it is indispensable for the drugs, which are transdermally absorbed alone with the expectation of satisfactory pharmacological action, to meet several conditions: appropriate physicochemical properties (e.g., low molecular weight, low melting point, and optimum partition coefficient with the skin) and potent pharmacological actions. However, the drugs capable of meeting such conditions are currently limited, as represented by nitroglycerin and others. Therefore, the need for a penetration enhancer that is applicable to a broader range of drugs and preparations for the purpose of making full use of the merits of the transdermal preparations has been elevated.

Therefore, we synthesized a new penetration enhancer, pirotiodecane, by analyzing the constituents and functions of the skin and investigated the compound from several points. The *in vitro* and *in vivo* studies on the penetration-enhancing action and safety of pirotiodecane have led to the consideration that the concentration at which pirotiodecane is adequately used is 3%. Furthermore, studies using several drugs with different lipophilicities showed that pirotiodecane possesses a penetration-enhancing action on all drugs examined; pirotiodecane tended to indicate a potent action, especially on water-soluble drugs. The factors on the side of the preparations (solvents) also were investigated, and pirotiodecane was suggested to be applicable to a relatively broad range of uses, e.g., ointment and patch.

In terms of safety, on the other hand, any systemic or local toxicity findings which may be problematic have not been recognized. This fact has been also suggested by the data on the absorption, distribution, metabolism, and excretion by intravenous and topical administrations. It has been elucidated that the bioavailability of pirotiodecane after topical application in rats is as low as about 10%, and that pirotiodecane is rapidly excreted or metabolized after transfer to blood. In addition, the major proportion of pirotiodecane is excreted to the urine, and accumulability after consecutive administration has not been recognized. Although the data are not shown in this chapter, no general pharmacological actions of pirotiodecane were indicated at concentrations used in the experiments.

Hyperpermeability of the hydrophilic route in the SC was suggested as one of the mechanisms of action for pirotiodecane. Further studies are required.

Because pirotiodecane possesses relatively high solubilizing action, the compound allows its application as a solubilizing agent for the slightly soluble drugs. In addition, pirotiodecane was recently discovered to possess a penetration-enhancing action in routes for other topical uses than on the skin (e.g., nasal mucosa and buccal mucosa); therefore, pirotiodecane can be applied to a broad range of field. Further investigation is expected.

REFERENCES

1. **Yano, T., Higo, N., Furukawa, K., Tsuji, M., Noda, K., and Otagiri, M.,** Evaluation of a new penetration enhancer 1-[2-(decylthio)ethyl]azacyclopentan-2-one (HPE-101), *J. Pharmacobio-Dyn.*, 15, 527, 1992.
2. **Saita, M., Shimozono, Y., Sakai, M., Okayama, A., Furuta, K., and Tsuji, M.,** Evaluation of a new penetration enhancer HPE-101 (3), *Ther. Res.*, 10, 971, 1989.
3. **Saita, M., Shimozono, Y., Sakai, M., Deguchi, Y., Okayama, A., and Tsuji, M.,** Evaluation of a new penetration enhancer HPE-101 (4), *Ther. Res.*, 10, 972, 1989.
4. **Taniguchi, Y., Shimozono, Y., Okayama, A., Sakai, M., Hamanaka, S., Hori, M., Manako, T., and Saita, M.,** Evaluation of a new penetration enhancer HPE-101 (9), *Ther. Res.*, 11, 638, 1990.
5. **Teruto, N., Manako, T., Shimozono, Y., Noda, M., and Tsuji, M.,** Evaluation of a new penetration enhancer HPE-101 (5), in *Proc. 109th Annu. Meet. Pharm. Soc. Jpn.*, II-153, 1989.
6. **Adachi, H., Irie, T., Uekama, K., Manako, T., Yano, T., and Saita, M.,** Inhibitory effect of prostaglandin E1 on laurate-induced peripheral vascular occlusive sequelae in rabbits: optimized topical formulation with β-cyclodextrin derivative and penetration enhancer HPE-101, *J. Pharm. Pharmacol.*, 44, 1033, 1992.
7. **Saita, M., Shimozono, Y., Sakai, M., Okayama, A., and Tsuji, M.,** in *Proc. 109th Annu. Meet. Pharm. Soc. Jpn.*, II-157, 1989.
8. **Irie, T., Abe, K., Adachi, H., Uekama, K., Manako, T., Yano, T., and Saita, M.,** Potential use of 2-hydroxypropyl-β-cyclodextrin in designing nasal preparation of insulin involving lipophilic absorption enhancer HPE-101, *Drug Deliv. Syst.*, 7, 91, 1992.
9. **Yano, T., Fukuda, K., Furukawa, K., Gondo, H., and Tsuji, M.,** Evaluation of a new penetration enhancer HPE-101 (6), in *Proc. 109th Annu. Meet. Pharm. Soc. Jpn.*, II-83, 1989.
10. **Yano, T., Furukawa, K., Fukuda, T., Gondo, H., and Saita, M.,** Evaluation of a new penetration enhancer HPE-101 (11), in *Proc. 110th Annu. Meet. Pharm. Soc. Jpn.*, 4–151, 1990.

Chapter 8.1

Surfactants

Stephen B. Ruddy

CONTENTS

I. INTRODUCTION

The stratum corneum (SC), the outermost layer of mammalian epidermis, has long been recognized as the principal barrier to the percutaneous penetration of exogenous substances of chemical and biologic origin.[1] It has been demonstrated, however, that certain classes of compounds possess the unique ability to interact with various lipid and protein components within the membrane, resulting in a transient or permanent increase in skin permeability.[2] While the extent to which human skin is exposed to certain of these chemicals, such as organic solvents or strong alkali, is generally quite limited, exposure to other classes of percutaneous penetration enhancers, such as surface-active agents, is far more common. Accordingly, considerable efforts have been undertaken in recent years to resolve the mechanisms responsible for surfactant interaction with the skin, particularly those related to the disruption of cutaneous barrier function.

This chapter deals primarily with the putative mechanisms underlying surfactant-facilitated percutaneous penetration enhancement and the potential utility of surfactants for enhanced delivery of therapeutic agents via the transdermal route. Particular emphasis is placed on those surfactants whose effects are readily reversible and less likely to result in pronounced cutaneous irritation. Lesser attention is devoted to the biological consequences of topically applied surfactants. The latter topic was reviewed recently by Rhein and Simion.[3]

0-8493-2605-2/95/$0.00+$.50

II. MECHANISMS OF SURFACTANT–SKIN INTERACTION

A. PHYSICOCHEMICAL BASIS FOR CUTANEOUS BARRIER DISRUPTION

More than 30 years ago, Bettley and Donoghue[4] and Bettley[5] demonstrated that soaps could enhance the flux of water, glucose, and salicylate across isolated human epidermis. Shortly thereafter, Bettley[6] compared the penetration of ^{14}C-labeled potassium soaps of octanoic, dodecanoic, hexadecanoic, and *cis*-9-octadecenoic acids across the same membrane. Data from the study showed that 24.4% of the dodecanoate penetrated the epidermis after 7 d, while octanoate (5.29%), *cis*-9-octadecenoate (2.08%), and hexadecanoate (0.15%) penetrated the membrane in substantially smaller quantities over the same time period. Moreover, 48-h patch testing in human volunteers revealed a strong correlation between the irritant effects of the soaps and the extent to which they penetrated the excised epidermal tissue. Accordingly, these studies provided the first evidence that disruption of cutaneous barrier function is directly related to the degree of chemical and physical interaction between the enhancing agent and the skin.

Later, Scheuplein and Ross[7] reported that the capacity of the SC to retain significant quantities of membrane-bound water is markedly reduced in the presence of sodium dodecanoate and sodium dodecyl sulfate (SDS), an effect which is readily reversible upon removal of the surface-active agent. These investigators proposed that anionic surfactants alter the permeability of the skin by acting on the helical filaments of the SC, thereby resulting in the uncoiling and extension of α-keratin filaments to form β-keratin together with the overall expansion of the membrane. More than 20 years later, surfactants are still believed to increase the permeability of mammalian skin, in part, through transient or permanent denaturation of epidermal keratin. However, more recent findings suggest that impairment of the skin's barrier properties is unlikely to result from changes in protein conformation alone, and that additional mechanisms are undoubtedly operative in surfactant-facilitated percutaneous penetration enhancement.

Lodén[8] investigated the simultaneous penetration of tritiated water and ^{35}S-labeled SDS through excised, full-thickness human skin. This worker reported both concentration-dependent and time-dependent increases in the pseudosteady-state flux of surfactant and water, the results of which are summarized in Figures 1 and 2, respectively. Interestingly, apparent permeability coefficients for SDS were found to be nearly equivalent at the highest surfactant concentrations studied (1 and 10%), yet significantly greater than those obtained at low surfactant concentration (0.1%). Such results would be largely unexpected because the highest surfactant concentrations employed in the study reside well above the critical micelle concentration (CMC) for SDS in an aqueous vehicle (≈0.24%), and would presumably contain identical quantities of surfactant monomer. It is generally accepted that micelles do not penetrate the skin on account of excessive bulkiness and, in the case of SDS, excessive charge density. Accordingly, these results were initially attributed to the micelle-dependent solubilization of skin lipids.

Further support for a micelle-dependent solubilization mechanism resulted from observed temporal increases in the rate of SDS and water penetration during surfactant exposure, indicative of a time-dependent decrease in the skin's barrier function.

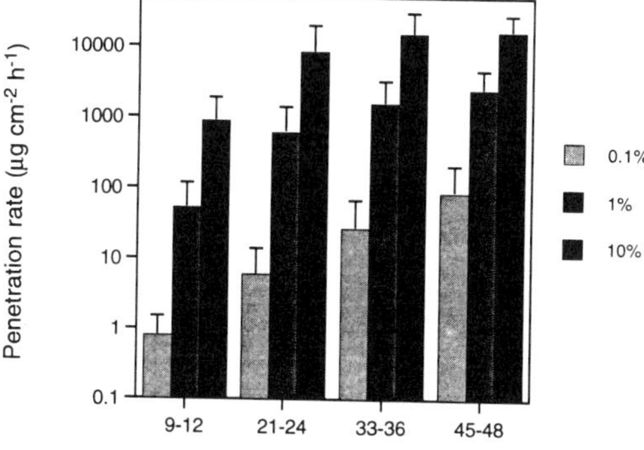

Figure 1 Influence of surfactant concentration on the rate of ^{35}S-labeled SDS penetration (mean ± SEM; $n = 5$) through excised, full-thickness human skin at selected time intervals. (Data from Lodén, M., *J. Soc. Cosmet. Chem.*, 41, 227, 1990.)

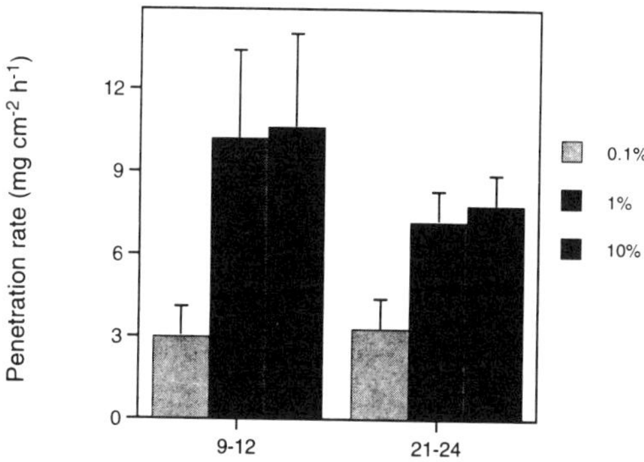

Figure 2 Influence of SDS concentration on the rate of tritiated water penetration (mean ± SEM; $n = 5$) through excised, full-thickness human skin at selected time intervals. (Data from Lodén, M., *J. Soc. Cosmet. Chem.*, 41, 227, 1990.)

Imokawa et al.[9] had reported earlier that cutaneous exposure to SDS results in the extraction of various components from the intercellular lipid matrix of the SC. However, Lodén's observed rates of penetration of tritiated water through the skin were not found to differ appreciably at high surfactant concentrations, and therefore appeared to be inconsistent with the observed flux of SDS under identical conditions. Accordingly, Lodén concluded that the activity of the SDS monomer does not remain constant above the CMC, as previously believed, but increases in proportion to the number of micelles present. Yet, a more tenable argument may be built around the selective extraction of skin lipids by SDS micelles, thereby resulting in the preferential disruption of a pathway through the SC in favor of SDS.

Takahashi et al.[10] observed complete disruption of isolated guinea pig SC secondary to immersion in a solution of SDS and *N,N*-dimethyl-dodecylamine oxide (C_{12}DMAO) 2:8 in the absence of ultrasonic energy or mechanical manipulation. These workers attributed the fragmentation of the membrane to the dissolution of "intercellular cement" or destruction of intercorneocyte bonds. The extent of fragmentation was found to be proportional to the total concentration of surfactant, and was not observed at concentrations lower than the CMC. These results provide additional evidence in support of micellar dissolution of intercellular components. It should be noted, however, that treatment of the SC with ether, ethanol, or chloroform:methanol (2:1) did not result in decomposition of the membrane. Such findings would further suggest that surfactant micelles solubilize specific components within the intercellular lipid matrix, and may serve to explain the observed differences in SDS and water flux reported previously by Lodén. Moreover, Triton® X-100, sodium dodecanoate, polyoxyethylene-(15)-dodecyl ether, sodium dodecylbenzenesulfonate, dodecyltrimethylammonium chloride, and *N*-dodecyl-*N,N*-dimethylaminoacetic acid failed to induce fragmentation of the membrane. These findings also serve to underscore potential differences in surfactant action on mammalian skin.

Additional evidence to support the micellar solubilization of SC lipids was provided more recently by Ridout et al.,[11] who studied the enhancing effects of various zwitterionic surfactants on the penetration of nicotinamide across excised hairless mouse skin. For each of three betaines studied (dodecyl betaine, hexadecyl betaine, and C_{16} propyl betaine), nicotinamide penetration was found to be proportional to surfactant concentration. Moreover, the enhancing effects of the three surfactants were determined to be equivalent, based upon normalization of each surfactant with respect to the CMC.

B. COMPARATIVE EFFECTS OF CATIONIC, ANIONIC, AND NONIONIC SURFACTANTS

While the ability of a surfactant to enhance the rate of drug penetration into and through the skin is desirable, it is equally critical that the task be accomplished in the absence of significant irritation or sensitization. Ideally, the effects should be of short duration and readily reversible upon removal of the enhancing agent. However, experience has shown that the extent to which the permeability of the skin is reduced is strongly correlated with the development of various, undesirable cutaneous responses. These include skin tightness and roughness as well as erythema and inflammation, the latter of which suggest some level of interaction between the surfactant and the various components of the viable epidermis. Ideally, the optimal surfactant for percutaneous penetration enhancement is one which acts primarily on the SC and to a minimal degree with the underlying tissue.[12] While such an agent has yet to be identified, the requirements for such an agent are not excessively prohibitive and, therefore, provide a reasonable target for future surfactant design.

As a general rule, cationic surfactants elicit greater irritation and skin "damage" than anionic surfactants which, in turn, are more damaging than nonionic surfactants. Not surprising, the ability of surfactants to alter skin permeability typically follows in similar fashion. Ashton et al.[13] compared the effects of dodecyltrimethylammonium

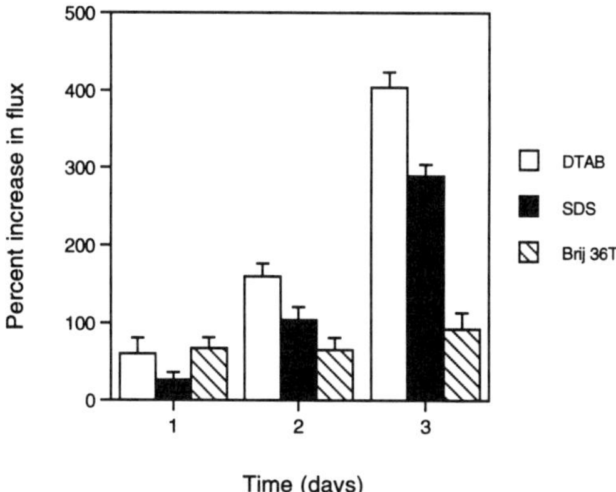

Figure 3 Influence of surfactant type on the observed flux enhancement of methyl nicotinamide (mean ± SD; $n \geq 5$) across excised, full-thickness human skin as a function of time. (Data from Ashton, P. et al., *Int. J. Pharm.*, 87, 261, 1992.)

bromide (DTAB), SDS, and Brij 36T™ on the *in vitro* flux of methyl nicotinamide across excised human skin. Results of the study confirmed the anticipated rank order of penetration enhancement: DTAB>SDS>Brij 36T™. Interestingly, however, it was observed that Brij 36T™ exhibited a smaller but more immediate effect on the penetration of methyl nicotinate, resulting in the highest degree of flux enhancement over the first 24-h period (see Figure 3). These observations were attributed to differences in the rate of surfactant penetration into the SC, thereby suggesting that nonionic surfactants penetrate the membrane more rapidly, but interact less extensively, than their ionic counterparts. Such findings should not be surprising, however, as a charged species is not expected to penetrate the skin as readily as an uncharged species of similar chemical structure. Moreover, these data are in good agreement with the earlier results of Prottey and Ferguson,[14] in which the nonionic surfactants, $C_{12}(EO)_3$ and $C_{12}(EO)_6$, were found to penetrate guinea pig skin far more rapidly than SDS. These investigators concluded that anionic surfactants bind extensively to components of the SC, thereby contributing to the lower than expected levels of surfactant in underlying (viable) tissues.

In a related study Ashton et al.[15] investigated the effects of DTAB, SDS, and Brij 36T™ on the thermotropic properties and birefringence of isolated SC. Results of the study revealed a correlation between the observed ability of a surfactant to increase the birefringence of the membrane and its reported ability to elicit a cutaneous response. Both DTAB and SDS produced substantial increases in the intensity of transmitted light (approximately 50%), while the effects of Brij 36T™ were substantially reduced. Of equal importance, the observed ability of a surfactant to increase the birefringence of the SC followed the same rank order of methyl nicotinamide flux enhancement. Interestingly, the extraction of SC lipids failed to produce changes in the birefringence of the membrane. Yet, thermograms of SC treated with both DTAB and SDS resulted in the disappearance of two peaks between 70° and 90°C, regions attributed to transitions of intercellular lipids and protein-bound lipids of the corneocyte envelope,[16] respectively. Such findings would suggest that the ability of DTAB and

SDS to impair cutaneous barrier function cannot be attributed to surfactant interaction with proteins alone. Interestingly, thermograms of SC treated with Brij 36T™ revealed four peaks at 55°, 62°, 67°, and 100°C. While the apparent shifting of the first three thermotropic transitions to lower temperatures would indicate some type of surfactant interaction with the membrane, it can be argued that the presence of the peaks is nonetheless indicative of weaker overall interaction of nonionic surfactants with the membrane.

C. INHIBITION OF SURFACTANT–SKIN INTERACTION

A number of investigations have demonstrated the utility of various "mild" surfactants in minimizing the interactions of certain ionic surfactants with the skin. Rhein and co-workers[17] reported the ability of alkyl ethoxy sulfates (AEOS) and certain amphoteric surfactants to reduce the swelling of isolated human SC secondary to SDS exposure. Treatment with a mixture of 1% SDS and 1% AEOS-$(EO)_3$ resulted in a marked decrease in swelling as compared to 1% SDS alone, despite a twofold increase in the quantity of surfactant applied to the membrane. Moreover, the substitution of AEOS-$(EO)_6$ for AEOS-$(EO)_3$ demonstrated a further reduction in SC swelling, as illustrated in Figure 4. Comparable results were obtained with the amphoteric surfactants, dodecyldimethylamine oxide and cocoamidopropyl betaine, in which swelling was reduced by as much as 85%. In the latter case the extent of membrane swelling was found to be dependent upon the concentration of the amphoteric surfactant, the results of which are summarized in Figure 5. Such findings were confirmed in a later series of experiments in which the swelling of a collagen film was determined to be inversely related to the degree of ethoxylation of the same alkyl ether sulfates (see Figure 6).[18]

Rhein and Simion[3] have suggested that the observed reduction in SC swelling is dependent upon two principal mechanisms which may operate individually or jointly to produce a synergistic effect. The first mechanism is based upon surfactant interaction with components of the membrane. Accordingly, the inhibition of membrane swelling may result from competition with the irritating surfactant for binding sites or binding surfaces within the membrane itself. Such an effect was demonstrated in a previous study by Dominguez et al.,[19] who showed the ability of alkyl betaines to inhibit the binding of SDS to skin callus. The second mechanism is based upon physicochemical interaction between surfactant monomers in solution, resulting in the formation of mixed micelles. Such interactions may result in a lowering of the CMC of the irritating surfactant, thereby reducing the concentration of free monomer which is available to interact with the membrane. Evidence to support the latter hypothesis may be obtained from the previous investigations of Faucher and Goddard,[20] who observed a decrease in SDS binding to human hair keratin following addition of the nonionic surfactant, Tergitol 15-S-9™, and of Miyazawra et al.,[21] who studied the protein denaturing ability of surfactant mixtures.

While the previous results clearly demonstrate the ability of certain nonionic and amphoteric surfactants to inhibit the irritation potential of anionic surfactants, the impact of surfactant mixtures on percutaneous drug absorption has not been reported. However, insight into the effects of surfactant blends on cutaneous barrier function and vascular events may be obtained from a recent series of investigations by

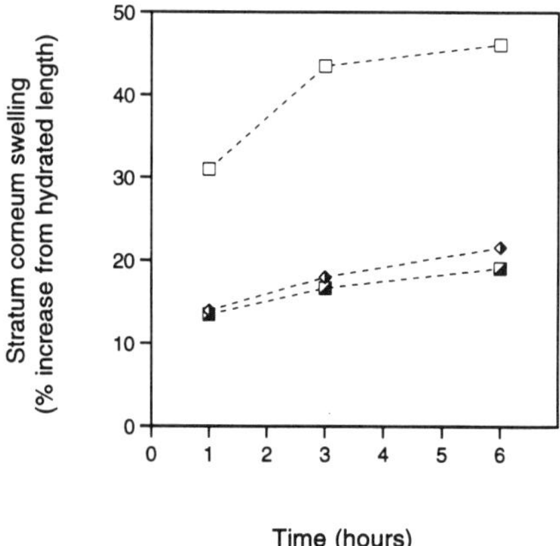

Figure 4 Influence of alkyl ethoxy sulfates on the extent of SDS-induced swelling of isolated human SC (□, 1% SDS; ◆, 1% SDS + 1% AEOS-EO_3; ◪, 1% SDS + 1% AEOS-EO_6). (Data from Rhein, L. et al., *J. Soc. Cosmet. Chem.*, 37, 125, 1986.)

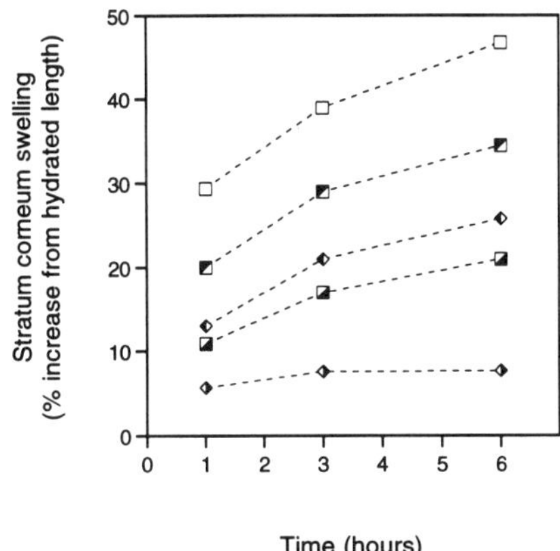

Figure 5 Influence of selected amphoteric surfactants on the extent of SDS-induced swelling of isolated human SC (□, 1% SDS; ◪, 1% SDS + 0.5% cocoamidopropyl betaine; ◆, 1% SDS + 0.5% dodecyldimethylamine oxide; ◩, 1% SDS + 1% cocoamidopropyl betaine; ◆, 1% SDS + 1% dodecyldimethylamine oxide). (Data from Rhein, L. et al., *J. Soc. Cosmet. Chem.*, 37, 125, 1986.)

Zehnder et al.[22] in which the effects of ether carboxylate–SDS mixtures on transepidermal water loss, electrical conductance, cutaneous blood flow, skin color reflectance, and clinical erythema were examined. Measurements were obtained following 2-h occlusive patch testing on each of five consecutive days. Resulting data revealed a marked reduction in transepidermal water loss and a marked increase in cutaneous electrical resistance with increasing molar ratios of both ether carboxylates, indicative of a concentration-dependent decrease in cutaneous barrier impairment. A reduction in cutaneous blood flow, skin color reflectance, and erythema was also observed with increasing molar ratios of the carboxylates. Consistent with the

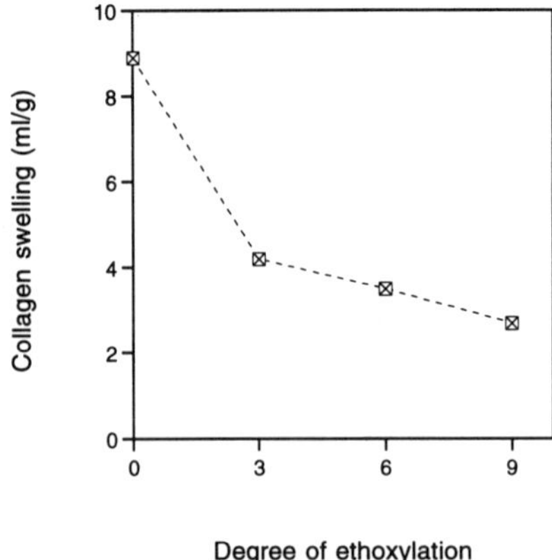

Figure 6 Influence of ethoxylation (as average mole addition of EO) of alkyl ether sulfates on the extent of swelling of a collagen film substrate. (Data from Blake-Haskins, J. C. et al., *J. Soc. Cosmet. Chem.*, 37, 199, 1986.)

results of Blake-Haskins and co-workers,[18] the ability to minimize the deleterious effects of SDS were more pronounced with increasing ethoxylation.

Accordingly, the preceding results offer an attractive strategy for surfactant-facilitated percutaneous enhancement in which the enhancing effects may be modulated not only by the concentration of the "active" surfactant, but also by adjustment of molar ratios of secondary, nonirritating or "mild" surfactants. Such an approach could potentially provide for a satisfactory level of barrier impairment together with an acceptable level of cutaneous effects, both of which would be readily reversible upon removal of the surfactant mixture.

III. SURFACTANT-FACILITATED PENETRATION ENHANCEMENT

A. INFLUENCE OF SURFACTANT CHARGE AND STRUCTURE

Despite the ability of many ionic surfactants to increase the permeability of the skin to a variety of substances, the overall utility of such agents as percutaneous penetration enhancers is potentially limited. In addition to their tendency to induce irritation and numerous other cutaneous responses, the enhancing effects of ionic surfactants have been shown to be poorly reversible *in vitro.* Kushla and Zatz[23] investigated the effects of various cationic surfactants on the penetration of radiolabeled water and lidocaine through excised human epidermis. The surfactants studied comprised three primary classes: alkyl dimethylbenzylammonium halides, alkyl trimethylammonium halides, and alkyl pyridinium halides. In order to gain insight into the reversibility of surfactant action, these workers adopted a study design in which each skin sample served as its own control. Individual samples were initially exposed to a control formulation (containing no surfactant) for the first of three 24-h periods, followed by a test formulation and a repeat control formulation over the second and third 24-h periods, respectively. Steady-state fluxes of both radiolabeled permeants were determined for each of the three 24-h periods, thereby allowing for the determination of the magnitude and duration of surfactant-induced effects.

As expected, the presence of surfactant resulted in a two- to fourfold increase in the mean steady-state flux of water and lidocaine as compared to the initial control period. However, the permeability of the epidermis to both compounds remained artificially high throughout the second control period, despite the absence of surfactant in the control formulation. Accordingly, the observed persistence in barrier disruption was attributed to two primary mechanisms: (1) the extraction of lipids from the SC and (2) the penetration of surfactant into the intercellular lipid matrix of the cornified layer. Both mechanisms would be expected to result in the prolonged impairment of cutaneous barrier function, particularly in the case of excised tissue in which repair mechanisms are known to be inoperative.

It is important to note, however, that no significant differences in the enhancing effects of three unique hexadecyl derivatives were observed, thereby suggesting that the nature of the surfactant head group exerts little influence on cutaneous barrier impairment. Such a finding conflicts with Laughlin's[24] proposed relationship between barrier disruption and the hydrophilicity of the surfactant head group. According to Laughlin's hypothesis, surfactants with hydrophilic head groups should be more effective at enhancing the percutaneous penetration of polar molecules, while those of lesser hydrophilicity (such as alcohols) should be considerably less effective. Therefore, in the present case one might expect enhancement potential to follow the following rank order: trimethylammonium > dimethylbenzyl > pyridinium.

Of additional significance, Kushla and Zatz also demonstrated that maximum flux enhancement resulted from those derivatives with an alkyl chain length of 12 to 14 carbons. Such results are in good agreement with the previous findings of Scheuplein and Dugard,[25] who studied the electrical conductance of the skin secondary to treatment with a homologous series of alkyl sulfates. These investigators observed the maximum disruption of the skin's electrical barrier to coincide with a chain length of 12 carbons. Cooper and Berner[26] have argued that the optimal chain length for cutaneous barrier impairment (and therefore for percutaneous penetration enhancement) may be attributed to a number of factors, including the solubility of the surfactant in the donor vehicle, the CMC, the SC–vehicle partition coefficient, and the binding affinity of the surfactant for epidermal keratin. Accordingly, an optimum chain length of 12 to 14 carbons may represent compromise between aqueous solubility and lipophilic character. Moreover, SC keratin may bind preferentially with carbons chains of specific length, beyond which no thermodynamic advantage is offered.

B. POTENTIAL ROLE OF NONIONIC SURFACTANTS

It is generally recognized that nonionic surfactants are less damaging to the skin than ionic surfactants. Unfortunately, however, the former are also known to exhibit relatively weak effects on cutaneous barrier function. The limited ability of nonionic surfactants to alter the permeability of the skin to test substances was recently demonstrated by Cappel and Kreuter, who examined the enhancing effects of polysorbates[27] as well as poloxamer and poloxamine surfactants[28] on the penetration of methanol and octanol across excised hairless mouse skin.

In an initial series of studies[27] these workers compared the enhancement potential of polysorbates 20, 21, 80, and 81. Data from these studies clearly demonstrated that

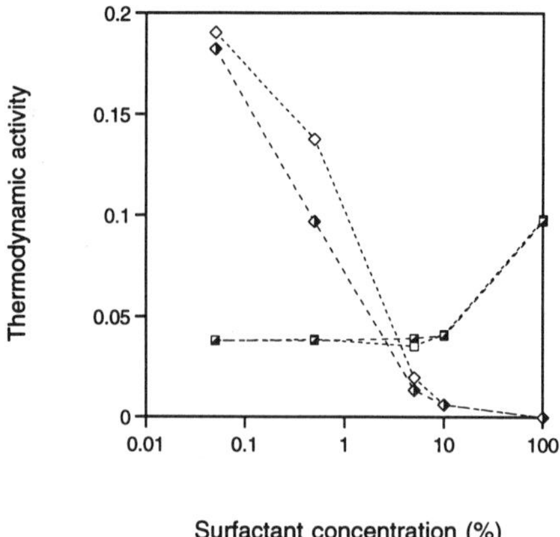

Figure 7 Influence of polysorbate 20 and polysorbate 80 on the thermodynamic activity of methanol (diamonds) and octanol (squares) as a function of surfactant concentration. (◇ and □, polysorbate 20; ◆ and ◪, polysorbate 80.) (Data from Cappel, M. J. and Krenter, J., *Int. J. Pharm.*, 69, 143, 1991.)

polysorbates had a limited impact on the transdermal penetration of methanol. Maximum flux enhancement of two- to threefold was achieved in the presence of polysorbates 21 and 81, indicating that the more lipophilic polysorbates alter the barrier properties of the skin to a greater extent than their hydrophilic analogues. In comparison, the presence of polysorbates had a negative impact on octanol penetration through the same membrane, an effect that was attributed to the concentration-dependent decrease in octanol thermodynamic activity secondary to micellar solubilization of the lipophilic permeant (see Figure 7).

It is interesting to note, however, that neat polysorbate surfactants produced significant increases in methanol penetration, resulting in fluxes nearly 13-fold greater than those observed in the absence of surfactant. While these findings were related to an increase in the thermodynamic activity of the permeant, it is possible that additional mechanisms further contributed to the unexpected increase in methanol transport across the skin. Such results also may have reflected an increase in the SC–vehicle partition coefficient as well as the disruption of the skin's barrier properties on account of the high concentration of surfactant monomer at the skin surface.

Sarpotdar and Zatz[29] demonstrated the enhancing effects of selected polysorbates on the penetration of lidocaine through excised hairless mouse skin from propylene glycol (PG):water vehicles. These workers discovered that polysorbate 20 and polysorbate 80 successfully enhanced the rate of drug transport into and through the skin, the magnitude of which was proportional to the concentration of PG in the donor vehicle. A nearly threefold increase in lidocaine flux resulted from solutions of the polysorbates in donor vehicles comprising 80% PG. Similar results were achieved in the subsequent study of polysorbate effects on hydrocortisone transport across the same membrane.[30] These investigators attributed the observed PG-dependent action of the polysorbates to changes in surfactant CMC and attendant changes in the concentration of surfactant monomer in solution. Surface tension studies confirmed that the CMC of the polysorbates increases with increasing proportions of PG in an aqueous vehicle. Accordingly, it was hypothesized that the presence of PG in the donor vehicle results in higher levels of surfactant monomer free to penetrate the SC and interact with components within the membrane.

More recently, Pandey et al.[31] reported that incorporation of 10% PG and 20% polysorbate 20 into a hydrophilic ointment base produced a marked increase in the *in vitro* transport of piroxacam across full-thickness rat skin. Interestingly, at early time points (30 min to 12 h), the flux of the drug was greater from the ointment containing polysorbate 20 alone. However, 24-h data revealed a twofold increase in piroxacam flux from the ointment containing both PG and polysorbate 20 as compared to polysorbate alone. An explanation for the apparent time-dependent synergy between the two components was not offered.

In contrast to the enhancing effects of polysorbates, however, other classes of nonionic surfactants have been shown to have little effect on cutaneous barrier disruption. Dalvi and Zatz[32] evaluated the transport properties of benzocaine across excised hairless mouse skin in the presence and absence of various polyoxyethylene nonylphenols with polyoxyethylene chain lengths ranging from 9 to 50 subunits. Data from the study revealed that benzocaine flux across the membrane was not favorably influenced by any of the surfactants studied. More recently, Cappel and Kreuter[28] investigated the effects of poloxamer and poloxamine surfactants on the penetration of methanol and octanol across hairless mouse skin *in vitro.* With the exception of poloxamer 188, which was found to enhance the penetration of octanol but not methanol, neither class of surfactants was found to alter the permeability of the skin, despite large differences in molecular weight (2900 to 14,000 D) and Hydrophilic-Lipophilic Balance (HLB) values (15 to 25). These findings may reflect the block-copolymer structure of the surfactants, in which a hydrophobic polypropylene oxide backbone is "sandwiched" between adjacent polyethylene oxide chains. Such a structure is unlikely to favor the penetration of surfactant monomer into the SC. Indeed, the effects of poloxamer 188 on octanol flux were observed to be immediately reversible, and were attributed solely to a surfactant-induced change in the vehicle–SC partition coefficient in favor of the skin.

On the other hand, Nishiyama et al.[33] investigated the *in vivo* transport of radiolabeled polyoxyethylene dodecyl ether surfactants into and through hairless mouse skin. These workers reported that the amount of each surfactant which successfully traversed the membrane increased linearly with time. Furthermore, the percent of each surfactant which completely penetrated the skin was found to be inversely related to the length of the polyoxyethylene chain, while the percent retained by the skin was found to increase with increasing ethoxylation (see Figure 8). Not surprisingly, rates of surfactant penetration through the skin were determined to be inversely related to the degree of ethoxylation, as illustrated in Figure 9. Accordingly, these results provide insight into the requisite structural requirements for successful interaction between nonionic surfactants and the skin.

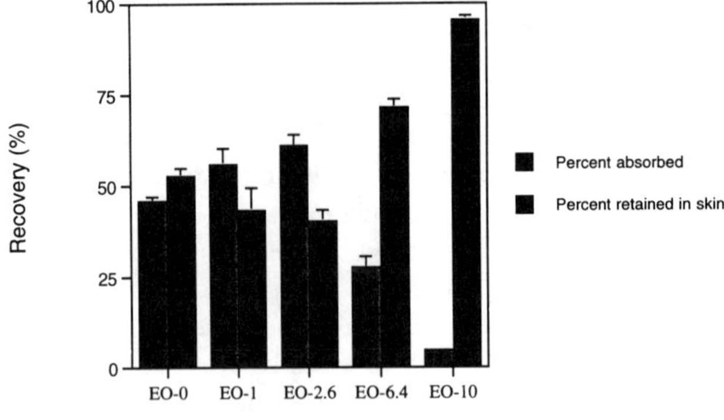

Figure 8 Influence of ethoxylation (as average mole addition of EO) on the *in vivo* recovery of radiolabeled polyoxyethylene dodecyl ether surfactants (mean ± SD; n = 3) following topical application to hairless mice. (Data from Nishiyama, T. et al., *J. Soc. Cosmet. Chem.*, 34, 263, 1983.)

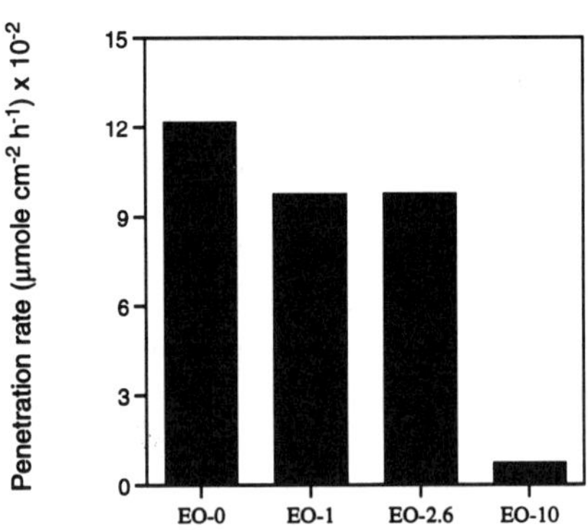

Figure 9 Influence of ethoxylation (as average mole addition of EO) on the *in vivo* flux of radiolabeled polyoxyethylene dodecyl ether surfactants (mean ± SD; n = 3) across hairless mouse skin. (Data from Nishiyama, T. et al., *J. Soc. Cosmet. Chem.*, 34, 263, 1983.)

REFERENCES

1. **Scheuplein, R. J. and Blank, I. H.,** Permeability of the skin, *Physiol. Rev.,* 51, 702, 1971.
2. **Barry, B. W.,** Lipid-protein-partitioning theory of skin penetration enhancement, *J. Control. Rel.,* 15, 237, 1991.
3. **Rhein, L. D. and Simion, F. A.,** Surfactant interactions with skin, in *Interfacial Phenomena in Biological Systems,* Bender, M., Ed., Marcel Dekker, New York, 1991, 33.
4. **Bettley, F. R. and Donoghue, E.,** Effect of soap on the diffusion of water through isolated human epidermis, *Nature,* 17, 185, 1960.
5. **Bettley, F. R.,** The influence of soap on the permeability of the epidermis, *Br. J. Dermatol.,* 73, 448, 1961.
6. **Bettley, F. R.,** The irritant effect of soap in relation to epidermal permeability, *Br. J. Dermatol.,* 75, 113, 1963.

7. **Scheuplein, R. and Ross, L.,** Effects of surfactants and solvents on the permeability of the epidermis, *J. Soc. Cosmet. Chem.*, 21, 853, 1970.
8. **Lodén, M.,** The simultaneous penetration of water and sodium lauryl sulfate through isolated human skin, *J. Soc. Cosmet. Chem.*, 41, 227, 1990.
9. **Imokawa, G., Akasaki, S., Minematsu, Y., and Kawai, M.,** Importance of intercellular lipids in water-retention properties of the SC: induction and recovery study of surfactant dry skin, *Arch. Dermatol. Res.*, 281, 45, 1989.
10. **Takahashi, M., Aizawa, M., Miyazawa, K., and Machida, Y.,** Effects of surface active agents on SC cell cohesion, *J. Soc. Cosmet. Chem.*, 38, 21, 1987.
11. **Ridout, G., Hinz, R. S., Hostynek, J. J., Reddy, A. K., Wiersema, R. J., Hodson, C. D., Lorence, C. R., and Guy, R. H.,** The effects of zwitterionic surfactants on skin barrier function, *Fund. Appl. Toxicol.*, 16, 41, 1991.
12. **Cooper, E. R. and Berner, B.,** Penetration enhancers, in *Transdermal Delivery of Drugs,* Vol. 2, Kydonieus, A. F. and Berner, B., Eds., CRC Press, Boca Raton, FL, 1987, 57.
13. **Ashton, P., Walters, K. A., Brain, K. R., and Hadgraft, J.,** Surfactant effects in percutaneous absorption. I. Effects on the transdermal flux of methyl nicotinate, *Int. J. Pharm.*, 87, 261, 1992.
14. **Prottey, C. and Ferguson, T.,** *J. Soc. Cosmet. Chem.*, 26, 29, 1975.
15. **Ashton, P., Walters, K. A., Brain, K. R., and Hadgraft, J.,** Surfactant effects in percutaneous absorption. II. Effects on protein and lipid structure of the SC, *Int. J. Pharm.*, 87, 265, 1992.
16. **Potts, R. R., Golden, G. M., Guzek, D. B., Harris, R. R., and McKie, J. E.,** Lipid thermotropic transitions in human SC, *J. Invest. Dermatol.*, 86, 255, 1986.
17. **Rhein, L. D., Robbins, C. R., Fernee, K., and Cantore, R.,** Surfactant structure effects on swelling of isolated human SC, *J. Soc. Cosmet. Chem.*, 37, 125, 1986.
18. **Blake-Haskins, J. C., Scala, D., Rhein, L. D., and Robbins, C. R.,** Predicting surfactant irritation from the swelling response of a collagen film, *J. Soc. Cosmet. Chem.*, 37, 199, 1986.
19. **Dominguez, J. G., Balaguer, F., Parra, J. L., and Pelejero, C. M.,** The inhibitory effect of some amphoteric surfactants on the irritation potential of alkylsulphates, *Int. J. Cosmet. Sci.*, 3, 57, 1981.
20. **Faucher, J. A. and Goddard, E. D.,** Interaction of keratinous substrates with sodium lauryl sulfate. I. Sorption, *J. Soc. Cosmet. Chem.*, 29, 323, 1978.
21. **Miyazawra, M., Ogawa, M., and Mitsui, T.,** The physico-chemical properties and protein denaturation potential of surfactant mixtures, *Int. J. Cosmet. Sci.*, 6, 33, 1984.
22. **Zehnder, S., Mark, R., Manning, S., Sakr, A., Lichtin, J. L., and Gabriel, K. L.,** A human *in vivo* method for assessing reduction of the irritation potential of sodium lauryl sulfate by mild surfactants: validation with an ether carboxylate with two different degrees of ethoxylation, *J. Soc. Cosmet. Chem.*, 43, 313, 1992.
23. **Kushla, G. P. and Zatz, J. L.,** Correlation of water and lidocaine flux enhancement by cationic surfactants *in vitro*, *J. Pharm. Sci.*, 80, 1079, 1991.
24. **Laughlin, R. G.,** Relative hydrophilicities among surfactant hydrophilic groups, in *Advances in Liquid Crystals,* Brown, G. H., Ed., Academic Press, New York, 1978, 41.
25. **Scheuplein, R. J. and Dugard, P. H.,** Effects of ionic surfactants on the permeability of human epidermis: an electrometric study, *J. Invest. Dermatol.*, 60, 263, 1973.
26. **Cooper, E. R. and Berner, B.,** Interactions of surfactants with epidermal tissues — physicochemical aspects, in *Surfactants in Cosmetics,* Rieger, M. M., Ed., Marcel Dekker, New York, 1984, 195.
27. **Cappel, M. J. and Kreuter, J.,** Effect of nonionic surfactants on transdermal drug delivery. I. Polysorbates, *Int. J. Pharm.*, 69, 143, 1991.
28. **Cappel, M. J. and Kreuter, J.,** Effect of nonionic surfactants on transdermal drug delivery. II. Poloxamer and poloxamine surfactants, *Int. J. Pharm.*, 69, 155, 1991.
29. **Sarpotdar, P. P. and Zatz, J. L.,** Evaluation of penetration enhancement of lidocaine by nonionic surfactants through hairless mouse skin *in vitro*, *J. Pharm. Sci.*, 75, 176, 1986.
30. **Sarpotdar, P. P. and Zatz, J. L.,** Percutaneous absorption enhancement by nonionic surfactants, *Drug Dev. Ind. Pharm.*, 12, 1625, 1986.
31. **Pandey, R. K., Ganga, S., Jayaswal, S. B., and Singh, J.,** Transdermal transport of piroxacam from ointment bases, *Pharmazie,* 47, 800, 1992.
32. **Dalvi, U. G. and Zatz, J. L.,** Effect of nonionic surfactants on penetration of dissolved benzocaine through hairless mouse skin, *J. Soc. Cosmet. Chem.*, 32, 87, 1981.
33. **Nishiyama, T., Iwata, Y., Nakajima, K., and Mitsui, T.,** *In vivo* percutaneous absorption of polyoxyethylene lauryl ether surfactants in hairless mice, *J. Soc. Cosmet. Chem.*, 34, 263, 1983.

Chapter 8.2

Benzalkonium Chloride Polymers

Takao Aoyagi and Yu Nagase

CONTENTS

I. INTRODUCTION

This chapter deals with a novel type of transdermal penetration enhancer that itself permeates with difficulty through the skin. That is, a "polymerized" surfactant was studied to establish that it could be applied to a skin permeation enhancer. Surfactants are well known to exhibit strong enhancing activity, but they are generally very irritating to the skin.[1] However, if the surfactant was polymerized and thus turned into a macromolecule, it was expected to be impermeable through the skin, and not to be an irritant. A surfactant monomer, *p*-vinylbenzyldimethylalkylammonium chloride, having a long alkyl chain, was polymerized and the enhancing activities of the monomer and the resulting polymer were estimated.[2] Moreover, in order to confirm that a structurally alternative cationic surfactant polymer would enhance drug penetration, another polymeric enhancer, cetylpyridinium bromide polymer, was prepared by the reaction of poly(4-vinylpyridine) with cetyl bromide, and the enhancing activity was also evaluated.[3] Additionally, to estimate whether the polymeric enhancers irritate the skin, the Draize test was carried out.

II. PREPARATION OF BENZALKONIUM CHLORIDE POLYMERS

A. PREPARATION OF MONOMERS

In general, a quaternary ammonium salt is easily prepared by the reaction of tertiary amine with alkyl halide (Menschutkin reaction). Surfactant monomers were synthesized by the reaction of chloromethylstyrene with *N,N*-dimethylalkylamine, as shown in Figure 1. The structures of the monomers are similar to that of benzalkonium chloride (the structure is shown in Figure 1), which is a typical cationic surfactant. Monomers of this type were easily radically polymerized, and the molecular weights of the corresponding homopolymers were controlled by using appropriate amounts

0-8493-2605-2/95/$0.00+$.50

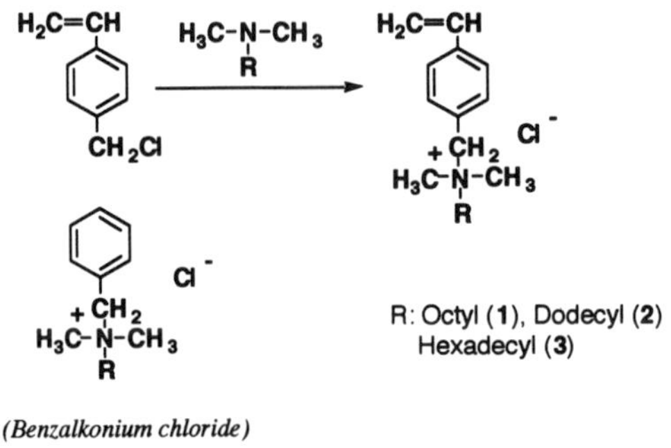

Figure 1 Preparation of benzalkonium chloride monomers. **1, 2,** and **3** contained octyl, dodecyl, and hexadecyl groups, respectively.

of chain transfer agent in radical polymerization, as described below. Three kinds of monomers, which had octyl, dodecyl, and cetyl groups, respectively, were synthesized in order to estimate the effect of the alkyl chain length upon the extent of enhancing activity of drug absorption. Based on the structure-activity relationship of the penetration enhancers, alkyl chain length seemed to be one of the important factors in the enhancing activity.[4–6]

B. POLYMERIZATION AND CHARACTERIZATION

The benzalkonium chloride polymers were prepared according to the scheme shown in Figure 2. The results of preparation of cationic surfactant polymers having a hexadecyl group were summarized in Table 1. The reason this monomer was chosen was that it showed the most effective enhancement of the drug permeation, as described below. The molecular weights of the polymers were determined by gel permeation chromatography, and the absence of the residual unpolymerized monomer was also confirmed by the same chromatographic chart. In radical polymerization using a chain transfer agent, so-called "oligomerization", the relationship between $1/DP_n$ (DP_n = degree of polymerization) and $[S]/[M]$ ($[S]$ = concentration of chain transfer agent, $[M]$ = concentration of monomer) is expressed by the following equation:

$$1/DP_n = 1/DP_0 + C_{tr}[S]/[M]$$

DP_0 is the degree of polymerization in bulk (without solvent) and C_{tr} is the chain transfer constant. As $1/DP_0$ and C_{tr} are constant, molecular weight can be easily controlled by changing the $[S]/[M]$ value.

Figure 3 shows the relationship between $[S]/[M]$ and the reciprocal of the degree of the polymerization. The good relationship between $[S]/[M]$ and $1/DP_n$ demonstrated the successful preparation of the polymers having various molecular weights.

III. PREPARATION OF CETYLPYRIDINIUM BROMIDE POLYMERS

Another type of cationic surfactant polymer, cetylpyridinium bromide polymer, was prepared. The procedure is shown in Figure 4, and the results are summarized in Table 2. In this reaction use of a polar solvent, such as formamide, ethylene glycol,

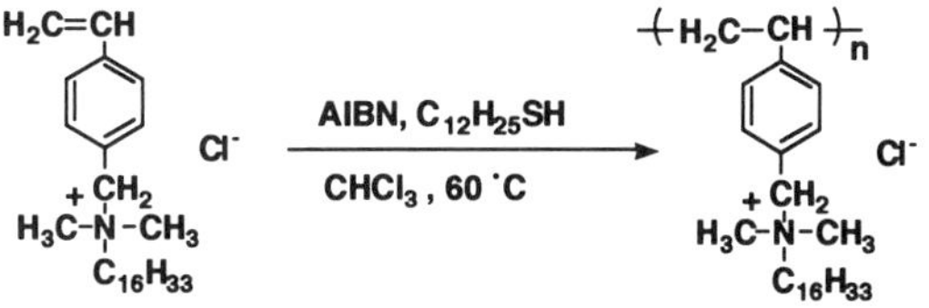

H2C=CH
Cl-
+CH2
H3C-N-CH3
C16H33
AIBN, C12H25SH
CHCl3, 60 °C
H2C-CH
n

Figure 2 Polymerization of benzalkonium chloride monomer.

Table 1 Preparation of Benzalkonium Chloride Polymers

Sample	[*S*]/[*M*][a]	Yield (%)	Mol wt[b]
P-1	0.025	72.5	32,100
P-2	0.050	71.4	14,900
P-3	0.100	68.4	12,300
P-4	0.125	52.0	8,800
P-5	0.150	57.4	7,500
P-6	0.250	39.4	4,800
P-7	0.300	39.8	2,900

[a] [*S*] indicates concentration of chain transfer agent (mol/l); [*M*] indicates concentration of monomer (1.0 mol/l).

[b] Determined by gel permeation chromatography (GPC) measurement.

0.20
0.15
0.10
0.05
0
1/DPn
0
0.1
0.2
0.3
[S]/[M]

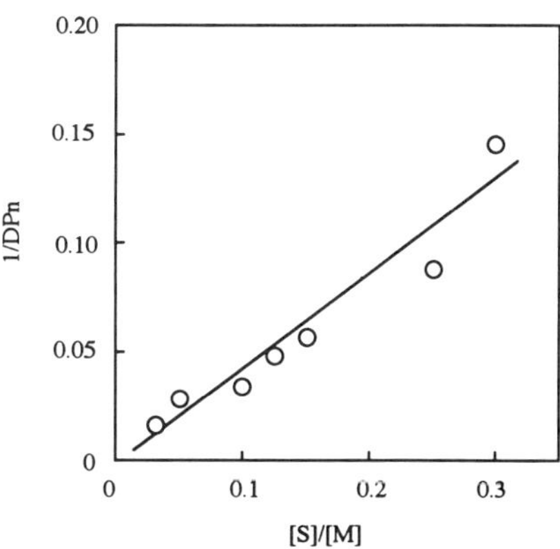

Figure 3 Relationship between [*S*]/[*M*] value and reciprocal of degree of polymerization.

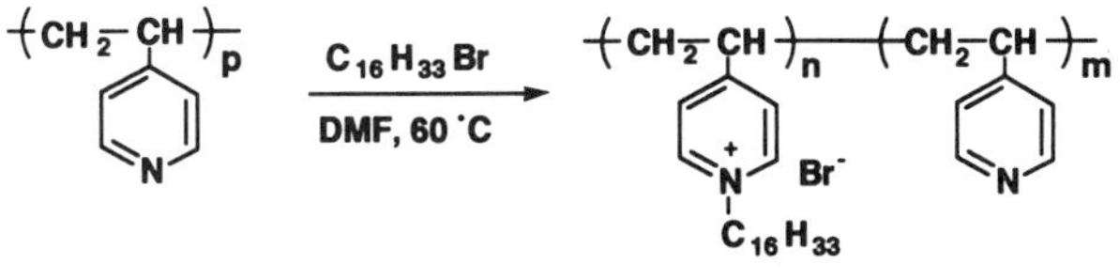

CH2-CH
p
N
C16H33Br
DMF, 60 °C
n
m
Br-
C16H33

Figure 4 Preparation of cetylpyridinium bromide polymer.

Table 2 Preparation of Cetylpyridinium Bromide Polymers

Sample No.	Poly(4-VP) (g)	Cetyl bromide/ poly(4-VP) (molar ratio)	Content of pyridinium group (mol%)[a]	Yield (g)
PVP-1	1.5[b]	1/5	11	1.85
PVP-2	1.5[b]	1/2	19	1.36
PVP-3	1.5[b]	1/1	28	1.06
PVP-4	2.5[b]	2/1	54	4.15
PVP-5	2.5[b]	3/1	62	5.43
PVP-6	1.5[c]	1/2	20	1.79
PVP-7	1.5[c]	1/1	40	2.44
PVP-8	1.5[c]	2/1	47	2.69
PVP-9	2.5[c]	3/1	56	5.20

[a] Determined from elemental analysis.

[b] Number average molecular weight (Mn) and weight average molecular weight (Mw) of starting poly(4-VP) were 11,500 and 22,500, respectively.

[c] Mn and mol wt of starting poly(4-VP) were 9,800 and 15,200, respectively.

and DMF are preferable, and in this study, DMF was suitable. The content of cetylpyridinium bromide in the polymer was in a range of 11 to 62 mol%, which could be controlled by changing the molar ratio of cetyl bromide to poly(4-VP) from 1:5 to 3:1.

IV. ENHANCEMENT OF 5-FLUOROURACIL PERMEATION

A. BY BENZALKONIUM CHLORIDE-TYPE POLYMERS

The drug penetration-enhancing activities of the polymeric enhancers were evaluated via an *in vitro* drug permeation experiment using excised rabbit abdominal skin and a two-chamber diffusion cell. The donor phase was the ethanolic solution containing 5% polymers and saturated 5-fluorouracil (5-FU). The receiver phase was phosphate buffer solution adjusted to pH 7.4. Figure 5 shows the permeation profiles of 5-FU through the skin with three kinds of monomers used as penetration enhancers. All the monomers, especially **2** and **3,** effectively enhanced drug penetration. The values of permeation coefficients (mean over 6 to 12 h) of 5-FU were as follows: **1,** 2.36×10^{-6} (cm/s), **2,** 1.27×10^{-5} (cm/s), **3,** 1.30×10^{-5} (cm/s), that with no enhancer, 2.86×10^{-7} (cm/s). The enhancing effect on drug penetration evidently increased in the order **1, 2,** and **3.** The polymerization of the monomers is predicted to lower mobility and surfactant activity and, as a result, to decrease their enhancing activity. Therefore, the most effective monomer, i.e., the compound having hexadecyl group **(3),** was chosen as a monomer to be polymerized.

Figure 6 indicates the permeation profiles of 5-FU through the skin using the polymers as penetration enhancers. The polymers also effectively enhanced drug absorption through the skin. The enhancing activity increased with decreasing molecular weight of the polymers, as shown in the figure. This tendency is shown more clearly in Figure 7, which represents the relationship between the molecular weights of polymers and the permeation coefficients of 5-FU. The molecular weight was a very important factor in drug penetration enhancement of these benzalkonium chloride polymers.

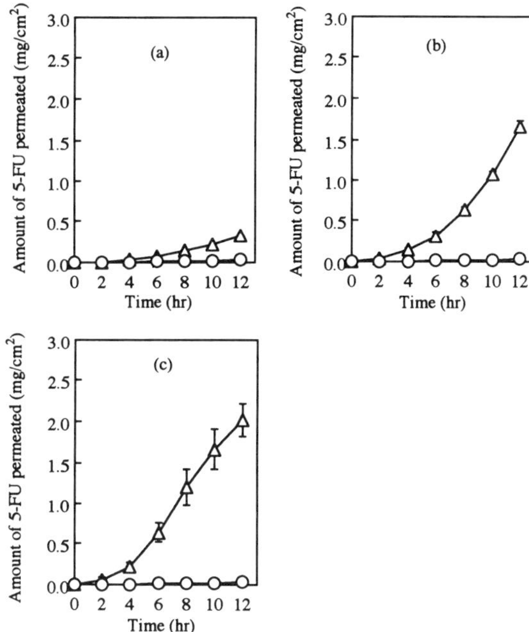

Figure 5 Permeation profiles of 5-FU through rabbit abdominal skin using benzalkonium chloride monomers. (a) **1**, (b) **2**, and (c) **3**.

The solubility of 5-FU before and after addition of the polymeric enhancers was determined. The concentration of 5-FU was almost unchanged in both cases. Therefore, the thermodynamic activity of the drug was held constant in all the donor solutions of the diffusion experiment. The high enhancing activities of the polymers may not be due to the increase of thermodynamic activity of the drug. Proportionality between the molecular weight of the polymer and permeation coefficient also indicated that the mobility and/or the activity as enhancer decreased with an increase in the molecular weight.

B. BY CETYLPYRIDINIUM BROMIDE POLYMERS

Figure 8 shows the permeation profiles of 5-FU using cetylpyridinium bromide polymers. The contents of the cetylpyridinium group were more than about 30 mol% for these polymers. The addition of PVP-1, PVP-2, and PVP-6 depressed the permeability of the drug. These polymers, which showed no enhancement, have a relatively small amount of pyridinium moiety. For each polymer used, the enhancing activity intensified steeply with an increase in the contents of pyridinium moiety. The polymers derived from the starting material, having lower molecular weights, showed larger enhancing activities. Therefore, this indicates that penetration enhancement is probably affected by not only the content of cetylpyridinium bromide in the polymer but also the molecular weight of the polymer. Regarding the benzalkonium chloride polymers, the enhancement also depended on the molecular weight of the polymer. The enhancing activities of the cetylpyridinium bromide polymers in this study were smaller than that of benzalkonium chloride polymers, which may be due to the difference in molecular weight rather than the molecular structure.

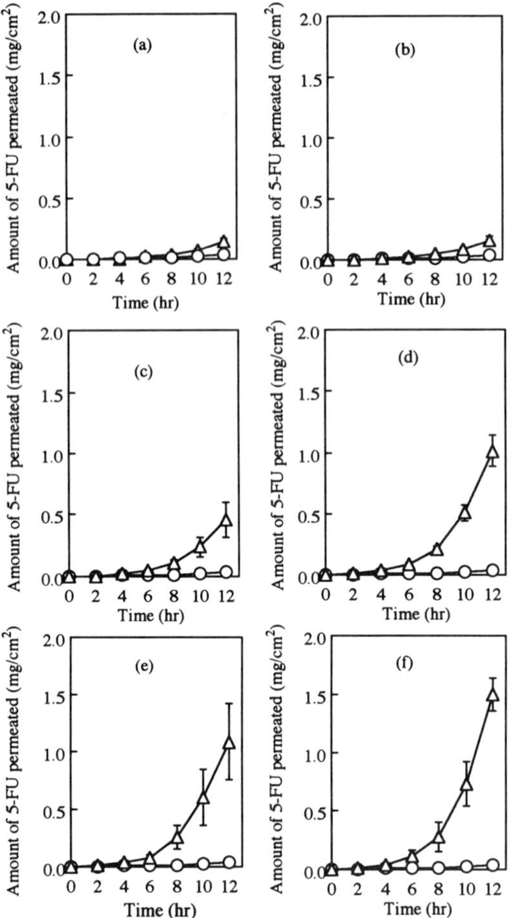

Figure 6 Permeation profiles of 5-FU through rabbit abdominal skin using benzalkonium chloride polymers. (a) P-1, (b) P-2, (c) P-3, (d) P-4, (e) P-5, and (f) P-7.

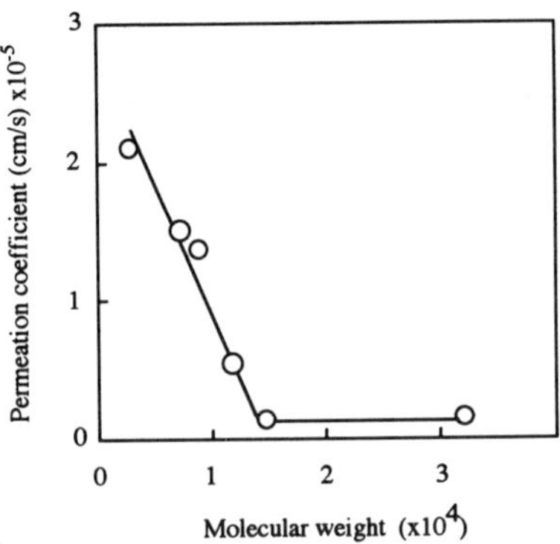

Figure 7 Relationship between molecular weight of benzalkonium chloride polymers and permeation coefficient of 5-FU.

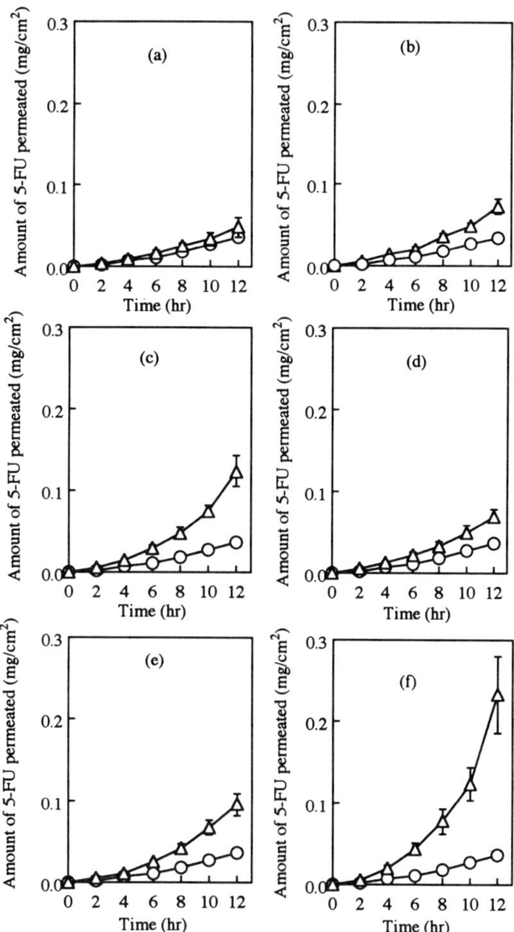

Figure 8 Permeation profiles of 5-FU through rabbit abdominal skin using cetylpyridinium bromide polymers. (a) PVP-3, (b) PVP-4, (c) PVP-5, (d) PVP-7, (e) PVP-8, and (f) PVP-9.

Solubilities of 5-FU in the donor solution in the presence or absence of the polymers were measured. The solubilities of the drug were almost unchanged by adding the polymers. Thus, the solubilities were kept almost constant in all the donor solutions through the diffusion experiments. Also, in the case of the cetylpyridinium bromide polymer, its drug penetration-enhancing capability may not owe to the increase in the thermodynamic activity of 5-FU.

V. IRRITATION TO THE SKIN

The Draize test was carried out on the polymeric enhancer in order to estimate skin irritation. In the experiment benzalkonium chloride type P-7 and cetylpyridinium bromide type PVP-9 were evaluated, because these compounds showed a larger effect in the enhancement of drug penetration. The results of the Draize test are summarized in Table 3. The *PII* value of these polymeric enhancers was smaller than 0.5 and the value was almost equal to that without enhancer. This indicated that the

Table 3 Results of Draize Test for Polymeric Enhancers

Enhancer	Normal skin	Damaged skin	*PII*
P-7	0.5 ± 0.4	0.1 ± 0.3	0.3 ± 0.3
PVP-9	0.5 ± 0.4	0.0	0.3 ± 0.2
Control[a]	0.1 ± 0.3	0.1 ± 0.3	0.1 ± 0.3

[a] Only solvent (1,3-butylene glycol was used).

polymers may not irritate the skin and would be safe as transdermal penetration enhancers in practical use.

Consequently, it was demonstrated that cationic surfactant polymers may be responsible for the high enhancing activity of drug penetration and also that such polymeric enhancers showed low skin irritation owing to its large molecular weight.

REFERENCES

1. **Woodford, R. and Barry, B. W.,** Penetration enhancers and the percutaneous absorption of drugs: an update, *J. Toxicol. Cut. Ocul. Toxicol.,* 5, 167, 1986.
2. **Aoyagi, T., Terashima, O., Suzuki, N., Matsui, K., and Nagase, Y.,** Polymerization of benzalkonium chloride-type monomer and application to percutaneous drug absorption enhancer, *J. Control. Rel.,* 13, 63, 1990.
3. **Aoyagi, T., Terashima, O., Suzuki, N., Nagase, Y., and Matsui, K.,** Preparation of a polymer containing hexadecylpyridinium bromide groups and its utilization as a transdermal drug penetration enhancer, *Polymer,* 32, 2106, 1991.
4. **Aoyagi, T., Yamamura, M., Matsui, K., and Nagase, Y.,** Preparations of phosphate, phosphoramidate and phosphate derivatives and their evaluation as transdermal penetration enhancers, *Drug Des. Discov.,* 8, 47, 1991.
5. **Aoyagi, T., Yamamura, M., Matsui, K., and Nagase, Y.,** Preparations of cyclic sulfoxide derivatives and their evaluation as transdermal penetration enhancers, *Chem. Pharm. Bull.,* 40, 1961, 1992.
6. **Aungst, B. J., Rogers, N. J., and Shefter, E.,** Enhancement of naloxone penetration through human skin *in vitro* using fatty acids, fatty alcohols, surfactants, sulfoxides and amides, *Int. J. Pharm.,* 33, 225, 1986.

Chapter 8.3

Silicone-Based Polymers

Takao Aoyagi and Yu Nagase

CONTENTS

I. INTRODUCTION

Polydimethylsiloxane (PDMS) has been known to possess distinctive physicochemical properties, for example, high flexibility, hydrophobicity, good biocompatibility and physiological inertness. From these features, this material is chemically or physically modified, and has been used in the pharmaceutical field as pressure-sensitive adhesives.[1,2] Also, regarding molecular design of penetration enhancers, a compound containing PDMS is expected to be less irritating to the skin. Furthermore, for the siloxane bond, the angle of the Si–O–Si bond is 130° and the distance of the Si–O bond is 0.163 nm. Compared to the bond that includes carbon rather than silicon, the angles of C–O–C and C–C–C are 111° and 112°, respectively. Additionally, the distances of the bonds of C–O and C–C are 0.142 and 0.154 nm, respectively. The rotational energy of –Si–O–Si– is almost zero. The polymeric compound with dimethylsiloxane chain seems bulkier, and the polymeric enhancer including PDMS is expected to be difficult to permeate through the skin.

II. PREPARATION OF POLYDIMETHYLSILOXANES (PDMSs) CONTAINING CATIONIC GROUP AT THE CHAIN END

A. METHYLPYRIDINIO-TERMINATED PDMS

According to the scheme in Figure 1, methylpyridinio-terminated PDMS (MePy-PDMS) was prepared. Prepolymer pyridyl-terminated PDMS (Py-PDMS)

0-8493-2605-2/95/$0.00+$.50

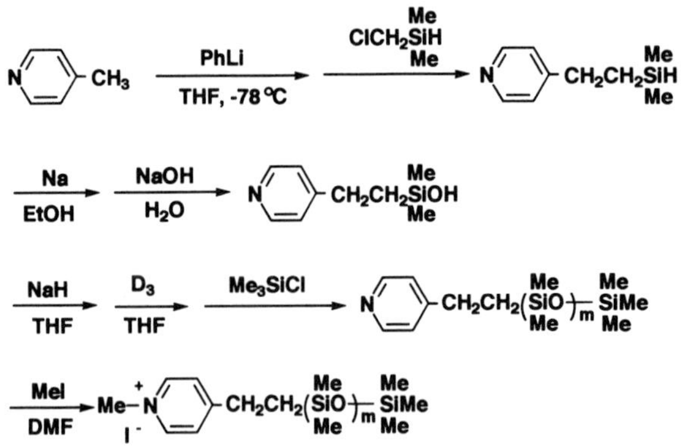

Figure 1 Preparation of methylpyridinio-terminated PDMS.

Table 1 Results of Preparation of Py-PDMS and MePy-PDMS

Code	D_3: initiator[a] (mole ratio)	m^b of Py-PDMS Theoretical	m^b of Py-PDMS Observed	Mn[c] of MePy-PDMS	Mw/Mn[c] of MePy-PDMS
MP-1	1.0	4.0	3.2	—[d]	—[d]
MP-2	1.5	5.5	5.1	460	1.14
MP-3	3.0	10.0	9.5	1000	1.15
MP-4	5.0	16.0	15.0	1400	1.18
MP-5	7.0	21.0	19.8	2200	1.25
MP-6	10.0	31.0	34.0	3000	1.07

[a] Molar ratio of hexamethylcyclotrisiloxane (D_3) and sodium 2-(4-pyridyl)-ethyldimethylsilanolate in the polymerization.

[b] The theoretical value of the average degree of polymerization, m was calculated from the equation, m=3[D_3]/[initiator]+1, and the observed value of m was determined on the basis of the ^{1}H-nuclear magnetic resonance spectrum.

[c] Determined by GPC.

[d] Insoluble in tetrohydrofuran (THF) used as GPC eluent.

was synthesized by the ring-opening polymerization of hexamethylcyclotrisiloxane (D_3) initiated with sodium 2-(4-pyridyl)ethylsilanolate[4] followed by termination with trimethylchlorosilane. Then, quaternization of the pyridyl group was carried out using methyl iodide. The average degree of polymerization of PDMS could be controlled easily by changing the ratio of the initiator and D_3. As listed in Table 1, MePy-PDMSs having various degrees of polymerization were successfully prepared.

B. PYRIDINIO- OR AMMONIO-TERMINATED PDMSs

The procedures used to prepare pyridinio- and ammonio-terminated PDMSs (PDMS-Py$^+$ and PDMS-Am$^+$)[5] are shown in Figure 2. The prepolymer, α-(3-chloropropyl)-PDMS (PDMS-Cl) was prepared by ring-opening polymerization of D_3 initiated with lithium trimethylsilanolate and terminating with 3-chloropropyldimethylchlorosilane. The chloropropyl group at the chain end was converted to the iodopropyl group by the substitution of halogen with sodium iodide to afford α-(3-iodopropyl)-PDMS

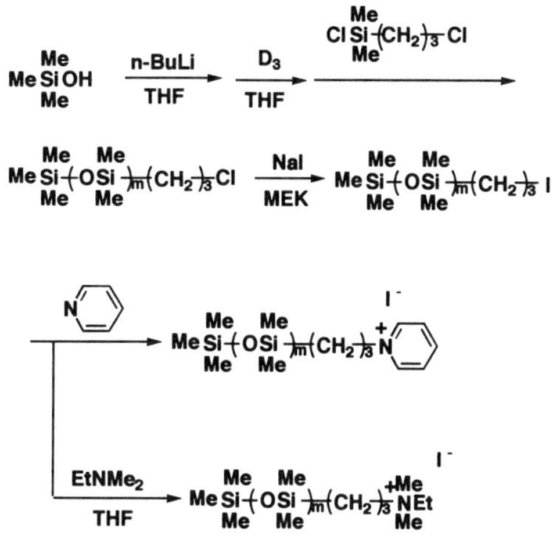

Figure 2 Preparation of pyridinio- or ammonio-terminated PDMS.

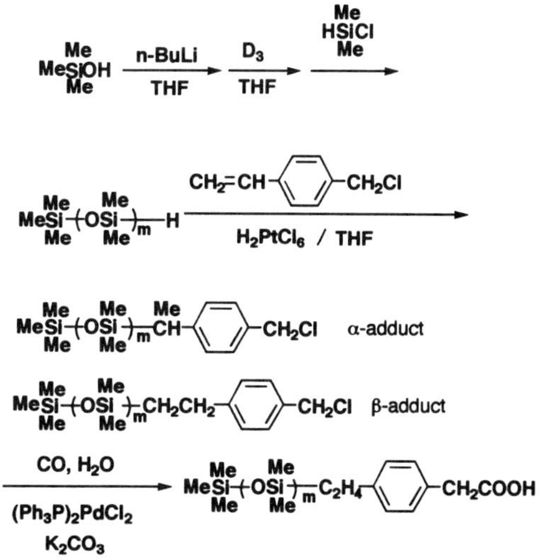

Figure 3 Preparation of carboxy-terminated PDMS.

(PDMS-I), because the iodoalkyl group reacts with tertiary amines much easier than chloroalkyl group under mild conditions. The quaternizing reaction of PDMS-I with pyridine or *N,N*-dimethylethylamine easily resulted in PDMS-Py$^+$ and PDMS-Am$^+$.

III. PREPARATION OF PDMSs CONTAINING ANIONIC GROUP AT THE CHAIN END

Polydimethylsiloxanes having carboxyl at the chain end[6] were prepared according to the procedure shown in Figure 3. First, prepolymer PDMSs containing the hydrosilyl group at the chain end was synthesized, second, hydrosilylation with chloromethylstyrene

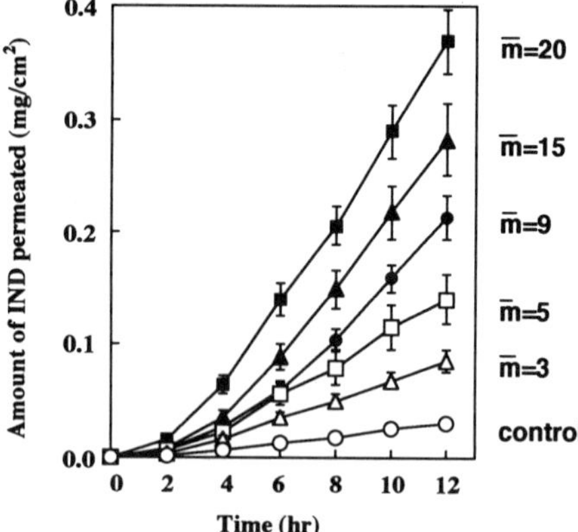

Figure 4 Permeation profiles of IND through rabbit abdominal skin using methylpyridinio-terminated PDMS.

was carried out, and third, the desired polymer was obtained by carbonylation using palladium catalyst.

VI. ENHANCEMENT OF INDOMETHACIN PERMEATION

A. BY PDMSs CONTAINING CATIONIC GROUP

The enhancing activity of indomethacin (IND) permeation was evaluated in an *in vitro* experiment using excised rabbit abdominal skin and a two-chamber diffusion cell. The donor phase was the ethanolic aqueous solution (50 wt%) containing 2 w/vol% enhancer and saturated drug, and the receiver phase was phosphate buffer solution adjusted to pH 7.4. Figure 4 shows the permeation profiles of IND through the skin with MePy-PDMSs as penetration enhancers. All MePy-PDMSs showed the effective enhancing activity of drug penetration through the skin. As described in Chapter 8.2, on the benzalkonium chloride polymers, the enhancing activities increased proportionally with the decrease in molecular weight in the range between 3000 and 15,000 Da. The activities of MePy-PDMSs also depended on the degree of polymerization, *m,* however, the enhancing activity increased with increase of *m,* contrary to the case of the benzalkonium chloride polymer. Also, regarding the permeation of IND with PDMS-Py$^+$ and PDMS-Am$^+$, the same behavior as that of MePy-PDMS was observed. This "chain length-dependence" suggested that the hydrophobicity of the enhancer might play an important role on the transdermal drug penetration enhancement because the hydrophobicity of the PDMS-bearing cationic group becomes larger with an increase of *m.*

To discuss the enhancing mechanism of PDMS-containing cationic groups, permeation parameters, such as permeation, diffusion, and partition coefficients in the transdermal drug permeation were calculated. Table 2 lists these coefficients using MePy-PDMSs as enhancers. In this permeation experiment the drug was saturated in the donor phase; therefore, the concentration (C_v) of the drug remained constant

Table 2 Effect of Addition of MePy-PDMS on IND Permeation Through the Skin

Code	m	Permeation coefficient, P ($\times 10^{-6}$ cm/s)	Diffusion coefficient, D ($\times 10^{-11}$ cm^2/s)	Partition coefficient, K
MP-1	3	0.69	2.57	27.0
MP-2	5	1.02	2.20	46.3
MP-3	10	2.09	1.23	169.3
MP-4	15	2.88	1.42	202.3
MP-5	20	3.55	1.87	190.2
Control[a]	—	0.22	2.01	11.0

[a] Without enhancer.

throughout the experiment. On this polymeric enhancer, P- and K-values increased with an increase in m. For example, the K-value on MP-4 and MP-5 (m was 15 and 20, respectively) was about 20-fold of that without enhancer. However, the diffusion coefficients of the drug remained constant, regardless of m. Similar behavior was observed on PDMS-Py$^+$ and PDMS-Am$^+$. Polydimethylsiloxanes containing cationic groups may not change the diffusivity of the drug at the skin barrier, and high enhancing effects of the polymers are exactly due to the considerable increase of the drug partition from the vehicle to the skin.

Some kinds of penetration enhancers which have relatively low molecular weights penetrate the skin barrier and stratum corneum (SC), and change the diffusivity of the drug in them. Dimethylsulfoxide permeates the lipid phase of the SC and interacts with lipid polar head group, and finally the hydrocarbon chain is lost.[7] Furthermore, the same literature suggests that the action of Azone® is its insertion between the lipid phase and prevention of chain crystallization. These existing penetration enhancers surely induce change of drug diffusivity by interaction with the components in the skin barrier. The results that PDMSs containing cationic groups did not change the drug diffusivity evidently meant the difference in the enhancing mechanism of these low molecular weight penetration enhancers. Further investigation was conducted in order to confirm the distinction on the enhancement (described below).

B. BY PDMSs CONTAINING AN ANIONIC GROUP

Figure 5 shows the permeation profiles of IND through the skin using the carboxy-terminated PDMSs as enhancers. All the polymers showed the enhancing activities of the drug penetration, however, the compound whose m was 1 showed the most effective enhancement. This result is the reverse of the cases of PDMSs bearing cationic groups. Although the carboxyl group is able to dissociate in aqueous medium, its dissociation constant is very small. As the donor phase in the permeation experiment was the mixture of water and ethanol, it was considered that the carboxyl group at the PDMS chain end might scarcely dissociate in the medium. As a result, the polarity of the compounds may be small. The reason that the carboxy-terminated PDMS, having a larger degree of polymerization, showed lesser enhancement is probably to be due to the small polarity of the compounds. This fact supported the consideration that the hydrophobicity of the penetration enhancer might play a very important role in enhancing the drug penetration.

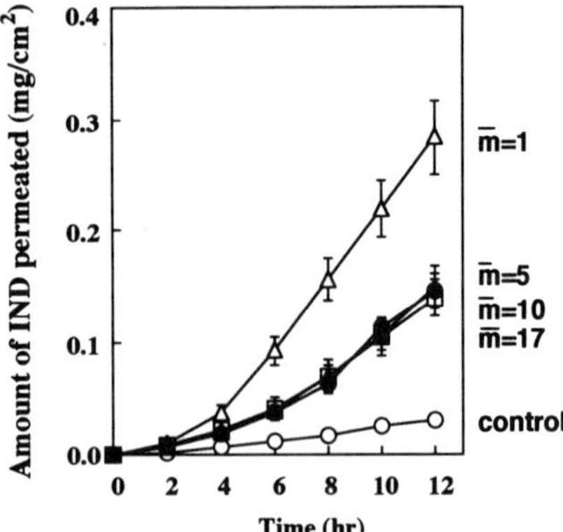

Figure 5 Permeation profiles of IND through rabbit abdominal skin using carboxy-terminated PDMS.

V. DIFFERENCE BETWEEN POLYMERIC AND LOW MOLECULAR WEIGHT PENETRATION ENHANCER

A. EFFECT ON LIPID ASSOCIATION

The differential scanning calorimetry (DSC) method revealed that Azone® rearranges the association of lipids in the SC, and therefore, shows the high enhancing effect on the drug penetration.[7] To investigate whether the polymeric enhancer influences the lipid association or not, the change of Tc (phase transition temperature) of a model lipid against adding the enhancers was observed by DSC. The measurement was carried out using 50 wt% ethanolic aqueous solution containing 50 wt% of dihexadecyldimethylammonium bromide. This compound does not exist naturally in the skin, however, it was used for the reason that it showed very clear Tc in the solution.[8] Figure 6a shows the DSC curves of the lipid solution containing PDMS-Py^+. Phase transition temperature of the lipid remained constant by even addition of the polymeric enhancer up to 30%. The intrusion of the polymeric enhancer into the lipid phase may be obstructed by the bulkiness of its dimethylsiloxane chain, even though the same investigation is carried out using natural lipids in the skin. The DSC curve of the lipid solution, including 1-propyl-3-dodecyl-2-pyrrolidone, is shown in Figure 6b. This derivative acted as a more effective enhancer of IND penetration than Azone®.[9] In the case of this compound Tc shifted to a lower temperature with increasing concentration of the added compound. Such an enhancer probably permeates the lipid region and rearranges the lipid in the SC.

B. EFFECT OF PRETREATMENT

For the purpose of clarifying the function of the polymeric and low molecular weight penetration enhancers to the skin, drug permeation experiments using the enhancer-pretreated skin were carried out. The skin used was treated with ethanolic aqueous solution (composition was 50 wt%) containing only enhancer (2 wt%) for 12 h in advance. Figure 7 shows the permeation profiles of IND in the cases of pretreatment

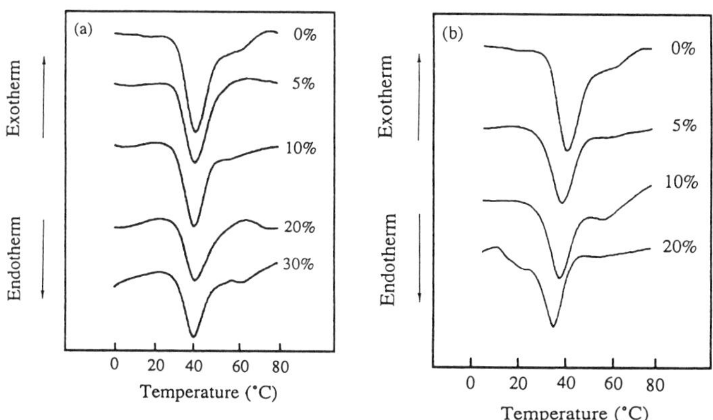

Figure 6 DSC curves of 50 wt% ethanolic aqueous solution containing dihexadecyldimethylammonium bromide. (a) PDMS-Py+ was added to the solution in the range of 0 to 30%. (b) 1-Propyl-3-dodecyl-2-pyrrolidone was added to the solution in the range of 0 to 20%.

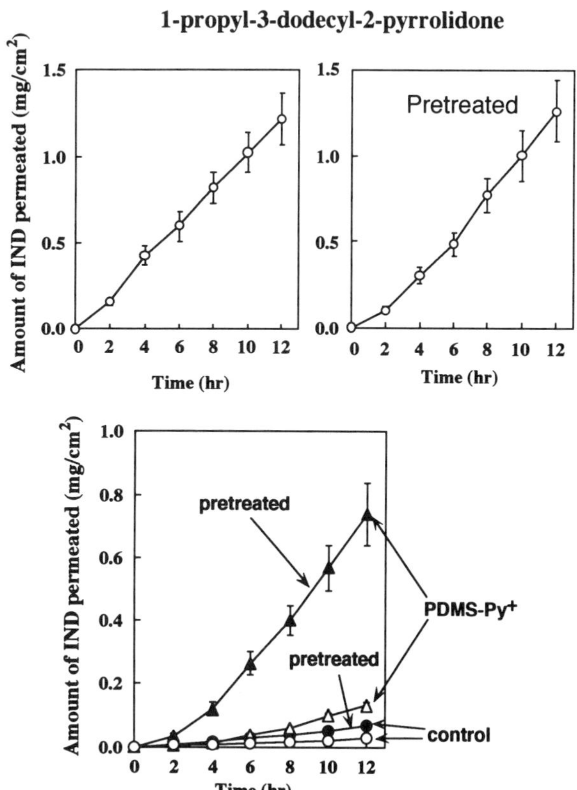

Figure 7 Effect of pretreatment with enhancer on IND permeation through the skin.

Table 3 Effect of Pretreatment with PDMS-Py+ on IND Permeation Through the Skin

Enhancer	Permeation coefficient, *P* ($\times 10^{-6}$ cm/s)	Diffusion coefficient *D* ($\times 10^{-11}$ cm²/s)	Partition coefficient, *K*
PDMS-Py+	1.01	0.99	110.1
Control	0.24	1.17	20.8
Pretreated PDMS-Py+	5.34	1.40	381.4
Control	0.49	1.47	33.4

with PDMS-Py+ and 1-propyl-3-dodecyl-2-pyrrolidone, respectively. Table 3 lists the permeation parameters on PDMS-Py+ that were obtained from the profiles. In the case of the pyrrolidone derivative pretreatment with the compound did not influence the permeation behavior of the drug through the skin. It was considered that the compound may immediately contact the surface of the skin and penetrate into the SC. Because this action occurred very quickly, pretreatment may not affect the manner of permeation.

On the other hand, pretreatment with PDMS-Py+ made the permeability of the drug much greater as compared to cases in which the enhancer and the drug were used together. In cases of diffusion coefficient of the drug, the value almost corresponded to that without enhancer. Only the partition coefficient increased, and the enlarged permeability was evidently due to the improvement of drug partition to the skin. Concerning the penetration-enhancing mechanism of the polymeric enhancers, we considered the following. First, the polymeric enhancer adsorbed onto the surface of the SC and the surface became more hydrophobic. Second, the partition of the hydrophobic drug to the modified surface increased more than it did to the original surface. Consequently, the large permeation was brought about by an improvement in drug partition. Enlargement by pretreatment with the polymeric enhancer may contribute to make the enhancer-adsorbed layer stable.

REFERENCES

1. **Pfister, W. R.,** Customizing silicone adhesives for transdermal drug delivery systems, *Pharm. Tech.,* 13, 126, 1989.
2. **Pfister, W. R., Woodard, J. T., and Grigoras, S.,** Silicone adhesives for transdermal drug delivery, *Chem. Br.,* 27, 43, 1991.
3. **Aoyagi, T., Takamura, Y., Nakamura, T., Yabuchi, Y., and Nagase, Y.,** Novel silicones for transdermal therapeutic system. I. Synthesis of 1-methyl-4-pyridinio-terminated polydimethylsiloxane and the evaluation as transdermal penetration enhancer, *Polymer,* 33, 2203, 1992.
4. **Aoyagi, T., Takamura, Y., Nakamura, T., and Nagase, Y.,** Preparations of pyridyl-terminated polydimethylsiloxane and siloxane-grafted copolymers containing pyridyl group at the side chain end, *Polymer,* 33, 1530, 1992.
5. **Aoyagi, T., Nakamura, T., Yabuchi, Y., and Nagase, Y.,** Novel silicones for transdermal therapeutic system. III. Preparation of pyridinio or ammonio-terminated polydimethylsiloxane and the evaluation as transdermal penetration enhancers, *Polym. J.,* 24, 545, 1992.
6. **Aoyagi, T., Akimoto, T., and Nagase, Y.,** Preparations of polydimethylsiloxanes containing cationic or anionic group at the chain end and their transdermal penetration enhancement, *Kobunshi Ronbunshu,* 49, 839, 1992 (in Japanese).

7. **Barry, B. W.,** Mode of action of penetration enhancers in human skin, in *Advances in Drug Delivery Systems, Vol. 3,* Anderson, J. M. and Kim, S. W., Eds., Elsevier, Amsterdam, 1987, 85.
8. **Okahata, Y., Lim, H., Nakamura, G., and Hachiya, S.,** A large nylon capsule coated with a synthetic bilayer membrane. Permeability control of NaCl by phase transition of the dialkylammonium bilayer coating, *J. Am. Chem. Soc.,* 105, 4855, 1983.
9. **Aoyagi, T., Yamamura, M., Suzuki, N., Matsui, K., and Nagase, Y.,** Preparation of alkyl-substituted pyrrolidone derivatives and their evaluation as transdermal penetration enhancers, *Drug Design Discovery,* 8, 37, 1991.

Chapter 9.1

Fatty Acids as Skin Permeation Enhancers

Bruce J. Aungst

CONTENTS

I. OVERVIEW OF FATTY ACID EFFECTS ON SKIN PERMEATION

Fatty acids and fatty acid salts, or soaps, have been known to increase skin permeability since at least 1961, when Bettley[1] reported that epidermis exposed to potassium oleate had increased permeability. More recently, much work has been done to characterize the effects of fatty acids on skin. The majority of this work was stimulated by the desire to reproduce the success that was achieved by the transdermal drug delivery systems initially introduced more than a decade ago, and the attempts to deliver other drugs transdermally. These attempts for transdermal delivery have often reaffirmed that the skin is an excellent barrier to foreign substances, and that the transdermal delivery of most compounds at therapeutic doses is not feasible unless skin permeation is increased in some way. Skin permeation enhancement has also been used to improve topical drug delivery.

Fatty acids have potential utility as skin permeation enhancers to improve the transdermal or topical delivery of drugs. The critical questions in assessing this utility are

- How effective are fatty acids as enhancers, and for what types of compounds?
- Which fatty acids are most effective?
- What is the role of the vehicle?
- What are the mechanisms involved in enhanced skin permeation?
- Will toxicity occur?

This chapter attempts to answer these questions.

0-8493-2605-2/95/$0.00+$.50

Table 1 Examples of the Effects of Fatty Acids as Skin Permeation Enhancers for Various Permeants

Permeant	Fatty acid	Vehicle	Skin Source	Enhancement Ratio	Ref.
Acyclovir	1% oleic acid	PG[a]	Human	9-144	2
	5% oleic acid			55-166	
5-Fluorouracil	5% oleic acid	PG	Human	8	3
			Hairless mouse	33	
Tetrahydro-cannabinol	3–10% oleic acid	PG:ethanol (1:1)	Hairless mouse	7	4
Oxymorphone	10% linoleic acid	Aqueous	Hairless mouse	63	5
		Triacetin:PG (2:1)		41	
Naloxone	0.5 *M* lauric acid	PG	Human	38	6
Testosterone				5	
Benzoic acid				1.3	
Indomethacin				102	
5-Fluorouracil				58	
Methotrexate				1.4	
Mannitol	5% oleic acid	PG	Human	84	7
Hydrocortisone				233	
Progesterone				8	
Dihydro-ergotamine	6% oleic acid	PG	Rabbit	207	8
	6% lauric acid			3	
Leuprolide	2% lauric acid	Ethanol:water (4:1)	Nude mouse	675	9
	2% capric acid			383	

Note: The fatty acid structure, vehicle, and skin source are important variables impacting the enhancement ratio.

[a] Propylene glycol.

Some examples of studies in which fatty acids were used to increase skin permeation are given in Table 1. The enhancement ratio is a ratio of the skin permeability coefficient or the flux for skin exposed to the fatty acid vs. a control value for skin not exposed to a fatty acid enhancer. Skin permeation enhancement with fatty acids is drug dependent. As shown in Table 1, fatty acids increased the skin permeation rates of some compounds by as much as two to three orders of magnitude, whereas under similar experimental conditions the skin permeation of other compounds was not affected much at all. Table 1 includes both lipophilic and hydrophilic compounds whose skin permeation was enhanced by fatty acids. The extent of permeation enhancement is greatly dependent upon the vehicle used and the structure of the fatty acid. These factors are reviewed in subsequent sections.

Fatty acids can be as effective or more effective than other types of skin permeation enhancers. In our work on naloxone skin permeation, in which we used vehicles containing 10% adjuvant in propylene glycol (PG), several fatty acids were more effective enhancers than nonionic surfactants, sodium lauryl sulfate, dimethylsulfoxide or decylmethylsulfoxide, dodecylazocycloheptanone (Azone®), or alkylpyrrolidones.[10] Similarly, in a comparison of the effects of various enhancers on 5-fluorouracil (5-FU) permeation through hairless mouse or human skin pretreated with aqueous or PG vehicles, oleic acid was as effective or more effective than dodecylazocycloheptanone or decylmethylsulfoxide.[3] Similar conclusions were obtained for estradiol permeation of human epidermis.[11]

Table 2 *In Vitro* Permeability Coefficients (K_p) of 5-Fluorouracil for Skin Pretreated with Various Vehicles

	K_p (×10⁴ cm/hr, mean ± SD)		
Vehicle	**Human**	**Hairless mouse**	**Black rat snake**
Saline	0.35 ± 0.55	0.96 ± 0.86	3.18 ± 1.5
PG	1.23 ± 1.4	8.83 ± 5.6	8.09 ± 4.8
5% oleic acid in PG	10.9 ± 10	177 ± 60	7.20 ± 1.8

Adapted from Rigg, P. C. and Barry, B. W., *J. Invest. Dermatol.*, 94, 235, 1990.

In considering fatty acids or any other skin permeation enhancer, it should be emphasized that rodent skin, which has been used often as a model for human skin, is more sensitive to the effects of fatty acids and other skin permeation enhancers than is human skin. This was clearly shown in a comparison of hairless mouse and human skin by Bond and Barry.[3] Oleic acid in a PG vehicle increased 5-FU permeation 8-fold using human skin, and 33-fold using hairless mouse skin. We have done *in vitro* studies comparing oxymorphone permeation through human skin and hairless guinea pig skin. The permeation-enhancing effect of a myristic acid/PG vehicle was much greater for hairless guinea pig skin than for human skin.[12] Shed snake skin also was used recently as a model to evaluate permeation enhancers. A comparison of the effects of oleic acid and PG on permeation of 5-FU through human, hairless mouse, and black rat skin is given in Table 2. While hairless mouse skin was more sensitive to the effects of permeation enhancers, snake skin was less sensitive than human skin and thus will provide a conservative prediction.

II. INFLUENCE OF FATTY ACID STRUCTURE

Structurally fatty acids consist of an aliphatic hydrocarbon chain and a terminal carboxyl group. Fatty acids could differ in their chain length, in the number, position, and configuration of double bonds, and have branching and other substituents. The influences of these structural variations on their effects as skin penetration are discussed. In this discussion the symbolic notation used to represent fatty acid structures is according to the following example. Oleic acid is $18{:}1^{\Delta 9}$, or 18 carbons and 1 double bond at carbons 9 and 10. Unless otherwise stated, double bonds should be assumed to have *cis* configuration.

A. EFFECT OF CHAIN LENGTH

The skin permeation-enhancing effects of saturated fatty acids are consistently greatest for C_{10} and C_{12} fatty acids. Figure 1 represents a compilation of data from four independent studies[10,14–16] comparing the effects of various saturated fatty acids on skin permeation. These results cover four compounds, three species, and used different vehicles, but in each case the maximum enhancement was observed with lauric acid. A final example is a study of the effects of saturated fatty acids on molsidomine percutaneous absorption *in vivo* in rats, wherein lauric acid (12:0) was much more effective than capric acid (10:0) and myristic acid (14:0), and 6:0, 8:0, and 16:0 were relatively ineffective.[17]

Longer chain fatty acids have higher melting points and lower solubilities in PG, which was used often as the vehicle in such studies. These factors probably contribute

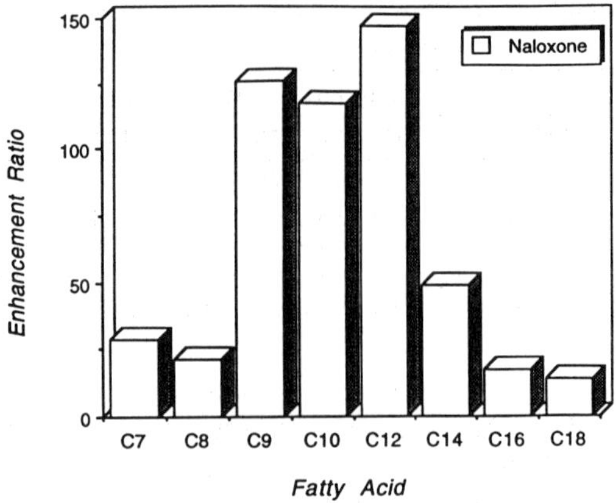

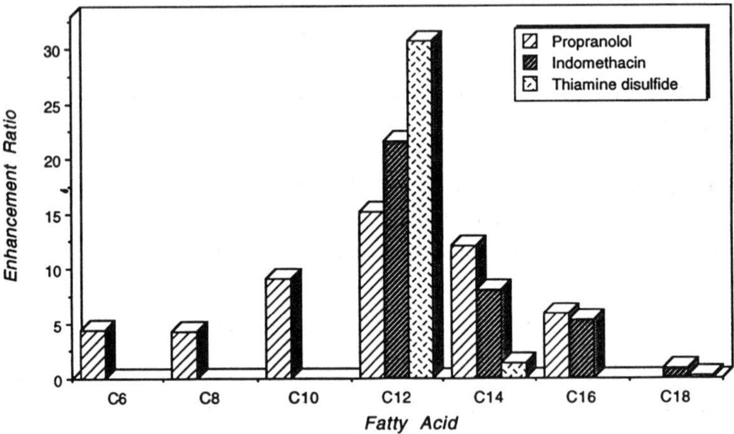

Figure 1 Influence of chain length of saturated fatty acids on their effectiveness as skin permeation enhancers for various compounds. The enhancement ratio is the skin permeation rate for fatty acid-exposed skin relative to skin treated with the same vehicle without fatty acid. (Data obtained from References 10 and 14 to 16.)

to their relatively poor permeation-enhancing effects. Short-chain fatty acids seem to affect the structure and barrier properties of the skin less than do medium-chain fatty acids. It is known that the effects of other permeation enhancers on skin, and the effects of fatty acids or other enhancers on permeabilities of mucosal and other cell membranes, often are greatest when the aliphatic hydrocarbon portion of the agent is C_{10} or C_{12}.

B. SATURATED VS. UNSATURATED

Oleic acid ($18{:}1^{\Delta 9}$) has been shown in numerous studies to be an effective skin permeation enhancer, whereas stearic acid (18:0) usually has not had skin permeation-enhancing effects. Other long-chain unsaturated fatty acids are also effective enhancers, including myristoleic (14:1), palmitoleic (16:1), vaccenic ($18{:}1^{\Delta 11}$), petroselenic ($18{:}1^{\Delta 6}$), eicosenoic ($20{:}1^{\Delta 11}$), linoleic (18:2), linolenic (18:3), and linoelaidic ($18{:}2^{trans}$).[18] Whereas unsaturated long-chain fatty acids ($\geq C_{18}$) are clearly more effective at increasing skin permeation than the analogous saturated fatty acids, few studies have compared saturated and unsaturated short- and medium-chain fatty acids.

The number, position, and configuration of the double bonds of unsaturated fatty acids could also influence their effectiveness as skin permeation enhancers. Some studies showed that increasing the number of double bonds increased the skin permeation-enhancing effects, i.e., oleic acid (18:1) < linoleic acid (18:2) and linolenic acid (18:3).[10,19] In other studies, however, oleic acid and linoleic acid have had similar magnitudes of enhancing effects.[17,18,20]

The effects of position and configuration of 18:1 fatty acids were evaluated by Golden et al.[21] using porcine stratum corneum (SC) and vehicles containing 0.15 *M* fatty acid in ethanol. The *cis* isomers of $18{:}1^{\Delta 9}$ and $18{:}1^{\Delta 11}$ were effective permeation enhancers, whereas the corresponding *trans* isomers had less or no enhancing effect. Neither $18{:}1^{\Delta 6cis}$ nor $18{:}1^{\Delta 6trans}$ enhanced salicylic acid flux. However, in another study using human skin and PG vehicles, salicylic acid flux was greatly enhanced by the *cis* isomers of $18{:}1^{\Delta 11}$ and $18{:}1^{\Delta 6}$.[18] Our laboratory evaluated three pairs of *cis/trans* isomers as permeation enhancers for naloxone, using human skin and PG vehicles containing 10% fatty acid. There were no differences between the cis and trans forms of $16{:}1^{\Delta 9}$, $18{:}1^{\Delta 9}$, and $18{:}2^{\Delta 9,12}$ fatty acids.[22]

C. BRANCHING AND OTHER SUBSTITUENTS

Very few studies exist of how branched or substituted fatty acids affect skin permeability. In one study various C_6, C_7, C_8, C_9, C_{10}, C_{12}, C_{14}, and C_{18} branched and linear fatty acids were compared using human skin and PG vehicles.[22] No differences between branched and linear fatty acids of the various chain lengths were observed except for C_{18}. Isostearic acid of the structure $(CH_3)_2CH(CH_2)_{14}COOH$ was a more effective permeation enhancer than was stearic acid. This branched fatty acid also had a lower melting point and apparently greater solubility in PG than stearic acid, factors which could be related to its permeation-enhancing effects.

Another type of possible skin permeation enhancer is hydroxy fatty acids. These are known to plasticize and increase the flexibility of skin,[23] but none have been explored for their effects on skin permeation of drugs.

III. EFFECTS OF VEHICLE AND FATTY ACID CONCENTRATION

The permeation-enhancing effects of fatty acids are greatly influenced by the vehicle used to deliver the permeant and fatty acid. This is illustrated by the results presented in Figure 2. In this example, as in other works,[12,18] fatty acids were most effective as enhancers when PG was used as the vehicle. The inclusion of fatty acids in vehicles comprised of polyethylene glycols, alcohols, glycerin, water, or oily solvents such as isopropyl myristate and mineral oil, may provide skin permeation enhancement, but not to the extent attained with PG.

Maximum effects of fatty acid enhancers using PG as the vehicle usually were observed at enhancer concentrations of 2 to 20%. This was true for lauric acid enhancement of naloxone permeation of human skin,[10] linoleic acid enhancement of morphine permeation of hairless mouse skin,[5] oleic acid and lauric acid enhancement

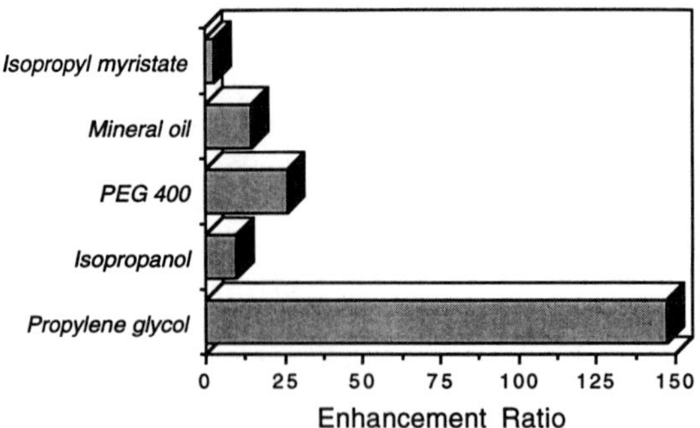

Figure 2 Enhancement ratios for naloxone skin permeation using various vehicles containing 10% lauric acid, relative to the lauric acid-free control vehicle. PEG = polyethyleneglycol. (Adapted from Aungst, B. J., Rogers, N. J., and Shefter, E., *Int. J. Pharm.*, 33, 225, 1992.)

of molsidomine permeation of rat skin *in vivo*,[17] and oleic acid enhancement of indomethacin absorption through rat skin *in vivo*.[24]

As discussed later, PG was shown to have its own skin permeation-enhancing effects.[7] Another effect of oleic acid was to increase the absorption of PG, and the greatest enhancement of absorption was at oleic acid concentrations of 5 to 10%.[24,25] Polyethylene glycol 200 and glycerin were absorbed much less than PG, either in the presence or absence of oleic acid.[25] Propylene glycol penetration into the skin might promote drug absorption by increasing drug partitioning into solvent-soaked skin, a mechanism similar to solvent drag.[6,11,25] The effect of a permeation enhancer on the absorption of PG, and the combined effects of the fatty acid and solvent on permeation of the drug, also depend on the drug being investigated.[6] Vehicles containing a high concentration of a fatty acid (20 to 100%) are generally less effective as absorption enhancers. This could be because these vehicles are less effective than PG as solvents for the drug, and because the fatty acid does not penetrate skin as rapidly as when the vehicle is comprised primarily of propylene glycol.

IV. MECHANISMS

The possible routes of drug permeation are through the keratinocytes, a tortuous pathway around the keratinocytes and through the intercellular lipid material, and through the appendages, the hair follicles, sweat glands, and sebaceous glands. The appendages are generally believed to contribute little to percutaneous drug absorption. Thus, the barriers to skin permeation are the keratinocytes and the intercellular lipids of the multilayered SC.

Barry and co-workers[11,26,27] proposed that three mechanisms can account for the actions of various types of skin permeation enhancers:

- Disruption of the barrier properties of SC lipids
- Interaction with cellular proteins
- Increased partitioning of the drug or solvent into the SC

This has been referred to as the 'lipid protein partitioning' theory of skin permeation enhancement. The effects of fatty acids can be described according to this classification.

A. EFFECTS ON BARRIER PROPERTIES OF SC LIPIDS

The intercellular lipids are arranged in an ordered structure of multiple bilayers of polar and nonpolar regions.[28,29] The structure of the intercellular lipids can be monitored using thermal analytical and various spectroscopic methods. Golden et al.[30] used differential scanning calorimetry (DSC) to analyze human SC, and identified four thermal transitions, two of which were associated with intercellular lipids. Changes in the temperature or in the heat flow associated with these transitions are indicative of changes in the lipid structures. Complementary analysis using infrared spectroscopy (IR) suggested that thermally induced changes in C-H stretching absorbances are associated with increased freedom and motion of the intercellular lipid hydrocarbon chains.[30,31] Such a decreased packing order of the alkyl chains is often referred to as increased fluidity. Fatty acid-treated skin showed increased fluidity of the intercellular lipids by DSC and IR, and the increases in fluidity were correlated with changes in permeability to salicylic acid.[21] This is strongly supportive of the hypothesis that these fatty acids increase skin permeability by increasing the fluidity or disrupting the packing of the intercellular lipids. The effects of oleic acid were further correlated with the amount of oleic acid taken up by the SC.[32] Electron spin resonance of model lipid bilayers also showed that oleic acid increased the rotational movement of the hydrocarbon chains, decreasing the order of the bilayer structure.[33]

The hydrocarbon chains of the SC lipids primarily have chain lengths of 16 or more carbon atoms, and are saturated.[28] These long, saturated hydrocarbon chains are able to pack together tightly within the bilayer structure. It was proposed that oleic acid disrupts the packed structure of the intercellular lipids because of the incorporation of its kinked structure (the kink is due to the *cis* double bond).[21,26] This helps explain why oleic acid is a much more effective permeation enhancer than is stearic acid. Studies with model lipid membranes suggested that packed lipid structures of long, saturated hydrocarbon chains are also disrupted by the incorporation of shorter, saturated hydrocarbon chains, or those with branched side chains.[34,35] It is reasonable to assume that this also applies to the packing of the intercellular lipids of the SC. This is then consistent with the observations that C_{10} to C_{12} saturated fatty acids are more effective in enhancing permeability than longer-chain saturated fatty acids, and that a branched C_{18} fatty acid was more effective than a linear fatty acid.[22]

Another recently proposed concept is that oleic acid permeates the SC, but does not homogenously mix with the SC lipids. Thermal analytical methods and microscopy suggested that oleic acid may exist as pools of fluid within the SC, forming defects in the permeability barrier.[36,37] Those defect areas also may be associated with water or coadministered solvent to account for the increased permeation of polar and charged permeants after oleic acid treatment.

Finally, Takeuchi et al.[38] reported evidence, obtained using IR spectroscopy, that oleic acid/PG treatment of rat skin produced a time-dependent extraction of SC lipids. This essentially would create a void volume to allow permeation of solutes or solvents. Lipid extraction was not seen when skin was treated with oleic acid in ethanol.

B. EFFECTS ON STRATUM CORNEUM PROTEINS

Oleic acid and lauric acid treatments of SC affected the conformation of SC proteins, as measured using DSC[26] and IR.[16] However, PG, which was used as the vehicle, also affects the SC proteins. In these studies the fatty acid/PG effects on SC proteins could have been due solely to the PG.[26] Fatty acid enhancement of PG skin penetration is one possible explanation for the synergistic effects of fatty acids and PG. Another is the separate mechanisms by which fatty acids and PG increase skin permeability.

C. INCREASED PARTITIONING OF DRUG OR SOLVENT

Partitioning of a drug into the SC is influenced by the permeation of the solvent into the SC and the affinity of the drug for the solvent. If the solvent permeates skin readily, and the drug has a high affinity for the solvent, the partitioning into and permeation through the skin can be increased by a solvent drag mechanism (drug and vehicle permeating together). The permeation rates of drug and PG were correlated for molsidomine,[25] indomethacin,[24] and narcotic analgesics,[5] using vehicles containing fatty acids. This indicates the possible involvement of a solvent drag mechanism. Fatty acids can increase the skin penetration rate of PG.[5] The effect of an enhancer on the permeation rate of the solvent can also be influenced by the inclusion of the drug in the vehicle. For example, PG skin permeation was increased by lauric acid and dodecylamine, but the effect of dodecylamine was totally negated when methotrexate was added to the vehicle.[6]

Another mechanism proposed to contribute to the enhancement of skin permeation with fatty acids is ion pairing of a basic drug with the fatty acid. Oleic acid and lauric acid greatly increased the partition coefficient (isopropyl myristate–buffer) of naphazoline, a cationic compound, but not that of caffeine, a neutral compound.[39] An ion-pairing mechanism would contribute the most for hydrophilic compounds that permeate the skin slowly. Thus, oleic acid had little effect on the skin permeation rates of several beta-blockers, even though their oil–water partitioning was increased.[40] Drug–fatty acid ion pairing also could influence the permeation rate of the fatty acid. Lauric acid permeation of shed snake skin was reduced by the addition of propranolol to the vehicle.[14]

V. TOXICITY

Fatty acids clearly have the potential to cause skin irritation. Application of a 5% oleic acid/PG vehicle to the skin of six human subjects for 6 h resulted in minor irritation; severe irritation occurred with a 20% oleic acid/PG vehicle.[41] An aqueous vehicle containing 10% oleic acid was applied to the skin of nude mice for 24 h under occlusion, and resulted in ulcerative eruptions, hyperplasia, and edema of the epidermis, and inflammation of the dermis.[42] In rabbits, skin treated with 10% oleic acid in PG for 18 h exhibited exfoliation, although a 12-h treatment had less serious effects.[43] Medium chain length saturated fatty acids are also potential skin irritants.[44]

Can the irritation-inducing and permeation-enhancing effects of fatty acids be separated? One approach to accomplish this would be to carefully control the concentration and delivery of a potentially irritating fatty acid. Oleic acid at 0.5 and 1% concentrations caused no changes or only minor damage to guinea pig skin, but these concentrations were still effective in enhancing physostigmine transdermal absorption.[45]

Another approach to reduce the irritation potential would be to select a less irritating fatty acid. Myristic acid is known to be much less irritating than lauric acid,[44] and while it is a less effective permeation enhancer than lauric acid, it

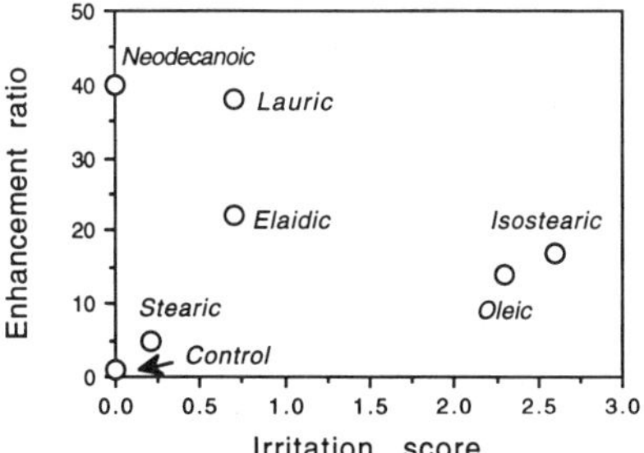

Figure 3 Correlation of irritation potential and permeation enhancement for PG vehicles containing 10% concentrations of various fatty acids. The enhancement ratio is for naloxone permeation of human skin *in vitro*. The irritation score represents the erythema and edema observed after a 6-h application under occlusion to shaved rabbit skin. A score of 8 would represent maximum irritation. (Adapted from Aungst, B. J., *Pharm. Res.*, 6, 244, 1989.)

provided significant absorption enhancement.[12] We have shown that the irritation potential of fatty acids does not necessarily correlate with their permeation-enhancing effects.[22] Figure 3 shows the permeation-enhancing and irritation-inducing effects of various fatty acids when applied in 10% fatty acid/PG vehicles. These results suggest that some fatty acids may be effective permeation enhancers, but not irritants.

Irritation of fatty acid/PG vehicles also might be minimized by the inclusion of other ingredients in the vehicle. It was claimed that an oleic acid/PG/glycerin (5/70/25) vehicle was much less irritating than an oleic acid/PG/water (5/70/25) vehicle, while maintaining the same skin penetration rate of estradiol.[46] Similarly, vitamin E and squalene reduced the irritation due to lauroylsarcosine, while maintaining as enhanced percutaneous absorption of isosorbide dinitrate.[47]

VI. SUMMARY

Fatty acids are broadly effective in enhancing skin permeation of drugs. Medium chain length, saturated fatty acids, and unsaturated fatty acids are the most effective. They work primarily by disrupting the packed structure of the intercellular lipids of the SC. The effects of fatty acids are highly dependent on the vehicle, with PG generally providing maximum permeation enhancement. Possible interactions among drug, fatty acid, and vehicle exist, in that each can influence the permeation of the other. The major challenge in successfully utilizing fatty acids for delivering drugs through skin will be in avoiding skin irritation.

REFERENCES

1. **Bettley, F. R.,** The influence of soap on the permeability of the epidermis, *Br. J. Dermatol.*, 73, 448, 1961.
2. **Cooper, E. R., Merritt, E. W., and Smith, R. L.,** Effect of fatty acids and alcohols on the penetration of acyclovir across human skin *in vitro*, *J. Pharm. Sci.*, 74, 688, 1985.
3. **Bond, J. R. and Barry, B. W.,** Hairless mouse skin is limited as a model for assessing the effects of penetration enhancers in human skin, *J. Invest. Dermatol.*, 90, 810, 1988.
4. **Touitou, E. and Fabin, B.,** Altered skin permeation of a highly lipophilic molecule: tetrahydrocannabinol, *Int. J. Pharm.*, 43, 17, 1988.

5. **Mahjour, M., Mauser, B. E., and Fawzi, M. B.,** Skin permeation enhancement effects of linoleic acid and Azone® on narcotic analgesics, *Int. J. Pharm.*, 56, 1, 1989.
6. **Aungst, B. J., Blake, J. A., and Hussain, M. A.,** Contributions of drug solubilization, partitioning, barrier disruption, and solvent permeation to the enhancement of skin permeation of various compounds with fatty acids and amines, *Pharm. Res.*, 7, 712, 1990.
7. **Barry, B. W. and Bennett, S. L.,** Effect of penetration enhancers on the permeation of mannitol, hydrocortisone and progesterone through human skin, *J. Pharm. Pharmacol.*, 39, 535, 1987.
8. **Niazy, E. M.,** Influence of oleic acid and other permeation promoters on transdermal delivery of dihydroergotamine through rabbit skin, *Int. J. Pharm.*, 67, 97, 1991.
9. **Lu, M. F., Lee, D., and Rao, G. S.,** Percutaneous absorption enhancement of leuprolide, *Pharm. Res.*, 9, 1575, 1992.
10. **Aungst, B. J., Rogers, N. J., and Shefter, E.,** Enhancement of naloxone penetration through human skin *in vitro* using fatty acids, fatty alcohols, surfactants, sulfoxides, and amides, *Int. J. Pharm.*, 33, 225, 1986.
11. **Goodman, M. and Barry, B. W.,** Lipid-protein-partitioning (LPP) theory of skin enhancer activity: finite dose technique, *Int. J. Pharm.*, 57, 29, 1989.
12. **Aungst, B. J., Blake, J. A., Rogers, N. J., and Hussain, M. A.,** Transdermal oxymorphone formulation development and methods for evaluating flux and lag times for two skin permeation-enhancing vehicles, *J. Pharm. Sci.*, 79, 1072, 1990.
13. **Rigg, P. C. and Barry, B. W.,** Shed snake skin and hairless mouse skin as model membranes for human skin during permeation studies, *J. Invest. Dermatol.*, 94, 235, 1990.
14. **Ogiso, T. and Shintani, M.,** Mechanism for the enhancement effect of fatty acids on the percutaneous absorption of propranolol, *J. Pharm. Sci.*, 79, 1065, 1990.
15. **Komata, Y., Inaoka, M., Kaneko, A., and Fujie, T.,** *In vitro* percutaneous absorption of thiamine disulfide from a mixture of propylene glycol and fatty acid, *J. Pharm. Sci.*, 81, 744, 1992.
16. **Takeuchi, Y., Yasukawa, H., Yamaoka, Y., Kato, Y., Morimoto, Y., Fukumori, Y., and Fukuda, T.,** Effects of fatty acids, fatty amines and propylene glycol on rat SC lipids and proteins *in vitro* measured by Fourier transform infrared/attenuated total reflection (FT-IR/ATR) spectroscopy, *Chem. Pharm. Bull.*, 40, 1887, 1992.
17. **Yamada, M. and Uda, Y.,** Enhancement of percutaneous absorption of molsidomine, *Chem. Pharm. Bull.*, 35, 3390, 1987.
18. **Cooper, E. R.,** Increased skin permeability for lipophilic molecules, *J. Pharm. Sci.*, 73, 1153, 1984.
19. **Carelli, V., Di Colo, G., Nannipieri, E., and Serafini, M. F.,** Enhancement effects in the permeation of alprazolam through hairless mouse skin, *Int. J. Pharm.*, 88, 89, 1992.
20. **Lee, C. K., Uchida, T., Noguchi, E., Kim. N.-S., and Goto, S.,** Skin permeation enhancement of tegafur by ethanol/panasate 800 or ethanol/water binary vehicle and combined effect of fatty acids and fatty alcohols, *J. Pharm. Sci.*, 82, 1155, 1993.
21. **Golden, G. M., McKie, J. E., and Potts, R. O.,** Role of SC lipid fluidity in transdermal drug flux, *J. Pharm. Sci.*, 76, 25, 1987.
22. **Aungst, B. J.,** Structure/effect studies of fatty acid isomers as skin penetration enhancers and skin irritants, *Pharm. Res.*, 6, 244, 1989.
23. **Hall, K. J. and Hill, J. C.,** The skin plasticisation effect of 2-hydroxyoctanoic acid. I. The use of potentiators, *J. Soc. Cosmet. Chem.*, 37, 397, 1986.
24. **Nomura, H., Kaiho, F., Sugimoto, Y., Miyashita, Y., Dohi, M., and Kato, Y.,** Percutaneous absorption of indomethacin from mixtures of fatty alcohol and propylene glycol (FAPG bases) through rat skin: effects of oleic acid added to FAPG base, *Chem. Pharm. Bull.*, 38, 1421, 1990.
25. **Yamada, M., Uda, Y., and Tanigawara, Y.,** Mechanism of enhancement of percutaneous absorption of molsidomine by oleic acid, *Chem. Pharm. Bull.*, 35, 3399, 1987.
26. **Barry, B. W.,** Mode of action of penetration enhancers in human skin, *J. Control. Rel.*, 6, 85, 1987.
27. **Williams, A. C. and Barry, B. W.,** Skin absorption enhancers, *Crit. Rev. Ther. Drug Carrier Syst.*, 9, 305, 1992.
28. **Downing, D. T., Stewart, M. E., Wertz, P. W., Colton, S. W., Abraham, W., and Strauss, J. S.,** Skin lipids: an update, *J. Invest. Dermatol.*, 88, 2s, 1987.
29. **Swartzendruber, D. C., Wertz, P. W., Kitko, D. J., Madison, K. C., and Downing, D. T.,** Molecular models of the intercellular lipid lamellae in mammalian SC, *J. Invest. Dermatol.*, 92, 251, 1989.

30. **Golden, G. M., Guzek, D. B., Harris, R. R., McKie, J. E., and Potts, R. O.,** Lipid thermotropic transitions in human SC, *J. Invest. Dermatol.,* 86, 255, 1986.
31. **Knutson, K., Krill, S. L., Lambert, W. J., and Higuchi, W. I.,** Physicochemical aspects of transdermal permeation, *J. Control. Rel.,* 6, 59, 1987.
32. **Francoeur, M. L., Golden, G. M., and Potts, R. O.,** Oleic acid: its effects on SC in relation to (trans)dermal drug delivery, *Pharm. Res.,* 7, 621, 1990.
33. **Gay, C. L., Murphy, T. M., Hadgraft, J., Kellaway, I. W., Evans, J. C., and Rowlands, C. C.,** An electron spin resonance study of skin penetration enhancers, *Int. J. Pharm.,* 49, 39, 1989.
34. **Small, D. M.,** Lateral chain packing in lipids and membranes, *J. Lipid Res.,* 25, 1490, 1984.
35. **Lewis, R. N. A. H. and McElhaney, R. N.,** Thermotropic phase behavior of model membranes composed of phosphatidylcholines containing iso-branched fatty acids. I. Differential scanning calorimetric studies, *Biochemistry,* 24, 2431, 1985.
36. **Ongpipattanakul, B., Burnette, R. R., Potts, R. O., and Francoeur, M. L.,** Evidence that oleic acid exists in a separate phase within SC lipids, *Pharm. Res.,* 8, 350, 1991.
37. **Walker, M. and Hadgraft, J.,** Oleic acid — a membrane "fluidiser" or fluid within the membrane?, *Int. J. Pharm.,* 71, R1, 1991.
38. **Takeuchi, Y., Yasukawa, H., Yamaoka, Y., Takahashi, N., Tamura, C., Morimoto, Y., Fukushima, S., and Vasavada, R. C.,** Effects of oleic acid/propylene glycol on rat abdominal SC: lipid extraction and appearance of propylene glycol in the dermis measured by Fourier transform infrared/attenuated total reflectance (FT-IR/ATR) spectroscopy, *Chem. Pharm. Bull.,* 41, 1434, 1993.
39. **Green, P. G., Guy, R. H., and Hadgraft, J.,** *In vitro* and *in vivo* enhancement of skin permeation with oleic and lauric acids, *Int. J. Pharm.,* 48, 103, 1988.
40. **Green, P. G., Hadgraft, J., and Ridout, G.,** Enhanced *in vitro* skin permeation of cationic drugs, *Pharm. Res.,* 6, 628, 1989.
41. **Loftsson, T., Gildersleeve, N., and Bodor, N.,** The effect of vehicle additives on the transdermal delivery of nitroglycerin, *Pharm. Res.,* 4, 436, 1987.
42. **Lashmar, U. T., Hadgraft, J., and Thomas, N.,** Topical application of penetration enhancers to the skin of nude mice: a histopathological study, *J. Pharm. Pharmacol.,* 41, 118, 1989.
43. **Hsu, L.-R., Tsai, Y.-H., and Huang, Y.-B.,** The effect of pretreatment by penetration enhancers on the *in vivo* percutaneous absorption of piroxicam from its gel form in rabbits, *Int. J. Pharm.,* 71, 193, 1991.
44. **Stillman, M. A., Maibach, H. I., and Shalita, A. R.,** Relative irritancy of free fatty acids of different chain length, *Contact Dermatitis,* 1, 65, 1975.
45. **Meshulam, Y., Kadar, T., Wengier, A., Dachir, S., and Levy, A.,** Transdermal penetration of physostigmine: effects of oleic acid enhancer, *Drug Dev. Res.,* 28, 510, 1993.
46. **Patel, D. C. and Ebert, C. D.,** U.S. Patent 4,855,294, 1989.
47. **Aioi, A., Kuriyama, K., Shimizu, T., Yoshioka, M., and Uenoyama, S.,** Effects of vitamin E and squalene on skin irritation of a transdermal absorption enhancer, lauroylsarcosine, *Int. J. Pharm.,* 93, 1, 1993.

Chapter 10.1

Urea and Its Derivatives as Penetration Enhancers

Adrian C. Williams

CONTENTS

I. INTRODUCTION

Urea (carbamide, NH_2CONH_2) is an odorless, colorless slightly hygroscopic crystalline powder which is soluble in water (approximately 1 g/ml). It is weakly basic, forming salts with strong acids, and it undergoes hydrolysis in the presence of acids, bases, or the enzyme urease (generated by many bacteria such as *Micrococcus ureae*). Urea is an osmotic diuretic and has been used intravenously in the treatment of acute increases in intracranial pressure due to cerebral edema and to decrease intraocular pressure in acute glaucoma. However, because urea produces side effects, including nausea, vomiting, headache, and mental confusion, it has largely been replaced as a diuretic by mannitol.

Urea is used more commonly as a hydrating agent and is employed in the treatment of scaling conditions such as ichthyosis, psoriasis, and other hyperkeratotic skin conditions.[1,2] Used as commercially available 10% creams, urea was effective in the treatment of 17 ichthyotic patients and 10 of 11 patients with hyperkeratosis of the hands and feet.[1] Ichthyotic skin scales treated with the 10% urea cream also were shown to have an increased water retention (of about 100%) as compared to the placebo cream base, while having little effect on the epidermal water barrier.[2] The effect of urea in the treatment of ichthyosis is probably due to its hygroscopic nature, although urea is also a mild keratolytic agent and hence may affect stratum corneum (SC) corneocytes, particularly after prolonged contact.

In a double-blind trial involving 50 patients with atopic eczema a cream containing 10% urea and 1% hydrocortisone was as effective as 0.1% betamethasone valerate cream, although six patients who had excoriated skin reported initial smarting when the urea-containing cream was first applied.[3] Prolonged contact of the skin with urea also was reported to provoke epidermal thinning, associated with a decreased number of DNA-synthesizing cells.[4] The authors suggested that additional or preliminary treatment with urea may enhance the effectiveness of topical drugs.

0-8493-2605-2/95/$0.00+$.50

II. PERCUTANEOUS ABSORPTION OF UREA

The percutaneous absorption of (among others) urea from a petrolatum vehicle through rat skin *in vitro* and *in vivo* was studied by Bronaugh and co-workers,[5,6] who determined a permeability coefficient of 1.6×10^{-5} cm/h (equal to 7.2% of the applied dose). Urea was selected to allow a comparison of the values on rat skin with those from Feldman and Maibach,[7] who studied urea absorption across human skin *in vivo* from urinary excretion data. Franz[8] also examined the percutaneous absorption of urea across human skin *in vitro,* and despite differences in experimental protocols, such as duration of contact, choice of skin membranes, and vehicles, the values from these three groups of workers showed good agreement.

Evidence that the permeability coefficient of urea may be species dependent has been provided. Wahlberg and Swanbeck[9] reported a very low permeability for urea through human skin, whereas Wohlrab and Schiemann[10] found very rapid penetration of urea through mini pig skin *in vivo,* although the amount of urea detected in the serum was very small. The permeation of urea through hairless mouse skin *in vitro* was studied by Ackermann et al.,[11] who found that the permeation of carbamide increased over the first 100 h of the experiment. Subsequent studies showed that the integrity of hairless mouse skin over this length of time is questionable.[12–14]

III. PERMEATION ENHANCEMENT BY UREA

Numerous studies employing urea as an enhancer of drug permeation have been reported in the literature, summarized here as those improving steroid permeation and those enhancing nonsteroidal agents.

A. IMPROVEMENT OF STEROID PERMEATION

Some of the earliest studies of transdermal permeation enhancement used urea to improve the efficacy of topically applied corticosteroids. Hydrocortisone permeation was improved by urea in a study which also showed that urea itself possessed a very low permeation through human skin.[9] The effects of urea on the diffusion of hydrocortisone acetate from a cream vehicle across the skin of volunteers *in vivo* were investigated by Feldman and Maibach.[15] These studies followed the urinary excretion of a radiolabeled marker from the drug (^{14}C) in a crossover experimental protocol, and concluded that the presence of 10% urea in the cream formulation increased steroid permeation approximately twofold. Other clinically controlled studies also demonstrated that incorporation of urea (typically around 10%) into hydrocortisone cream bases improves efficacy of the corticosteroid.[16–18] A study using a commercially available preparation of urea and hydrocortisone, applied to the skin of pigs *in vivo,* was claimed to show that carbamide improved the steroid permeation.[19] However, criticisms of this experimental protocol have been raised.[20]

As described earlier, urea can act to hydrate the SC. Using a vasoconstrictor assay in human volunteers, Barry and Woodford[21] studied the bioavailability of hydrocortisone in six commercial cream formulations, of which two contained urea. When the creams were applied to the skin for 6 h under occlusion, no significant increase in the skin penetration of hydrocortisone was observed from the urea-containing creams. Possible reasons for this effect included the use of an occlusive dressing which may have caused the SC water content to increase dramatically, thereby obscuring any hydrating effects that the urea may have induced. Additionally, the creams were applied for a relatively short time, and hence the full effects of carbamide on the nature of the SC may not have been attained. A subsequent study by the same workers[22] used a protocol to avoid these potential problems; the corticosteroids were applied in a multiple dosage regimen over a period of 5 d with no occlusive dressing. The results clearly demonstrated that a formulation including urea provided a significantly greater activity and bioavailability of the steroid as compared to non-urea-containing creams. The extended time period for urea to act on the skin and exert its keratolytic properties and the nonocclusion allowing carbamide to hydrate the skin probably accounts for the differences in these two study results.

B. IMPROVEMENT OF NONSTEROIDAL DRUG PERMEATION

The widespread use of carbamide as a penetration enhancer may be restricted by the acidity of typical urea-containing creams;[20] this may lead to problems of irritancy (particularly in excoriated skin) or problems with product stability. Indeed, problems with stability were found in a delivery system using urea and starch to promote dithranol penetration.[23–25]

More recently, urea was used as a penetration enhancer for hexyl nicotinate.[26,27] The study examined the effects of various urea concentrations on the release of the nicotinate from simple aqueous and oily cream formulations. *In vivo* studies were then performed on human volunteers by an assessment of the time to onset of erythema following application of the creams to the flexor aspect of forearms. While concluding that urea (10% in an oily base) decreased the time to onset of erythema, the approach used by these investigators to analyze the data allowed a proposal for the mechanism of action of carbamide as a penetration enhancer. In contrast, urea did not improve the permeation of benzyl nicotinate in human volunteers *in vivo,*[28] as assessed by the onset of erythema. The authors reported that this may have been due to the fact that urea crystallized visibly on the skin after drying, thus hindering the observation of redness.

Urea also was evaluated as an enhancer for the opioid antagonist naloxone.[29] The *in vitro* experiments used human skin (0.4-mm thick membranes incorporating the SC, epidermis, and some dermal tissue) and applied the test enhancer as a 10% admixture in propylene glycol (PG). The authors reported that urea and dimethylacetamide had no effect on naloxone flux, but examination of their data shows that the drug flux decreased when urea was included in the glycol vehicle to 25% of that in the control experiments (no adjuvant added).

A recent study employed urea to improve the penetration of the nonsteroidal anti-inflammatory drug, ketoprofen, through rat skin *in vitro.*[30] The effects of the accelerant were apparently dependent on the vehicle composition. When urea was included at 20% in an aqueous vehicle the permeability coefficient for ketoprofen decreased to 3.67×10^{-3} cm/h from a control value of 32.9×10^{-3} cm/h when urea was not present. This was attributed to a large reduction in the partition coefficient of the drug between the vehicle and the skin when urea was present. However, when PG or PG/ethanol/water vehicles were used the effects of urea on ketoprofen permeation were not pronounced, although effects on partition coefficients and diffusion coefficients were described. Pretreatment of the skin with a 20% aqueous urea solution or normal saline provided a slight increase in the permeability coefficient of the drug. However, no comment was made as to the integrity of the rat skin during these studies, and animal skins may not be entirely reliable for assessments of the action of an enhancer which possesses keratolytic properties.

Percutaneous absorption of indomethacin was improved by the addition of urea to an ointment base.[31] The study, using rabbit skin *in vivo,* analyzed the plasma concentration of the drug after topical application of indomethacin from ointment bases with urea concentrations varying from 0.5 to 5%. A marked increase in drug absorption was reported with 0.5% urea in the formulation, but a decreased absorption was noted on increasing the carbamide concentration to 2.5 or 5% in the ointment. This decreased absorption was correlated with the pH of the aqueous phase of the absorption ointment. A subsequent study using mefenamic acid demonstrated that urea did not promote this nonsteroidal anti-inflammatory drug across rabbit skin.[32]

We also looked at the effects of vehicle selection on the activity of urea and a series of analogues as penetration enhancers.[33] Because many effective penetration enhancers possess a C_{12} (or other) alkyl chain, we synthesized 1-dodecylurea and 1,3-didodecylurea with the aim of combining the keratolytic or hydrating properties of urea with the lipid-disrupting abilities associated with some fatty acids. We also evaluated 1,3-diphenylurea as an enhancer, again looking at the effects of adding a C_{12} moiety to the carbamide. These enhancers were then evaluated from a range of vehicles: light liquid paraffin, dimethylisosorbide, and PG. The structural formulas of these analogues and vehicles are in Figure 1.

Our experiments looked at the activities of the enhancers toward the model polar permeant 5-fluorouracil (5-FU) in human epidermal membranes *in vitro.* The pseudo steady-state permeability coefficient of the drug permeating the membranes from a saturated aqueous solution was measured as a control value. The test enhancers were then applied to the membranes for 12 h saturated in the various vehicles, and the vehicles were used without analogues to act as further controls. By applying the enhancers saturated in the vehicles the urea analogues were delivered from a system at their maximum thermodynamic activities. After this treatment the enhancers were removed from the membranes and the pseudo steady-state diffusion of a fresh saturated aqueous solution of 5-FU was assessed. The activities of the enhancers were expressed as an enhancement ratio (ER) where:

$$\mathrm{ER} = \frac{\text{permeability coefficient after enhancer treatment}}{\text{permeability coefficient before enhancer treatment}}$$

The results of our study are illustrated in Figure 2, which shows the mean enhancement ratios for the analogues toward 5-FU when applied from the different vehicles.

The results demonstrated that urea saturated in the vehicles, and the vehicles alone produced no significant increase ($p = 0.05$) in the permeability coefficient of 5-FU through human epidermal membranes *in vitro.* Also, the analogues showed no significant difference ($p = 0.05$) in penetration-enhancing activities from a given vehicle. However, the influence of the choice of vehicle on the activities of the enhancers was marked; delivery as saturated solutions from PG was more effective than delivery when saturated in dimethylisosorbide, while delivery from light liquid paraffin was ineffective for promoting the polar drug permeation.

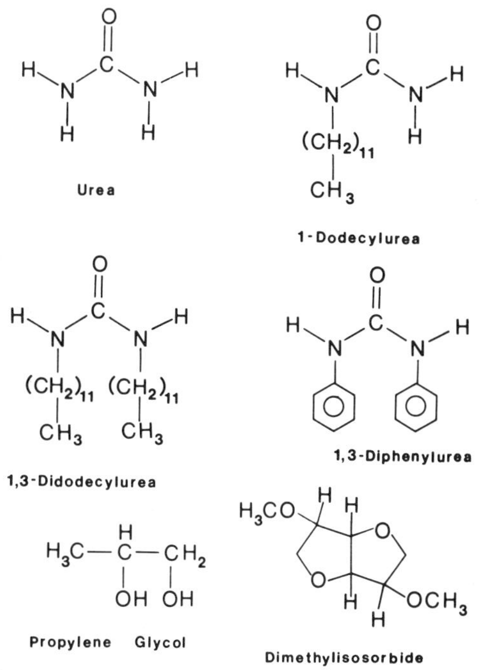

Figure 1 The structural formulas of some urea analogues and vehicles which were evaluated as penetration enhancers in human skin.

IV. MECHANISMS OF ACTION FOR UREA AS A PENETRATION ENHANCER

Urea has several possible mechanisms for penetration enhancement. As previously indicated, carbamide has keratolytic properties.[34] However, for the material to exert appreciable effects from interaction with the corneocytes sufficient time must be allowed for urea to act. Most of the studies employing urea to date have applied the material for short time periods during which appreciable breakdown of keratin would not be expected (although this may not be the case with some more fragile animal skins used to model human tissue in some studies).

The principal mode of action of urea as a penetration enhancer probably arises from its effects on the water content of the SC. Urea is a component (approximately 7%) of natural moisturizing factor (NMF) and has been shown to increase the water content of the skin.[34] This action of carbamide was also illustrated in the *in vivo* vasoconstrictor studies of Barry and Woodford.[21,22]

An additional mode of action for urea as an enhancer also was proposed in which carbamide may alter the integrity of the lipid bilayers in the SC.[27,35] Beastall et al.[27] suggested that urea may lower the phase transition temperature of the lipid component to such an extent that they are fluidized at the ambient temperatures of the skin. Alternatively, they suggest that the increase in tissue hydration obtained by employing urea may increase the water content of the lipid bilayers, thus disrupting their structure and rendering them more permeable. Subsequent work using X-ray diffractometry showed that this is an unlikely scenario.[36,37] What is also clear from

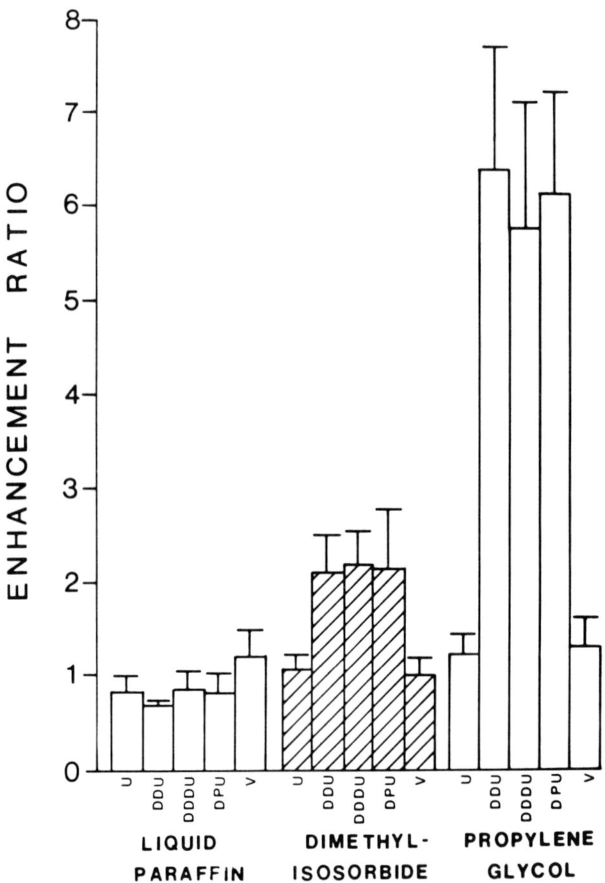

Figure 2 The penetration enhancing activities toward 5-FU of some urea analogues applied from different vehicles to human skin *in vitro.* U = urea; DDU = 1-dodecylurea; DDDU = 1,3-didodecylurea; DPU = 1,3-diphenylurea; V = vehicle alone.

these studies is that urea can exert its effects very rapidly, and that the effects arise from an interaction with skin components because in the study of Beastall et al. no influence of urea on the partitioning of hexyl nicotinate between its vehicle and the skin was found.

The recent study by Kim et al.[30] speculated that pretreatment with urea (and hydration with normal saline) may alter the ultrastructure of the SC, leading to the formation of large and extensive hydrophilic diffusion channels. However, the integrity and validity of some animal skins for such studies have been questioned. Clearly, the vehicle selected for application of urea to the rat skin was an important factor in the enhancer's efficacy, possibly resulting from variations in the thermodynamic activity of urea in the different solvent mixtures. In our own studies the activity of the enhancers in their vehicles was maximized, and we concluded that some urea analogue altered the lipid structure of the SC. However, our work used C_{12} moieties substituted into the structure of urea, and hence it is likely that the enhancers may have acted in a manner different than that of the simple carbamide. In our studies the choice of vehicle was an important consideration in determining the enhancer activities; PG provided a synergistic effect with the urea analogues, although urea itself showed no significant activity toward 5-FU permeation.

One further effect of urea on drug permeation in general appears to be a decrease in the lag time to steady-state drug diffusion. This may indicate that urea interacts with the protein component of the skin to decrease drug–keratin binding.

In summary, while urea can act on the skin in a variety of ways (keratolytic, hydration, lipid disruption, binding), its widespread use may be limited due to its proteolytic actions. However, urea is one of a very few penetration enhancers currently used in marketed dermatological formulations.

REFERENCES

1. **Rosten, M.,** The treatment of ichthyosis and hyperkeratotic conditions with urea, *Aust. J. Dermatol.,* 11, 142, 1970.
2. **Grice, K., Sattar, H., and Baker, H.,** Urea and retinoic acid in ichthyosis and their effect on transepidermal water loss and water holding capacity of SC, *Acta Derm. (Stockholm),* 53, 114, 1973.
3. **Almeyda, J. and Fry, L.,** Controlled trial of the treatment of atopic eczema with a urea-hydrocortisone preparation versus betamethasone 17-valerate, *Br. J. Dermatol.,* 88, 493, 1973.
4. **Wohlrab, W.,** Der einfluss von Harnstoff auf perkutane Permeationsmechanismen, *Dermatologica,* 155, 97, 1977.
5. **Bronaugh, R. L., Stewart, R. F., Congdon, E. R., and Giles, A. L.,** Methods for in-vitro percutaneous absorption studies. I. Comparison with *in vivo* results, *Toxicol. Appl. Pharmacol.,* 62, 474, 1982.
6. **Bronaugh, R. L., Stewart, R. F., and Congdon, E. R.,** Methods for in-vitro percutaneous absorption studies. II. Animal models for human skin, *Toxicol. Appl. Pharmacol.,* 62, 481, 1982.
7. **Feldman, R. and Maibach, H. I.,** Absorption of some organic compounds through the skin in man, *J. Invest. Dermatol.,* 54, 399, 1970.
8. **Franz, T. J.,** Percutaneous absorption. On the relevance of *in vitro* data, *J. Invest. Dermatol.,* 64, 190, 1975.
9. **Wahlberg, J. E. and Swanbeck, G.,** The effect of urea and lactic acid on the percutaneous absorption of hydrocortisone, *Acta Dermato-Venereol.,* 53, 207, 1973.
10. **Wohlrab, W. and Schiemann, S.,** Untersuchungen zum Mechanismus der Harnstoffwirkung auf die haut, *Arch. Dermatol. Forsch.,* 23, 225, 1976.
11. **Ackermann, C., Flynn, G. L., and Van Wyk, C. J.,** Percutaneous absorption of urea, *Int. J. Cosmet. Sci.,* 7, 251, 1985.
12. **Bond, J. R. and Barry, B. W.,** Damaging effect of acetone on the permeability barrier of hairless mouse skin compared with that of human skin, *Int. J. Pharm.,* 41, 91, 1988.
13. **Bond, J. R. and Barry, B. W.,** Limitations of hairless mouse skin as a model for *in vitro* permeation studies through human skin: hydration damage, *J. Invest. Dermatol.,* 90, 486, 1988.
14. **Bond, J. R. and Barry, B. W.,** Hairless mouse skin is limited as a model for assessing the effects of penetration enhancers in human skin, *J. Invest. Dermatol.,* 90, 810, 1988.
15. **Feldman, R. and Maibach, H. I.,** Percutaneous penetration of hydrocortisone with urea, *Arch. Dermatol.,* 109, 58, 1974.
16. **Swanbeck, G.,** A new treatment of ichthyosis and other hyperkeratotic conditions, *Acta Dermato-Venereol.,* 48, 123, 1968.
17. **Hindson, T. C.,** Urea in the topical treatment of atopic eczema, *Arch. Dermatol.,* 104, 284, 1971.
18. **Woodford, R. and Barry, B. W.,** Alphaderm cream (1% hydrocortisone plus 10% urea): investigation of vasoconstrictor activity, bioavailability and application regimens in human volunteers, *Curr. Theor. Res.,* 35, 759, 1984.
19. **Ayres, P. J. W. and Hooper, G.,** Assessment of the skin penetration properties of different carrier vehicles for topically applied cortisol, *Br. J. Dermatol.,* 99, 307, 1978.

20. **Barry, B. W.,** *Dermatological Formulations; Percutaneous Absorption,* Marcel Dekker, New York, 1983, chap. 4.
21. **Barry, B. W. and Woodford, R.,** Proprietary hydrocortisone creams — vasoconstrictor activities and bioavailabilities of six preparations, *Br. J. Dermatol.,* 95, 423, 1976.
22. **Barry, B. W. and Woodford, R.,** Vasoconstrictor activities and bioavailabilities of seven proprietary corticosteroid creams assessed using a non-occluded multiple dosage regimen; clinical implications, *Br. J. Dermatol.,* 97, 555, 1977.
23. **Hooper, G.,** Psoradrate cream, *Pharm. J.,* 222, 303, 1979.
24. **Thorne, N.,** Psoradrate cream, *Pharm. J.,* 222, 395, 1979.
25. **Yarrow, H.,** Psoradrate cream, *Pharm. J.,* 222, 413, 1979.
26. **Hadgraft, J.,** Penetration enhancers in percutaneous absorption, *Pharm. Int.,* 5, 252, 1984.
27. **Beastall, J., Guy, R. H., Hadgraft, J., and Wilding, I.,** The influence of urea on percutaneous absorption, *Pharm. Res.,* 3, 294, 1986.
28. **Lippold, B. C. and Hackemüller, D.,** The influence of skin moisturizers on drug permeation *in vivo, Int. J. Pharm.,* 61, 205, 1990.
29. **Aungst, B. J., Rogers, N. J., and Shefter, E.,** Enhancement of naloxone penetration through human skin *in vitro* using fatty acids, fatty alcohols, surfactants, sulphoxides and amides, *Int. J. Pharm.,* 33, 225, 1986.
30. **Kim, C. K., Kim, J. J., Chi, S. C., and Shim, C. K.,** Effect of fatty acids and urea on the penetration of ketoprofen through rat skin, *Int. J. Pharm.,* 99, 109, 1993.
31. **Naito, S. I. and Tsai, Y. H.,** Percutaneous absorption of indomethacin from ointment bases in rabbits, *Int. J. Pharm.,* 8, 263, 1981.
32. **Naito, S. I., Nakamori, S., Awataguchi, M., Nakajima, T., and Tominaga, H.,** Observation on and pharmacokinetic discussion of percutaneous absorption of mefenamic acid, *Int. J. Pharm.,* 24, 127, 1985.
33. **Williams, A. C. and Barry, B. W.,** Urea analogues in propylene glycol as penetration enhancers in human skin, *Int. J. Pharm.,* 56, 43, 1989.
34. **Hellgren, L. and Larsson, K.** On the effect of urea on human epidermis, *Dermatologica,* 149, 289, 1974.
35. **Cooper, E. R.,** Vehicle effects on skin penetration, in *Percutaneous Absorption; Mechanisms-Methodology-Drug Delivery,* Bronaugh, R. L. and Maibach, H. I., Eds., Marcel Dekker, New York, 1985, chap. 39.
36. **Bouwstra, J. A., Gooris, G. S., van der Spek, J. A., and Bras, W.,** Structural investigations of human SC by small angle x-ray scattering, *J. Invest. Dermatol.,* 97, 1005, 1991.
37. **Bouwstra, J. A., Gooris, G. S., Salomons-de Vries, M. A., van der Spek, J. A., and Bras, W.,** Structure of human SC as a function of temperature and hydration: a small angle x-ray diffraction study, *Int. J. Pharm.,* 84, 205, 1992.

Chapter 10.2

Biodegradable Unsaturated Cyclic Ureas as Penetration Enhancers

Ooi Wong and J. Howard Rytting

CONTENTS

I. BACKGROUND

The transdermal route of administration is a superior way to deliver a drug in many circumstances.[1] However, most existing therapeutic agents do not penetrate the skin readily owing to the great resistance of the stratum corneum (SC) to absorption. One effective approach to this problem is to use penetration enhancers to reduce skin resistance. Azone®, oleic acid, dimethylsulfoxide, diethyltoluamide (DEET), cyclic ureas, long-chain sulfoxides, and pyrrolidones all show penetration enhancement for particular types of drugs. Recent reviews of penetration enhancers related to transdermal drug delivery are available.[2–4] Although many studies of chemical enhancers have been done, thus far enhancers have not been used much in transdermal drug delivery products. Recent literature shows ongoing intensive investigation on enhancers, and this may help transdermal product developers identify suitable enhancers for their products. Toxicity, both local and systemic, is one of the major reasons that hinders most chemical enhancers from being used in transdermal products.

An alternative approach is to prepare biodegradable enhancers to reduce the toxicity of the enhancers. Ibuki[5] investigated a series of nonbiodegradable cyclic ureas for transdermal penetration enhancement of indomethacin in a petrolatum ointment dosage form using the shed skin of the black rat snake *(Elaphe obsoleta)* as a skin model. The results indicate that one of these cyclic ureas shows enhancement that was two times better than that of Azone®. Unfortunately, this compound and Azone® exhibited LD_{50} = 136 and 232 mg/kg, respectively, when given intraperitoneally to mice.[5] Therefore, these compounds might not be suitable for practical use. This chapter discusses the implementation of a new concept to reduce the

0-8493-2605-2/95/$0.00+$.50

toxicity of cyclic ureas, and at the same time to modify the structures to increase their penetration enhancement. The transdermal penetration enhancers investigated consist mainly of two parts, a highly polar parent moiety, which is an unsaturated cyclic urea (1-alkyl-4-imidazolin-2-one),[6] and a long-chain alkyl ester group.

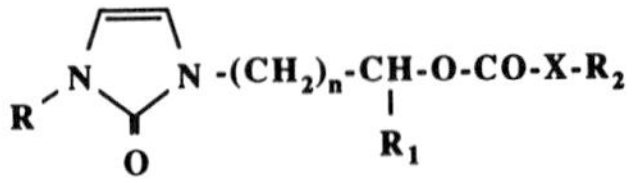

R–N(ring, C=O)N–$(CH_2)_n$–CH(R_1)–O–CO–X–R_2

(A)

(A1): $n=1$; $R=R_1=CH_3$; $X=CH_2$; $R_2=(CH_2)_9CH_3$

(A2): $n=0$; $R=R_1=CH_3$; $X=CH_2$; $R_2=(CH_2)_{11}CH_3$

(A3): $n=2$; $R=CH_3$; $R_1=H$; $X=CH_2$; $R_2=(CH_2)_9CH_3$

When X is CH_2, the compound is an ester derivative and when X is O it becomes a carbonate.

We evaluated the penetration-enhancing effects of these enhancers on the transport of indomethacin from petrolatum ointment through the shed skin of the black rat snake. As a substitute for human and animal skin, Ibuki,[5] Higuchi and Konishi,[7] and Itoh et al.[8] have investigated the use of shed snake skin for transdermal penetration studies. It was demonstrated that the shed skin of the black rat snake is suitable for this type of study. Most recently, the molecular structure of the shed skin of the black rat snake was compared to the human SC by Raman spectroscopy.[9] It was found that the spectra for both skins have similarities. The advantages of using snake skin as a model of the SC have been discussed by Higuchi and Konishi;[7] we, therefore, have adopted this technique in our evaluation of the biodegradable enhancers. Because biological membranes normally produce large variation in penetration results, it is advantageous to use a standard enhancer for comparing the new penetration enhancers. Azone® was chosen as the standard because it produces good penetration enhancement for a variety of drugs and has been studied extensively.

II. SYNTHESIS

The parent cyclic urea compounds were synthesized by acid-catalyzed cyclization of *N*-(2,2-dialkoxyl)-*N*-alkylureas, which were prepared by reaction of aminoacetaldehyde diethyl acetal with methyl or ethyl isocyanate in high yield (Scheme 1).

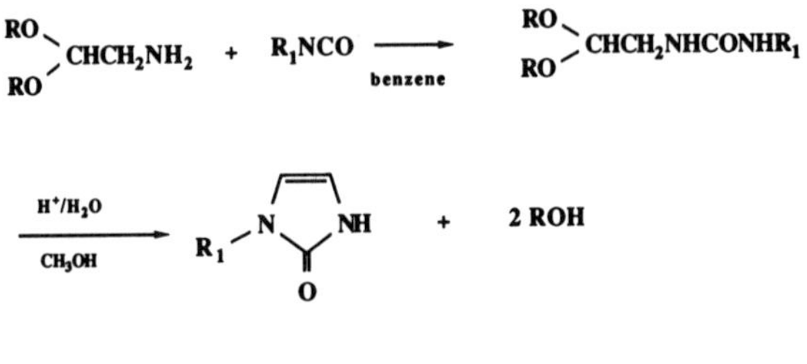

$$(RO)_2CHCH_2NH_2 + R_1NCO \xrightarrow{\text{benzene}} (RO)_2CHCH_2NHCONHR_1$$

$$\xrightarrow[CH_3OH]{H^+/H_2O} R_1\text{–N(ring, C=O)NH} + 2\ ROH$$

Scheme 1

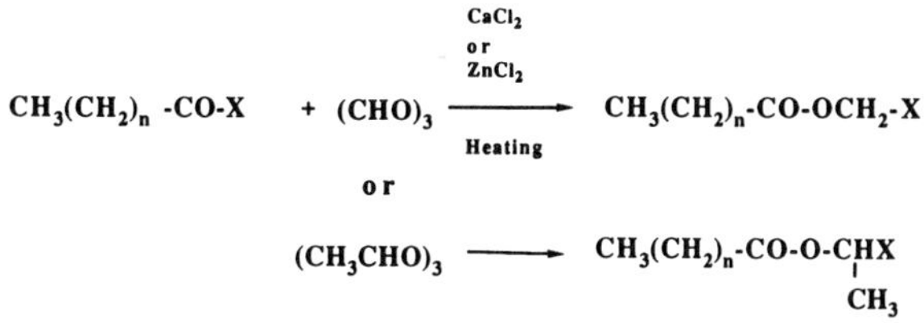

$$CH_3(CH_2)_n\text{-CO-X} + (CHO)_3 \xrightarrow[\text{Heating}]{CaCl_2 \text{ or } ZnCl_2} CH_3(CH_2)_n\text{-CO-OCH}_2\text{-X}$$

or

$$(CH_3CHO)_3 \longrightarrow CH_3(CH_2)_n\text{-CO-O-CH(CH}_3\text{)X}$$

Scheme 2

The soft alkylating reagents were synthesized, according to Scheme 2, by an insertion reaction of a formaldehyde or acetaldehyde group into alkyl halides by refluxing the corresponding acyl halides and paraformaldehyde in the presence of zinc chloride or calcium chloride. Some typical soft alkylating reagents were prepared by reaction of the corresponding halo alcohols with the appropriate acyl halides in chloroform in the presence of triethylamine. The enhancers were prepared by *N*-alkylation of the parent compound with soft alkylating reagents in chloroform in the presence of sodium hydride. In cases in which *N*-alkylation of the parent compound using the above method is difficult or unsuccessful a phase transfer catalysis technique becomes effective (Scheme 3).

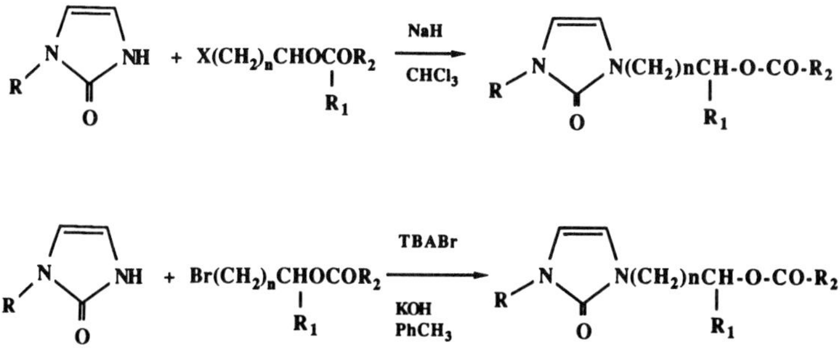

$$\text{R-N(imidazolinone)NH} + X(CH_2)_nCH(R_1)OCOR_2 \xrightarrow[CHCl_3]{NaH} \text{R-N(imidazolinone)N}(CH_2)_nCH(R_1)\text{-O-CO-}R_2$$

$$\text{R-N(imidazolinone)NH} + Br(CH_2)_nCH(R_1)OCOR_2 \xrightarrow[KOH,\ PhCH_3]{TBABr} \text{R-N(imidazolinone)N}(CH_2)_nCH(R_1)\text{-O-CO-}R_2$$

Scheme 3

The carbonate derivatives of the soft enhancers were prepared by reaction of 1-methyl-4-imidazolin-2-one with formaldehyde in the presence of sodium hydroxide to give the 3-*N*-hydroxymethyl product which was condensed with the alkyl chloroformates to yield the carbonate enhancers (Scheme 4). Details of synthesis for the enhancers were reported elsewhere.[10]

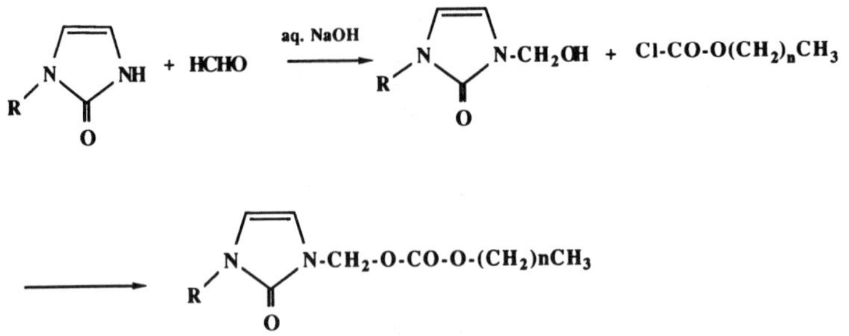

Scheme 4

III. HYPOTHESIS

The main reason for making these type of enhancers is first to allow them to exert their penetration-enhancing effects on the drug transport through the skin barrier, and then to allow them to be fragmentated by enzymes (in this case esterases) in the skin into the parent compound and the fatty acid while passing through the skin where esterase activity is known to exist (Scheme 5). In this way the toxicity of the enhancers can be reduced remarkably. Furthermore, a temperal limit can be placed on the action of the enhancer. At physiological pH, on the right-hand side of the reaction, the *N*-hydroxy compound might not revert to the parent compound depending on the number of methylene groups present. If n is zero and $R^1 = H$, k_1 is expected to be greater than k_{-1} and the parent compound becomes the major species in the equilibrium reaction. Examples are numerous in the literature showing fast reversion of the *N*-hydroxymethyl group of amides to their parent compound.[11] When n becomes larger the dissociation constant (k_1/k_{-1}) will become smaller or zero leaving the *N*-hydroxyalkyl compound as the major or the only species. This is due to the greater stability or nonreversibility of the *N*-hydroxyalkyl compound with a higher number of methylene groups.

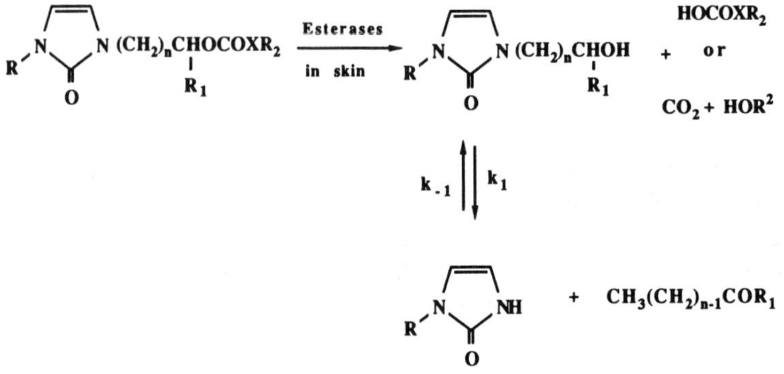

Scheme 5

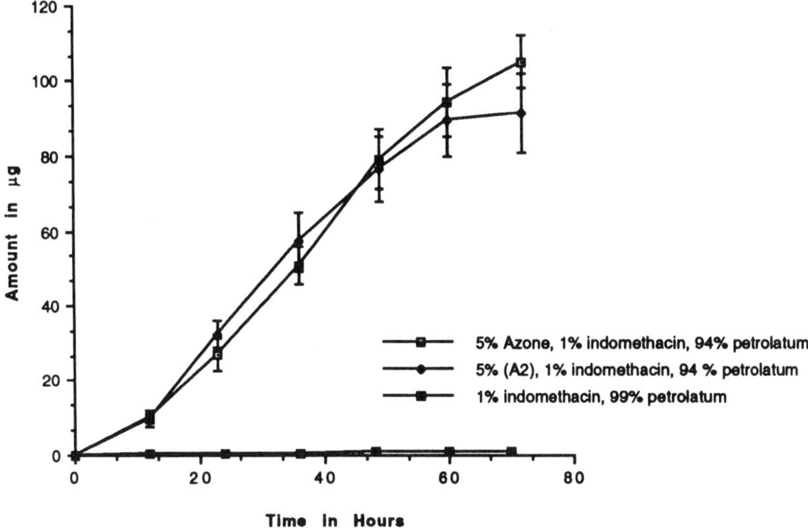

Figure 1 Time course penetration profiles of indomethacin through shed snake skin at 32°C using (A2) and Azone® as the enhancers. Data points represent the mean values obtained from four independent experimental runs. The amount of indomethacin (µg) on the *y*-axis was the cumulative amount detected in the receptor cells at the appropriate time.

IV. PENETRATION ENHANCEMENT

Because the area to which the ointments were applied was held constant at 1.77 cm^2, comparison of penetration enhancement of indomethacin by Azone® or the (A) series can be done by comparing the slope of the amount of indomethacin penetrating vs. time (Figure 1). Details of the penetration study were reported elsewhere.[12] After the first 12 h of the experiment, the same amount of indomethacin was detected in the receptor cells for both Azone® and (A2) ointments. The standard errors of the mean in both cases were relatively small. At the end of 72 h approximately 33% (100 g) of the total applied indomethacin penetrated through the skin. In this case the penetration fluxes of indomethacin for both Azone® and (A2) are regarded as equivalent. The flux of indomethacin in the control ointments without enhancer in all experiments was always very low. To compare the enhancement between the new enhancers and Azone®, we set a relative penetration enhancement (RPE) as:

$$\text{RPE} = \frac{\text{Steady-state slope of an (A) enhancer}}{\text{Steady-state slope of Azone}}$$

By this comparison, penetration enhancement of indomethacin due to Azone® is taken as 1. The results of all enhancers studied are shown in Table 1. The enhancer (A1) that shows the best penetration enhancement of indomethacin for ointments gave a RPE of 1.2 to 2.0 times of Azone®.

V. STRUCTURE-ACTIVITY RELATIONSHIP

The transdermal penetration enhancement by the (A) series enhancers appear to depend on the stability of the enhancers. 1-Methyl-4-imidazoline-3-methylenepivalate

Table 1 Transdermal Penetration Enhancement of Indomethacin Through Snake Skin at 32°C by the (A) Series Enhancers

	R	R[1]	*m*	*n*	*X*	RPE[a]	m.p.	Mol Wt
1	Me	Me	7	1	CH_2	0.5	liq.	310
2	Me	Me	9	1	CH_2	1.2–2.0	l.m.	338
3	Me	Me	11	1	CH_2	0.7	44.5	366
4	Me	Me	9	0	CH_2	0.6	38	324
5	Me	Me	11	0	CH_2	0.8–1.0	43	352
6	Me	H	9	1	CH_2	0.6	liq.	324
7	Me	H	9	2	CH_2	1.0	liq.	338
8	Me	H	7	0	CH_2	0.1	liq.	282
9	Me	H	9	0	CH_2	0.1	liq.	310
10	Et	Me	11	0	CH_2	0.5	42.5	366
11	Me	H	9	0	O	0.15	40	312
12	Me	H	11	0	O	0.5	44	340
13	Me	H	13	0	O	0.1	60	368

[a] RPE for Azone® was taken as 1. l.m. = low melting point.

was found to decompose in air after 1 week. The decanoate derivative also deteriorated after a period of several months, and this may account for the low penetration enhancement. Three possible ways to stabilize the molecules include: (1) making carbonate derivatives; (2) placing a methyl group on the 3-methylene group to increase the steric effects so that hydrolysis can be reduced; and (3) to elongate the methylene group to ethylene or propylene group.

The carbonate derivatives did not produce good penetration enhancement. For example, the dodecyl derivative enhances penetration only about 0.5 times that of Azone®. This moderate increase in enhancement over the corresponding ester analogues may be due to the more stable carbonate functional group. However, the higher polar carbonate group may at the same time dampen the activity of the enhancer.

The structure (A2), having an alpha methyl group at the 3-position of the imidazolin-2-one moiety, produces about the same penetration enhancement as Azone® which is a large improvement over the methylene derivatives. Also, this increment of enhancement over the carbonate series cannot be due to melting point and molecular weights because these two properties of the miniseries of compounds are similar.

By elongating the 3-methylene group, we see a steady increase in penetration enhancement from methylene, to ethylene and propylene derivative. This increment of enhancement may be attributed to the increase in both the chemical and enzymatic stability of (A3). It has been shown that the esterase stability of an ester group increases as its distance from a tertiary amino group increases.[11] Esterase activity in snake skin is high,[7,13] and the esterase stability of the enhancer may become a very important factor during the penetration processes to account for the higher penetration enhancement of (A3). At this point it would be advantageous to make the 3-isopropylene decanoate derivatives to see if they produce any further increase in enhancement. Indeed, (A1), the best of all compounds, shows enhancement as high as 2.0 times that of Azone®. A small change in structure could result in a dramatic change in enhancement. Comparing (A2) and compound 8, we see a drop in enhancement

Table 2 Preliminary Toxicity Results for (A2)

Group of Mice	Acute Dose (mg/kg)	Group of Mice	Chronic Daily Dose (mg/kg)
$n = 5$	100	$n = 6$	1000 for 14 d
$n = 5$	320	Control ($n = 5$)	0
$n = 5$	1000		
Control ($n = 5$)	0		
Results: No death		No death	

by extending the 1-methyl to 1-ethyl group, although the two compounds have similar melting points.

Penetration enhancement of indomethacin through snake skin has been shown to depend on the lipophilicity of the enhancer. When *n*-alkanols with chain numbers ranging from 4 to 16 carbons were used as enhancers,[14] the profile of penetration enhancement vs. lipophilicity of enhancer is a parabolic relationship with lauryl alcohol and tridecanol exhibiting the maximum effect. This type of profile was also seen in the penetration of a series of ester prodrugs of acetaminophen through snake skin[15] and in the penetration enhancement of indomethacin by a series of cyclic ureas with structures similar to the (A) series enhancers.[5]

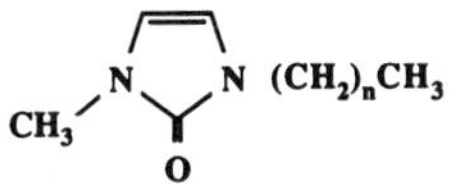

CH_3–N, N $(CH_2)_nCH_3$, O

We have noted similar enhancement profiles for the new enhancers we developed. Within the miniseries such as carbonate and (A1) series a lead or optimum compound shows the highest enhancement in the particular miniseries. The dependency of penetration enhancement on lipophilicity in the above examples is empirical and the explanation for this dependency may be related to a mixture of factors such as including interaction with the skin barrier.

VI. TOXICITY STUDIES

Detail of a preliminary study was reported elsewhere.[12]

1. Acute study: Three group of white mice were given subcutaneously an acute dose of (A2) of 100, 320, and 1000 mg/kg.
2. Chronic study: The mice were given subcutaneously a chronic dose of (A2) of 1000 mg/kg daily for 14 d.

One reason for injecting (A2) subcutaneously is to allow it to be cleaved by the enzymes in the subcutaneous tissues into fragments to reduce its toxicity. The toxicity results are shown in Table 2. Neither the acute nor chronic studies show any death of mice. The chronic toxicity study used a very high total dose of 14 g/kg (1.4% of the mice body weight) of (A2), but it did not cause any death of the mice or damage to the tissue at the injection site. The mice were kept for observation up to 39 d after the experiment and they appeared to be normal even at the injection site of the subcutaneous administration of the enhancer. This study demonstrates that the biodegradable concept is useful in reducing the toxicity of the nonbiodegradable enhancers studied by Ibuki.[5]

VII. CHEMICAL STABILITY

The ester enhancers with structures of (A), $n = 1$, $R^1 = H$ were found to be unstable upon standing in the air during synthesis. Two methods stabilize the compounds, either by elongating the methylene group or building up the steric group at R^1.

A preliminary stability study of (A3) was conducted by stirring the enhancer in a solution of isotonic phosphate buffer, pH 7.2, $I = 0.15\ M$ at 32°C and by following the disappearance of the enhancer with high-performance liquid chromatography analysis.[12] The plot of the log of the peak height of (A3) vs. time gave the pseudo-first-order hydrolysis rate of 0.00384/min ($t^1/_2 = 3$ h). (A3) has a propylene group between the parent cyclic urea and the ester functional group and it is more stable in anhydrous conditions. Steric effects have been known to hinder hydrolysis.[16] By building the steric group such as in (A1), it is expected the enhancer would become more chemically stable. The reason to choose (A3) in this study is to allow for a comparison of the chemical stability with the enzymatic stability discussed in the biodegradability section.

VIII. BIODEGRADABILITY

The (A) series enhancers are designed to be biodegradable, and it is important to demonstrate at least in *in vitro* experiments that they are fragmented by enzymes such as esterases. (A3) was chosen as the model enhancer for this study because it bears no chiral center in its structure. (A1) and (A2) both have a chiral center which may complicate the study by producing two hydrolysis rates due to their optical isomers. The reduction of intensity of the peak height for (A3) vs. time was obtained in the presence of 0.30 U of porcine esterase in an isotonic phosphate buffer (pH 7.2 and $I = 0.15\ M$) at 32°C. Because the enhancer shows low absorption in the ultraviolet region, the detection wavelength was set at 220 nm. The plot of logarithms of the peak heights vs. time indicates clearly that the esterase hydrolysis rate is psuedo-first-order for (A3), as shown in Figure 2, with $k_{obs} = 0.0952$/min and $t_{1/2} = 7.28$ min. The k_{obs} must represent contributions from hydrolysis due to the esterases and also to the isotonic phosphate buffer:

$$k_{obs} = k_{est} + k_{buff}$$

$$= k_{enz}[\text{esterase}] + k_{buff}[\text{buffer}] + k_{H}[\text{H}^+] + k_{OH}[\text{OH}^-] + k_0$$

where k_{obs} is the pseudo-first-order hydrolysis rate due to the esterase and the buffer solution and k_{buff} is the pseudo-first-order hydrolysis rate due to the buffer solution alone. $k_{buff} = k_{buff}$ [buffer] + k_H [H$^+$] + k_{OH} [OH$^-$] + k_0, where k_{buff} is the microscopic rate constant of buffer, and k_0 is the rate constant for H_2O. The term k_{est} is the pseudo-first-order hydrolysis rate due to k_{enz} [esterases], where k_{enz} is the microscopic rate constant for esterases. Because the hydrolysis rate constant (0.00384/min) due to the

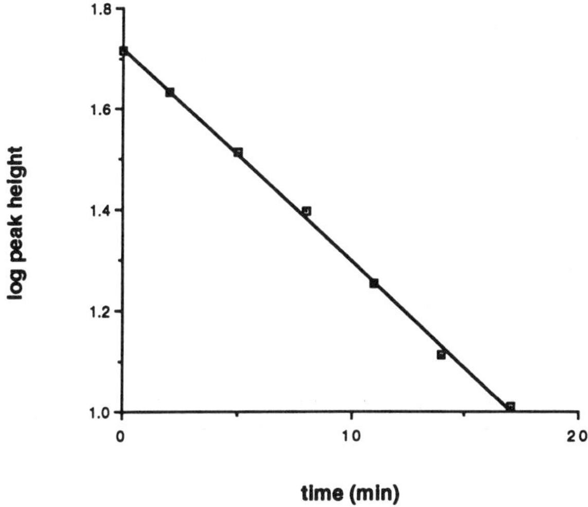

Figure 2 A linear first-order plot of the log peak heights of (A3) vs. time. k_{obs} = 0.0951/min; $t\frac{1}{2}$ = 7.29 min; r = 0.999.

buffer term determined in the chemical stability study is much smaller than that (0.0952/min) due to the esterases, the biodegradable of (A3) by esterases is confirmed. The hydrolysis rate constants, k_{obs} and k_{buff}, are comparable because the experimental conditions for determining the rates are the same.

IX. POSSIBLE MECHANISM

To confirm our hypothesis that the enhancers interacted with the skin, we carried out an electron micrograph study to gain physical evidence of the morphological changes in the skin caused by enhancer. The shed skin of *Elaphe obsoleta* has three different layers containing mainly keratin and lipids. The outermost layer is called the β-layer (β-keratin rich), the middle layer is called the meso layer (α-keratin and lipid rich), and the innermost layer is called the α-layer (α-keratin rich).[5] By treating the snake skin with (A1), we would expect a morphological change in the middle layer if the skin interacts with (A1). The scanning electron and light transmission micrographs of shed snake skin for control, and skin treated with (A1) indicated that (A1) has changed the morphology of the middle layer of the snake skin.[12] This study confirms that the role of this series of new enhancers includes an increase in skin permeability.

The electron micrograph study clearly shows that (A1) interacted with the snake skin and changed the morphology of the skin. (A1) swelled the keratin-rich layers, and in particular, the lipid-rich meso layer, thus reducing the density of the barrier. However, not all enhancers work in this way. We developed another series of biodegradable enhancers made of amino acetates. This type of enhancers fused the lipid-rich meso layer instead of swelling it.[17]

The release of indomethacin from ointments is expected to occur generally under sink conditions. Figure 3 shows a plot of the release rates of indomethacin from ointments vs. the loading concentration of indomethacin. From this study, it is estimated that the saturated concentration of indomethacin in petrolatum base is

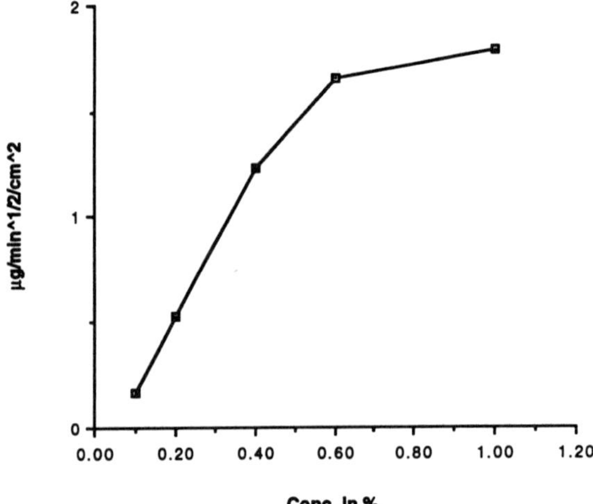

Figure 3 Plot of release rates of indomethacin vs. concentration of indomethacin in the ointments.

about 0.6% of indomethacin, and, therefore, at a 1% level of indomethacin, the thermodynamic activity of indomethacin in petrolatum is expected to be constant, producing a constant release rate. The release rate of indomethacin from ointment made of 1% indomethacin, 5% (A1), and 94% petrolatum base was 13.6 g/h/cm^2. Comparing the release rate to the steady-state shed snake skin fluxes (0.61 g/h/cm^2) of indomethacin, using the same ointment, obtained from the penetration studies for snake skin, we can suggest that penetration of the skin barrier is the rate-limiting step. This information further supports the hypothesis that the role of the new enhancers includes an increase in skin permeability.

X. CONCLUSION

This chapter demonstrated that the concept of biodegradability is useful in reducing the toxicity of a series of cyclic ureas and at the same time maintaining the penetration effectiveness of the enhancers. This concept has found usefulness in other enhancer development.[17–19] This biodegradable approach may be applicable to a change of the polar head group so that nontoxic starting materials can be chosen to synthesize enhancers that may have low toxicity, both local and systemic, or enhancers that have specific physical chemical properties required for a specific use.

REFERENCES

1. **Kydonieus, A. F. and Berner, B.,** Eds., *Transdermal Delivery of Drugs,* Vol. 1 to 3, CRC Press, Boca Raton, FL, 1987.
2. **Pfister, W. and Hsieh, D. S. T.,** Permeation enhancers compatible with transdermal drug delivery systems. I. Selection and formulation consideration, *Pharm. Technol.,* 14(9), 132, 1990.
3. **Pfister, W. and Hsieh, D. S. T.,** Permeation enhancers compatible with transdermal drug delivery systems. II. System design consideration, *Pharm. Technol.,* 14(10), 54, 1990.

4. **Ghosh, T. K. and Banga, A. K.,** Methods of enhancement of transdermal drug delivery. IIB. Chemical permeation enhancers, *Pharm. Technol.,* 17(5), 68, 1993.
5. **Ibuki, R.,** Use of Shed Snake Skin as Model Membrane for Percutaneous Absorption Studies: Behaviour of Several Penetration Enhancers in the System, Ph.D. thesis, University of Kansas, Lawrence, 1985.
6. **Wong, O., Tsuzuki, N., Richardson, M., Rytting, J. H., Konishi, R., and Higuchi, T.,** *Heterocycles,* 26, 3153, 1987.
7. **Higuchi, T. and Konishi, R.,** *In vitro* testing and transdermal delivery, *Ther. Res.,* 6, 280, 1987.
8. **Itoh, T., Xia, J., Magavi, R., Nishihata, T., and Rytting, J. H.,** Use of shed snake skin as model membrane for *in vitro* percutaneous penetration studies: comparison with human skin, *Pharm. Res.,* 7, 1042, 1990.
9. **Williams, A. C. and Barry, B. W.,** Snake Skin as a Model for Human Skin in Permeation Studies; Molecular Evaluation by Raman Spectroscopy, presented at the 8th Annu. Meet. Am. Assoc. Pharm. Sci., Orlando, FL, November 14 to 18, 1993.
10. **Wong, O., Huntington, J., Konishi, R., Rytting, J. H., and Higuchi, T.,** Unsaturated cyclic ureas as new non-toxic biodegradable transdermal penetration enhancers. I. Synthesis, *J. Pharm. Sci.,* 77, 967, 1988.
11. **Bodor, N.,** Soft drugs: principles and methods for the design of safe drugs, *Med. Res. Rev.,* 4, 449, 1984.
12. **Wong, O., Tsuzuki, N., Nghiem, B., Keuhnhoff, J., Itoh, T., Masaki, K., Huntington, J., Konishi, R., Rytting, J. H., and Higuchi, T.,** Unsaturated cyclic ureas as new non-toxic biodegradable transdermal penetration enhancers. II. Evaluation study, *Int. J. Pharm.,* 52, 191, 1989.
13. **Nghiem, B. T. and Higuchi, T.,** Esterase activity in snake skin, *Int. J. Pharm.,* 44, 125, 1988.
14. **Tsuzuki, N., Wong, O., and Higuchi, T.,** Effect of primary alcohols on percutaneous absorption, *Int. J. Pharm.,* 46, 19, 1988.
15. **Nghiem, B. T., Wong, O., Masaki, K., Kuehnhoff, J., Konishi, R., and Higuchi, T.,** Effects of Esterase Activity in Snake Skin on Ester Prodrugs of Acetaminophen, presented at the Japan and United States Congress of Pharmaceutical Sciences, poster number N-04-w-53, Honolulu, December 1987.
16. **Newman, M. S.,** Ed., *Steric Effects in Organic chemistry,* John Wiley & Sons, New York, 1956.
17. **Wong, O., Huntington, J., Nishihata, T., and Rytting, J. H.,** New alkyl N,N-dialkyl-substituted amino acetates as transdermal penetration enhancers, *Pharm. Res.,* 6, 286, 1989.
18. **Lambert, W. J., Kudla, R. J., Holland, J. M., and Curry, J. T.,** A biodegradable transdermal penetration enhancer based on N-(2-hydroyxethyl)-2-pyrrolidone. I. Synthesis and characterization, *Int. J. Pharm.,* 95, 181, 1993.
19. **Dolezal, P., Hrabalek, A., and Semecky, V.,** ε-Aminocaproic acid esters as transdermal penetration enhancing agents, *Pharm. Res.,* 10, 1015, 1993.

Chapter 11.1

Terpenes as Penetration Enhancers

Mitsuru Hashida and Fumiyoshi Yamashita

CONTENTS

I. INTRODUCTION

The use of penetration enhancers is one of the more promising approaches to improving skin penetration of poorly absorbed drugs.[1,2] Compounds such as sulfoxides,[3] pyrrolidones,[4] fatty acids,[5,6] and alcohols[6] have been evaluated as penetration enhancers. An ideal penetration enhancer would be pharmacologically inert, nontoxic, and nonirritating, while reversibly modifying the barrier properties of the skin. However, most experimentally established enhancers have not yet been adopted because of suspected pharmacological activities or unclarified problems in safety. By using natural products as an enhancer, some side effects may be avoided.

Terpenes are constituents of essential oils that are the volatile and fragrant substances found mainly in the flowers, fruits, and leaves of plants. The compounds have been used as flavoring, perfumes, and medicines; for example, *d*-limonene, the main component of orange or lemon oils, is approved by the U.S. Food and Drug Administration for food use and is employed in fragrances and as a flavoring agent. Recently, the terpenes were reported to show an enhancement effect on percutaneous drug absorption.[7–9] Prior to these studies on terpenes, synthetic compounds with terpene moieties had been developed as safe enhancers.[10–12] The purpose of this chapter is to discuss the enhancing activities of terpenes and their related compounds in conjunction with their modes of action.

II. TERPENES AND ESSENTIAL OILS AS PENETRATION ENHANCERS

A. CLASSIFICATION OF TERPENES

Terpenes are a series of naturally occurring compounds which consist of isoprene (C_5H_8) units. In addition to unsaturated hydrocarbons, oxygen-containing structures

0-8493-2605-2/95/$0.00+$.50

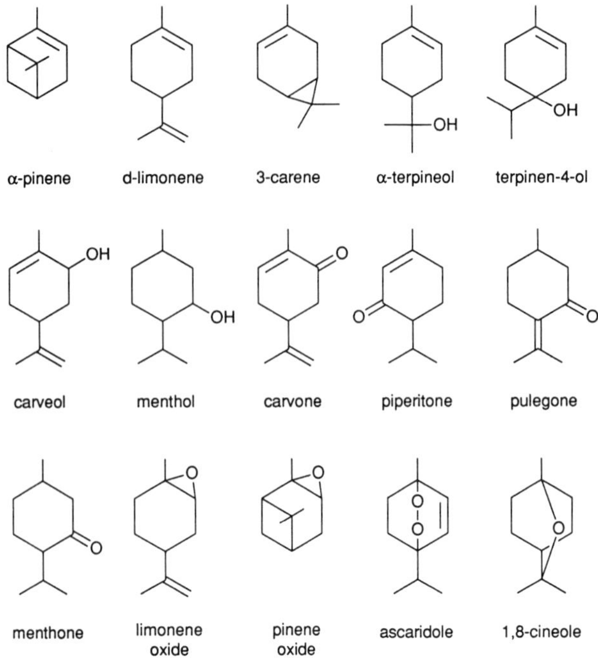

Figure 1 The structural formulas of cyclic monoterpenes tested as percutaneous penetration enhancers.

such as alcohols, ketones, and oxides have been naturally found to occur. The terpenes are classified according to the number of isoprene units; for example, monoterpenes (C_{10}), sesquiterpenes (C_{15}), and diterpenes (C_{20}). They are also subdivided into acyclic, monocyclic, bicyclic, and so forth.

The structural formulas of some cyclic monoterpenes which have been assessed as skin penetration enhancers are shown in Figure 1. A great majority of monocyclic monoterpenes have a *p*-methane carbon skeleton, including a six-membered ring. Bicyclic compounds such as α-pinene and 3-carene also exist in the group of cyclic monoterpenes. Physicochemical properties of the cyclic terpenes widely differ from one another. Fundamentally, they are highly lipophilic compounds showing high lipophilic index values[7,13] and large partition coefficients between octanol and water.[8]

B. ENHANCING ACTIVITY OF TERPENES

In recent years it has been revealed that terpenes and essential oils have an ability to enhance percutaneous drug absorption. As a first step, an enhancement activity of essential oils was reported.[14,15] The acetone extract of cardamon seeds which contains terpineol and acetyl terpineol improved the transdermal absorption of prednisolone more effectively than Azone®.[14] The oils of chenopodium, eucalyptus, anise, and ylang ylang were investigated as penetration enhancers in human skin by Williams and Barry.[15] The highest efficacies were observed for eucalyptus and chenopodium, containing primarily 1,8-cineole and ascaridole, respectively. The subsequent study revealed that the essential oils were less effective than the corresponding isolated terpenes, probably because these active constituents are not at high thermodynamic activities in the oils.[8]

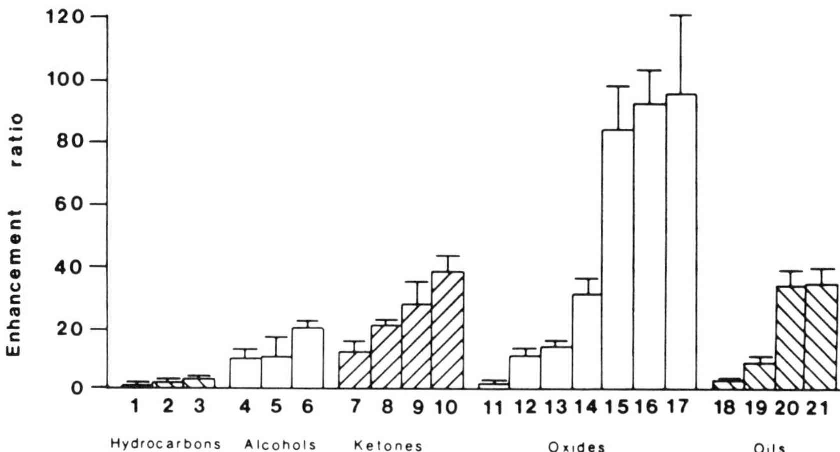

Figure 2 The penetration-enhancing activities of the terpenes expressed as enhancement ratios with S.E. The enhancement ratio (ER) is calculated as follows: ER = permeability coefficient after application of penetration enhancer/permeability coefficient before application of penetration enhancer. Key: 1, α-pinene; 2, *d*-limonene; 3, 3-carene; 4, α-terpineol; 5, terpinen-4-ol; 6, carveol; 7, carvone; 8, pulgone; 9, piperilone; 10, menthone; 11, cyclohexane oxide; 12, limonene oxide; 13, pinene oxide, 14, cyclopentene oxide; 15, ascaridole; 16, 7-oxabicyclo[2.2.1]heptane; 17, 1,8-cineole; 18, anise oil; 19, oil of ylang ylang; 20, oil of chenopodium; 21, oil of eucalyptus. (From Williams, A. C. and Barry, B. W., *Pharm. Res.*, 8, 17, 1991.)

The enhancing activities of a series of terpenes were evaluated for various drugs. Okabe et al.[7] evaluated ten cyclic monoterpenes as penetration enhancers toward lipophilic indomethacin in rats. *In vivo* absorption of indomethacin from gel ointment was remarkably enhanced by hydrocarbon terpenes such as *d*-limonene, while it was not affected by oxygen-containing terpenes. They concluded that cyclic monoterpenes with lipophilic indices of >0 were most effective for indomethacin. On the other hand, alcohol and ketone terpenes were less effective toward lipophilic drugs such as diazepam[9] and estradiol.[16] On the other hand, the enhancing activities of terpenes on hydrophilic drugs also was evaluated.[8,17] Williams and Barry[8] found that hydrocarbon terpenes show minimal activity as compared to the oxygen-containing terpenes (alcohols, ketones, epoxides, and cyclic ethers) for 5-fluorouracil (5-FU) (Figure 2). Obata et al.[17] also found that percutaneous absorption of hydrophilic diclofenac sodium was remarkably enhanced in the presence of *l*-menthol and *dl*-menthone, while it was little enhanced by *d*-limonene and *p*-menthane. Thus, the effects of monocyclic terpenes vary according to physicochemical properties of the drugs. Apparently, hydrocarbon terpenes are effective for lipophilic drugs and oxygen-containing terpenes are effective for hydrophilic drugs (Table 1).

In cyclic monoterpenes the ring conformation and side chain also seem to affect their enhancing activities.[8] Among oxide terpenes, the enhancement effects of 1,2-oxygen-bridged terpenes (epoxides) were considerably lower than those of the longer oxygen-bridged terpenes (cyclic ethers) such as 1,8-cineole (Figure 2). The six-membered ring of cyclic terpenes is essentially flat, being in the thermodynamically stable chair conformation, while the longer oxygen-bridged terpenes such as 1,8-cineole and ascaridole are in a less stable boat conformation. Thus, structural conformations might be an important factor in determining enhancing activity of terpenes.

Table 1 Penetration Enhancement Activity of Various Types of Cyclic Monoterpenes Reported in Recent Studies

Drug	No. of tested terpenes	Enhancer conc and vehicle	Animal (tested system)	Enhancement Ratio					Ref.
				Hydrocarbons	Alcohols	Ketones	Epoxides	Cyclic ethers	
5-Fluorouracil	14	Water (pretreatment)	Human *(in vitro)*	3.2 (3-carene)	20 (carveol)	38 (menthone)	14 (pinene oxide)	95 (cineole)	8
Estradiol	14	Water (pretreatment)	Human *(in vitro)*	4.4 (3-carene)	0.45 (terpinen-4-ol)	0.36 (menthone)	1.9 (pinene oxide)	4.8 (ascaridole)	16
Indomethacin	10	1% gel ointment	Rat *(in vivo)*	(210) (terpinolene)	N.D.	N.D.	—	N.D.	7
Ketoprofen	5	1% gel ointment	Rat *(in vivo)*	110 (limonene)	1.3 (menthol)	2.6 (menthone)	—	1.5 (cineole)	18
Diclofenac	5	1% gel ointment	Rat *(in vivo)*	2.6 (limonene)	5.6 (menthol)	5.1 (menthone)	—	1.3 (cineole)	17
Propranolol	6	10% *N*-methylpyrrolidone	Rat *(in vitro)*	42 (terpinene)	38 (menthol)	30 (menthone)	—	—	9
Diazepam	6	10% *N*-methylpyrrolidone	Rat *(in vitro)*	6.3 (menthane)	2.1 (menthol)	2.5 (menthone)	—	—	9

Note: Enhancement ratios to the control experiment (without enhancers) were calculated based on permeability (5-fluorouracil and estradiol), area under plasma concentration profile (AUC) within 8 h (ketoprofen and diclofenac), or amount of penetration within 24 h (propranolol and diazepam). The values showing the largest enhancement in each group are listed. For indomethacin, the value in parentheses shows AUC value within 8 h and N.D. means that drug penetration was not detected.

In fact, 7-oxabicyclo[2.2.1]heptane, which has a boat conformation, also shows a large enhancing activity for 5-FU. In contrast, it was reported that 1,8-cineole has minimal promoting activity for some drugs in rats.[7,18] The diversity may be explained by the differences in types of model drugs and/or formulations. On the other hand, a "bulky" side chain of terpenes is also relevant to their enhancing activity.[8] The hydrocarbon side chains increase the steric bulk of limonene oxide and α-pinene oxide, which are significantly better than unsubstituted cyclohexene oxide in penetration enhancement.

Lipophilicities of enhancers are considered to affect their enhancing activities because they determine the transfer to skin as well as in that of drugs. In a group of ketone or epoxide terpenes a linear relationship was observed between enhancement ratios for 5-FU permeation and logarithms of their octanol–water partition coefficients.[8] The authors concluded that the concentration of the terpenes retained in the barrier will in part determine the extent of lipid disruption and hence drug diffusivity. On the other hand, Takayama et al.[13] evaluated the enhancing activities of monoterpenes, sesquiterpenes, and diterpenes and found that the terpenes with relatively high lipophilic index values exhibited absorption promoting effects, whereas too much high lipophilicity led to the lower enhancing activities. Obata et al.[19] suggested that the difference in the promoting efficiency of terpenes arose from the difference in their thermodynamic activities in the vehicle.

Synergistic effects with ethanol were investigated by Obata et al.[20] for some terpenes. At lower concentrations of ethanol, the enhancement effects of hydrophilic terpenes such as 1,8-cineole and L-menthol were much greater than those of the lipophilic terpenes. Kobayashi et al.[21] reported that an aqueous vehicle containing L-menthol and ethanol shows a marked enhancement effect not only on water-soluble drugs, but also on lipophilic drugs. Similarly, the synergistic effect of terpenes with propylene glycol was reported by Barry and Williams.[22] It has been generally accepted that these solvents used with enhancers accumulate in the tissue and increase the partitioning of drugs due to large affinities of drugs for the solvents.[23,24]

An ideal penetration enhancer should have reversible action and show low irritation to skin. The irritancy of some cyclic monoterpenes to skin was evaluated according to the Draize scoring method.[18] All terpenes have much lower irritancy than Azone® at an equivalent concentration in gel ointment. A certain extent of recovery of the skin surface from the erythema is observed in the case of the treatment with terpenes at all concentrations. The skin irritation caused by these compounds is observed in the following order: α-terpinene ≤ *trans-p*-menthane = *d*-limonene < terpinolene ≪ Azone®. In these terpenes the enhancing activity for ketoprofen increased with increasing skin irritation. The authors concluded that *d*-limonene was a promising candidate as a penetration enhancer. It was also reported that D-limonene allowed a reversible change in the skin structure when administered with a pretreatment method.[7] In another study the reversibility of the action of terpenes was verified from the observation that drug flux in the terpene-treated membranes fell with time after the washout of the accelerants from the skin surface.[8]

C. MECHANISM OF ACTION OF TERPENES

Penetration enhancers improve drug permeation by interacting with the stratum corneum (SC), which is the most impermeable barrier in the skin. The lipid protein partitioning theory was introduced by Barry[24] to describe the modes of action of penetration enhancers. According to the theory, enhancers would act by one or more of three main mechanisms: (1) disruption of the highly ordered structure of SC lipid, (2) interaction with intracellular protein, and (3) improvement in partitioning of a drug, coenhancer, or cosolvent into the SC. For terpenes, the enhancer-protein interaction might play a relatively small role because they are highly lipophilic compounds.[8]

Diffusion coefficients and partition coefficients of 5-FU through the human skin pretreated with 17 monoterpenes were evaluated in the same report.[8] The results showed that the increase in diffusion coefficient apparently related to the penetration enhancement ratio (Figure 3), suggesting that the terpenes act, at least in part, by modifying intercellular lipids and disrupting their highly ordered structure to increase drug diffusivity. It is unclear whether the terpenes increase drug partitioning or not. The analysis of the penetration profiles suggested that the terpenes also increased partitioning of 5-FU into skin. However, the experimentally determined partition coefficients using SC membrane showed that the terpenes exert no positive effect to increase partitioning of the drug. The authors concluded that the terpenes do not increase the partitioning of hydrophilic drugs such as 5-FU because the drugs are less soluble in the terpenes than in water. They also suggested that partition phenomena might be more important in the acceleration of highly lipophilic drugs. In their subsequent study they showed that cyclic ether-type terpenes such as ascaridole increased the partitioning of highly lipophilic estradiol.[16]

Differential scanning calorimetry (DSC) study showed that cyclic terpenes decreased the transition temperatures associated with SC lipids.[25,26] The DSC result supports the speculation that the enhancers mainly increase drug diffusivity by disrupting intercellular lipids of the SC. However, shifts in the lipid phase transition temperatures following the terpene treatment did not correlate with changes in skin permeability. For example, *d*-limonene dramatically decreases the transition temperatures, while it shows little enhancement effect for 5-FU. The lack of correlation may suggest that terpenes have additional action. The electrical conductivities of human epidermis before and after the treatment with terpenes were determined.[27] The significant increases in conductivity following the treatment with terpenes suggested that the enhancers open new polar channels across the SC. It was also revealed that increases in conductivity are correlated with increases in skin permeability for 5-FU, suggesting that terpenes would create new polar pathways through which both ions and polar drugs pass. The authors concluded that the most likely site for polar pathway formation was the lipid bilayers based on the observation in DSC studies that terpenes disrupted the intercellular lipids in the SC.

III. SYNTHETIC ENHANCERS WITH TERPENE MOIETIES

A. ENHANCING ACTIVITY OF TERPENE DERIVATIVES

Compounds containing azacycloalkanone rings similar to Azone® and acyclic terpene chains were evaluated as penetration enhancers by Okamoto and co-workers[10-12] (Figure 4). The structure-activity relationship in the enhancement action of these 1-alkyl- or 1-alkenylazacycloalkanone derivatives was examined using 6-mercaptopurine as a model drug in a guinea pig skin pretreated with the enhancers.[12] With respect to tail chain length, compounds with monoterpene (C_{10}) or sesquiterpene

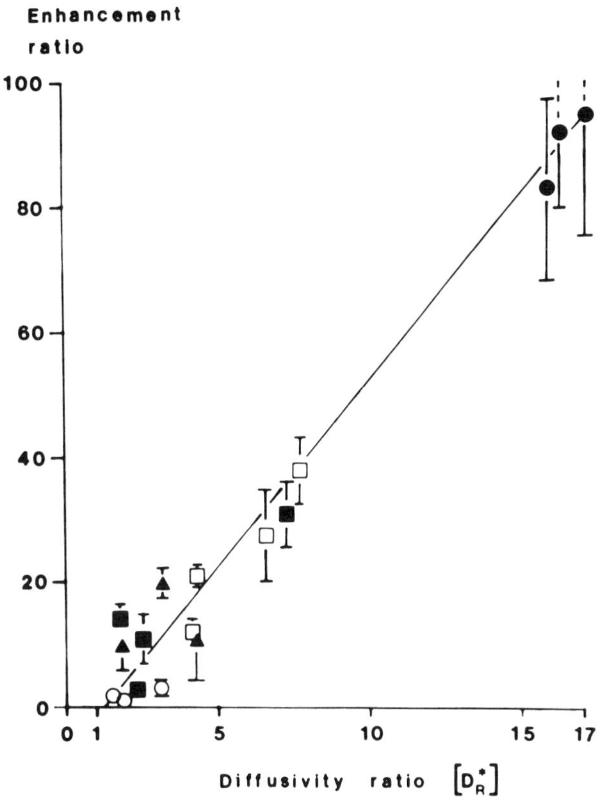

Figure 3 The relationship between the increased diffusivity of 5-FU in human epidermal membranes following terpene treatment and enhancement ratios. (•) Cyclic ethers; (□) ketones; (■) epoxides; (▲) alcohols; (○) hydrocarbons. From Williams, A. C. and Barry, B. W., *Pharm. Res.*, 8, 17, 1991.

(C_{15}) chains show greater enhancement effects than those with a longer chain (C_{20}). The saturation of the alkenyl chain has no significant effect. The size of azacycloalkanone ring from five- to seven-member ring little affects the enhancing activity, while the compound with two carbonyl groups in a polar head is less effective than the other enhancers with one carbonyl group. This study also revealed that enhancers with *trans* double bonds in the tail chain have low irritancy in spite of their high enhancing activities. Among nine tested enhancers, 1-geranylaza-cycloheptan-2-one had high enhancing activity, while it showed much lower skin irritation than Azone®. Analysis based on a one-layer diffusion model revealed that the enhancers accelerate skin permeation of the drug by increasing its partitioning into the skin.[28]

The effects of combinations of vehicle and the terpene derivatives on skin penetration of acyclovir were investigated by the same group using the excised hairless mouse and rat skin.[29] The penetration of acyclovir through hairless mouse skin from isopropanol was remarkably enhanced by 1-geranylazacycloheptan-2-one, whereas that from isopropyl myristate was not affected. Further, the effect of each enhancer on acyclovir penetration through rat skin was highly affected by the type of vehicle,

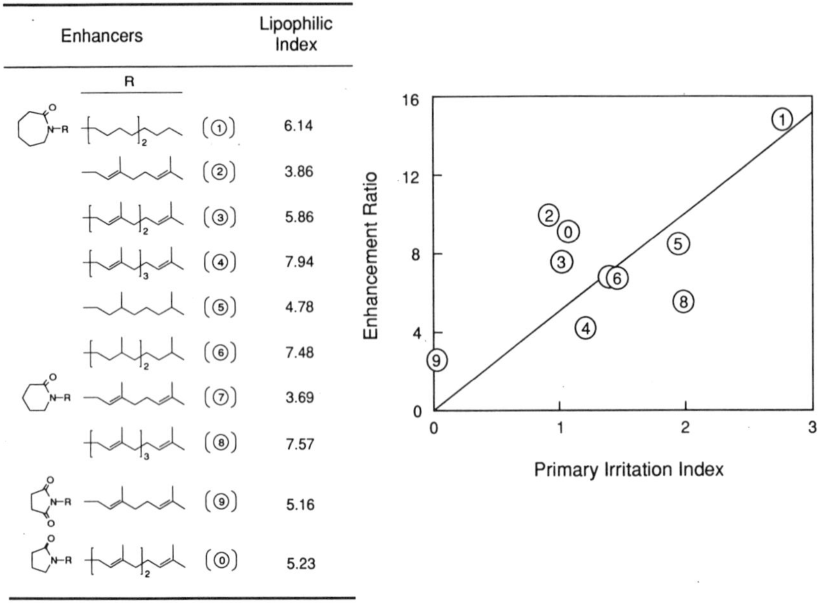

Figure 4 Relationship between enhancing ratios and primary irritation indices of 1-alkyl- or 1-alkenylazacycloalkanone derivatives. The enhancing ratios were evaluated using 6-mercaptopurine in guinea pig skin. The primary irritation indices on both erythema and edema in rabbits were averaged for 7 d. Key: 1, 1-dodecylazacycloheptan-2-one(Azone); 2, 1-geranylazacycloheptan-2-one; 3, 1-farnesylazacycloheptan-2-one; 4, 1-geranylgeranylazacycloheptan-2-one; 5, 1-(3,7-dimethyloctyl)azacycloheptan-2-one; 6, 1-(3,7,11-trimethyldodecyl)-azacycloheptan-2-one; 7, 1-geranylazacyclohexan-2-one; 8, 1-geranylgeranylazacyclohexan-2-one; 9,1-farnesylazacyclopentan-2,5-dione; 10, 1-farnesylazacyclopentan-2-one.

and it was suggested that the vehicles determined the transfer of the enhancer itself to skin. For example, isopropyl myristate prevented the lipophilic enhancers from transferring to the skin because it has similar polarity to the enhancers. Consequently, the combination of a relatively hydrophilic vehicle and a lipophilic enhancer is the most potent. It was also indicated that the great enhancing effect was caused by some synergistic actions of the enhancers and the vehicle, in addition to the increased higher escaping tendencies (thermodynamic activities) of the enhancers in the vehicle.

Okamoto et al.[30] further investigated the effect of 1-alkyl- or 1-alkenylazacycloalkanone derivatives on the penetration of drugs with different lipophilicities. Large penetration enhancement was observed for the drugs, such as 5-FU and 6-mercaptopurine with octanol–water partition coefficient of approximately unity, in both aqueous and ethanolic vehicles. In addition, the dose-dependent effect of 1-geranylazacycloheptan-2-one on seven drugs with different lipophilicities was investigated in detail.[31] In Figure 5 the enhancing effects on drug penetration and drug amounts in the skin after the *in vitro* diffusion experiment are shown as a function of drug lipophilicity when the skin was pretreated with different amounts of the enhancer. A bell-shaped relationship existed between the enhancement effect of the accelerant and drug lipophilicity (Figure 5A). On the other hand, the enhancer dose-dependently increased the amount of drug in the skin (Figure 5B).

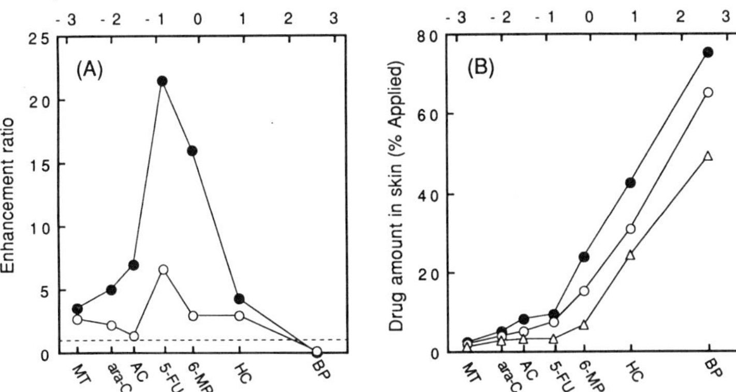

Figure 5 The relationship between drug lipophilicities and enhancement ratio (A) and drug amount in skin (B) at 24 h under pretreatment with 0 (Δ), 6.4 (○), and 25.5 (•) μmol of 1-geranylazacycloheptan-2-one. Enhancement ratios were calculated by dividing the drug amount penetrated through the enhancer-pretreated skin within 24 h by that of ethanol-pretreated control experiment. (From Yamashita, F. et al., *Biol. Pharm. Bull.*, 16, 690, 1993.)

B. MECHANISM OF ACTION OF SYNTHETIC TERPENE DERIVATIVES

The effectiveness of enhancers essentially depends on the action site of the enhancers and transport pathways of drug. Therefore, the action mechanism of enhancers should be discussed based on a comprehensive understanding of the penetration pathway of the drug. Yamashita et al.[31] constructed a two-layer skin model with polar and nonpolar routes in the SC (Figure 6), and derived the Laplace transforms for the amounts of drug penetrating through skin ($\overline{Q}$) and remaining in the vehicle ($\overline{X}$) and the skin ($\overline{M}$) in the *in vitro* diffusion experiment:

$$\overline{Q} = Z_d X_0 \left(Z_{np} \sinh d_p + Z_p \sinh d_{np} \right) / s / k(s)$$

$$\overline{X} = V_v X_0 \left(Z_p \cosh d_p \sinh d_{np} \sinh d_d + Z_{np} \sinh d_p \cosh d_{np} \sinh d_d + Z_d \sinh d_p \sinh d_{np} \cosh d_d \right) / s / k(s)$$

$$\overline{M} = \overline{M}_p + \overline{M}_{np} + \overline{M}_d$$

$$\overline{M}_p = Z_p X_0 \left[\left\{ Z_p \sinh d_p \sinh d_{np} + Z_{np} \left(\cosh d_p - 1 \right) \left(\cosh d_{np} + 1 \right) \right\} \sinh d_d + Z_d \left(\cosh d_p - 1 \right) \sinh d_{np} \cosh d_d \right] / s / k(s)$$

$$\overline{M}_{np} = Z_{np} X_0 \left[\left\{ Z_{np} \sinh d_p \sinh d_{np} + Z_p \left(\cosh d_p + 1 \right) \left(\cosh d_{np} - 1 \right) \right\} \sinh d_d + Z_d \left(\cosh d_{np} - 1 \right) \sinh d_p \cosh d_d \right] / s / k(s)$$

$$\overline{M}_d = Z_d X_0 \left(Z_{np} \sinh d_p + Z_p \sinh d_{np} \right) \left(\cosh d_d - 1 \right) / s / k(s)$$

where s is the Laplace operator with respect to time and X_0 is the initially applied dose; subscripts s, p, np, and d express the SC, the polar route, the nonpolar route, and the second viable layer, respectively, and

$$d_p = L_s\sqrt{s/D_p}$$

$$d_{np} = L_s\sqrt{s/D_{np}}$$

$$d_d = L_d\sqrt{s/D_d}$$

$$Z_p = K_p V_p / d_p$$

$$Z_{np} = K_{np} V_{np} / d_{np}$$

$$Z_d = K_d V_d / d_d$$

$$\begin{aligned}
k(s) = {} & V_v\left(Z_p \cosh d_p \sinh d_{np} \sinh d_d + Z_{np} \sinh d_p \cosh d_{np} \sinh d_d\right. \\
& \left. + Z_d \sinh d_p \sinh d_{np} \cosh d_d\right) \\
& + Z_p\left\{Z_p \sinh d_p \sinh d_{np} \sinh d_d + Z_{np} \sinh d_d\left(\cosh d_p \cosh d_{np} - 1\right)\right. \\
& \left. + Z_d \cosh d_p \sinh d_{np} \cosh d_d\right\} \\
& + Z_{np}\left\{Z_{np} \sinh d_p \sinh d_{np} \sinh d_d + Z_p \sinh d_d\left(\cosh d_p \cosh d_{np} - 1\right)\right. \\
& \left. Z_d \sinh d_p \cosh d_{np} \cosh d_d\right\}
\end{aligned}$$

where V_v is the volume of the vehicle and L_s and L_d are diffusion length of the SC and the second layer, respectively; D_i, K_i, and V_i ($i = p$, np, or d) are the diffusion coefficient, the partition coefficient, and the effective volume for diffusion. The inversion of the Laplace transforms to real time course was numerically performed by use of the fast inverse Laplace transform (FILT) algorithm.[32,33]

The curve fitting to penetration profiles of drugs through the skin pretreated with 1-geranylazacycloheptan-2-one were performed using a regression program, MULTI(FILT), combined with the FILT algorithm.[31] Analysis revealed that the enhancer mainly acts on the nonpolar route in the SC by increasing the drug partitioning into the route. The bell-shaped relationship between the effect of the enhancer and drug lipophilicities (Figure 5) can be theoretically explained by this analysis. Because the lipophilic enhancers affect the nonpolar route, their activities are considered to be retained low for highly hydrophilic drugs which predominantly penetrate the aqueous polar route. As the lipophilicity of drugs increase, the larger enhancements are obtained because they mainly pass the nonpolar route and their affinity to it increased as the enhancer affects it. However, the enhancer apparently

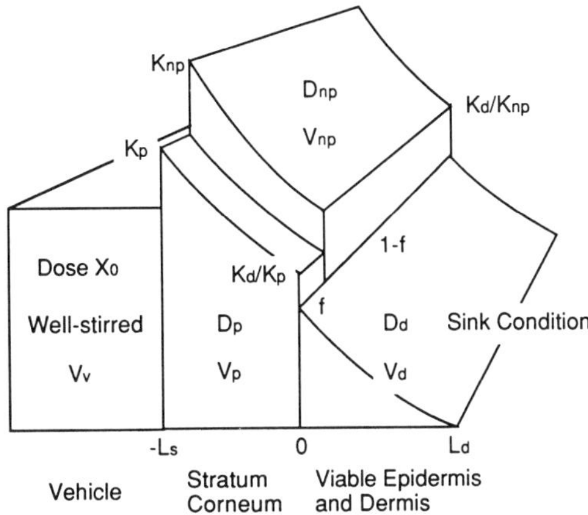

Figure 6 A two-layer skin model with polar and nonpolar routes in the SC. Well-stirred and sink conditions are assumed in the vehicle and the receptor, respectively. Key: *K*, partition coefficient; *D*, diffusion coefficient; *V*, volume; *L*, distance; *f*, area fraction; *v*, vehicle; *p*, polar domain; *np*, nonpolar domain; *d*, viable epidermis and dermis. (From Yamashita, F., et al., *Biol. Pharm. Bull.*, 16, 690, 1993.)

shows less effect for highly lipophilic drugs such as butylparaben because their penetration is mainly limited by the second aqueous viable layer regardless of a change in the solvent nature of the SC. Furthermore, the analysis based on a free-energy relationship suggested that the increase in drug partitioning into the nonpolar route resulted from increasing polarity of the SC with treatment by the enhancer. It was also suggested that the same mechanism of action stood both *in vitro* and *in vivo*.[34]

In the subsequent paper the effects of 1-geranylazacycloheptan-2-one on penetration of drugs with different lipophilicities were compared to those of D-limonene and oleic acid using guinea pig skin based on the same analysis.[35] All enhancers showed the largest enhancing effect for 6-mercaptopurine. The analysis revealed that all the enhancers affected the nonpolar route in the SC, while their mechanisms were different from one another. D-Limonene mainly increases drug diffusivity, while 1-geranylazacycloheptan-2-one predominantly enhances drug partitioning into the skin, as shown previously. On the other hand, oleic acid moderately increases both diffusion and partition parameters. Thus, the analysis based on a two-layer skin model with parallel routes in the SC clearly characterized the action site and mechanism of enhancers with terpene moieties.

IV. CONCLUSION

Terpenes and azacycloalkanone derivatives with terpene side chains are promising candidates for percutaneous penetration enhancers from the aspects of both enhancing activity and skin irritation. They show a wide variety of penetration-enhancing activities, depending on their chemical structures and their physicochemical characteristics. In addition, the enhancement effects remarkably differ for drugs with different physicochemical properties such as lipophilicity. These findings suggest that their activities are determined by a combination of drug transport pathways and enhancer action sites. Consequently, the potential and action mechanism of enhancers should be discussed based on a comprehensive understanding of the transport pathways and the mass balance of drugs in skin penetration.

REFERENCES

1. **Hadgraft, J.,** Penetration enhancers in percutaneous absorption, *Pharm. Int.,* 5, 252, 1984.
2. **Williams, A. C. and Barry, B. W.,** Skin absorption enhancers, *Crit. Rev. Ther. Drug Carrier Syst.,* 9, 305, 1992.
3. **Sekura, D. L. and Scala, J.,** The percutaneous absorption of alkyl methyl sulfoxides, *Adv. Biol. Skin,* 12, 257, 1972.
4. **Sasaki, H., Kojima, M., Nakamura, J., and Shibasaki, J.,** Enhancing effect of pyrrolidone derivatives on transdermal drug delivery. I., *Int. J. Pharm.,* 44, 15, 1988.
5. **Cooper, E. R.,** Increased skin permeability for lipophilic molecules, *J. Pharm. Sci.,* 73, 1153, 1984.
6. **Aungst, B. J., Rogers, N. J., and Shefter, E.,** Enhancement of naloxone penetration through human skin *in vitro* using fatty acids, fatty alcohols, surfactants, sulfoxides and amides, *Int. J. Pharm.,* 33, 225, 1986.
7. **Okabe, H., Takayama, K., Ogura, A., and Nagai, T.,** Effect of limonene and related compounds on the percutaneous absorption of indomethacin, *Drug Design Deliv.,* 4, 313, 1989.
8. **Williams, A. C. and Barry, B. W.,** Terpenes and the lipid-protein-partitioning theory of skin penetration enhancement, *Pharm. Res.,* 8, 17, 1991.
9. **Hori, M., Satoh, S., Maibach, H. I., and Guy, R. H.,** Enhancement of propranolol hydrochloride and diazepam skin absorption *in vitro*: effect of enhancer lipophilicity, *J. Pharm. Sci.,* 80, 32, 1991.
10. **Okamoto, H., Tsukahara, H., Hashida, M., and Sezaki, H.,** Effect of 1-alkyl- or 1-alkenylazacycloalkanone derivatives on penetration of mitomycin C through rat skin, *Chem. Pharm. Bull.,* 35, 4605, 1987.
11. **Okamoto, H., Ohyabu, M., Hashida, M., and Sezaki, H.,** Enhanced penetration of mitomycin C through hairless mouse and rat skin by enhancers with terpene moieties, *J. Pharm. Pharmacol.,* 39, 531, 1987.
12. **Okamoto, H., Hashida, M., and Sezaki, H.,** Structure-activity relationship of 1-alkyl- or 1-alkenylazacycloalkanone derivatives as percutaneous penetration enhancers, *J. Pharm. Sci.,* 77, 418, 1988.
13. **Takayama, K., Kikuchi, K., Obata, Y., Okabe, H., Machida, Y., and Nagai, T.,** Terpenes as percutaneous absorption promoters, *S.T.P. Pharm. Sci.,* 1, 83, 1991.
14. **Yamahara, J., Kashiwa, H., Kishi, K., and Fujimura, H.,** Dermal penetration enhancement by crude drugs: *in vitro* skin permeation of predonisolone enhanced by active constituents in cardamon seed, *Chem. Pharm. Bull.,* 37, 855, 1989.
15. **Williams, A. C. and Barry, B. W.,** Essential oils as novel human skin penetration enhancers, *Int. J. Pharm.,* 57, R7, 1989.
16. **Williams, A. C. and Barry, B. W.,** The enhancement index concept applied to terpene penetration enhancers for human skin and model lipophilic (oestradiol) and hydrophilic (5-fluorouracil) drugs, *Int. J. Pharm.,* 74, 157, 1991.
17. **Obata, Y., Takayama, K., Okabe, H., and Nagai, T.,** Effect of cyclic monoterpenes on percutaneous absorption in the case of a water-soluble drug (diclofenac sodium), *Drug Design Del.,* 6, 319, 1990.
18. **Okabe, H., Obata, Y., Takayama, K., and Nagai, T.,** Percutaneous absorption enhancing effect and skin irritation of monocyclic monoterpenes, *Drug Design Del.,* 6, 229, 1990.
19. **Obata, Y., Takayama, K., Maitani, Y., Machida, Y., and Nagai, T.,** Effect of pretreatment of skin with cyclic monoterpenes on permeation of diclofenac in hairless rat, *Biol. Pharm. Bull.,* 16, 312, 1993.

20. **Obata, Y., Takayama, K., Machida, Y., and Nagai, T.**, Combined effect of cyclic monoterpenes and ethanol on percutaneous absorption of diclofenac sodium, *Drug Design Del.*, 8, 137, 1991.
21. **Kobayashi, D., Matsuzawa, T., Sugibayashi, K., Morimoto, Y., Kobayashi, M., and Kimura, M.**, Feasibility of use of several cardiovascular agents in transdermal therapeutic systems with *l*-menthol-ethanol system on hairless rat and human skin, *Biol. Pharm. Bull.*, 16, 254, 1993.
22. **Barry, B. W. and Williams, A. C.**, Human skin penetration enhancement: the synergy of propylene glycol with terpenes, *Proc. Int. Symp. Control. Rel. Bioact. Mater.*, 16, 33, 1989.
23. **Barry, B. W.**, Mode of action of penetration enhancers in human skin, *J. Control. Rel.*, 6, 85, 1987.
24. **Barry, B. W.**, Lipid-protein-partitioning theory of skin penetration enhancement, *J. Control. Rel.*, 15, 237, 1991.
25. **Williams, A. C. and Barry, B. W.**, Permeation, FTIR and DSC investigations of terpene penetration enhancers in human skin, *J. Pharm. Pharmacol.*, 41(Suppl.), 12P, 1989.
26. **Williams, A. C. and Barry, B. W.**, Differential scanning calorimetry dose not predict the activity of terpene penetration enhancers in human skin, *J. Pharm. Pharmacol.*, 42(Suppl.), 156P, 1990.
27. **Cornwell, P. A. and Barry, B. W.**, The route of penetration of ions and 5-fluorouracil across human skin and the mechanisms of action of terpene skin penetration enhancers, *Int. J. Pharm.*, 94, 189, 1993.
28. **Hashida, M., Okamoto, H., and Sezaki, H.**, Analysis of drug penetration through skin considering donor concentration decrease, *J. Pharmacobio-Dyn.*, 11, 636, 1988.
29. **Okamoto, H., Muta, K., Hashida, M., and Sezaki, H.**, Percutaneous penetration of acyclovir through excised hairless mouse and rat skin: effect of vehicle and percutaneous penetration enhancer, *Pharm. Res.*, 7, 64, 1990.
30. **Okamoto, H., Hashida, M., and Sezaki, H.**, Effect of 1-alkyl- or 1-alkenylazacycloalkanone derivatives on the penetration of drugs with different lipophilicities through guinea pig skin, *J. Pharm. Sci.*, 80, 39, 1991.
31. **Yamashita, F., Yoshioka, T., Koyama, Y., Okamoto, H., Sezaki, H., and Hashida, M.**, Analysis of skin penetration enhancement based on a two-layer skin diffusion model with polar and nonpolar routes in the SC: dose-dependent effect of 1-geranylazacycloheptan-2-one on drugs with different lipophilicities, *Biol. Pharm. Bull.*, 16, 690, 1993.
32. **Hosono, T.**, Numerical inversion of Laplace transform and application to wave optics, *Radio Sci.*, 16, 1015, 1981.
33. **Yano, Y., Yamaoka, K., and Tanaka, H.**, A nonlinear least squares program, MULTI(FILT), based on fast inverse Laplace transform for microcomputers, *Chem. Pharm. Bull.*, 37, 1035, 1989.
34. **Yamashita, F., Bando, H., Koyama, Y., Kitagawa, S., Takakura, Y., and Hashida, M.**, *In vivo* and *in vitro* analysis of skin penetration enhancement based on a two-layer diffusion model with polar and nonpolar routes in the SC, *Pharm. Res.*, 11, 185, 1994.
35. **Koyama, Y., Bando, H., Yamashita, F., Takakura, Y., Sezaki, H., and Hashida, M.**, Comparative analysis of percutaneous absorption enhancement by d-limonene and oleic acid based on a skin diffusion model, *Pharm. Res.*, 11, 377, 1994.

Chapter 12.1

Liposomes as Penetration Enhancers and Controlled Release Units

Monika-Hildegard Schmid and Hans C. Korting

CONTENTS

I. INTRODUCTION

It is well known that the permeability of the skin depends on the condition of the stratum corneum (SC), which functions as the main barrier. In the last decade morphological, histochemical, and biochemical research pointed to the fact that intercellular lipids are important for permeability regulation.[1]

Different classes of epidermal lipids have been differentiated in the last few years.[2] The epidermal ceramides, a large and heterogeneous group of polar lipids, in particular, take part in the process of regulating the water content and the water loss of the epidermis. Epidermal lipids are a major component of membrane-coating granules, which may play a decisive role in maintaining the barrier function.[3,4] These granules are ovoid organelles appearing in the upper strata of living epidermis. They consist of stacks of parallel lipid disks which are extruded by keratinocytes and fuse to intercellular lamellae.

Concerning the transdermal absorption, conventional topically applied drugs have the following problem: their application on the skin surface does not necessarily mean the drug gets to the site of action to an adequate extent in all cases. For this reason penetration enhancers have been introduced for topical therapy of skin diseases. More than 200 patents on the general topic of skin penetration enhancement are reported in the pertinent literature.[5] To gain insight into the mechanism of

0-8493-2605-2/95/$0.00+$.50

enhancement of transdermal drug absorption experiments have been performed using indomethacin as the model drug in a triglyceride ointment base with different potential penetration enhancers added.[6] Those drug enhancers leading to higher drug levels in the dermis have chemical characteristics which are believed to disturb the packing of the intercellular lipid bilayers and to liquify intercellular lipid sheets.[7] Because conventional penetration enhancers often exhibit overt toxic or irritant side effects, their use in improved drug targeting must be questioned.

Recently liposomes were suggested as a special form of "penetration enhancers".[8] These lipid vesicles, which are similar to biological membranes, have been known since the early 1960s. The advantages of liposomes are that they are potentially nontoxic, degradable, and nonimmunogenic.[8] Moreover, they can store water-soluble and lipophilic substances due to their amphipathic structure. Liposomes made of skin ceramides may be more successful in penetrating the horny layer than conventional vehicles and conventional drug enhancers. Because it has been suggested that the deposition of liposomes into the SC would create a "drug reservoir", one may consider liposomes to be "localizers" rather than "transporters".

II. INTERACTION OF LIPOSOMES WITH EPIDERMAL STRUCTURE

A. MORPHOLOGICAL ASPECTS

Conflicting experimental results have been reported concerning liposomes as drug penetration enhancers. For this reason Bouwstra et al.[9] carried out several studies to investigate the interactions among three different types of liposomes and human SC using freeze-fracture electron microscopy. The liposomes, which were all unilamellar and of comparable size, differed in their hydrophilicity and charge. Depending on the liposomes' physicochemical properties changes in the intercellular lipid structure were either limited to the interface or extended to deeper parts of the SC. With the help of transmission electron microscopy further insight into the interaction between liposomes and skin could be obtained. Korting et al.[10] exposed human keratinocytes grown *in vitro* to large oligolamellar liposomes mainly made of phospholipids. They found evidence for the attachment of these particles to keratinocytes, followed by an invagination process (Figure 1). Finally, the incorporated liposomes could be found both inside and outside the lysosomes (Figure 2). Moreover, evidence exists for the disintegration of the liposomal lipids after incorporation into lysosomes.

However, the same type of liposomes applied topically to epidermis reconstructed *in vitro* was not phagocytosed.[11] Instead, a dose-dependent alteration of the morphology of both the SC and the living part of the epidermis occurred. With increased incubation periods and increased lipid concentrations higher amounts of lipid droplets could be found between corneocytes and keratinocytes. Remnants of intact liposomes or even intact liposomes were seen only rarely. Moreover, the appearance of particularly osmophilic membranes in the SC and in deeper strata of the living epidermis indicated lipid transfer.

B. FUNCTIONAL ASPECTS

Boddé et al.[12] chose another approach to gain insight into liposome–skin interaction. They monitored *in vivo* skin hydration in the presence of liposomal suspensions containing deuterium oxide and compared it to a preparation with free deuterium

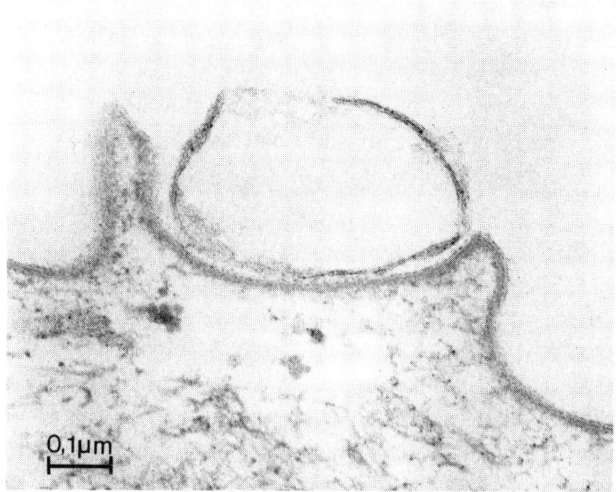

Figure 1 Attachment of a liposome to a keratinocyte, which begins the process of engulfment. (From Korting, H. C., Schmid, M. H., Hartinger, A., Maierhofer, G., Stolz, W., and Braun-Falco, O., *J. Microencapsulation,* 10, 223, 1993. With permission.)

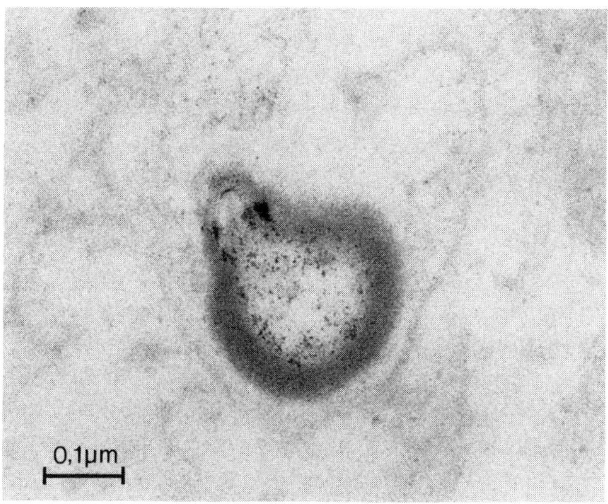

Figure 2 Liposomes within the cytoplasm of a keratinocyte close to the cytoplasmic membrane surrounded by a lysosomal membrane at high magnification. (From Korting, H. C., Schmid, M. H., Hartinger, A., Maierhofer, G., Stolz, W., and Braun-Falco, O., *J. Microencapsulation,* 10, 223, 1993. With permission.)

oxide using infrared spectroscopy in conjunction with tape stripping.[12] The main results were that the liposomal form increased the "driving-rate" of deuterium oxide into the SC but decreased the accumulated amount of hydrogen oxide. These phenomena may be explained by the penetration of phospholipids from the liposomal preparation into the SC, thus leading to a higher permeability due to an increased disorder of the genuine skin lipids.

Röding et al.[13] focused on another aspect concerning the interaction between liposomes and epidermal structures, by investigating the influence of the chemical composition of liposomes on the humidity of normal skin both after single application and over the long term. The results clearly demonstrated the superiority of liposomes with a high content in zwitterionic and lipophilic phosphatidylcholine over those with negative charge and hydrophilic phospholipids. The maximum in skin humidity was reached after about one 1 week's treatment followed by a steady state. Accordingly, liposomes containing adequate amounts of the suitable phospholipids might be capable not only of transporting water into the epidermis, but also to other chemical entities.

From ultrastructural and biochemical analyses it may be concluded that the incorporation of liposomal phospholipids into a topical leads to a reformation of intercellular lipid structures, resulting in an increased fluidity.[14] Drug penetration *sensu strictus* may take place in the short time period during the interaction between liposomal lipids and epidermal lipids.

C. KINETIC ASPECTS CONCERNING CARRIER COMPONENTS

Kreuter et al.[15] performed experiments using radioactive-labeled cholesterol- or sitosterol-containing liposomes and two-chamber side-by-side diffusion cells separated by artificial silicone membranes. The measurement of the radioactivity in the receiver chamber was necessary for the determination of the permeability coefficients. The results showed a reduced permeability coefficient of sitosterol as compared to cholesterol, suggesting the involvement of an interfacial barrier in the liposomal delivery of cholesterol and sitosterol. Free diffusion of the sterols through the water phase to the membrane was not indicated.

Other evidence for the value of liposomes as a drug carrier system for topical application was forwarded by Artmann et al.[16] For their experiments they used five liposome dispersions of differing concentrations labeled with tritium. These liposome dispersions were applied topically to a defined area of shorn dorsal piglet skin for 30, 60, and 180 min. For radioactive measurements 20 skin strips were taken from each treated area. They found that the content of radioactive phospholipids of the SC increased with time, which was not the case after increasing the applied concentration. This means that the amount of liposomes penetrating the skin per time unit is already reached at the concentration of 1.0 mg phospholipid per square centimeter. Moreover, the experimental results suggest that the concentration jump among SC, epidermis, and subcutaneous fat is significant 3 h after one-time application of the liposomal dispersion.

These findings are in accordance with the results of Egbaria et al.,[17] who examined the extent of drug accumulation in the various skin strata after topical application of liposomal or conventional formulations containing a water-soluble marker in excised animal skin using the stripping technique. Summing up the results the following trends are reported:

1. The ratio of liposomal lipids to water-soluble marker was not altered in the various skin layers, indicating the ability of liposomes to carry water-soluble molecules even into the deeper skin strata.
2. The ratio of the radiolabeled liposomal lipids was maintained throughout the skin strata, suggesting a mixing up of the liposomal and SC lipids (Figure 3).

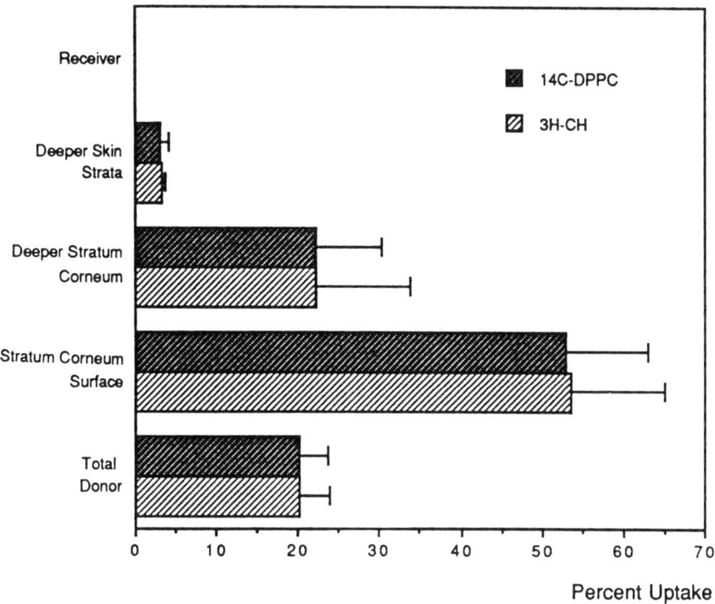

Figure 3 The 24-h *in vitro* distribution of ^{3}H-CH and ^{14}C-DPPC (dipalmitoylphosphatidylcholine) from MLVs multi lamellar vesicles in various skin strata of the hairless mouse. (From Egbaria, K. and Weiner, N., in *Liposome Dermatics,* Springer-Verlag, Heidelberg, 1992, 179. With permission.)

3. The uptake of cyclosporine was greater after topical application of the liposome formulation than after the application of a conventional emulsion with similar lipid composition.[18]

D. KINETIC ASPECTS CONCERNING ACTIVE INGREDIENTS

Concerning the pharmacokinetics of liposomally entrapped drugs, investigations for the absorption and disposition of encapsulated active ingredients were performed by Mezei et al.[19] They designed animal experiments with guinea pigs and compared the effectiveness of drug delivery after the application of radiolabeled liposomal and conventional formulations to defined hairless areas of the animals. Different active ingredients such as triamcinolone acetonide (TRMA), econazole, minoxidil, tetracaine, and vitamin A acid were tested. Concerning the topical glucocorticoids the following results were important: the liposomal form delivered 4.5 times more TRMA to the epidermis and 3 times less TRMA to the thalamic region as compared to the ointment form, suggesting that the percutaneous absorption, and therefore the systemic effects, of the glucocorticoids are reduced with the liposomal method of application. Lieb et al.[20] performed experiments using the hamster ear as a model for sebaceous glands to investigate the delivery of carboxyfluorescin (CF) via the follicular route. For this reason quantitative measurements were performed with two different fluorescent techniques. The ears were treated for 24 h with various test formulations, each containing the same amount of CF. In summary, the topical application of liposomal formulation resulted in a significantly higher accumulation of CF in the pilosebaceous glands as compared to all other nonliposomal preparations. These results may indicate

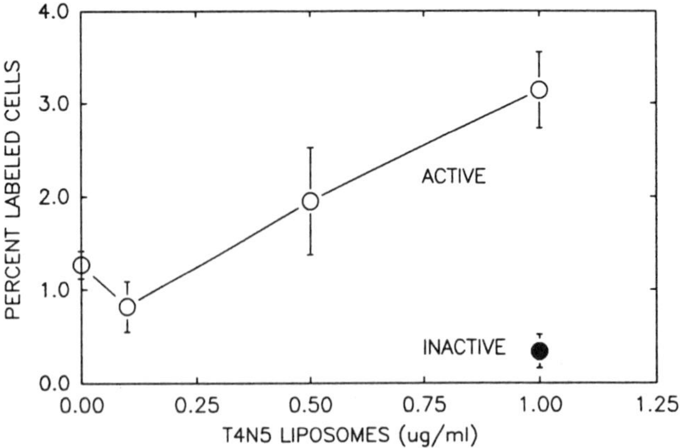

Figure 4 Skin cancer in UV-irradiated mice treated with T4N5 liposomes. (From Yarosh, D. B., in *Liposome Dermatics,* Springer-Verlag, Heidelberg, 1992, 266. With permission.)

the possibility of an increased effect in the treatment of follicular diseases with the liposomal method of application.

Other pharmacokinetic investigations were performed by Yarosh et al.[21] Knowing that the epidermal DNA plays an important role in the solar ultraviolet (UV) damage of skin they designed experiments with DNA-repair enzymes encapsulated in liposomes (T4N5 liposomes) for the topical treatment of sun exposure in human or mice skin. Penetration of the repair enzymes into the epidermis was observed after staining skin sections with antibodies to these enzymes. The enzyme-containing liposomes were localized in the skin even after 24 h, and <0.1% of the original dose was found systemically.

E. DYNAMIC ASPECTS ACCORDING TO ANIMAL EXPERIMENTS

Yarosh et al.[22] also performed experiments concerning the repair of UV damage in the skin of humans and mice as described above to focus on several dynamic aspects. The use of T4N5 liposomes in mice enhanced the removal of UV-DNA photoproducts from epidermal DNA in a dose-dependent manner, reaching a plateau at about 0.5 μg/ml (Figure 4). The same dose response relationship was found for human skin. The development of skin cancer in UVB-irradiated mice, however, was delayed with the topical application of T4N5 liposomes after each UV exposure. Thus, one may conclude that liposomally applied DNA-repair enzymes at least protect the skin from this chronic effect of sun exposure.

Meybeck et al.[23] reported that liposomally encapsulated retinoic acid is very effective in reducing the size of comedones in hairless rhino mice. Indeed, the liposomal vitamin A acid formulation was able to reduce the comedones at a dose five to ten times smaller than conventional preparations of vitamin A acid. Moreover, the percutaneous penetration of retinoic acid is two times less with liposomes than with an alcoholic gel formulation. Thus, the following conclusions can be drawn: the reduced effective dose combined with the reduced percutaneous penetration rate of active ingredients may lead to an attenuation of long- and short-term side effects. In other words, the benefit:risk ratio may be increased.

III. MAIN FIELDS FOR CLINICAL APPLICATION IN DERMATOLOGY

A. GLUCOCORTICOSTEROIDS

In a clinical trial the effect of liposomally encapsulated betamethasone dipropionate (BDP; 0.039%) was compared to that of 0.064% conventional BDP gel, including a penetration enhancer.[24] Korting et al. tested both preparations in a double-blind, randomized, paired trial lasting 14 d in 20 patients suffering from atopic eczema or psoriasis vulgaris. Despite the lower content of active ingredient the liposomal preparation reduced erythema and scaling in eczema to a higher extent than the conventional preparation. Yet the opposite was true for psoriasis vulgaris. There, the commercial BDP formulation proved more efficacious. These results indicate that liposomal formulations may also affect the pharmacodynamics of topical glucocorticoids. Possibly, the anti-inflammatory activity in atopic eczema is increased, while this is not the case with the antiproliferative activity essential to psoriasis vulgaris. Although it is well known that patients with atopic eczema suffer from a defect of the permeability barrier, this is controversial for psoriasis vulgaris.[25,26] Hence, the alteration of the permeability barrier function in eczema may explain the increase of glucocorticoid activity. This would lead to the conclusion that liposome encapsulation probably increases the benefit to risk ratio for this type of inflammatory skin disease.

B. HAMAMELIS DISTILLATE

The superiority of liposomal preparations for clinical use was demonstrated for another active ingredient. Korting et al.[27] focused on the anti-inflammatory activity of Hamamelis distillate in a liposomal formulation as compared to that of a conventional oil-in-water emulsion. To a conventional oil-in-water emulsion the "preliposome system" Phosal® and Hamamelis distillate were added (concentration of active ingredients: 5.35%). This liposomal formulation was compared to other nonliposomal formulations, such as a verum preparation with a higher drug concentration and a corresponding oil-in-water-emulsion without Phosal®. It was found that the use of a "preliposome system" can enhance the activity of Hamamelis distillate. Moreover, liposomally encapsulated Hamamelis distillate can be defined as a "true active", which does not apply to the oil-in-water cream formulation in clinical use previously.

C. TRETINOIN

Because it is well known that the main problem in treating acne vulgaris with conventional topical tretinoin preparations is the poor patient compliance due to skin irritancy or flare-up reactions, Frosch[28] focused on an improved topical application. In a clinical trial recently performed by Schäfer-Korting and co-workers 20 patients with uncomplicated acne vulgaris were treated daily with liposomal tretinoin (0.01%) on one side of the body and with a commercial gel preparation with either 0.025 or 0.05% tretinoin on the other side.[29] In this double-blind study comedones, papules, and pustules were counted and skin irritancy reactions were rated for 10 weeks. The results indicated that a less concentrated liposomal tretinoin formulation has an efficacy equal to their higher concentrated conventional counterparts available so far. What also matters is that due to less adverse effects the acceptance of the topical treatment was improved.

IV. OTHER FIELDS OF APPLICATION

With respect to the topical treatment of psoriasis vulgaris, investigations on anthralin were performed by Gehring et al.[30] They compared the quality of the dithranol erythema after application of two different liposomal dithranol gels to the quality after application of dithranol vaseline in healthy skin. The marked increase of the dithranol erythema using both liposomal formulations led to the assumption that the liposomal gel can promote drug penetration. This, indeed, may be especially interesting in the forms of psoriasis vulgaris with possibly increased epidermal barrier function, e.g., psoriasis inversa.[30]

Due to the limited penetration rate and the short residence time, most of the commercially available local anesthetic products show poor effectiveness.[31] For this reason the development of liposomal formulations containing local anesthetics has looked promising. Gesztes and Mezei[32] evaluated the anesthetic effects of tetracaine and lidocaine either in conventional formulations or in liposomal forms. Pontocaine® cream, which contains 1% tetracaine, and a half-concentrated liposomal tetracaine "cream" were tested on the arms of healthy volunteers. Using the pinprick method, the superiority of the liposomal form could be demonstrated, which was also true for the corresponding experiments with lidocaine. This effect may be in part due to the capability of the liposomes to act as slow release vehicles within the skin. However, an improvement of activity by liposomally encapsulated active ingredients cannot be found in all cases. For example, in the skin pigmentation product kaempferol no improvement of activity occurred after liposomal encapsulation.[33] Hence, it seems necessary to determine the *in vivo* efficacy of liposome cosmetics in a case-by-case comparison to conventional formulations.

V. SCALING-UP AND MASS PRODUCTION

It was not until 1984 that Cilag, a Swiss company, focused on the development and large-scale production of a galenically improved liposome dermatic.[34] The antifungal drug econazole was suggested as a suitable candidate for liposomal encapsulation due to its solubility in ethanol and in ethanol–lecithin mixtures which are commonly used for liposome preparation by the ethanol injection method. For scaling-up, the ethanol injection method, first described by Batzri and Korn[35] in 1973, was changed in some regard. Moreover, the problems concerning the stability of liposomal econazole could finally be solved. Today, the liposomal econazole drug can fulfill the pharmaceutical quality requirements in terms of liposome size, encapsulation efficiency, and stability. It has been approved by several drug registration authorities in Europe and is marketed under the brand name Pevaryl®-Lipogel.

Recently, preliposome systems were introduced for the production of loaded liposomes. In contrast to the usual way of liposome preparation, starting with phospholipids and the active ingredient using various preparation methods, the preliposome systems Natipide®-II and Phosal 75 SA® offer new possibilities for commercial liposome production based on phospholipid concentrates.[36,37] The advantages of Natipide®-II are the constant liposome quality (no changes during the loading process) and the simple handling. Phosal 75 SA® consists of a liquid phospholipid solution (natural phosphatidylcholine in vegetable oil) in which lipophilic active ingredients can be dissolved easily after the addition of water. Thus, both preliposome systems offered to the pharmaceutical industry by RPR-Nattermann-Phospholipid (Cologne, Germany) can be used for the easy manufacture of liposomal systems without the usual difficulties in technical processing.

VI. OUTLOOK

Summing up the facts mentioned above, liposomes for topical application of active ingredients show promise and warrant further studies. Concerning the advantages and disadvantages of these vesicles, the following holds true: the safety and the possibilities of influencing drug disposition are advantageous, while the relatively high production costs and the difficulties in long-term stability are the main disadvantages. However, they may be overcome by improvements in technology in the near future. Generally speaking, at least the following groups of active compounds can be considered candidates for liposomal topical application:

1. Drugs such as cyclosporins, which are known to have an effect after systemic application, but disappoint after topical application in conventional dosage forms.[38]
2. Drugs such as hamamelis distillate, which currently show no or insufficient effects after topical application.[27]
3. Drugs such as topical glucocorticoids (betamethasone dipropionate), which may show an improved benefit:risk ratio when applied in a liposomal formulation as compared to conventional preparations (e.g., creams and ointments).[24]

However, much basic research must be performed to obtain complete insight into the field of liposomes. Moreover, clinical trials in patients suffering from various skin diseases are important in defining the practical use of topical liposomal drugs in external dermatotherapy in comparison to corresponding conventional formulations. Considering the experimental results reported above, it already seems obvious that liposomes are far more than penetration enhancers in the conventional sense; rather they act as controlled release units.

REFERENCES

1. **Elias, P. M.,** Lipids and the epidermal permeability barrier, *Arch. Dermatol. Res.,* 270, 95, 1981.
2. **Kerscher, M., Korting, H. C., and Schäfer-Korting, M.,** Skin ceramides: structure and function, *Eur. J. Dermatol.,* 1, 39, 1991.
3. **Schmid, M. H. and Korting, H. C.,** Liposomes for atopic dry skin: the rationale for a promising approach, *Clin. Invest.,* 71, 5, 1993.
4. **Fartasch, M., Bassuhas, I. D., and Diepgen, T. C.,** Structural relationship between epidermal lipid lamellae, lamellar bodies and desmosomes in human epidermis: an ultrastructural study, *Br. J. Dermatol.,* 128, 221, 1993.
5. **Santus, G. C. and Baker, R. W.,** Transdermal enhancer patent literature, *J. Control. Rel.,* 25, 1, 1993.
6. **Blasius, S.,** Sorptionsvermittler: Einfluss auf die Liberation von Indometacin aus Salben und auf die Arzneistoffaufnahme durch exzidierte Haut, Thesis, Universität des Saarlandes, Saarbrücken, 1985, 1.
7. **Loth, H.,** Skin permeability, *Methods Find. Exp. Clin. Pharmacol.,* 11, 155, 1989.
8. **Egbaria, K. and Weiner, N.,** Topical application of liposomal preparations, *Cosmet. Toilet.,* 136, 79, 1991.
9. **Bouwstra, J. A., Hofland, H. E. J., Spies, F., Gooris, G. S., and Junginger, H. E.,** Changes in the structure of human SC induced by liposomes, in *Liposome Dermatics,* Braun-Falco, O., Korting, H. C., and Maibach, H. I., Eds., Springer-Verlag, Heidelberg, 1992, 122.

10. **Korting, H. C., Schmid, M. H., Hartinger, A., Maierhofer, G., Stolz, W., and Braun-Falco, O.,** Evidence for the phagocytosis of intact oligolamellar liposomes by human keratinocytes *in vitro* and consecutive intracellular disintegration, *J. Microencapsulation,* 10, 223, 1993.
11. **Korting, H. C., Stolz, W., Schmid, M. H., and Maierhofer, G.,** Interaction of liposomes with human epidermis reconstructed *in vitro, Br. J. Dermatol.,* 1995.
12. **Boddé, H. E., Pechtold, L. A. R. M., Subnel, M. T. A., and de Haan, F. H. N.,** Monitoring *in vivo* skin hydration by liposomes using infrared spectroscopy in conjunction with tape stripping, in *Liposome Dermatics,* Braun-Falco, O., Korting, H. C., and Maibach, H. I., Eds., Springer-Verlag, Heidelberg, 1992, 137.
13. **Röding, J. and Ghyczy, M.,** Control of skin humidity with liposomes: stabilization of skin care oils and lipophilic active substances with liposomes, *Seifen, Oele, Fette, Wachse,* 10, 372, 1991.
14. **Juninger, H. E., Hofland, H. E., and Bouwstra, J. A.,** Liposomes and niosomes: interaction with human skin, *Cosmet. Toilet.,* 106, 45, 1991.
15. **Kreuter, J., Higuchi, W. I., Ganesan, M. G., and Weiner, N. D.,** Delivery of liposome membrane-associated sterols through silastic membranes, *Biochim. Biophys. Acta,* 676, 181, 1981.
16. **Artmann, C., Röding, J., and Ghyczy, M.,** Liposomes from soya phospholipids as percutaneous drug carriers. 2nd Communication. Qualitative *in vivo* investigations by macromolecules and salt loaded liposomes with radioactive labeling, *Drug Res.,* 40(II), 12, 1965.
17. **Egbaria, K. and Weiner, N.,** Topical delivery of liposomally encapsulated ingredients evaluated by *in vitro* diffusion studies, in *Liposome Dermatics,* Braun-Falco, O., Korting, H. C., and Maibach, H. I., Eds., Springer-Verlag, Heidelberg, 1992, 172.
18. **Egbaria, K., Ramachandran, C., and Weiner, N.,** Topical delivery of cyclosporin: evaluation of various formulations using in-vitro diffusion studies in hairless mouse skin, *Skin Pharmacol.,* 3, 21, 1990.
19. **Mezei, M. and Gulasekharam, V.,** Liposomes — a selective drug delivery system for the topical route of administration: lotion dosage form, *Life Sci.,* 26, 1473, 1980.
20. **Lieb, L. M., Ramachandran, C., and Weiner, N.,** Liposomally encapsulated active ingredients penetrate through the follicle, in *Liposome Dermatics,* Braun-Falco, O., Korting, H. C., and Maibach, H. I., Eds., Springer-Verlag, Heidelberg, 1992, 200.
21. **Yarosh, D. B., Tsimis, J., and Yee, V.,** Enhancement of DNA repair of UV damage in mouse and human skin by liposomes containing a DNA repair enzyme, *J. Soc. Cosmet. Chem.,* 41, 856, 1990.
22. **Yarosh, D. B., Kibitel, J., Green, L., and Spinowitz, A.,** Enhanced unscheduled DNA synthesis in UV-irradiated human skin explants treated with T4N5 liposomes, *J. Invest. Dermatol.,* 97, 147, 1990.
23. **Meybeck, A., Bonte, F., and Redzinak, G.,** Improvement of Comedolytic Activity and Tolerance of Vitamin A Acid in Topical Liposome Formulation, presented at 5th Int. Conf. Pharmaceutical Technology, Paris, May 30 to June 1, 1989, 399.
24. **Korting, H. C., Zienicke, H., Schäfer-Korting, M., and Braun-Falco, O.,** Liposome encapsulation improves efficacy of betamethasone dipropionate in atopic eczema but not in psoriasis vulgaris, *Eur. J. Clin. Pharmacol.,* 29, 349, 1991.
25. **Wester, R. C., Bucks, D. A. W., and Maibach, H. I.,** *In vivo* percutaneous absorption of hydrocortisone in psoriatic patients and normal volunteers, *J. Am. Acad. Dermatol.,* 8, 646, 1983.
26. **Wester, R., Mobayen, M., Ryatt, K., Bucks, D., and Maibach, H. I.,** *In vivo* percutaneous absorption of dithranol in psoriatic and normal volunteers, in *Psoriasis,* Farber, E., Ed., Elsevier, Amsterdam, 1987, 429.
27. **Korting, H. C., Schäfer-Korting, M., Hart, A., Laux, P., and Schmid, M.,** Antiinflammatory activity of hamamelis distillate applied topically to the skin. Influence of vehicle and dose, *Eur. J. Clin. Pharmacol.,* 44, 315, 1993.
28. **Frosch, P. J.,** Irritative und kontaktallergische Nebenwirkungen von Akne-Externa, *Hautarzt (Suppl.),* 36, 179, 1985.
29. **Schäfer-Korting, M., Korting, H. C., and Ponce-Pöschl, E.,** Liposomal tretinoin for uncomplicated acne vulgaris, *CCinvestig.,* 72, 1086, 1994.
30. **Gehring, W., Ghyczy, M., Gloor, M., Scheer, T., and Röding, J.,** Enhancement of the penetration of dithranol on the skin by liposomes, *Drug Res.,* 42, 983, 1992.
31. **Dalili, H. and Adrian, J.,** The efficacy of local anesthetics in blocking the sensation of itch, burning and pain in normal and sunburned skin, *Clin. Pharmacol. Ther.,* 12, 913, 1971.

32. **Gesztes, A. and Mezei, M.,** Topical anesthesia of the liposome-encapsulated tetracaine, *Anesth. Analg.,* 67, 1079, 1988.
33. **Meybeck, A., Bonte, F., and Dumas, M.,** Use of Kaempferol and Certain Derivatives Thereof for the Preparation of a Cosmetic or Pharmaceutical Composition, FR Patent, No. 88.15770, 1 December 1988.
34. **Kriftner, R. W.,** Liposome production: the ethanol injection technique and the development of the first approved liposome dermatic, in *Liposome Dermatics,* Braun-Falco, O., Korting, H. C., and Maibach, H. I., Eds., Springer-Verlag, Heidelberg, 1992, 91.
35. **Batzri, S. and Korn, E. D.,** Single bilayer liposomes prepared without sonication, *Biochim. Biophys. Acta,* 298, 1015, 1973.
36. **Röding, J.,** Natipide®-II: A new easy liposome system, *Seifen, Oele, Fette, Wachse,* 14, 509, 1990.
37. **Röding, J.,** Stabilität, physialische Eigenschaften und Charakterisierung von Liposomen in flüssigen und halbfesten Zubereitungen, *Parfüm. Kosmet.,* 2, 80, 1990.
38. **Hermann, R. C., Taylor, R. S., Ellis, C. N., Williams, M. A., Weiner, N. D., Flinn, G. L., Annesly, T. M., and Voorhees, J. J.,** Topical cyclosporine for psoriasis, *Skin Pharmacol.,* 1, 246, 1988.

Chapter 13.1

Effect of Cyclodextrins on Percutaneous Transport of Drugs

Thorsteinn Loftsson and Nicholas Bodor

CONTENTS

I. INTRODUCTION

Cyclodextrins are natural products formed by the action of bacterial enzymes on starch. They were first isolated over 100 years ago by Villiers from a culture medium of *Bacillus amylobacter,*[1] and Schardinger discovered their cyclic structure and laid the foundations of the cyclodextrin chemistry.[2,3] Much of the old literature refers to cyclodextrins as Schardinger's dextrins. In the beginning only small amounts of cyclodextrins could be produced in the laboratory and high production costs prevented their industrial usage. Recent biotechnological advancements have resulted in dramatic improvements in the cyclodextrin production which has lowered their production costs.[4] Cyclodextrins now have multiple uses in the pharmaceutical, food, cosmetic, agrochemical, and toiletry industries.

A. CYCLODEXTRIN STRUCTURE

The three major, industrially produced cyclodextrins are α-cyclodextrin (or cyclohexaamylose), β-cyclodextrin (or cycloheptaamylose), and γ-cyclodextrin (or cyclooctaamylose), consisting of six, seven, or eight α-1,4 linked glucopyranose units, respectively (Figure 1). All the nonbonding electron pairs of the glucosyl-O-bridges are directed to the center of the molecule, resulting in a torus shape and a somewhat lipophilic central cavity with a high electron density. The size of the cavity is determined by the number of glucopyranose units forming the cyclodextrin molecule. The primary hydroxyl groups are located on the narrow side while the secondary hydroxyl groups are located on the wider side. In an effort to improve the biological and/or physiochemical properties of the parent cyclodextrins numerous cyclodextrin derivatives have been synthesized. Thus, methyl and ethyl derivatives are formed by alkylation of the hydroxyl groups, hydroxypropyl and hydroxyethyl derivatives by hydroxyalkylation, and glucosyl and maltosyl derivatives (i.e., branched

0-8493-2605-2/95/$0.00+$.50

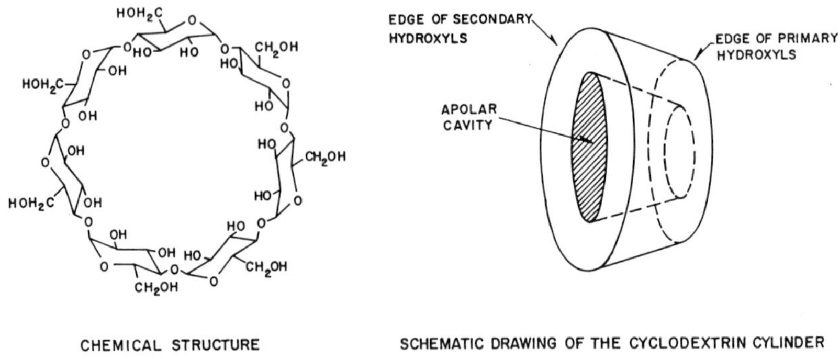

Figure 1 The chemical structure of β-cyclodextrin and the torus shape of the cyclodextrin cylinder.

cyclodextrins) by substituting the primary hydroxyl groups with saccharides.[5,6] Various ionizable cyclodextrin derivatives have also been synthesized.[5–7] Over 50 cyclodextrin derivatives are now commercially available. The effects of only a few of these cyclodextrins and cyclodextrin derivatives on dermal and transdermal delivery of drugs have been investigated: β-cyclodextrin (βCD), 2-hydroxypropyl-β-cyclodextrin (HPβCD), diethyl-β-cyclodextrin (DEβCD), triethyl-β-cyclodextrin (TEβCD), dimethyl-β-cyclodextrin (DMβCD), carboxymethylethyl-β-cyclodextrin (CMEβCD), and γ-cyclodextrin (γCD) (see Table 1).

B. PHYSICOCHEMICAL PROPERTIES OF CYCLODEXTRINS

Cyclodextrins are capable of forming inclusion complexes with many molecules by taking up a whole molecule or some part of it into the central cavity.[5–7,19,26,27] No covalent bonds are formed or broken during complex formation, and in aqueous solutions the free guest molecules are in rapid equilibrium, with guest molecules bound within the cavity of the cyclodextrin host molecules. The polarity of the βCD cavity has been estimated to be similar to that of ethanol,[28] and the high electron density inside the cavity gives it some Lewis-base character. However, the main driving force for the complex formation is thought to be the release of enthalpy-rich water from the cavity. The water molecules inside the cavity cannot satisfy their hydrogen bonding abilities in the same way as those in the bulk of the solution, and therefore they are of higher enthalpy.[5,29] The energy of the system is lowered when these enthalpy-rich water molecules in the cavity are replaced by suitable hydrophobic guest molecules. Relatively weak van der Waals forces, hydrogen bonds, and hydrophobic interactions keep the complex together. The size and chemical structure of the guest molecules are also of importance. Only relatively hydrophobic molecules of appropriate size are able to enter the cyclodextrin cavity. Too-large or too-polar molecules will not form inclusion complexes. However, it is often sufficient for complex formation that some hydrophobic part of a large molecule fits into the cavity.[26,30] The size of the cyclodextrin cavity is also important. For example, the α-cyclodextrin (αCD) cavity is too small for naphthalene, and only the γCD cavity can accommodate anthracene.[5] β-Cyclodextrin is the most useful for complexation of

Table 1 Investigations of the Effect of Cyclodextrins on the Release of Drugs from Topical Vehicles and Their Percutaneous Transport

Cyclodextrin	Drug
β-Cyclodextrin	Betamethasone[8]
	4-Biphenylylacetic acid[9]
	Butylparaben[10]
	Ethyl 4-biphenylyl acetate[11]
	Indomethacin[10]
	Nitroglycerin[12,13]
	Prednisolone[14]
	Prostaglandin E_1[15–18]
	Sulfanilic acid[10]
β-Cyclodextrin-epichlorohydrin polymer	Nitroglycerin[13]
Hydroxypropyl-β-cyclodextrin	4-Biphenylylacetic acid[9]
	17β-Estradiol[19,20]
	Ethyl 4-biphenylyl acetate[11]
	Hydrocortisone[20,21]
	Itraconazole[22]
	Prostaglandin E_1[16]
	Testosterone[20]
Dimethyl-β-cyclodextrin	4-Biphenylylacetic acid[9]
	Butylparaben[10]
	Ethyl 4-biphenylyl acetate[11]
	Hydrocortisone[20]
	Indomethacin[10]
	Loteprednol etabonate[23]
	Nitroglycerin[12]
	Prostaglandin E_1[16]
	Sulfanilic acid[10]
Carboxymethylethyl-β-cyclodextrin	Prostaglandin E_1[15–18]
Diethyl-β-cyclodextrin	Indomethacin[24]
	Nitroglycerin[12]
	Prostaglandin E_1[16]
Triethyl-β-cyclodextrin	Prostaglandin E_1[16]
γ-Cyclodextrin	Betamethasone[8]
	Beclomethasone dipropionate[25]
	Prednisolone[14]

average size molecules such as most drugs. Unfortunately, βCD is poorly water soluble (only 1.85 g/100 ml) as compared to α- and γCD (14.5 and 23.3 g/100 ml, respectively), but many βCD derivatives (e.g., HPβCD, DMβCD, and CMEβCD) have excellent solubility in water.

II. CYCLODEXTRINS AS PERMEABILITY ENHANCERS

The cyclodextrin molecules are relatively large (molecular weight of about 1000 to over 2000), with a hydrated outer surface, and under normal conditions, cyclodextrin molecules will only permeate biological membranes with some difficulty. For example, numerous *in vitro* and *in vivo* experiments demonstrated that only insignificant amounts of orally administered cyclodextrins are absorbed unmetabolized from the intestinal tract.[5] Cyclodextrins, e.g., DMβCD, are poorly absorbed transdermally,[31] and pretreatment of the skin with cyclodextrins does not enhance dermal drug absorption.[11] However, under certain conditions, such as coadministration of a lipophilic penetration enhancer and usage of occlusive dressing, cyclodextrins are able to penetrate into the skin and affect its barrier.[9,11,18] Hydrophobic cyclodextrin derivatives, such as DMβCD, are able to modify the skin barrier by extraction of components such as cholesterol and triglycerides from the skin.[10] In most cases, however, the effects of cyclodextrins on the skin and its barrier have only a minor influence on drug transport into and through the skin. It is believed that cyclodextrins act as true carriers by keeping the hydrophobic drug molecules in solution and delivering them to the skin surface where they partition into the skin barrier.[5,20] The skin has a much lower affinity for the large hydrophilic cyclodextrin molecules and therefore they will remain in the aqueous vehicle system.

A. PERMEATION THROUGH SEMIPERMEABLE MEMBRANES

The dermal and transdermal availability of drugs in dermatological preparations depends on several factors such as the release of the drug from the vehicle system, partition of the drug into the skin barrier, and permeation of the drug molecules through the barrier into the viable layers of the skin. One way of studying the effects of vehicle components on the release of drugs from vehicle systems is to measure the flux of a drug from vehicles of different composition through semipermeable cellophane membranes. Figure 2 shows the effect of HPβCD on the flux of hydrocortisone. Cellophane membrane was placed in a Franz diffusion cell and aqueous vehicle containing 1% hydrocortisone and 0 to 15% HPβCD in the donor chamber of the cell.[21] At low HPβCD concentrations, when hydrocortisone was in suspension, the flux of hydrocortisone through the membrane increased with increasing HPβCD concentration. After all hydrocortisone dissolved (at about 5% HPβCD) further addition of HPβCD decreased the hydrocortisone flux through the membrane. At low concentrations increasing amounts of HPβCD in the aqueous vehicle increase the amount of dissolved hydrocortisone. Because the rate of hydrocortisone release from the hydrocortisone-HPβCD complex is much faster than the rate of dissolution, this consequently leads to larger flux through the membrane. When all hydrocortisone is in solution, an increasing amount of HPβCD results in a decreasing amount of free hydrocortisone in the solution, and because the hydrocortisone-HPβCD complex permeates much slower through the membrane than the free drug molecules, this leads to a smaller flux. Similar results were obtained when the flux of hydrocortisone was measured through a semipermeable cellophane membrane from an oil-in-water cream containing 0 to 10% HPβCD (Table 2). Initially, when the HPβCD concentration is increased the flux increases, reaching maximum when just enough HPβCD is added to dissolve all hydrocortisone (at 5% HPβCD), but then the flux levels off and even decreases upon further addition of HPβCD.

Both the free drug and the complex permeated through the membrane, but the complex permeated at a much slower rate. The total flux of hydrocortisone through the membrane (I_t) is the sum of the flux of the free drug (I_D) and the flux of the drug-cyclodextrin complex ($I_{D\cdot CD}$):[20]

$$I_t = I_D f_D + I_{D\cdot CD}\left(1 - f_D\right)$$

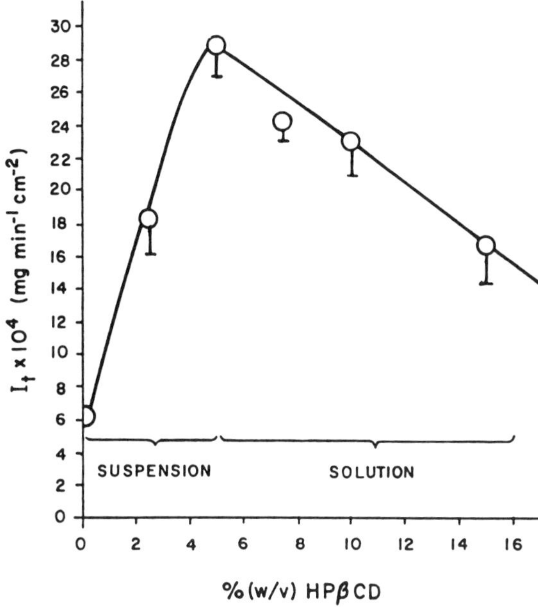

Figure 2 The relationship between the HPβCD concentration and the total flux *(I_t)* of hydrocortisone through a semipermeable cellophane membrane. Each experiment was repeated four times and the error bars represent the standard deviation.[21]

Table 2 The Effect of HPβCD on the Flux of Hydrocortisone from an Oil-In-Water Cream Containing 1% Hydrocortisone Through Semipermeable Cellophane Membrane[21]

HPβCD conc (% w/v)	Flux (μg/h/cm^{-2})
0.0	70.8
2.5	99.6
5.0	143
7.5	123
10	127

where f_D is the fraction of free drug and $(1–f_D)$ is the fraction of the drug in the complex. The value of f_D can be calculated from the stability constant of the hydrocortisone-HPβCD complex. For hydrocortisone the values of I_D and $I_{D \cdot CD}$ were determined to be 9.0×10^{-7} and 7.2×10^{-8} mol/cm^2/h, respectively.[20] In aqueous solution the radius of the hydrated hydrocortisone-HPβCD complex is much larger than the radius of the free hydrophobic hydrocortisone molecule. Larger radius gives a smaller diffusion coefficient and, hence, slower diffusion of the complex through the membrane. This supports the previously mentioned notion that under normal conditions only the free drug molecules and not the drug-cyclodextrin complexes permeate the skin barrier.

Table 3 Effect of HPβCD Concentration on Permeability of Drugs in Aqueous Suspensions Through Hairless Mouse Skin *In Vitro*[20]

Drug	HPβCD conc (% w/v)	Solubility[a] (mg/ml)	Flux ± SE × 10^{3b} (μg h/cm^{-2})
17β-Estradiol	20	10.7	172 ± 5
	25	14.3	330 ± 29
	40	30.1	207 ± 9
	50	40.5	60 ± 3
Hydrocortisone	20	23.7	174 ± 19
	40	47.1	94 ± 4
Testosterone	20	17.0	505 ± 41
	40	19.9	619 ± 10
	60	30.9	501 ± 9

[a] Solubility of hydrocortisone in the HPβCD vehicle.
[b] SE: standard error of the mean.

B. PERMEATION THROUGH SKIN

It is obvious from the permeability studies that simple introduction of cyclodextrins to a vehicle through semipermeable membranes will not automatically lead to greater drug permeability through the skin barrier. The drug:cyclodextrin ratio will always be important. In this sense cyclodextrins are different from other skin penetration enhancers. Table 3 shows the effect of HPβCD on the transdermal delivery of drugs from aqueous suspensions through hairless mouse skin.[20] Initially, as the HPβCD concentration increases more drug is available to the skin (i.e., the drug solubility in the vehicle increases) and the flux of the drug through the skin becomes larger. At higher HPβCD concentrations the flux decreases. This decrease could be partly due to increased viscosity of the aqueous vehicle. Aqueous solutions containing over 30 to 40% (w/v) HPβCD are very viscous, and the viscosity will slow down both the dissolution of the solid drug in the vehicle and the diffusion of the drug molecules and their HPβCD complexes to the skin surface. As for semipermeable membranes it is important to use just enough HPβCD to keep all the drug in the vehicle, or almost all of it in solution. In fact, maximum flux from an aqueous HPβCD vehicle containing 1% hydrocortisone, through excised hairless mouse skin, was obtained when the HPβCD concentration was kept low so that only 97% of the drug was in solution (Table 4).

2-Hydroxypropyl-β-cyclodextrin is a very hydrophilic βCD derivative which, under normal conditions, does not penetrate into the skin and does not irritate tissues.[11] Thus, this cyclodextrin derivative may be particularly useful as a penetration enhancer for dermal and transdermal delivery of drugs, but other cyclodextrin derivatives can also be used (see Table 1). For example, it has been shown that DMβCD and CMEβCD are equally or even more effective penetration enhancers than is HPβCD.[7,11,20]

As discussed previously, cyclodextrins act as penetration enhancers by making drug molecules more available to the skin surface. By combining cyclodextrins and penetration enhancers, which act directly on the skin barrier, such as some lipophilic enhancers, it is possible to obtain greater enhancement than if either enhancer is used alone. Uekama et al.[17,18] demonstrated that combined usage of a cyclodextrin such as CMEβCD and a lipophilic penetration enhancer such as HPE-101 (1-[2-(decylthio)-

Table 4 Effect Of HPβCD on the Flux of Hydrocortisone from Aqueous HPβCD Solution Containing 1% (w/v) Hydrocortisone Through Hairless Mouse Skin[21]

Vehicle composition	Solubility[a] (mg/ml)	Flux ± SE × 10^3[b] (μg/h/cm^{-2})
6% (w/v) aqueous HPβCD solution containing 1% (w/v) hydrocortisone in suspension	9.7	139 ± 54
8% (w/v) aqueous HPβCD solution containing 1% (w/v) hydrocortisone in solution	10.0	75 ± 27

[a] Solubility of hydrocortisone in the HPβCD vehicle.
[b] SE: standard error of the mean.

ethyl]aza-cyclopentane-2-one) or Azone® in topical vehicles enhances the transdermal delivery of prostaglandin E_1 in a synergistic manner.

III. CONCLUSIONS

Cyclodextrin molecules are relatively large, with a hydrated outer surface and, under normal conditions they are unable to penetrate the skin barrier. In aqueous vehicles cyclodextrins act as penetration enhancers by solubilizing lipophilic water-insoluble drugs and constantly supplying dissolved drug molecules to the skin surface, where they partition into the skin barrier. Optimum penetration enhancement is obtained when just enough cyclodextrin is used to solubilize all or almost all the drug in the vehicle. It is possible to enhance dermal and transdermal delivery of drugs even further by adding lipophilic penetration enhancers, which act directly on the skin barrier, to the cyclodextrin-containing vehicles.

REFERENCES

1. **Villiers, A.,** Sur la fermentation de la fécule par l'action du ferment butyrique, *C. R. Acad. Sci.*, 112, 536, 1891.
2. **Schardinger, F.,** Azetongärung, *Wien Klin. Wochenschr.*, 17, 207, 1904.
3. **Schardinger, F.,** Bildung kristallisierter Polysaccharide (Dextrine) aus Stärke kleister durch Mikrobien, *Zentralbl. Bakteriol. Parasitenkd. Infektionskr. Hyg. II*, 29, 188, 1911.
4. **Sicard, P. J. and Saniez, M.-H.,** Biosynthesis of cycloglycosyltransferase and obtention of its enzymatic reaction products, in *Cyclodextrins and Their Industrial Uses*, Duchêne, D., Ed., Editions de Santé, Paris, 1987, chap. 2.
5. **Szejtli, J.,** *Cyclodextrin Technology*, Kluwer Academic Publishers, Dordrecht, Netherlands, 1988, chap. 1 to 3.
6. **Szejtli, J.,** Cyclodextrins in drug formulations. I. *Pharm. Tech. Int.*, 3(2), 15, 1991.
7. **Uekama, K., Hirayama, F., and Irie, T.,** Modifications of drug release by cyclodextrin derivatives, in *New Trends in Cyclodextrins and Derivatives*, Duchêne, D., Ed., Editions de Santé, Paris, 1991, chap. 12.
8. **Otagiri, M., Fujinaga, T., Sakai, A., and Uekama, K.,** Effects of β- and γ-cyclodextrins on release of betamethasone from ointment bases, *Chem. Pharm. Bull.*, 32, 2401, 1984.
9. **Arima, H., Adachi, H., Irie, T., and Uekama, K.,** Improved drug delivery through the skin by hydrophilic β-cyclodextrins. Enhancement of anti-inflammatory effect of 4-biphenylylacetic acid in rats, *Drug Invest.*, 2, 155, 1990.
10. **Okamoto, H., Komatsu, H., Hashida, M., and Sezaki, H.,** Effects of β-cyclodextrin and di-O-methyl-β-cyclodextrin on the percutaneous absorption of butylparaben, indomethacin and sulfanilic acid, *Int. J. Pharm.*, 30, 35, 1986.

11. **Arima, H., Adachi, H., Irie, T., Uekama, K., and Pitha, J.,** Enhancement of the antiinflammatory effect of ethyl 4-biphenylyl acetate in ointment by β-cyclodextrin derivatives: increased absorption and localized activation of the prodrug in rats, *Pharm. Res.,* 7, 1152, 1990.
12. **Umemura, M., Ueda, H., Tomono, K., and Nagai, T.,** Effect of diethyl-β-cyclodextrin on the release of nitroglycerin from formulations, *Drug Design Deliv.,* 6, 297, 1990.
13. **Tomono, K., Gotoh, H., Okamura, M., Horioka, M., Ueda, H., and Nagai, T.,** Effect of β-cyclodextrins on sustained release of nitroglycerin from ointment bases, *Yakuzaigaku,* 51, 22, 1991.
14. **Uekama, K., Arimori, K., Sakai, A., Masaki, K., Irie, T., and Otagiri, M.,** Improvement in percutaneous absorption of prednisolone by β- and γ-cyclodextrin complexation, *Chem. Pharm. Bull.,* 35, 2910, 1987.
15. **Adachi, H., Irie, T., Uekama, K., Manako, T., Yano, T., and Saita, M.,** Inhibitory effect of prostaglandin E_1 on laureate-induced peripheral vascular occlusive sequelae in rabbits: optimized topical formulation with β-cyclodextrin derivative and penetration enhancer HPE-101, *J. Pharm. Pharmacol.,* 44, 1033, 1992.
16. **Adachi, H., Irie, T., Hirayama, F., and Uekama, K.,** Stabilization of prostaglandin E_1 in fatty alcohol propylene glycol ointment by acidic cyclodextrin derivative, O-carboxymethyl-O-ethyl-β-cyclodextrin, *Chem. Pharm. Bull.,* 40, 1586, 1992.
17. **Uekama, K., Adachi, H., Irie, T., Yano, T., Saita, M., and Noda, K.,** Improved transdermal delivery of prostaglandin E_1 through hairless mouse skin: combined use of carboxymethyl-ethyl-b-cyclodextrin and penetration enhancers, *J. Pharm. Pharmacol.,* 44, 119, 1992.
18. **Adachi, H., Irie, T., Uekama, K., Manako, T., Yano, T., and Saita, M.,** Combination effects of O-carboxymethyl-O-ethyl-β-cyclodextrin and penetration enhancer HPE-101 on transdermal delivery of prostaglandin E_1 in hairless mice, *Eur. J. Pharm. Sci.,* 1, 117, 1993.
19. **Loftsson, T. and Bodor, N.,** Effects of 2-hydroxypropyl-β-cyclodextrin on the aqueous solubility of drugs and transdermal delivery of 17β-estradiol, *Acta Pharm. Nord.,* 1, 185, 1989.
20. **Loftsson, T., Ólafsdóttir, B. J., and Bodor, N.,** The effects of cyclodextrins on transdermal delivery of drugs, *Eur. J. Pharm. Biopharm.,* 37, 30, 1991.
21. **Loftsson, T., Fridriksdóttir, H., Ingvarsdóttir, G., Jónsdóttir, B., and Sigurdardóttir, A. M.,** The influence of 2-hydroxypropyl-β-cyclodextrin on diffusion rates and transdermal delivery of hydrocortisone, *Drug Dev. Ind. Pharm.,* 20, 1699, 1994.
22. **Van Cutsem, J.,** Oral, topical and parenteral antifungal treatment with itraconazole in normal and in immunocompromised animals, *Mycoses,* 32(Suppl. 1), 14, 1989.
23. **Bodor, N., Loftsson, T., and Wu, W.,** Metabolism, distribution, and transdermal permeation of a soft corticosteroid, loteprednol etabonate, *Pharm. Res.,* 9, 1275, 1992.
24. **Kawahara, K., Ueda, H., Tomono, K., and Nagai, T.,** Effect of diethyl-β-cyclodextrin on the release and absorption behaviour of indomethacin from ointment bases, *S. T. P. Pharm. Sci.,* 2, 506, 1992.
25. **Uekama, K., Otagiri, M., Sakai, A., Irie, T., Matsuo, N., and Matsuoka, Y.,** Improvement in the percutaneous absorption of beclomethasone dipropionate by γ-cyclodextrin complexation, *J. Pharm. Pharmacol.,* 37, 532, 1985.
26. **Szejtli, J.,** Cyclodextrins in drug formulations. II., *Pharm. Tech. Int.,* 3(3), 16, 1991.
27. **Loftsson, T., Brewster, M. E., Derendorf, H., and Bodor, N.,** 2-Hydroxypropyl-β-cyclodextrin: properties and usage in pharmaceutical formulations, *Pharm. Ztg. Wiss.,* 4/136, 5, 1991.
28. **Heredia, A., Requena, G., and García Sánchez, F.,** An approach for the estimation of the polarity of the β-cyclodextrin cavity, *J. Chem. Soc., Chem. Commun.,* 24, 1814, 1985.
29. **Bergeron, R. J.,** Cycloamylose-substrate binding, in *Inclusion Compounds,* Vol. 3, Attwood, J. L., Davies, J. E. D., and MacNicol, D. D., Eds., Academic Press, London, 1984, chap. 12.
30. **Brewster, M. E., Simpkins, J. W., Hora, M. S., Stern, W. C., and Bodor, N.,** Use of cyclodextrins in protein formulations, *J. Parenteral. Sci. Tech.,* 43, 231, 1989.
31. **Gerlóczy, A., Antal, S., and Szejtli, J.,** Percutaneous absorption of heptakis-(2,6-di-O-^{14}C-methyl)-β-cyclodextrin in rats, in *Proc. 4th Int. Symp. Cyclodextrins,* Huber, O. and Szejtli, J., Eds., Kluwer Academic Publishers, Dordrecht, Netherlands, 1988, 415.

Chapter 14.1

Triple Therapy: Multiple Dosing Enhances Hydrocortisone Percutaneous Absorption *In Vivo* in Humans

Ronald C. Wester, Joseph Melendres, Fred Logan, and Howard I. Maibach

CONTENTS

I. INTRODUCTION

On a historic and empiric basis, topical applications of hydrocortisone and other corticosteroids frequently use repeated, rather than single, bolus applications of drug to the skin. It is commonly assumed that multiple applications of hydrocortisone effectively increase its bioavailability and absorption. A long-term, multidose rhesus monkey study by Wester et al.[1] indicated that this was true. However, short-term experiments in the rhesus monkey by Wester et al.[2] and long-term pharmacokinetic assays by Bucks et al.[3] did not show an increase in hydrocortisone absorption following multiple dosing. An investigation was designed to determine if multiple dose therapy (dosing the same site three times in the same day) would increase drug bioavailability in human skin. The study was done *in vivo* using male volunteers (from whom informed consent had been obtained) and *in vitro* with human skin. Hydrocortisone was in either a solvent (acetone) vehicle or in a cream base vehicle.

II. METHODS

A. *IN VIVO*

In each procedure in this crossover study the subjects were healthy male volunteers, 25 to 85 years old, from whom informed consent had been obtained. The treatments were performed on two adjacent sites on each forearm. Each site received a different treatment; each was performed 2 to 3 weeks apart, alternating forearms between the treatments to allow for systemic and dermal clearance of residual hydrocortisone and radioactivity.

0-8493-2605-2/95/$0.00+$.50

[4-^{14}C]-Hydrocortisone purchased from Research Products International (Mount Prospect, IL) was administered in three vehicle formulations produced by dissolving a predetermined amount of unlabeled crystalline hydrocortisone (Sigma Chemicals, St. Louis, MO) in vehicle and mixing with an appropriate amount of ^{14}C-labeled material. Test material, 20 µl, was applied per application to 2.5 cm^2 of ventral forearm skin and protected by a modified nonocclusive, complete 25-mm polypropylene chamber (Hilltop Research, Inc., Miamiville, OH).[4] The chamber adhered to the skin by application of an adhesive dressing (Tegaderm, 3M Medical Surgical Division, St. Paul, MN) to the periphery of the complete chamber. The test material was washed off the treated area with soap and water after a 24-h dosing period. Urine was collected and measured every 24 h for 7 d, and duplicate 5-ml aliquots were collected and combined with 10 ml of liquid scintillation cocktail (Universol ES, ICN Biomedical, Costa Mesa, CA). ^{14}C content was measured using a liquid scintillation counter (Packard 4640, Arlington Heights, IL). The percentage of the dose secreted was calculated from the amount recovered in the urine. The urinary excretion data were corrected for radiolabeled hydrocortisone clearance through other routes by inclusion of intravenous data (mean = 76.55%) from previously reported rhesus monkey experiments. This was accomplished by dividing the average percentage of the applied dose recovered in the subjects' urine by the average percentage of the applied dose recovered in urine from rhesus monkeys following intravenous administration of radiolabeled hydrocortisone.[5,6] Percentage excretion was based upon the total amount of hydrocortisone applied during the first 24 h, specifically, the percentage of the single dose applied or the percentage from the cumulative total of the multiple doses applied, wherever appropriate. All data were calculated to percentage absorption and mass of hydrocortisone absorbed based on penetration through a 2.5-cm^2 area.

B. *IN VITRO*

Three separate human donor skin sources with replicates for each experiment were used. Small cells were of the flow-through design with 1-cm^2 surface area. Buffered saline at a rate of 1.25 ml/h (1 reservoir volume) served as a receptor fluid. Human cadaver skin was dermatomed to 500 µm and stored refrigerated at 4°C in Eagle's minimum essential medium. The skin was used within 5 d. This preservation/use regimen follows that used by the human skin transplant bank.

Radiolabeled hydrocortisone in either acetone or cream base vehicle was applied to the skin per the study design.

At the end of a 24-h period, the system was stopped. The residual fluid in the cells was collected and analyzed. The skin surface was washed once with liquid soap (soap:water, 1:1 v/v) (Ivory Liquid, Procter and Gamble, Cincinnati, OH) and rinsed with distilled water, using cotton balls. Cells were disassembled. The skin itself was completely solubilized in Soluene 350 (Packard Instruments, Downers Grove, IL) and 80% acetic acid was added to neutralize the homogenate. The receptor phase samples from the permeation cells and the skin itself were assayed for radioactivity by liquid scintillation counting.

C. STUDY DESIGN

The study was specifically designed to compare a single low dose (13.33 µg/cm^2) to a single, larger dose (40.0 µg/cm^2; three times the amount) and to three multiple-application therapy (13.33 µg/cm^2 × 3 = 40.0 µg/cm^2) treatments. Student two-tailed, paired *t*-tests were employed to compare the percentage of the applied dose absorbed and observed mass absorbed per square centimeter between each of the treatments.

Treatment 1 — One bolus application of 1.0 μCi/13.33 μg/cm² on the right arm, 3 in. from the antecubital fossa. The dose was exposed to the skin for 24 h, followed with removal by washing, and the chamber was replaced with a new one.

Treatment 2 — One bolus application of 1.0 μCi/40.0 μg/cm² on the left arm, 3 in. from the antecubital fossa. The dose was exposed to the skin for 24 h, followed with removal by washing, and the chamber was replaced with a new one.

Treatment 3 — Three repeat applications of 0.33 μCi/13.33 μg/cm² on the left ventral forearm, 1 in. from the antecubital fossa. One dose was applied, followed by identical doses 5 and 12 h after the initial dose. The site was washed and the chamber replaced with a new one 24 h after the initial dose was applied.

Hydrocortisone Dosing Sequence

Treatment	Dose per application (μg/cm²)	Cumulative dose (μg/cm²)	Total vehicle volume (μl)	
			Acetone	Cream
1[a]	13.33	13.33	20	100
2[b]	40.00	40.00	20	100
3[c]	13.33	40.00	60	100

[a] Single dose of 13.33 μg/cm², administered in 20 μl of vehicle.
[b] Single dose of 40.0 μg/cm², administered in 20 μl of vehicle.
[c] Three serial 13.33 μg/cm² doses, each administered in 20 μl of vehicle (total 60 μl).

III. RESULTS

Table 1 gives the predicted and observed hydrocortisone *in vivo* percutaneous absorption in acetone or cream vehicles dosed at 13.3 μg/cm² × 1 (single low dose), 40.0 μg/cm² × 1 (single high dose and an amount three times that of the low dose), and 13.3 μg/cm² × 3 (multiple dose, which is three times the single low dose and equal in total amount to the 40 μg/cm² in the single high dose). The predicted amounts are multiples (three times) of that of the observed single dose value.

With acetone vehicle 0.056 ± 0.073 μg/cm² hydrocortisone was absorbed for the low dose. The single high dose absorption was 0.140 ± 0.136 μg/cm², a value near its predicted linear amount of 0.168. The multiple dose absorption should have been the same predicted 0.168; however, the absorption was 0.372 ± 0.304 μg/cm², a value statistically ($p < 0.05$) greater than that of the single high dose (Figure 1).

With the cream vehicle, the same pattern emerged. The single high dose absorbed (0.91 ± 1.66 μg/cm²) was three times that of the low dose absorbed (0.31 ± 0.43 μg/cm²). The multiple dose absorbed (1.74 ± 0.93 μg/cm²) exceeded the predicted amount and was statistically ($p < 0.006$) greater than that of the single high dose (Figure 2).

Different volunteers were used in the acetone and in the cream studies; therefore absolute amounts absorbed cannot be directly compared. Note that individual variation is a large variant in percutaneous absorption, and is mostly responsible for the large standard deviations in the data. This is why statistical analyses were done on a paired basis. This is illustrated in Table 2, which lists the individual hydrocortisone values. Distinction can be made for "low absorbers" and "high absorbers", and this remains fairly true through the various dosing intervals.

Table 1 Predicted and Observed Hydrocortisone Absorption: *In Vivo*

Vehicle	Dosing sequence	Hydrocortisone absorbed (μg/cm²) Predicted	Observed
Acetone[a]	13.3 μg/cm² × 1	—	0.056 ± 0.073
	40.0 μg/cm² × 1	0.168[b]	0.140 ± 0.136[c]
	13.3 μg/cm² × 3	0.168	0.372 ± 0.304[c]
Cream[d]	13.3 μg/cm² × 1	—	0.31 ± 0.43
	40.0 μg/cm² × 1	0.93[b]	0.91 ± 1.66[e]
	13.3 μg/cm² × 3	0.93	1.74 ± 0.93[e]

Note: Different volunteers were used for each formulation; therefore, comparison of absolute bioavailability across vehicle is not justified.

[a] $n = 6$; mean ± S.D.

[b] 0.168 μg/cm² is 3× the measured value of 0.056 μg/cm²; 0.93 μg/cm² is 3× the measured value of 0.31 μg/cm².

[c] Statistically different ($p < 0.05$) paired *t*-test.

[d] $n = 5$; mean ± S.D.

[e] Statistically different ($p < 0.006$) paired *t*-test.

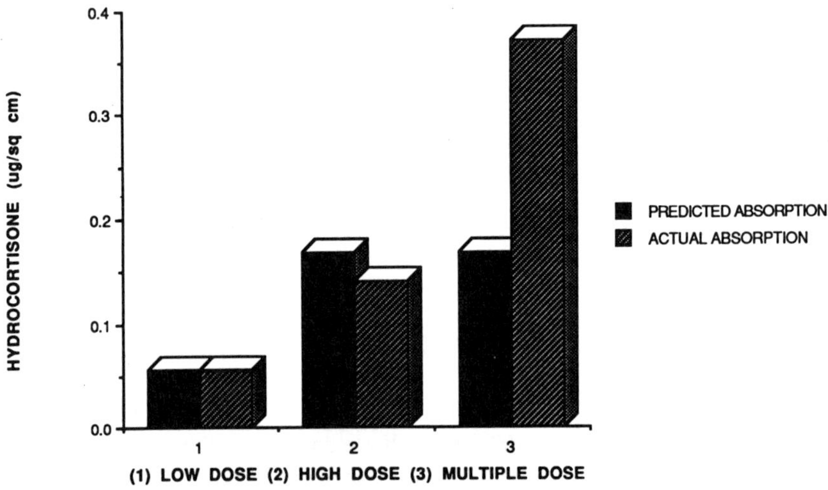

Figure 1 Hydrocortisone *in vivo* percutaneous absorption in humans with acetone vehicle and single and multiple dosing. The multiple dosing (triple therapy) exceeded predicted absorption and was statistically ($p < 0.05$) greater than the single high dose.

Table 3 and Figures 3 and 4 give the data for predicted and observed *in vitro* hydrocortisone percutaneous absorption. The receptor fluid accumulations (absorbed amounts) show the same trend as that seen *in vivo*. *In vitro* studies also allowed the human skin to be assayed for hydrocortisone content following the 24-h dosing interval. The skin content values markedly reflect those seen with the receptor fluid values. Only three observations were made per dosing sequence, so statistically no differences exist. The same human skin sources were used for both acetone and

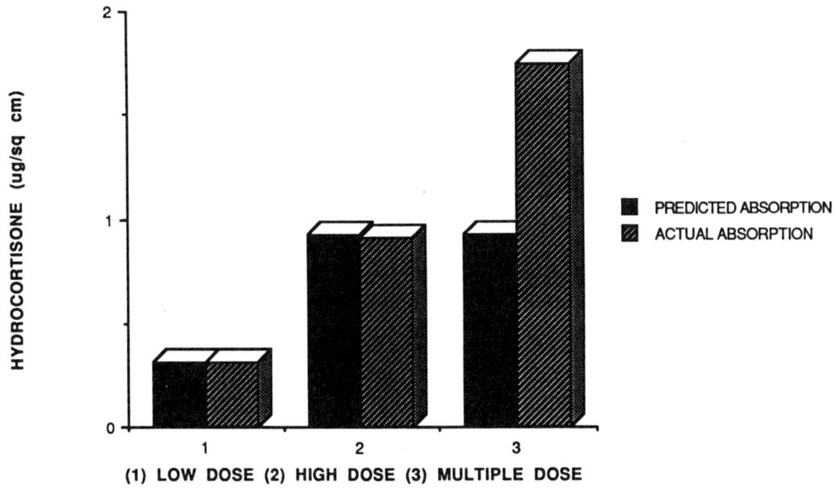

Figure 2 Hydrocortisone *in vivo* percutaneous absorption in humans with cream vehicle and single and multiple dosing. The multiple dosing (triple therapy) exceeded predicted absorption and was statistically ($p < 0.006$) greater than the single high dose.

Table 2 Individual Variation in Hydrocortisone Percutaneous Absorption

	Hydrocortisone absorption (μg/cm²)		
	Treatment		
Volunteer	**13.3 μg/cm² × 1**[a]	**40.0 μg/cm² × 1**[a]	**13.3 μg/cm² × 3**[a]
1	0.18	0.12	0.59
2	0.00	0.00	0.63
3	1.04	3.88	4.77
4	0.01	0.18	1.09
5	0.33	0.38	1.83
Mean ± S.D.	0.31 ± 0.43	0.91 ± 1.66	1.74 ± 0.93

Note: Absorbed hydrocortisone for 13.3 μg/cm × 1 is 0.31 ± 0.43 μg, and that the absorption for the 40 μg/cm² is the expected linear triple amount of 0.91 μg/cm². With "triple therapy" absorption is significantly ($p < 0.006$) enhanced. Also, crossover study design is necessary because of wide individual variation.

[a] Statistically significant $p < 0.006$ (paired *t*-test).

cream vehicles, so these absorption amounts can be compared. Hydrocortisone absorption is greater with the acetone vehicle.

IV. DISCUSSION

Little information is available on the most effective topical corticosteroid or other topical formulation dosing regimen regarding the number of skin applications in 1 d. Multiple applications for an ambulatory patient with a readily accessible skin site are common practice. However, for hospitalized patients, patients with less accessible

Table 3 Predicted and Observed Hydrocortisone Absorption: *In Vitro*

		Hydrocortisone (μg/cm²)			
		Receptor fluid		Skin	
Vehicle	**Dosing sequence**	**Predict**	**Observe**	**Predict**	**Observe**
Acetone[a]	13.3 μg/cm² × 1	—	0.13 ± 0.05	—	0.87 ± 0.23
	40.0 μg/cm² × 1	0.39[b]	0.35 ± 0.22	2.61[b]	2.21 ± 2.05
	13.3 μg/cm² × 3	0.39	0.55 ± 0.75	2.61	2.84 ± 2.05
Cream[a]	13.3 μg/cm² × 1	—	0.053 ± 0.029	—	0.30 ± 0.24
	40.0 μg/cm² × 1	0.16[b]	0.23 ± 0.03	0.90[b]	0.86 ± 0.53
	13.3 μg/cm² × 3	0.16	0.27 ± 0.21	0.90	1.19 ± 0.43

[a] $n = 3$; mean ± S.D.

[b] 0.39 μg/cm² is 3× the measured value of 0.13 μg/cm²; 2.61 μg/cm² is 3× the measured value of 0.87 μg/cm²; 0.16 μg/cm² is 3× the measured value of 0.053 μg/cm²; 0.90 μg/cm² is 3× the measured value of 0.30 μg/cm².

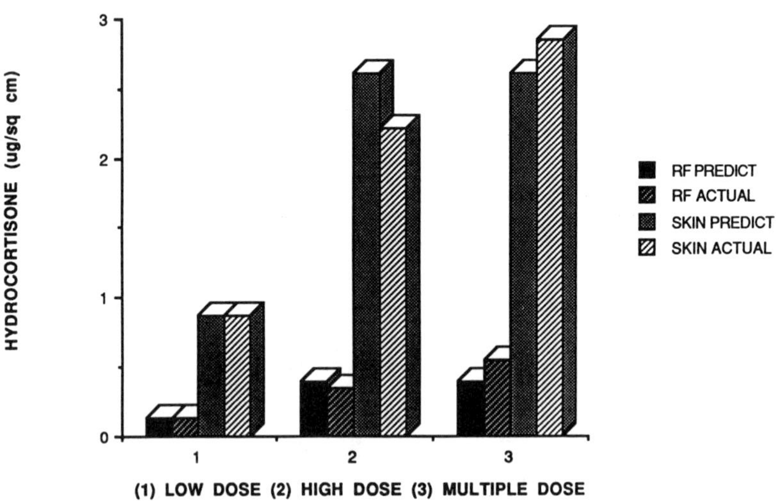

Figure 3 Hydrocortisone *in vitro* percutaneous absorption in human skin with acetone vehicle. Both absorbed amounts (receptor fluid) and skin content reflect dosing sequence. RF refers to receptor fluid accumulation.

skin sites, or patients with occluded skin sites, a single daily dose may be more practical. Along with cost, a single daily dose may be the most efficient if therapy is not compromised. Earlier animal studies using the same vehicle, acetone, suggest that drug bioavailability is not changed with increased daily application.[2] This study suggests that triple therapy in humans may have some advantage.[6] If increased bioavailability is desired, then multiple-application therapy may be the answer, if patient convenience is not an issue. Our data suggest the possibility that increased bioavailability is related to reapplication of vehicle; hence, a case may be made for

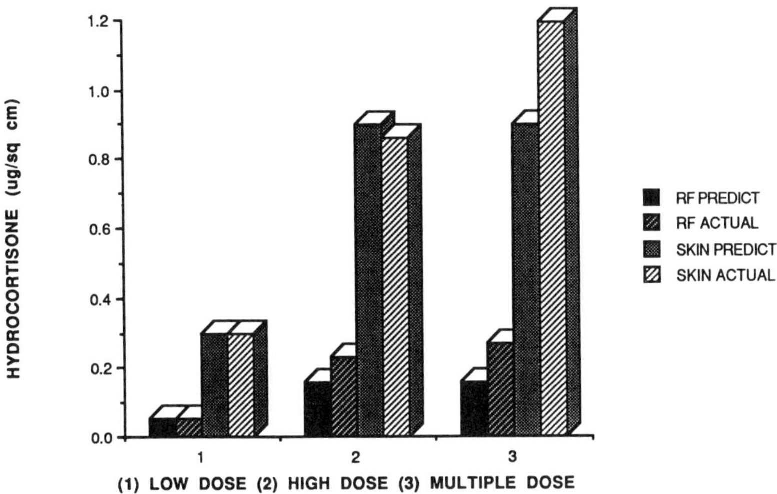

Figure 4 Hydrocortisone *in vitro* percutaneous absorption in human skin with cream vehicle. Both absorbed amounts (receptor fluid) and skin content reflect dosing sequence (i.e., both receptor fluid accumulation and skin content hydrocortisone increase when dose goes from 13.3 to 40 μg/cm^2). RF refers to receptor fluid accumulation.

increasing hydrocortisone bioavailability merely by applying serial doses of vehicle to a previously applied single dose of hydrocortisone at the skin surface. Such an experiment would verify whether the solvent-vehicle effect was the only component by which multiple application of hydrocortisone in acetone increased its bioavailability in human skin. The amount of cream vehicle was equal for each treatment. Reapplication of cream in triple therapy may have "activated" any hydrocortisone bound up in the stratum corneum (SC) reservoir.

REFERENCES

1. **Wester, R. C., Noonan, P. K., and Maibach, H. I.,** Percutaneous absorption of hydrocortisone increases significantly with long-term administration: *in vivo* studies in the rhesus monkey, *Arch. Dermatol.,* 116, 186, 1980.
2. **Wester, R. C., Noonan, P. K., and Maibach, H. I.,** Frequency of application on percutaneous absorption of hydrocortisone, *Arch. Dermatol.,* 113, 620, 1977.
3. **Bucks, D. A. W., Maibach, H. I., and Guy, R. H.,** Percutaneous absorption of steroids: effect of repeated applications, *J. Pharm. Sci.,* 74, 1337, 1985.
4. **Wester, R. C. and Maibach, H. I.,** Relationship of topical dose and percutaneous absorption in rhesus monkey and man, *J. Invest. Dermatol.,* 67, 518, 1976.
5. **Wester, R. C. and Maibach, H. I.,** Rhesus monkey as an animal model for percutaneous absorption, in *Animal Models in Dermatology,* Maibach, H., Ed., Churchill Livingstone, London, 1975, 133.
6. **Melenderes, J. L., Bucks, D. A. W., Camel, E., Wester, R. C., and Maibach, H. I.,** *In vivo* percutaneous absorption of hydrocortisone: multiple-application dosing in man, *Pharm. Res.,* 9, 1164, 1992.

Chapter 15.1

Iontophoresis

Burton H. Sage, Jr.

CONTENTS

I. INTRODUCTION AND HISTORICAL PERSPECTIVE

That ions are transported in an electric field has been known since the time of Faraday. This natural phenomenon has long been exploited in the field of electrophoresis to separate charged molecules. The use of an impressed electric field to transport therapeutic molecules across the skin has also been known for over a century. On August 19, 1862, the U.S. Patent Office issued specification 36,231, entitled "Electrical Apparatus for Medical Use," which describes a pair of fluid-filled electrodes conducting current through the body, with one of the electrodes containing medicament placed on the diseased portion of the body.

While iontophoresis may have been "invented" in the U.S., some of the best known early work was done by Sefan Leduc[1] in Europe. In his famous experiment a solution containing strychnine sulfate was placed in the anode of an iontophoresis system on one rabbit, and a solution of potassium cyanide was placed in the cathode

0-8493-2605-2/95/$0.00+$.50

of the system on a second rabbit. The rabbits were connected to each other, with water-filled electrodes serving as a cathode on the first rabbit and anode on the second rabbit. When current was applied, both rabbits died. When current was applied with the polarity of the battery reversed, neither rabbit died. The inescapable conclusion was that the electric current administered lethal ions in the first setup, but did not when the polarity was reversed.

Since the time of Leduc, iontophoresis has resurged in interest every generation or so. In the 1920s Cumberpatch[2] and colleagues advocated medicinal therapy using iontophoresis. In the 1950s and 1960s considerable advances in technology were made in the former Soviet Union by Komarova,[3] Samarin,[4] and Ulashik.[5] To this day, the methods developed by these researchers are routinely used to treat patients there. More recently, Gangarosa[6] and Jacobsen et al.[7] "rediscovered" iontophoresis for drug delivery. The major improvement in this case was the development of constant current power sources which were marketed in the late 1970s by Motion Control Corp. (now Iomed) and others. Still, iontophoresis was limited to use by physicians in an office environment to treat local conditions.

With the 1980s came the concept of controlled release and the unit dose transdermal patch for continuous administration of a systemically active drug. Shortly thereafter, the drug-filled unit dose iontophoresis system was conceived. Given the commercial success of passive transdermal systems and the commercial attractiveness of noninvasive delivery of drugs not deliverable by passive techniques, such as insulin and other new biotech drugs, a major research and development effort was initiated in the early to mid 1980s to develop iontophoresis products. This effort continues today.

A literature search of computerized databases using the single key word "iontophoresis" will identify over 4000 references. However, such searches miss much of the actual body of literature on iontophoresis because the technology is so old and much of the work was done in the Soviet Union before the fall of Communism. It is not the purpose here to review this extensive literature. Excellent reviews were published recently by others.[8–10] The intent here is to describe a method whereby the attractiveness of iontophoresis as a delivery modality for a candidate drug can be determined.

II. BASIC THEORIES OF IONTOPHORESIS

A diagram of a typical unit dose iontophoresis reservoir system is shown in Figure 1. The essential components of this system are the current source, including electronics for current control, the anode reservoir system, which includes the anode electrode, and the cathode reservoir system, which includes the cathode electrode. If the drug to be delivered were cationic, it would be placed in the anode reservoir system, and if the drug were anionic, it would be placed in the cathode reservoir system. If, for a given therapeutic indication two drugs are required, one of which is anionic and the other cationic, it is possible for an iontophoresis system to deliver both drugs simultaneously.

In the system shown in Figure 1 the object is to move the drug out of the reservoir and into or through the skin, depending on the desired site of action of the drug, with eventual absorption of the drug by the vasculature for distribution throughout the body and eventual elimination. Because the system is electrical in nature, it can be

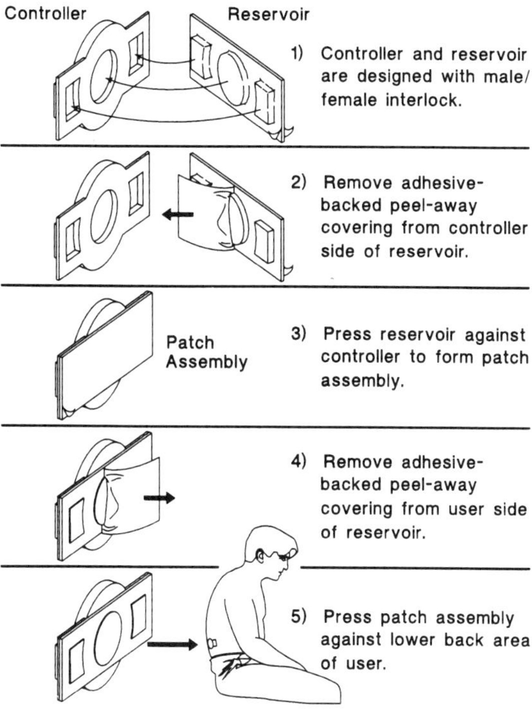

Figure 1 Iontophoresis system with reusable controller and disposable reservoir.

characterized by a voltage drop across the skin and a current running through the circuit which includes the skin. Theories for predicting the rate of drug delivery were developed using both the skin voltage drop and the current as the independent variable. Summaries of these theories are presented below. Further, because the skin is a barrier to penetration of the drug and iontophoresis is a method for enhancing the drug flux across this barrier, it is desirable to determine which, if any, of the various membranes and structures of skin serve as the rate-limiting barrier.

A. NERNST-PLANCK THEORY OF DRUG DELIVERY BY IONTOPHORESIS

The basic relationship known as the Nernst-Planck flux equation asserts that the flux of an ion across a membrane under the influence of an electric field is due to three components: an electroosmotic component, a diffusive component, and an iontophoretic component. Symbolically, it is written as:

$$J = Cu - D\left(\frac{dC}{dx}\right) + D\frac{zEFC}{kT} \tag{1}$$

where J = molar flux
C = molar concentration
u = convective water flow
D = diffusivity coefficient

dC/dx = molar concentration gradient in direction of flux
z = ionic valence
E = electric field
F = Faraday's constant
k = Boltzman's constant
T = temperature (Kelvin)

Most treatments of the problem of drug flux across skin using the Nernst-Planck approach ignore the first or electroosmotic term, although Pikal[11] predicted that under certain circumstances the electroosmotic term may predominate even when the molecule is ionized. Given this assumption, then, the Nernst-Planck flux equation becomes:

$$J = -D\left(\frac{dC}{dx}\right) + D\frac{zEFC}{kT} \tag{2}$$

In principle, this equation allows the prediction of drug flux through the membrane with the knowledge of only one experimental parameter — the drug diffusivity coefficient D. Unfortunately, this equation does not have a closed form solution unless certain simplifying assumptions are made. Planck assumed that the membrane was electrically neutral, however, this assumption fails when the membrane has fixed charges. Goldman assumed that the electric field was constant everywhere in the membrane, but this assumption fails when the membrane has shunt pathways. Because the membrane of interest is skin and skin has both fixed charges and shunt pathways, it is expected that the closed form solutions will have limited validity in predicting drug flux through skin. This is borne out in practice,[12] in which good agreement is shown for voltages up to about 0.5 V. For larger voltages, this theory underpredicts the flux, with the magnitude of underprediction increasing as the voltage increases. The theory might be more predictive if the resistance of the membrane did not decrease with time.[13] Under constant voltage conditions and a decreasing resistance, the ionic content of the skin changes, changing both the fixed charge distribution and the electric field distribution. Kasting and Kiester[12] reviewed the application of the Nernst-Planck flux equation to drug delivery by iontophoresis.

B. FARADAY'S LAW THEORY OF DRUG DELIVERY BY IONTOPHORESIS

While the Nernst-Planck flux equation describes drug flux through a membrane using an impressed voltage, and hence an impressed electric field as the independent variable, Faraday's law describes the flux in terms of the electric current flowing in the circuit. In its simplest form, Faraday's law states that the quantity of material transported in an aqueous solution is proportional to the electric current and the time the current is applied. Faraday himself measured the proportionality constant, appropriately called Faraday's constant, allowing the relationship to be written as:

$$M = \frac{IT}{zF} \tag{3}$$

where M = moles of compound transported
I = electric current (C/s)
T = time of current application (s)
z = molecule valence
F = Faraday's constant (C/mol)

When more than one ion is flowing in the aqueous circuit, each species of ion carries a fraction of the current. This fraction of the current is called transference number; the sum of the transference numbers for all the ions flowing in the circuit must add to 1.0. In an iontophoresis system, letting t_d = drug transference number, the moles of drug transported during the period of current application is predicted by:

$$M = t_d \frac{IT}{z_d F} \tag{4}$$

In terms of the formula weight (FW) of the drug, knowing that the mass of drug is related to moles of drug through the FW, the dose of drug administered by iontophoresis can be predicted by:

$$\text{Dose} = t_d \frac{FWIT}{z_d F} \tag{5}$$

As in the case of the Nernst-Planck flux equation, Equation 5 permits prediction of drug delivery in terms of just one experimentally determined parameter, the drug transference number. Unlike the Nernst-Planck flux equation, Equation 5 does not have to be solved (if current is a function of time, then, given I as provided by the current control circuit, Equation 5 must be integrated) to determine the dose.

The use of Equation 5 can be demonstrated with the following example. Pyridostigmine bromide is a compound which inhibits acetylcholinesterase in a reversible way, and is hence useful as a prophylactic for soldiers in a battle zone where nerve gas may be used. Further, it has been shown that a dose of about 2.5 mg/h can accomplish the prophylaxis. If a current of 1 mA is well tolerated, using Equation 5, the required drug transport number, t_d, can be calculated. Using the FW of 181, a drug transport number of 0.37 is calculated. While a transport number of 0.37 is relatively high, it is not impossible (a calculated transport number >1.0 would be impossible). Using an appropriate laboratory model system,[14] the actual transport number can be measured. Depending on the measured transport number, the current can be adjusted to provide the required dose.

For molecules of therapeutic interest, then, a first estimate of feasibility of an iontophoresis dosage form can be obtained using the required dosing and a current of 1 mA. If the calculated transference number is >1.0, feasibility should be considered low. If the calculated transference number is less than about 0.3, the next step of actually measuring the transference number is reasonable. Once the measured transference number is known, the required current can be calculated. Depending on the magnitude of current required (see Section IV for practical limitations), a better estimate of feasibility can be obtained. For further development of the Faraday's law approach, including a discussion of appropriate model systems for determining the drug transference number, see Sage and Riviere.[14]

C. RATE-LIMITING BARRIER IN IONTOPHORESIS

Conventional wisdom holds that for transdermal drug delivery, the stratum corneum (SC) is the rate-limiting barrier.[15,16] That this is the case for passive transdermal delivery seems beyond dispute. For active transdermal delivery by iontophoresis, then, is it safe to assume that the SC is still the rate-limiting barrier? This is an important consideration because therapeutic compounds may be either locally therapeutic or systemically therapeutic, and they may have vasoactivity as a side effect. If the SC is the rate-limiting barrier, then dilative action on the skin microcirculation will have little effect on increasing the systemic flux. However, if the SC is not the rate-limiting barrier, then any method whereby the microvasculature is dilated will result in a higher systemic flux. (The process of iontophoresis is naturally vasodilative, as shown by the modest erythema apparent after saline iontophoresis.) Similarly, if the SC is not the rate-limiting barrier and iontophoresis is vasodilative and local action of the drug is desired, then vasoconstrictive steps should be taken, such as co-iontophoresis of a vasoconstrictor.

The experiments to demonstrate that the SC is the rate-limiting barrier in passive transdermal delivery used the tape-stripping method to remove the SC from the epidermis. Drug flux with the SC intact is compared to drug flux with the SC tape-stripped away. When this is done, the flux is many times higher through the pieces of skin with the SC removed.

Using the isolated perfused porcine skin flap (IPPSF), developed by Jim Riviere at North Carolina State University,[17] a similar iontophoresis experiment was performed using lidocaine hydrochloride as the drug to be iontophoresed. The results are shown in Figure 2. As can be seen in the figure, the four flaps with intact SC achieved a delivery rate of nearly 30 μg/min with low variability, and an overall delivered dose of about 8.3 mg during the 4-h episode. However, the two flaps without SC each achieved a flux of only about 15 μg/min and an overall delivered dose of about 5.2 mg in 4 h. It is clear from this experiment that the SC is not the rate-limiting barrier, although the actual rate-limiting barrier is not clear from this experiment.

The data in Figure 2 immediately poses two further questions. First, how can the flux be lower when the SC is removed? One hypothesis is that the SC is permselective for cations, and that removing the SC removes this preference for transport of cations. Burnette and Ongpipattanakul[18] showed that the SC of nude mice is permselective, and that the permselectivity is roughly 1.6:1 (55/35) for cations. The datum shown in Figure 2 is 1.85:1 (65/35) for cations, which, given the difference in skin species, is reasonable agreement. The second question relates to the difference in clearance of lidocaine in the two cases. Because the drug reservoirs were not removed when the current was stopped, the most reasonable explanation is that the passive flux of lidocaine was higher when the SC was removed, which is expected.

III. RATIONALE FOR AN IONTOPHORETIC DOSAGE FORM

As seen in Figure 1, iontophoresis is a relatively sophisticated drug delivery technology as it relies on power from a battery to deliver the drug. Given the simplicity of

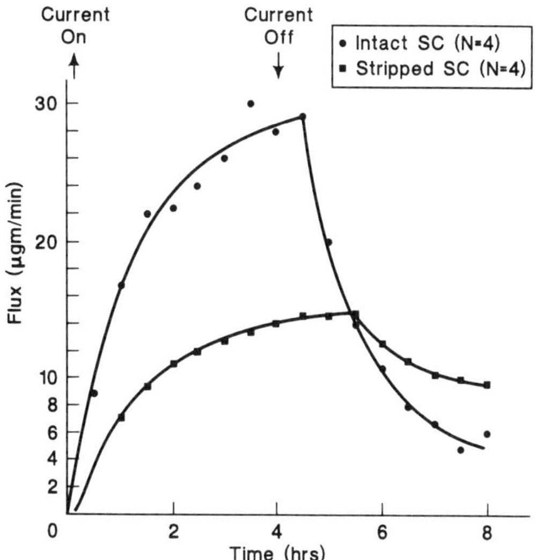

Figure 2 Lidocaine flux in porcine skin flap with and without intact SC.

pills, tablets, ointments, injections, and now passive transdermal patches, we must have good reasons to select iontophoresis as a drug delivery modality. These reasons are discussed below.

A. COMPLIANCE

A medicine developed, approved, and prescribed but not taken can do patients little good. Patients who miss doses and then double their dose to make up for the missed dose, or who take the proper amount of medicine, but at the wrong time fare somewhat better, but still do not reap the full benefits of their medicine.

Studies have shown that three basic reasons are given as to why patients do not comply with the specified dosing regimen. First, the dosing is so frequent that on-time dosing is unmanageable; for example, q.i.d. (every 6 h) makes a good night's sleep nearly impossible. Second, the dosing requires additional constraints besides timing; for example, take with food. Third, the dosing may involve discomfort, such as an injection. These same studies have shown that optimal compliance is obtained when the dosage form is quick, comfortable, and convenient. Once-a-day dosage forms which can be integrated into a patient's normal daily routines have been shown to have the highest compliance. Experience has shown[19] that passive transdermal patches are superior to once-a-day pills. Apparently patients like to wear their medicine.

In principle, iontophoresis should be a high compliance dosage form. It can easily be designed as a once-a-day system. It is also a system that is worn. However, its biggest advantage may arise from its ability to deliver drugs which are normally given by injection, for example, local anesthetics such as lidocaine[20] and other analgesics, and the newer biotech drugs such as peptides[21] and proteins.[22] Thus, one situation in which iontophoresis dosage forms may have overall therapeutic advantage is for medicines for which compliance is low.

B. PROGRAMMABILITY

While a prescribed medicine not taken does a patient no good, the true value of a medicine is not realized unless the medicine is provided as the patient needs it. For the pill, the tablet, the ointment, the injection, and even the transdermal patch, once administered, release of the medicine follows natural laws. Control of the administration rate of the drug has been lost.

For most oral dosage forms and injections, extended action of the drug usually includes early release of excessive amounts of the drug, with the result of varying types and degrees of side effects. As it is impractical to provide drugs in a large series of strengths, a dose which has optimal efficacy and safety in one individual may have no efficacy in another, and toxic side effects in a third. Further, certain drugs, such as theophylline and insulin, are more effective at certain times of the day than at others.

Many, if not all, therapeutic agents would be both safer and more efficacious if the rate of administration could be controlled. The only two known dosage forms in which the delivery rate is controlled are the infusion pump and iontophoresis. As discussed in Section II.B, the drug delivery rate in iontophoresis is proportional to the current. Thus, the peaks and valleys of blood levels that are inherent in pills and injections can be avoided simply by maintaining the current at a level known to provide the desired serum level. Because current can be changed easily, the drug administration rate can be adjusted to provide serum levels on an individual basis. Controlling the current to provide individualized and constant serum levels can go a long way to reduce and eliminate side effects and simultaneously enhance efficacy.

In the case in which more drug is needed at various times during the day, either the current can be programmed to change at these times or a button can be provided whereby the patient can "request" additional drug. Thus, a second situation in which iontophoresis may provide overall improved therapy is that for which control over the drug administration profile is needed, such as when the drug has a narrow therapeutic index, or has chronopharmacological properties, or where the drug is needed "on demand", or when individual titration of the drug is required.

C. INCREASED BIOAVAILABILITY

Besides providing the drug according to need (easily complied to administration regimen and dosing according to physiological need), steps to ensure utilization of as much of the loaded dose as possible should be taken. In oral dosing it is not uncommon to lose over half of the drug due to degradation in the stomach or to "first pass" metabolism in the liver. Following injections, it is not uncommon to have most of the dose merely cleared and excreted before it has a chance to interact with the receptor. For transdermal patches, for which the delivery rate is proportional to the concentration of drug in the patch, it is not uncommon for over 75% of the drug to still be in the patch when it is discarded and a new one placed. After nasal administration, it is not uncommon to swallow over half of the dose.

As increasing scrutiny is given to the overall cost of medicine, effective utilization of the drug in the dosage form will become increasingly important, especially for more expensive drugs such as peptides and proteins. In addition to being compliant and programmable, iontophoresis also has drug utilization advantages. First, as shown in Table 1, when the concentration of the drug in the reservoir, the level of the current, and the treatment episode are properly set, a very high proportion of the

Table 1 Mass of Lidocaine Recovered from Vasculature of Porcine Skin Flap

Flap	Loaded Dose (mg)	Recovered Dose (mg)	Residual Dose (mg)	Efficiency
186	17.2	14.7	2.5	0.85
189	17.2	12.6	4.6	0.73
190	17.2	16.1	1.1	0.93
191	17.2	13.7	3.5	0.80
192	17.2	17.0	0.2	0.98
197	17.2	12.7	4.5	0.74
198	17.2	12.1	5.1	0.70
Av.	17.2	14.1	3.1	0.70
S.D.		1.9	1.9	0.11
% C.V.		13%	61%	13%

loaded dose is delivered. Because these data were collected on the porcine skin flap, the delivered dose is that fraction which actually reaches the vasculature intact; i.e., it has crossed all of the biological barriers required to make it bioavailable. The data do not represent simply the fraction of the dose which is no longer in the patch.

Second, as shown in Figure 3, continuous administration of calcitonin results in a larger pharmacodynamic effect than an intravenous injection. The reduction of serum calcium, which is one of the biological effects of calcitonin, as measured by the area under the curve of calcium reduction is at least twice as high for the infusion as for the injection, resulting in more effective utilization of the dose of calcitonin. Continuous delivery of a drug is easily accomplished with iontophoresis.

Thus, a third situation in which iontophoresis may provide overall improved drug delivery is when the currently available dosage form provides very limited bioavailability.

IV. PRACTICAL LIMITATIONS TO IONTOPHORETIC DRUG DELIVERY

An examination of the U.S. Formulary reveals many situations in which the overall effectiveness of a drug may be improved, either by controlling the administration rate, by improving compliance, or by better overall utilization of the delivered dose. Further, the equations presented in Section II.C allow the calculation of currents and drug transference numbers to obtain a first estimate of the practicality of delivering a candidate drug using iontophoresis. Unfortunately, it is not possible to achieve a high transference number with every drug, and it is not possible to simply increase the current to compensate for a low transference number. At some level, a high current is no longer tolerated. The practical considerations which limit selection of an iontophoresis dosage form are discussed below.

A. PHYSICOCHEMICAL LIMITATIONS OF IONTOPHORETIC ADMINISTRATION

1. Ionic Drug Formulation

Many physicochemical properties influence efficient delivery of a candidate molecule by iontophoresis. The first and perhaps easiest property to ascertain is its

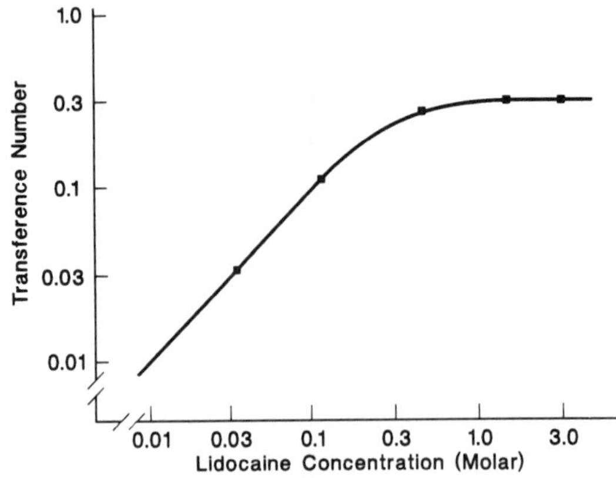

Figure 3 Rabbit responses to a calcitonin.

charge. The fundamental premise of iontophoresis is that the molecule is transported into and through the skin by the force on the molecule from the established electric field. If the molecule cannot be formulated as an ion, the prospects of its moving through the skin in sufficient quantity to be therapeutically effective are poor.

2. pH Range Where Drug Is Ionic

A second important physicochemical property relates to the pH ranges over which the molecule is charged. True salts dissociate freely and are charged at virtually all pH. The salts of weak acids and bases are characterized by a pH value known as its pK_a, at which half of the molecules in solution are dissociated and hence ionic. The other half are uncharged. For salts of weak bases, at pH above this critical pH most of the compound is neutral and at pH below this critical pH most of the compound is ionic. The reverse is true for salts of weak acids. Peptides and proteins and other amphoteric molecules are characterized by an isoelectric point (isoelectric range), a pH (pH range) above which the molecule is anionic, and below which the molecule is cationic.

It is the intent of iontophoresis to transport these molecules across skin. However, the pH of skin is highly variable; values range from 4 to 6 on the surface, drop to a minimum value ranging from about 4.0 to 4.5 at an unknown and variable distance below the surface of the skin,[23] and finally rise to about pH 7.3 in the well-hydrated portions of the epidermis. If the candidate molecule becomes uncharged at any of the pH encountered on its journey into the skin, the major effect of the electric field is lost. Further, as is the case for certain peptides and proteins which have an isoelectric point at a pH encountered in the skin further progress into the skin due to diffusion or electroosmosis can result in a charge reversal of the molecule. In this case the force of the electric field is now directed out of the skin, not into the skin. Thus, not only must the molecule be capable of existing in ionic form, it must exist in ionic form over a range of pH of about 4.0 to 7.3.[24] In reality, this means that the isoelectric point should be outside the range of about pH 3 to 8.3 to provide most of the molecules in the ionic form.

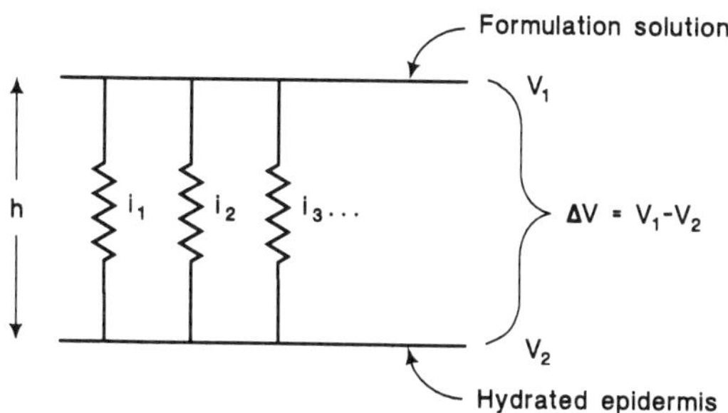

Figure 4 Electrical schematic of ions flowing through skin.

Once it has been determined that a molecule remains charged during its transport into and through the skin, it is possible to express the drug transport number, or current efficiency, in terms of the valence, mobility, and concentration of the drug and the other ions participating in the iontophoresis process.

3. Parasitic Ions and Drug Ion Valence, Mobility, and Concentration

In iontophoresis the drug ion is not the only ion flowing across the skin. There may be ions other than the drug in the drug reservoir which are charged similar to the drug ion. These ions also move out of the patch and into the skin. Because they carry charge, they account for a portion of the current. Many ions are also in the skin which are oppositely charged. These ions move from the skin into the drug reservoir, carrying charge and also accounting for a portion of the iontophoresis current.

Because the drug formulation is highly conducting, as is the well-hydrated portions of the tissue just below the SC, these fluids constitute virtual equipotential surfaces. In such a model the current carried by each of the different ionic species i_j can be interpreted as flowing through a resistor, as shown in Figure 4. Because all the current is flowing in a single loop,

$$\sum_j i_j = I \tag{6}$$

Because the current flows between two equipotential planes, the voltage causing the current to flow at any given time is a constant. (If the effective thickness, *h*, of the SC is known, the electric field, *E*, will be given by *E* over *h*.) Given a constant *E* and fixed current, by Ohm's law an apparent resistance of the path can be calculated:

$$R = E/I \tag{7}$$

Given the parallel flow of the currents as shown in Figure 4, a resistance for each ionic species can be defined:

$$R_j = \frac{E}{i_j} \tag{8}$$

Reversing the terms gives:

$$i_j = \frac{E}{R_j} \tag{9}$$

Combining Equations 6 and 9 gives:

$$I = \sum_j i_j = \sum_j E/R_j = E\sum_j 1/R_j \tag{10}$$

In Equation 10 the iontophoretic current is expressed as flowing through parallel resistors as shown in Figure 4. Because the inverse of resistance is conductance, Equation 10 can be written as:

$$I = E\sum_j \gamma_j \tag{11}$$

The conductivity of an ionic solution can be expressed as[25]

$$\gamma_j = KZ_j\mu_jC_j \tag{12}$$

where: K = geometric constant
u_j = mobility of jth species
C_j = molar concentration of jth species

Finally, the transference (of the drug or any one of the ions flowing through the skin) can be written as (because all the ions are flowing in precisely the same circuit, the geometric constant is the same for all ions, and hence the geometric constant K appears outside the summation and cancels):

$$t_j = \frac{i_j}{\sum_j i_j} = \frac{E\gamma_j}{\sum_j E\gamma_j} \tag{13}$$

$$t_j = \frac{Z_j\mu_jC_j}{\sum_j Z_j\mu_jC_j} \tag{14}$$

As can be seen from Equation 14, the transference (or current efficiency) depends upon four things: (1) the number of species flowing through the skin (removing terms from the denominator raises each of the remaining t_j), (2) the charge on the molecule, (3) the mobility of the species, and (4) molar concentration of the species.

In iontophoresis the transference number of interest is the drug transference number, t_d. As we are interested mostly in *in vivo* drug transport, the predominant species in the skin which can flow out of the skin and into the patch are known, as well as their concentrations and free solution mobilities. Finally, for many drugs, current carried by parasitic ions can be virtually eliminated. If it is assumed that the proportion of the current being carried out of the skin by ions other than saline is negligibly small, and that the saline ions are present at 0.15 *M* and have a mobility equal to their free solution mobility (given the size and concentration of the saline ions, these are not unreasonable initial assumptions), the drug transport can be estimated as, from Equation 14:

$$t_d = \frac{Z_d \mu_d C_d}{Z_d \mu_d C_d + A} \tag{15}$$

where $A = z^* u^* C$ for the saline ion.

Equation 15 has two interesting regimes:

$$Z_d \mu_d C_d \ll A \tag{16}$$

$$Z_d \mu_d C_d \gg A \tag{17}$$

In the first case (16), the denominator of the expression for t_d becomes approximately equal to the constant *A*, and the drug transference becomes directly proportional to the drug concentration, the mobility, and the valence. For a given drug, the valence and mobility are essentially constant, and hence t_d is directly proportional to concentration. Therefore, in general, drugs with larger valences and higher mobilities will have a transference advantage.

It is interesting to speculate on the range of drugs and drug concentrations for which the first case is appropriate. For the case of anodal iontophoresis, the skin ion is assumed to be chloride at 0.15 *M*. The valence is 1 and the free solution mobility is 7.8×10^{-4}, thus, $A = 1.2 \times 10^{-4}$. Assuming that the skin ion for cathodal delivery is sodium at a concentration of 0.15 *M* and a free solution mobility of 5.2×10^{-4}, an analogous value for the constant $A = 7.8 \times 10^{-5}$ can be calculated.

For a drug with a free solution mobility of 1×10^{-4}, a concentration of 0.1 *M*, and a valence of 1, the first case is valid. In a cursory review of the literature much of the experimentation is under conditions in which Equation 16 is appropriate. Hence, in general, more efficient delivery of the drug is expected when the concentration is increased.

Given Equation 15, however, as the concentration of the drug is increased, at some drug concentration, an equivalent percentage change in drug transport number will not be realized. Eventually the conditions shown in Equation 17 will be reached. If possible, however, reaching the conditions in Equation 17 has certain advantages: (1) knowledge that a higher transference number is unlikely, and the system is about as efficient as it can be made, and (2) as drug is delivered and the concentration in the

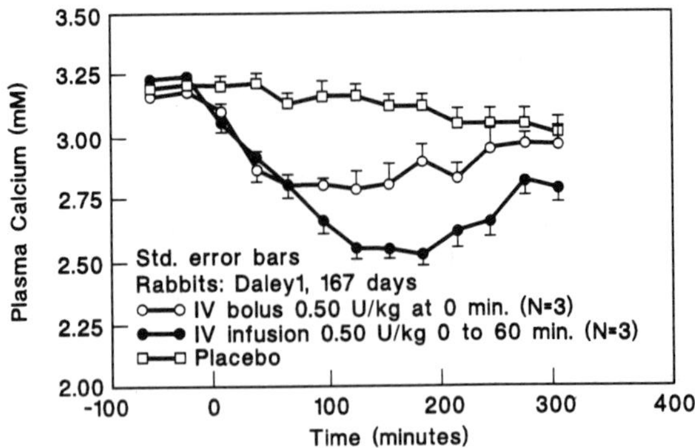

Figure 5 Transference number of lidocaine vs. lidocaine concentration in porcine skin flap model.

reservoir falls, the drug transference will remain steady, as will the rate of drug delivery.

As is apparent in the above development, several assumptions were made to simplify the analysis. The validity of these assumptions needs to be established. To test these relationships, a series of experiments were carried out using the porcine skin flap model. Lidocaine hydrochloride was used as the drug in a drug reservoir with a silver electrode. Such a reservoir system minimizes the number or extraneous reservoir ions to the point that they may be neglected. The concentration of lidocaine was varied over the range of 0.04 to 3.0 *M*. Given these concentrations, the lidocaine transference numbers should range from linear with concentration (Equation 16) to flat with concentration (Equation 17). The results of the experiments are shown in Figure 5.

As can be seen in Figure 5, the shape of the curve agrees with that predicted in Equation 15. Using the data in Figure 5, the theory can be tested in three ways. The first test is at the highest concentrations in which little change in drug transference occurs with concentration. The theory predicts that the drug transference should be very close to 1.0. However, the experimentally determined transference is only 0.3.

The second test can be made at the knee of the curve, i.e., at a lidocaine concentration of about 0.3 *M*. At this point, the lidocaine $z^*u^*C = A$, and the expression can be solved for u, and compared to the lidocaine-free solution $u = 1 \times 10^{-4}$. These data yield a lidocaine mobility of 4×10^{-5}, which is a about a factor of 2.5 low if the lidocaine is in fact passing through the skin with a mobility equivalent to its free solution mobility.

The third test occurs at the lower lidocaine concentration, or where Equation 16 should be a good approximation. Again, the data allow a direct calculation of the apparent lidocaine mobility for comparison to the free solution mobility. An experimental lidocaine mobility of 1.2×10^{-4} is calculated, which is in excellent agreement with the free solution mobility.

This experimentation with lidocaine shows qualitative agreement with the theory developed above, and perhaps semiquantitative agreement for Equation 16, in which the drug concentration is relatively low. The reasons for poorer agreement at high concentration are not known. Surprisingly, these results suggest that the mobility of the drug ion into and through the skin is not dramatically different from the free solution mobility, further suggesting that a reasonable estimate of drug transference number of iontophoretic delivery can be obtained by using the free solution mobility. Before such a general conclusion can be made, similar results should be obtained with other drugs, especially drugs with different physicochemical properties than lidocaine, e.g., drugs with different partition coefficients and drugs with higher molecular weights, especially peptides and proteins.

B. SKIN EFFECTS ARISING FROM IONTOPHORESIS

Equation 5 suggests that any required dose may be achieved in any treatment episode for any measured transference number simply by adjusting the current. This would be true if the motion of the ions through the skin did not cause secondary adverse effects. Unfortunately, the skin does limit the amount of current that can safely pass through the skin, first giving rise to uncomfortable sensations which, if the current is increased, causes a painful, burning sensation, and second, irritating the skin beyond the point of innocuous erythema to blister formation and skin necrosis.

Ledger[26] reviewed the skin effects resulting from drug delivery by iontophoresis. Citing the work of Molitor and Fernandez[27] and others, Ledger concluded that a determination of the maximum current that can be safely conducted through the skin "is subject to numerous conditions; one's definition of 'acceptable' (discernible or tolerable), the duration of current application, the electrode area, etc." Indeed, the data from Molitor and Fernandez[27] show that recommended maximum current levels range from about 4 mA with a 10 cm^2 electrode to 25 mA with a 250 cm^2 electrode.

In reality, skin effects due to iontophoresis can either arise from the process of iontophoresis; i.e., effects due to iontophoresis of physiological ions such as sodium and chloride, the drug which is being iontophoresed, or a synergistic effect from the combination of the drug and the process of iontophoresis. Because parameters such as electrode area and duration of current application can affect the tolerability of a system designed for a specific application, no substitute exists for complete testing of each system. However, for small systems, i.e., systems with skin contact areas of <50 cm^2 which can be conveniently worn on the skin, it seems unlikely that currents above a few milliamperes will be well tolerated.

C. ENERGY REQUIREMENTS FOR IONTOPHORESIS

Delivering a drug by iontophoresis requires electrical energy. It was concluded above that total currents in excess of a few milliamperes are unlikely. Our own work on humans has shown that the resistive load presented by the skin at currents of a few milliamperes is in the range of several thousand ohms. The power requirement is then on the order of 10 mW. If the current is constant over the treatment episode, the required energy (in joules) is the power times the episode length in seconds. For example, the 10-mW system for chronic, daily administration of a drug would require just under 1000 J (0.3 Wh) per day.

Several alternative battery technologies exist for portable equipment such as an iontophoresis system, and summaries which allow comparison have been published.[28] One of the better choices for iontophoresis equipment are the lithium/manganese dioxide coin cells. While these batteries are rated at about 8 Wh/in.^{3}, allowing for the need for higher power to overcome the initial higher impedance of skin, imperfect upconversion, and incomplete energy utilization of any battery, the effective rating of these batteries is on the order of 5 Wh/in.^{3}. Thus, 1 in.^{3} of this battery (a standard 9 V battery is roughly 0.5 in.^{3}) would last only 2 weeks. The much-touted "U.S. quarter"-sized cells have about 1500 J and need to be changed every day.

The energy required to power an iontophoresis device is thus a major consideration. Indications which require short-term application are preferred in terms of battery lifetime. For chronic applications, either new battery technologies must be developed, such as polymer batteries,[29] or innovative ways to use existing battery technologies such as the split air cathode battery[30] must be developed.

D. CONTROVERSIES IN IONTOPHORESIS

As in any field, the literature contains opposing views on aspects of iontophoresis. This final section presents the opposing views of two controversies: does pulsed current provide any advantage over direct current, and when the electric field is established across the skin, is the drug transport due to the force on the molecule because it is charged or to solution flow arising from the interaction of mobile ions with fixed charges on the surface of skin pores (electroosmosis)?

1. Does An Advantage of Pulsed Direct Current Over Continuous Exist?

This question implicitly relates to the rate of drug delivery. For small molecules at low frequencies, this question was effectively answered by Bagniefski and Burnette.[31] These results were repeated in our own laboratory using a different molecule (lidocaine) and a different model (the porcine skin flap). Up to a frequency of 1 kHz, within experimental error, no difference is found in the rate of delivery.

For larger molecules at higher frequencies, the answer is not so clear. Siddiqi and co-workers[23] reported significant enhancement of insulin iontophoresis at a frequency in excess of 10 kHz. It would be expected that such a significant result would be quickly confirmed by others, but no such confirmation has been reported. Questions that remain relate to the design of a pulsed DC power source operating at frequencies above 10 kHz (e.g., are current spikes available that may have electroporation effects?) and repeatability of the observations (the number of animals used in the different cohorts and the variability of the data).

Another example of a single report unconfirmed by publications from other laboratories is found in Okabe et al.[32] This is also a report of pulsed DC at a frequency above 10 kHz, so the same questions of power source design should be asked. Okabe further reports no skin irritation or sensation in spite of hours of operation at peak currents of hundreds of milliamperes over 50 cm^2 of skin contact.

One aspect of pulsed DC which can be quantitatively addressed is power utilization compared to continuous DC. In continuous DC the power is the resistance times the square of the current. In a pulsed DC system with a 50% duty which has the same average current as the continuous DC system, for the first half of the cycle the current is twice the continuous DC system, and during the second half of the cycle, the current is zero. Thus, during the first half of the cycle the power is four times the continuous DC system and zero during the second half of the cycle. Overall, a pulsed DC system with 50% duty consumes twice the power of a continuous DC system. As the duty cycle of the pulsed system decreases, it is even more at a disadvantage to the continuous DC system. From a power consumption point of view, then, the drug delivery rate of a pulsed system should be at least twice that of a continuous system in order to have an advantage.

The value of a pulsed system remains to be fully determined, especially in the frequency range above 1 kHz. The biggest need is confirmatory reports by independent workers.

2. Is It Iontophoresis or Electroosmosis?

In trying to deliver a dose of a therapeutic drug, the knee-jerk answer is, "Who cares?" On reflection, however, the question relates to an understanding of the mechanism by which molecules are transported across the skin. As improvements in performance usually follow improvements in understanding the process, the question is far from moot.

One of the first individuals to suggest that transport of a charged molecule in the presence of an electric field is primarily electroosmosis was Sibalis.[33] Transport of uncharged molecules by electroosmosis has been well known since the work of Rein.[34] Recently Pikal[11] published a review entitled "The Role of Electroosmotic Flow in Transdermal Iontophoresis". At issue is the path the ions take through the skin, and whether the path constitutes an aqueous "pore", the effective size of the "pore," and the distribution of charge in the "pore". The conclusion of this review from a drug delivery point of view is that as the size of the molecule increases, the contribution from electroosmosis increases, and for a Stokes radius >1 nm, the transport is predicted to be predominantly electroosmotic.

The primary difficulty in trying to answer this question experimentally using skin is that no way is known to answer the question, "was this molecule transported by an electrostatic force, an electroosmotic force, or a combination of both forces?". To date, an experimental technique which enables the variables to be successfully separated for transport of a charged molecule has not been devised. Final resolution of this question awaits development of the appropriate experimental technique.

REFERENCES

1. **Leduc, S.,** *Electronic Ions and Their Use in Medicine,* Rebman Ltd., Liverpool, U.K., 1908.
2. **Cumberpatch, E. P.,** Essentials in medical electricity, in *A Textbook of Actinotherapy,* Rosewarne, D. D., Ed., Henry Kimpton, London, 1933, chap. VIII and IX.
3. **Komarova, L. A.,** Deposition of electrophoresis-administered substances in the skin, in *Abstracts of Papers of All-Institute Scientific Conference,* S. M. Kirov Advanced Medical Institute, Leningrad, 1955, 61.
4. **Samarin, Y. N., Fredricksberg, D. A., and Tolkachev, S. S.,** Physicochemical study of iontophoresis, *Vopr. Kurortol. Fizioter. Lech. Fiz. Kultury.,* 4, 3, 1957.
5. **Ulashik, V. S.,** *Theory and Practice of Therapeutic Electrophoresis,* Belarus Pubishing, Minsk, 1976.
6. **Gangarosa, L. P.,** *Iontophoresis in Dental Practice,* Quintessence, Chicago, 1983.
7. **Jacobsen, S. C., Stephen, R. L., Johnson, R. T., Luntz, R., and Knutti, D.,** U.S. Patent 4, 141, 359, 1979.
8. **Banga, A. K. and Chien, Y. W.,** Iontophoretic delivery of drugs: fundamentals, developments and biomedical applications, *J. Control. Rel.,* 7, 1988.

9. **Lescure, F., Gurny, R., Doelker, E., and Augustynski, J.,** Utilisation du principe de l'iontophorese ou de l'ectrophorese pour le controle de la liberation de substances medicamenteuses, *Pharm. Acta Helv.* 64(8), 210, 1989.
10. **Guy, R. H.,** Ed., Iontophoresis, *Adv. Drug Deliv. Rev.,* 9(2/3), 119, 1992.
11. **Pikal, M. J.,** The role of electroosmotic flow in transdermal iontophoresis, *Adv. Drug Deliv. Rev.,* 9(2/3), 210, 1992.
12. **Kasting, G. B. and Keister, J. C.,** Application of electrodiffusion theory for a homogeneous membrane to iontophoretic transport through skin, *J. Control. Rel.,* 8, 195, 1989.
13. **Yamamoto, Y. and Yamamoto, T.,** Measurement of electrical bio-impedance and its applications, *Med. Prog. Technol.,* 12, 171, 1987.
14. **Sage, B. H. and Riviere, J. E.,** Model systems in iontophoresis, transport efficacy, *Adv. Drug Deliv. Rev.,* 9, 265, 1992.
15. **Berner, B.,** Pharmacokinetics of transdermal drug delivery, *J. Pharm. Sci.,* 74, 718, 1985.
16. **Brown, L. and Langer, R.,** Transdermal delivery of drugs, *Annu. Rev. Med.,* 39, 221, 1988.
17. **Riviere, J. E.,** The isolated perfused porcine skin flap (IPPSF). I. A novel *in vitro* model for percutaneous absorption and cutaneous toxicity studies, *Fund. Appl. Toxicol.,* 7, 444, 1986.
18. **Burnette, R. R. and Ongpipattanakul, B.,** Characterization of permselective properties of excised human skin during iontophoresis, *J. Pharm. Sci.,* 76, 765, 1987.
19. **Burris, J. F., Wallin, J. D., and Weidler, D. J.,** Therapeutic adherence in the elderly: transdermal clonidine compared to oral verapamil for hypertension, *Am. J. Med.,* 91(Suppl. 1A), 22S, 1991.
20. **Gangarosa, L. P.,** Defining a practical solution for iontophoretic local anesthesia of skin, *Methods Fund. Exp. Clin. Pharmacol.,* 3, 83, 1981.
21. **Meyer, R. B.,** Successful transdermal administration of therapeutic doses of a polypeptide to normal human volunteers, *Clin. Pharmacol. Ther. (St. Louis),* 44, 607, 1988.
22. **Haak, R.** Pulsatile Drug Delivery from Electrotransport Therapeutic Systems, presented at 3rd APV-CRS Joint Workshop: Pulsatile Drug Delivery — Current Applications and Future Trends, Koenigswinter, Germany, May 20 to 22, 1992.
23. **Siddiqi, O., Sun, Y., Liu, J. C., and Chien, Y. W.,** Facilitated transdermal transport of insulin, *J. Pharm. Sci.,* 76, 341, 1987.
24. **Sage, B. H.,** European Patent Appl. 0 552 878 A2, 1993.
25. **Bard, A. J. and Faulkner, L. R.,** *Electrochemical Methods,* John Wiley & Sons, New York, 1980, 66.
26. **Ledger, P. W.,** Skin biological issues in electrically enhanced transdermal delivery, *Adv. Drug Deliv. Rev.,* 9, 289, 1992.
27. **Molitor, H. and Fernandez, L.,** Studies on iontophoresis. I. Experimental studies on the causes and prevention of iontophoretic burns, *Am. J. Med. Sci.,* 198, 778, 1939.
28. **Bell, T. E.,** Choosing the best battery for portable equipment, *IEEE Spectrum,* 30, March 1988.
29. **Munshi, M. Z. and Owens, B. B.,** Flat polymer electrolytes promise thin-film power, *IEEE Spectrum,* 32, August 1989.
30. **Sage, B. H.,** U.S. Patent 5,037,381, 1991.
31. **Bagniefski, T. and Burnette, R. R.,** A comparison of pulsed and continuous current iontophoresis, *J. Control. Rel.,* 11, 113, 1990.
32. **Okabe, K., Yamaguchi, H., and Kawai, Y.,** New iontophoretic transdermal administration of the beta-blocker metoprolol, *J. Control. Rel.,* 4, 79, 1986.
33. **Sibalis, D.,** U.S. Patent 4,878,892, 1989.
34. **Rein, H.,** Experimental studies on electroosmosis in surviving human skin, *Z. Biol. (Zurich),* 81, 125, 1924.

Chapter 15.2

Ultrasound

Etienne Camel

CONTENTS

I. INTRODUCTION

The discovery of the piezoelectric effect of some crystalline materials by Pierre Curie made possible the use of ultrasound by humans. Since the work of Paul Langevin at the beginning of this century and the development of the SONAR instrument, considerable progress has been made in the development of new piezoelectric crystals and led to increased and diversified applications of ultrasound. Medical applications were the most rapidly increasing source of human exposure to ultrasound. In the 1950s interest in the use of ultrasound was demonstrated in physical medicine to treat localized skin conditions and delivery of drugs into inflamed joints.[1] Since this period, growing interest in percutaneous administration of drugs has stimulated efforts to develop ultrasound as a new technique for achieving controlled transdermal delivery. *In vivo* studies on animals have demonstrated the feasibility of phonophoresis (defined as the migration of drugs through living tissues, intact skin,

0-8493-2605-2/95/$0.00+$.50

under the influence of ultrasonic perturbation) in enhancing drug penetration into the systemic circulation.

This chapter attempts to present the technique of phonophoresis and its application to transdermal drug delivery with an overview of the most representative experimental and clinical studies. A review of the phonophoresis experimental variables and the possible mechanism of action are also presented.

II. PHYSICAL CHARACTERISTICS OF ULTRASOUND

Ultrasound is usually produced using a transducer incorporating a piezoelectric material (crystal).[2,3] When pressure is applied, a small voltage is generated across the crystal, and the effect can be detected and measured. Conversely, when an electric field is applied to a piezoelectric crystal, the crystal changes shape and returns to its resting state in an oscillating manner, generating pressure waves into the surrounding medium as soon as the electric field is removed. Selecting the physical size of the crystal allows vibrations at ultrasonic frequencies. Ultrasound can be generated as a continuous wave or as a pulsed beam.

The technique of phonophoresis depends on several physical and physiological variables that are discussed below. Ultrasound is defined by a number of parameters. *Frequency* is the number of times the wave is repeated in 1 s. The frequency is calculated by dividing the *period* (time it takes to complete a single cycle) into 1. Then, 1 Hz equals 1 cycle per second. Ultrasound is defined as any sound which is of a frequency beyond 20 kHz. Different applications are defined in the medical field with regard to their frequency:

- Diagnostic ultrasound (high frequencies): 2 to 10 MHz
- Therapeutic ultrasound (medium frequencies): 0.7 to 3 MHz
- Power ultrasound (low frequencies): 5 to 100 kHz

Intensity is a physical factor related to the absorption of ultrasonic energy and is defined as the rate of energy flux per unit area, watts or milliwatts per square centimeter. The intensity of ultrasound for phonophoresis ranges from 0 to 3 W/cm^2.[4]

Acoustic impedance represents the product of the density of the tissue and the speed of sound in the tissue. This is often given as:

$$Z = p \cdot c$$

where Z is the acoustic impedance, p is the density of the tissue, and c is the speed of sound. The speed of the sound is expressed by the relationship

$$c = \lambda \cdot f$$

where λ is wavelength and f is frequency.

Because of the total reflection of ultrasound by the air, a *coupling medium* or *contact agent* is needed to transfer energy between the ultrasound and the skin. Examples of coupling agents are mixtures of mineral oil and glycerin, water and propylene glycol, or aquasonic gels.[4]

III. PHONOPHORESIS AND SKIN PENETRATION ENHANCEMENT

A. FIRST REPORTED STUDIES ON PHONOPHORESIS

Considerable attention given over the past decade to the development of new techniques for achieving controlled transdermal delivery has motivated research on the use of ultrasound to limit the stratum corneum (SC) barrier function and enhance drug penetration. One of the first published works, reported by Fellinger and Schmid,[1] was related to percutaneous administration of hydrocortisone ointment to treat inflamed digital joints of the hands. Ultrasonic energy was widely used in the management of arthritis[5] because ultrasound by itself exhibits therapeutical effect. The successful results of Fellinger and Schmid has motivated many other investigations and hydrocortisone became the most widely studied drug associated with ultrasound treatment for several skin or clinical conditions.[6,7] It was demonstrated that combined with ultrasonic massage, injections of hydrocortisone improved results as compared to simple injections in bursitis therapy and post-traumatic lesions.[8] A double-blind study comparing hydrocortisone vs. a placebo demonstrated that 68% of the patients receiving hydrocortisone plus ultrasound (1 MHz, 1.5 W/cm^2) had a significant decrease in pain and an increase in range of motion as compared to 28% treated by ultrasound and a placebo.[9] Griffin et al.[10,11] reported that it was possible to inject a cortisol ointment onto pig skin *in situ* and to drive it into underlaying muscle and nerve with ultrasonic energy levels within the clinical range. Successful phonophoretic administration of lidocaine,[12] carbocaine,[13] phenylbutazone, benzidamine and other nonsteroidal anti-inflammatory drugs,[14–16] and antibiotics including tetracycline, biomycin, and penicillin,[17–19] also were reported. Treatment of herpes with zinc, urea, and tannic acid ointment ultrasound association was described.[20,21] A number of other clinical studies demonstrated an improvement of therapy with ultrasound, but part of them tend to be anecdotal rather than systematic. Phonophoresis studies have been quite well described.[22–24] Recent findings on phonophoresis are discussed in the following section.

B. RECENT FINDINGS ON THE EFFECTS OF PHONOPHORESIS

Some phonophoresis experiments attempted to accelerate the transdermal delivery of topically applied pharmaceutical compounds, such as corticosteroids, anti-inflammatories, analgesics, or anesthetics, for a local effect. McElnay et al.[25] demonstrated that ultrasound (870 kHz, 2 W/cm^2 for 5 min) increased the percutaneous absorption of fluocinolone acetonide in human volunteers to a significant extent from a gel base (Synalar gel). The percutaneous absorption of this corticosteroid was measured by the blanching test described by Barry and Woodford.[26] The authors concluded that the change in absorption was small and unlikely to make significant differences in clinical effect. The same authors also demonstrated successful enhancement of a lidocaine–prilocaine eutectic mixture topically applied on human volunteers.[27] This study suggested that pulsed-output ultrasound (1.5 and 3 MHz, 1.0 W/cm^2 for 5 min) was the most effective operating condition. Tachibana and Tachibanav recently demonstrated that a 5-min ultrasound exposure of topical lidocaine solution and gel (48 kHz, 0.17 W/cm^2), from an ultrasound-generating water tank, rapidly induced an anesthetic effect on hairless mice legs. A variety of topical medications, including anti-inflammatories (dexamethasone, salicylates) and local analgesics, was reported to be used in conjunction with ultrasound to treat localized conditions.[29,30] It is obvious that even with the use of fine needles, these administrations are sometimes painful. Therefore, phonophoresis is a useful technique to decrease patient discomfort and lag time associated with the absorption of the currently available topical mixture.

The feasibility of phonophoresis in enhancing drug penetration into the systemic circulation was suggested by *in vitro* studies with ibuprofen in human skin[31] and by the objective results obtained *in vivo* in the guinea pig and rat with inulin, physostigmine, and D-mannitol[32] with salicylic acid.[33] The total amount of ibuprofen penetrated through the epidermis after a 30-min ultrasound exposure (1 MHz at 1 W/cm^2) was elevated by about 15-fold as compared to passive diffusion on an *in vitro* Franz cell diffusion study.[31] At 4 h after the end of ultrasound treatment, the total amount of drug penetrated was 90 μg vs. 30 μg for the control samples. A second ultrasound exposure resulted in another elevation of ibuprofen delivery (110 μg penetrated vs. 40 μg by passive diffusion).

The lag time of D-mannitol and inulin after topical application was considerably shortened after a 1-MHz ultrasound exposure for 3 to 5 min at a 1.5 W/cm^2 intensity (continuous wave) or 3 W/cm^2 (pulsed wave).[32] Similar effects were observed with salicylic acid for which the diffusion lag time was reduced following phonophoresis.[33] Total amount of the absorbed drug was measured by evaluating the amount of salicylic acid recovered in SC tape strips and eliminated in urine. However, results demonstrated that phonophoresis for 20 min at 2 MHz caused no significant increase in the drug delivery as compared to a 10- and a 16-MHz exposure for 5 min. Significantly increased transdermal penetrations of, respectively, 4- and 2.5-fold were observed. Percutaneous absorption of three nicotinate esters was recently investigated in human volunteers in a double-blind, placebo-controlled crossover study.[34] Results indicated that a 5-min ultrasound exposure (3 MHz, 1.0 W/cm^2) led to significant enhancement of the vasodilator response to methyl and ethyl nicotinates, as measured by laser doppler velocimetry. Percutaneous absorption of hexyl nicotinate was also elevated, but was not found to be statistically significant, providing some clues with regard to the mechanism of action of ultrasound (discussed later).

The potential use of ultrasound as a means of improving therapy was also demonstrated in rats with indomethacin[35] and in alloxan-diabetic rabbits with insulin.[36] Miyazaki et al.[35] demonstrated that a 1-MHz ultrasound exposure for 10 min at intensity levels of 0.25, 0.5, and 0.75 W/cm^2 dramatically increased the indomethacin plasma concentration within 1 h; the 0.75 W/cm^2 intensity appeared to be the most effective intensity in improving the transdermal absorption of the drug, simultaneously increasing skin surface temperature from about 30° to 42°C. Interesting results were obtained by Tachibana[36] with a small piezoelectric element and a drug reservoir containing 3 ml of 40 U/ml neutral purified pork insulin to be administered in diabetic Japanese white rabbits. Ultrasound was delivered over a 1.5-hour period using the aqueous drug form instead of the cream or gel used in previous studies. The device was placed and fixed with the drug reservoir between the skin and the ultrasound element. The changes in the percentage of the initial blood glucose level were measured during the experiment as was the plasma insulin concentration. A gradually and marked decrease of blood glucose was observed after the end of ultrasound treatment, lasting about 4 h. The glucose level decreased to 85.8% at the endpoint of ultrasound exposure and reached a minimum of about 60% after 2 h. A return to the initial level was observed by 4 h following the end of ultrasound treatment. The lowest average blood glucose level obtained during the course of the experiment was reportedly 195 mg/dl. Plasma concentrations of insulin were significantly elevated by ultrasound treatment, with no lag time. The highest average value measured during the experiment was 120 μU/ml. This study is quite encouraging with regard to the observed results and its consequence on peptide delivery, but also because of the miniaturization and the practical convenience of the system placed on the skin due to the relatively low energy used (105 kHz).

C. LIMITS OF ULTRASOUND-ENHANCING EFFECTS

If some investigations have reported successful phonophoretic administration of a wide range of drugs, other did not report any transdermal enhancement. The effects of ultrasound are different according to the drug or the animal model used. Pratzel et al.[37] demonstrated the inefficiency of a 30-min ultrasound (with no specification of frequency) in increasing the percutaneous absorption of indomethacin from a gel in pig skin *in vivo.* McElnay et al., who reported that ultrasound leads to enhanced percutaneous absorption of fluocinolone acetonide in human volunteers,[25] conducted similar studies showing that ultrasound had no effect on the percutaneous absorption of lignocaine[38] or benzidamine.[39] Different magnitude enhancement responses were observed in humans, with a large interindividual variation, according to the physicochemical properties of nicotinate esters at a 3-MHz frequency for 5 min.[34]

Recent results suggested that a 1-MHz ultrasonic perturbation for 10 min was not effective in enhancing the excretion of acetylsalicylic acid in the rhesus monkey, nor did it modify the amount recovered in the SC.[40] Ultrasound was applied directly to the propylene glycol solution which functioned as the coupling agent after a 5-min contact time with the skin. The intensity (0.2 to 0.8 W/cm^2) had no significant effect on the profile and the penetration of the drug in the different SC layers. The diffusion profile of hydrocortisone, a more lipophilic molecule, in the SC was not modified by ultrasonic perturbation. The explanation given for the lack of effect on the enhancement of acetylsalicylic acid in the rhesus monkey may include the long urinary collection times because bladder catheterization was not employed. However, if ultrasound was effective in enhancing drug permeation and shortening the lag time, then a higher amount of drug should have been detected in the SC via the tape stripping experiment.

As a result of these negative findings, questions about the mechanism of action, influence of the formulation, the physicochemical properties of the molecule, the sensitivity of the method measuring the response, the phonophoretic experimental variables (frequency, power, duration), and the animal model need to be addressed in order to design an experimental protocol studying effect of ultrasound.

IV. PRACTICAL CONSIDERATIONS ABOUT EXPERIMENTAL VARIABLES OF PHONOPHORESIS

The different parameters related to ultrasound and described in Section II are of major importance in phonophoresis investigations with regard to the optimization of the desired effect. General directions may be given from the previous reported clinical studies with ultrasound, in terms of frequency, intensity, contact time, or coupling medium.

A. FREQUENCY

The frequency used for phonophoresis is typically from 20 kHz to 10 MHz. Different frequency values are reported in the literature, but no consistent correlation can be emphasized between these frequencies and the various observed results in terms of transdermal penetration enhancement. Kost and Langer[4] stated that the preferred range of frequency is from 0.5 to 1.5 MHz. Positive enhancement was observed with a 1-MHz transducer in rats and guinea pigs[32] or with a 3-MHz transducer in humans.[34] On the other hand, no significant increase in salicylic acid delivery was observed in guinea pigs with a 2-MHz frequency as compared to a 10- and a 16-MHz perturbation.[33] Positive enhancement was also recently observed with a 48- and a 105-kHz frequency with insulin and lidocaine.[35,36]

Explanations for the large range of frequency used in these studies may include bioavailability of commercial equipment, and part of the inconsistency in the obtained results may be related to transducer calibration and acoustic performance efficiency. However, the well-designed study conducted by Bommannan et al.[33] tends to give a better pattern of behavior with regard to the frequency and intensity to be used in phonophoresis studies. The results demonstrated that higher-frequency ultrasound (10 to 16 MHz) associated with a relatively low intensity (0.2 W/cm^2) for 5 min was more effective for transdermal enhancement of salicylic acid, supporting the hypothesis that higher-frequency ultrasound should increase energy deposition within the SC and render the membrane more permeable. Indeed, because the attenuation of ultrasound is directly related to the frequency,[3] the depth of penetration of ultrasonic energy into the skin is inversely proportional to the frequency. Therefore, the combination of high frequency and low intensity should tend to concentrate the effect of ultrasound on the superficial skin layers.

B. INTENSITY

Intensities ranging from 0.2 to 0.6 to 1.0 to 1.5 W/cm^2 are commonly used in the process of phonophoresis.[31–34] However, Bommannan et al.[33] demonstrated that a 0.2 W/cm^2 intensity, in combination with a high frequency, significantly enhanced transdermal penetration of salicylic acid. They also reported that a 0.35 W/cm^2 intensity, supplied to compensate for the low acoustic efficiency of the employed 16-MHz transducer, caused a considerable increase in the device temperature. To minimize heating and with regard to patient acceptability, physical therapists either use pulsed waves or move the probe transducer around the treated area. As discussed in Section V, a potential method of reducing interface heating is to increase the energy absorption in the focal zone by driving the transducer at high-power pulsed mode,[41] but also by reducing the ultrasound field intensity at the surface using higher frequencies. As sensations are not easy to evaluate in rats or guinea pigs, a well-designed animal (or human) studies must include experimental controls such as skin temperature measurements or transducer acoustic efficiency determination, to avoid using unacceptable and intolerable intensities.

C. COUPLING AGENT

An effective coupling agent is a major concern in transdermal studies in order to efficiently transfer ultrasound energy from the transducer into the skin. The acoustical impedance of air being very small compared to soft tissues,[42,43] all the acoustic energy incident to the interface is reflected back to the tissues; this results in a 100% increase in the absorbed power in tissues close to the interface, and induces elevated temperatures at the skin interface.[41] In physical therapy an aqueous coupling medium is used to exclude air between the transducer and the treated skin area to optimize the effect and patient acceptability with regard to induced heating sensation. Hynynen[41] demonstrated that the temperature elevation at the skin–air interface was about three times higher than when gel was used to prevent reflections following a 1-MHz exposure.

Ultrasonic gels and propylene glycol–water mixtures appear to be used commonly in phonophoresis studies for their contact agent properties.[31,32] The contact agent can also serve as a drug reservoir when the drug possesses appropriate solubility properties.[33,34] A good contact agent should have an absorption coefficient similar to that of water and its amount must be selected to optimize the efficiency of ultrasound energy transport to the skin during the whole experiment. McElnay et al.[25] reported that too much drug could mask any effect of the ultrasound and that the minimum amount of coupling agent required to produce an easily measurable response within a given time should be used. Gel formulations appear to be the most suitable coupling agent for phonophoresis experiments, as reported in a well-designed investigation studying percentage of transmission relative to water of ultrasound energy through topical pharmaceutical products.[44] The data indicated that transmission of ultrasound energy, at a 3-MHz frequency, was 0% (transmission relative to deionized degassed water) through a diethylamine salicylate cream, 22.84% through a triamcinolone acetonide cream, 43.47% through a hydrocortisone cream, and 120.27% through a benzocaine and salicylamide gel. Other topical corticosteroid products and ultrasound coupling agents were also studied, showing significant variations in ultrasound energy transmission. Therefore, determination of good ultrasound coupling characteristics of the preparation to be used should be conducted before any phonophoresis experiment in order to optimize ultrasound activity.

D. CONTACT TIME

Purpose of the initial contact time prior to expose the skin to ultrasound is to saturate the SC and induce better partitioning. A contact time of 5 min is often reported in phonophoresis studies.[23,25,32]

E. PHONOPHORESIS DURATION

Phonophoresis duration varies among studies from 3 min to 1.5 h, depending upon the frequency and the intensity. The most commonly reported total exposure time is 5 to 10 min.[23,25,33,34] Significant effects were observed following a 3-min exposure.[32]

F. CONCLUSION

No consensus on a standardized protocol to study ultrasound efficacy exists. The frequency, intensity, and time of exposure are interdependent, as is the nature of the molecule being studied. These parameters also depend on transducer acoustic efficiency and must be fixed in the range described for the desired application, taking into account induced patient sensations.

V. BIOPHYSICAL MECHANISMS OF ULTRASOUND

The mechanisms of action of ultrasound are complex because of the variety of the factors involved during phonophoresis. These mechanisms will be part of the future, better understanding and standardization of the use of ultrasound in clinical therapy. The pure molecular explanation, given over 30 years ago by Summer and Patrick,[45] suggesting that ultrasound induced oscillation of the molecules about a rest position, is not sufficient to explain ultrasound activity. Mechanical and thermal effects have been associated with phonophoresis.[46] Indeed, ultrasound can be transformed into several other forms of energy via a thermal mechanism, a cavitational mechanism, and stress mechanism, including streaming motions resulting from its interaction with living tissues.[3–46]

When an ultrasonic pulse is sent into soft tissue, the most significant change is attenuation, which is the progressive weakening of the sound beam as it travels through tissues.[3] Attenuation is dependent on the wavelength of the sound, the type, density, and heterogeneity of the tissue. The average attenuation of an ultrasound beam in human soft tissue is 1 dB/cm/MHz.[3–46] This means that an ultrasound beam with a frequency of 1 MHz loses 1 dB of amplitude for every centimeter it travels. The attenuation of ultrasound occurs primarily through three processes: *absorption,* in which energy is captured by the tissue. Most of this energy is converted in heat. *Reflection,* which is the redirection of part of the ultrasound beam back to its source. Finally, *scattering,* which is when the ultrasound beam hits an irregular or smaller medium than the sound beam.

A. MECHANICAL EFFECTS

Microstreaming and stable or transient cavitation are important parameters in cell interaction with ultrasound.[47–49] An ultrasound wave produces alternating areas of compression and rarefaction in the medium, and the resulting pressure changes can give rise to cavitation.[46] Cavitation appears as nucleation, bubble formation, and implosive collapse. Streaming motions and shearing stress can occur within the exposed system through stable cavitation. Acoustic streaming is defined as the time-independent circulation of fluid induced by a radiation force. These mechanical effects are difficult to assess and to quantify, but they were reported as the main factors contributing to the enhancing effect of ultrasound on synthetic membranes and on skin.[32,50,51]

Studies on the release of various molecules from bioerodible and nonerodible polymers also give an indication as to possible ultrasonically enhanced mechanisms.[52–55]

Micromassage is another mechanical effect of ultrasound, due mainly to the positive and negative pressure changes in the ultrasound beam involving the mechanical distortion of living tissues.

B. THERMAL EFFECTS

When an ultrasound beam passes through tissue, energy is partly absorbed and converted to heat, and hence causes a rise in tissue temperature.[3–46] Over the past few years, it has become clear that ultrasound can be used to heat deep-seated tumors at certain sites,[56] and some experimental studies conducted on the subject offer a better understanding of this effect.[41–57] Several reasons exist for enhanced temperature elevation at the skin–air interface.[41] One of these reasons is related to the acoustical impedance of the air (0.4×10^{-9} kg/m^2/s), which is very small compared to soft tissues (1.5×10^{-6} kg/m^2/s).[42,43] This causes all of the acoustic energy incident to the interface to be reflected back to the tissue, resulting in a 100% increase in the absorbed power in tissues close to the interface, as compared to a situation with no reflection. A second explanation is that the ultrasonic attenuation coefficient in the skin is much higher as compared to other soft tissues (14 to 66 Np/m at 1 MHz vs. 3 to 15 Np/m).[42,43] Experiments conducted by Hynynen[41] with a 1- and a 3.5-MHz transducer clearly demonstrated that skin temperature elevation was dominated by reflection and absorption. Results showed that a significant decrease was obtained by using a gel to prevent reflection, and by using a sharply focused transducer to allow the ultrasound power to diverge rapidly beyond the focal zone. Another technique to reduce heating is to increase the energy absorption in the focal zone by driving the transducer at high-power pulsed mode.[57] The study also demonstrated that hot spots on the outer surfaces can be eliminated by reducing the ultrasound field intensity at the surface by using higher-frequency fields which will be attenuated rapidly before the interface.

Thermal effects during the phonophoresis process were monitored by many authors. It was often concluded that a rise of 1° to 2°C was not likely to have any significant effect on skin permeability.[31–33] However, in a recent study showing successful enhancement of the transdermal absorption of indomethacin after ultrasound exposure at 1 MHz for 10 min a rise in skin temperature was demonstrated to be proportional to the ultrasound intensity. A 6°C elevation was observed with the lowest intensity (0.25 W/cm^2) and about 12°C with the highest intensity which remains in the therapeutic domain of the intensity currently used (0.75 W/cm^2).[35] Another study demonstrated that no correlation exists between a given ultrasound dose and skin temperature and blood flow.[58] Thus, other objective explorations of this effect need to be addressed for a better understanding of the phonophoresis mechanisms and its eventual influence on skin integrity for long-term transdermal treatment.

VI. SKIN BIOLOGICAL EFFECTS AND MECHANISM OF ACTION

Skin biological effects associated with phonophoresis have received little experimental attention despite the number of *in vitro* and *in vivo* studies on animals. If many studies concluded that it had a direct effect on the SC lipid structure, no evidence of it was demonstrated clearly. The mechanisms for ultrasonically enhanced skin permeation are not yet completely defined, but part of the mechanical and/or thermal effects previously described may explain the transport of drugs through tissues under the influence of ultrasound.[32] One study from 1958 had already indicated the possibility of permeability cell alteration under ultrasonic exposure.[59]

The few well-conducted studies available on the subject allow a better understanding of the effect of ultrasound on skin permeability. Levy et al.[32] suggested that ultrasound can temporarily and reversibly alter the permeability of the skin for both hydrophilic and lipophilic drugs. The reversibility of the effect of ultrasound on the skin was postulated because exposure of guinea pig skin to ultrasound for 1 h prior to drug application did not affect the penetration of the drug. Histologic analysis of skin sections exposed to ultrasound did not show any difference as compared to the nonexposed sections. The authors suggested that because both mixing and cavitation effects are involved in the diffusion phenomenon through membranes *in vitro,* and also play a significant role *in vivo,*[49] these factors may contribute to the enhanced permeability observed *in vivo* in animals. Tachibana[36] also demonstrated in his histological analysis that after a 1.5-h ultrasound exposure to insulin at a frequency of 105 kHz diabetic rabbit skin revealed no inflammation or destruction of tissue.

A recent study with nicotinate esters of different physicochemical properties provided some insight into the mechanism of action of phonophoresis.[34] Augmented response following ultrasound exposure was greatest in the case of more hydrophilic compounds. Preliminary study demonstrated that ultrasound treatment, prior to the application of one of the hydrophilic nicotinate esters (methyl nicotinate), enhanced percutaneous absorption of this ester.[60] Thus, Hadgraft et al. suggested that lipid fluidization may be a mechanism of skin structure interaction, resulting in improved percutaneous absorption by ultrasound.

Three years ago, one of the most representative studies on the effect of ultrasound on skin morphology was realized by Bommannan et al.[61] Electron microscopy was performed to follow the penetration of an electron-dense colloidal tracer (lanthanum hydroxide) on hairless guinea pig skin following sonophoresis. Results show that exposure to ultrasound for 5 min at either 10 or 16 MHz did not appear to alter cellular morphology. However, 20 min of exposure at 16 MHz seemed to induce significant structural alterations of the stratum granulosum and stratum basal cells. It was postulated, based on electron micrograph analysis, that cavitation may have produced this adverse finding by a possible repeated expansion and self-destruction of micronuclei in the skin. It must be emphasized that in a separate series of experiments Bommannan et al.[33] demonstrated that the release of salicylic acid from a gel formulation was not affected by an ultrasonic exposure, and that conversely to Levy et al.,[32] pretreating the skin with ultrasound enhanced salicylic acid skin penetration, suggesting a direct effect of ultrasound on the skin. As expressed by the authors, questions about reversibility and the adverse effects of different frequencies and exposure time need to be addressed. Therefore, an explanation for the lack of effect in the penetration of certain molecules in some skin models previously reported[37–40] may include a possible difference of the physical mechanisms of phonophoresis on the guinea pig or rat skin as compared to the rhesus monkey skin or the pig skin, due to skin structure and physiological differences. In previous transdermal studies the rhesus monkey and the pig showed a lower permeation rate to various compounds and the closest permeability characteristics to those of humans.[62,63] Also, longer duration and specific frequency with some particular drug models may be necessary to induce an effect and increase permeation on the rhesus monkey, pig, or human skin.

VII. EFFECTS OF ULTRASOUND ON DRUGS

Few direct studies have described the effect of ultrasound on drugs used phonophoretically. From these it can be concluded that ultrasonic exposure does not cause, in most cases, chemical changes in the drug molecule. Julian and Zentner[64] did not find any ultrasound-induced degradation of benzoic acid and hydrocortisone. These findings confirmed previous results indicating that hydrocortisone solutions exposed to ultrasonic intensities of 2 W/cm^2 for 10 min did not show any detectable decomposition.[7]

Kost et al.[52] assessed the effect of ultrasonic energy on the integrity of insulin samples by high-performance liquid chromatography. It was reported that ultrasound did not degrade the molecule released from polymeric systems and exposed to ultrasound. On the other hand, it was demonstrated that sodium dodecylbenzene sulfonate and sodium dodecyl sulfate were decomposed (benzene ring and alkyl group decomposition) by ultrasonic treatment at 304 kHz.[65]

VIII. PHONOPHORESIS AND CUTANEOUS TOLERANCE

Phonophoresis and long-term skin tolerance have received little experimental attention, but the long use of ultrasound in physical therapy may attest to the overall safety of this technique. When used improperly, this method does appear to be harmful. The burning of mouse skin exposed to ultrasound at a frequency of 1 MHz has been reported after a 5-min exposure at an intensity of 40 kW/m^2 at 4 d old and 10 kW/m^2 at 7 d.[66] Bilsters, edema, and congestion were also described in rats treated with 10 kW/m^2 for 1 min at 1 MHz. Greater skin damage was noted as the ultrasound intensity or duration was increased.[67] Patient discomfort related to ultrasound exposure is observed when ultrasound is specifically used to heat deep tumors at certain sites.[56] However, the power levels which produce these effects, ranging from slight warming of the tissue to total necrosis, are many orders of magnitude greater than the power levels used for clinical phonophoresis. Tachibana[36] demonstrated that a 1.5-h ultrasound exposure on diabetic rabbit skin, at a 105-kHz frequency, did not induce any sign of burns or erythema. Histological studies showed no alteration of the SC. McElnay et al.[25] reported that the procedure of phonophoresis was well tolerated by all volunteers after a 5-min ultrasound massage at a 2 W/cm^2 intensity and 870 kHz frequency.

When used at proper frequency, intensity, and duration the evidence is ample that phonophoresis is a safe technique.

IX. CONCLUSION

Several important issues about the theoretical basis have been solved since phonophoresis was used as a practical and therapeutic technique by Fellinger and Schmid. However, questions about mechanism of action, influence and optimization of the formulation/coupling medium, the physicochemical properties of the molecule associated with the practical phonophoretic conditions (frequency, power, duration), and the skin model still need to be addressed in order to design an experimental protocol for studying the effect of ultrasound. The importance of the positive findings in the rat and guinea pig with inulin, salicylic acid, indomethacin, and insulin suggest that further exploration of mechanisms be undertaken to define a standardized and effective procedure for drug therapy in humans.

Ultrasound appears to be an effective technique to enhance drug penetration across animal skin or improve the local effect of topical medications on human skin (e.g., analgesics, anti-inflammatories). The continuing use of phonophoresis for many years attests to the overall safety of this method and its lack of long-term effect on the skin when used properly. Nevertheless, important issues regarding long-term transdermal application have not been extensively investigated. The development of innovative electronics and controlled clinical studies are now required to prove the real improvement of this technique as an effective and safe long-term transdermal drug delivery method in humans.

REFERENCES

1. **Fellinger, K. and Schmid, J.,** *Klinick und therapie des chronischen Gelenkreurnatismus,* Maudrich, 1954, 549.
2. **Lutz, H. and Meudt, R.,** *Manual of Ultrasound,* Springer-Verlag, Berlin, 1984, 4.
3. **Bartrum, R. J. and Crow, H. C.,** *Gray-Scale Ultrasound: A Manual for Physicians and Technical Personnel,* W. B. Saunders, Philadelphia, 1977.
4. **Kost, J. and Langer, R.,** International Patent Appl. No. PCT/US87/01546, 1988.
5. **Aldes, J. H., Jadeson, W. J., and Grabinski, S.,** A new approach to the treatment of subdeltoid bursitis, *Am. J. Phys. Med.,* 33, 79, 1954.
6. **Belts, E. A. and Bondarenko, M. M.,** The use of ultrasound and phonophoresis with hydrocortisone in chronic psoriasis, *Vestn. Dermatol. Venerol.,* 45, 70, 1971.
7. **Popov, N. D., Kudryashov, V. V., and Pristupa, L. F.,** Level of 17-hydroxycorticosteroids in the blood and skin of rabbits during hydrocortisone phonophoresis, *Vopr. Kurortol. Fizioter. Lech. Fiz. Kult.,* 35, 295, 1970.
8. **Newman, M. L., Kill, M., and Frampton, G.,** Effects of ultrasound and combined with hydrocortisone injections by needle or hypospray, *Am. J. Phys. Med.,* 37, 206, 1958.
9. **Griffin, J. E., Echternach, J. L., Price, R. E., and Touchstone, J. C.,** Patients treated with ultrasonic driven hydrocortisone and with ultrasound alone, *Phys. Ther.,* 47, 594, 1967.
10. **Griffin, J. E. and Touchstone, J. C.,** Ultrasonic movement of cortisol into pig tissues. I. Movement into skeletal muscle, *Am. J. Phys. Med.,* 42, 77, 1963.
11. **Griffin, J. E., Touchstone, J. C., and Liu, A. C.** Ultrasonic movement of cortisol into pig tissues. II. Movement into paravertebral nerve, *Am. J. Phys. Med.,* 44, 20, 1965.
12. **Novak, E. J.,** Experimental transmission of lidocaine through intact skin by ultrasound, *Arch. Phys. Med. Rehab.,* 45, 1231, 1964.
13. **Cameroy, B. M.,** Ultrasound enhanced local anaesthesia, *Am. J. Orthoped.,* 8, 47, 1966.
14. **Brondolo, W.,** Phenylbutazone with ultrasonics in some cases of arthrosynovitis of the knee, *Arch. Ortop.,* 73, 532, 1960.
15. **Famaey, J. P.,** Sonophoresis with non-steroidal anti-inflammatory drugs. A survey of the problem, *J. Belg. Rhumatol. Med. Phys.,* 30, 129, 1975.
16. **Chatterjee, D. B.,** A double blind clinical study with benzydamine 3% cream on soft tissue injuries in an occupational health center, *J. Int. Med. Res.,* 5, 450, 1977.
17. **Parikov, V. A.,** Injection of tetracycline into the tissues of cow udders by ultrasonics, *Veterinaria,* 43, 88, 1966.
18. **Dynnik, T. K.,** Use of antibiotic phonophoresis in purulent inflammatory skin disease, *Vrach. Del.,* 115, 1977.
19. **Indkevich, P. A.,** Experience in the treatment of hidradenitis with biomycin phonophoresis, *Vestn. Dermatol. Venerol.,* 44, 75, 1971.
20. **Fahim, M.,** New treatment for herpes simplex virus type 2 (ultrasound and zinc, urea and tannic acid ointment). I. Male patients, *J. Med.,* 9, 245, 1978.
21. **Fahim, M.,** New treatment for herpes simplex virus type 2 (ultrasound and zinc, urea and tannic acid ointment). II. Female patients, *J. Med.,* 11, 143, 1980.
22. **Skauen, D. M. and Zentner, G.,** Phonophoresis, *Int. J. Pharm.,* 20, 235, 1984.
23. **Tyle, P. and Agrawala, P.,** Drug delivery by phonophoresis, *Pharm. Res.,* 6, 5, 1989.

24. **McElnay, J. C., Benson, H. A. E., Hadgraft, J., and Murphy, T. M.,** The use of ultrasound in skin penetration enhancement, *Pharmaceutical Skin Penetration Enhancement,* Walters, K. A. and Hadgraft, J., Ed., Marcel Dekker, New York, 1993, 293.
25. **McElnay, J. C., Kennedy, T. A., and Harland, R.,** The influence of ultrasound on the percutaneous absorption of fluocinolone acetonide, *Int. J. Pharm.,* 40, 105, 1987.
26. **Barry, B. W. and Woodford, R. K.,** Comparative bioavailability of proprietary topical corticosteroid preparations: vasoconstrictor essays on thirty creams and gels, *Br. J. Dermatol.,* 91, 323, 1974.
27. **Benson, H. A. E., McElnay, J. C., and Harland, R.,** Phonophoresis of lignocaine and prilocaine from Emla* cream, *Int. J. Pharm.,* 44, 65, 1988.
28. **Tachibana, K. and Tachibana, S.,** Use of ultrasound to enhance the local anesthetic effect of topically applied aqueous lidocaine, *Anesthesiology,* 78, 1091, 1993.
29. **Antich, T. J.,** Phonophoresis: the principles of the ultrasonic driving force and efficacy in treatment of common orthopaedic diagnoses, *J. Orthoped. Sports Phys. Ther.,* 4, 99, 1982.
30. **Williams, A. R.,** Phonophoresis: an in-vivo evaluation using three topical anaesthetic preparations, *Ultrasonics,* 28, 137, 1990.
31. **Brucks, R., Nanavaty, M., Jung, D., and Siegel, F.,** The effect of ultrasound on the *in vivo* penetration of ibuprofen through human epidermis, *Pharm. Res.,* 6, 697, 1989.
32. **Levy, D., Kost, J., Meshulam, Y., and Langer, R.,** Effect of ultrasound on transdermal drug delivery to rats and guinea pigs, *J. Clin. Invest.,* 83, 2074, 1989.
33. **Bommannan, D., Okuyama, H., Stauffer, P., and Guy, R. H.,** Sonophoresis. I. The use of high-frequency ultrasound to enhance transdermal drug delivery, *Pharm. Res.,* 9, 559, 1992.
34. **Benson, H. A. E., McElnay, J. C., Harland, R., and Hadgraph, J.,** Influence of ultrasound on the percutaneous absorption of nicotinate esters, *Pharm. Res.,* 8, 204, 1991.
35. **Miyazaki, S., Mizuoka, H., Oda, M., and Takada, M.,** External control of drug release and penetration: enhancement of the transdermal absorption of indomethacin by ultrasound irradiation, *J. Pharm. Pharmacol.,* 43, 115, 1991.
36. **Tachibana, K.,** Transdermal delivery of insulin to alloxan-diabetic rabbits by ultrasound exposure, *Pharm. Res.,* 9, 952, 1992.
37. **Pratzel, H., Dittrich, P., and Kukovetz, W.,** Spontaneous and forced cutaneous absorption of indomethacin in pigs and humans, *J. Rheumatol.,* 13, 1122, 1986.
38. **McElnay, J. C., Matthews, M. P., Harland, R., and McCafferty, D. F.,** The effect of ultrasound on the percutaneous absorption of lignocaine, *Br. J. Clin. Pharm.,* 20, 421, 1985.
39. **Benson, H. A. E., McElnay, J. C., and Harland, R.,** Use of ultrasound to enhance the percutaneous absorption of benzydamine, *Phys. Ther.,* 69, 113, 1989.
40. **Camel, E., Melendres, J., and Maibach, H. I.,** Effect of ultrasound on the *in vivo* percutaneous absorption of drugs in the rhesus monkey, unpublished data, 1990.
41. **Hynynen, K.,** Hot spots created at skin-air interfaces during ultrasound hyperthermia, *Int. J. Hyperthermia,* 6, 1005, 1990.
42. **Goss, S. A., Johnson, R. L., and Dunn, F.,** Comprehensive compilation of empirical ultrasonic properties of mammalian tissues, *J. Acoust. Soc. Am.,* 64, 423, 1978.
43. **Goss, S. A., Frizzell, L. A., and Dunn, F.,** Ultrasonic absorption and attenuation of high frequency sound in mammalian tissues, *Ultrasound Med. Biol.,* 5, 181, 1979.
44. **Benson, H. A. E. and McElnay, J. C.,** Transmission of ultrasound energy through topical pharmaceutical products, *Physiotherapy,* 74, 587, 1988.
45. **Summer, W. and Patrick, M. K.,** *Ultrasonic Therapy,* Elsevier, New York, 1964.
46. **Williams, A.R.,** *Ultrasound: Biological Effects and Potential Hazards,* Academic Press, New York, 1983.
47. **Hughes, D. E.,** The interaction of ultrasound with cells, in *Proc. Workshop Interaction of Ultrasound and Biological Tissues,* Reid, J. M. and Sikov, M. R., Eds., 1972, 61.
48. **Hill, C. R.,** The interaction of ultrasound with cells, in *Proc. Workshop Interaction of Ultrasound and Biological Tissues,* Reid, J. M. and Sikov, M. R., Eds., 1972, 57.
49. **Haar, G. R. and Daniels, S.,** Evidence for ultrasonically induced cavitation *in vivo, Phys. Med. Biol.,* 26, 1145, 1981.
50. **Kost, J., Machluf, M., and Langer, R.,** Effect of ultrasound on skin permeability, *Proc. Int. Symp. Control. Rel. Bioact. Mater.,* 16, 294, 1989.

51. **Kost, J.,** Ultrasound for controlled delivery of therapeutic, *Clin. Mater.,* 13, 155, 1993.
52. **Kost, J., Leong, K., and Langer, R.,** Ultrasound-enhanced polymer degradation and release of incorporated substances, *Proc. Natl. Acad. Sci. U.S.A.,* 86, 7663, 1989.
53. **Julian, T. N. and Zentner, G. M.,** Mechanism for ultrasonically enhanced transmembrane solute permeation, *J. Control. Rel.,* 12, 77, 1990.
54. **D'Emanuele, A., Kost, J., Hill, J. L., and Langer, R.,** An investigation of the effect of ultrasound on degradable polyanhydride matrices, *Macromolecules,* 25, 511, 1992.
55. **Liu, L. S., Kost, J., D'Emanuele, A., and Langer, R.,** Experimental approach to elucidate the mechanism of ultrasound-enhanced polymer erosion and release of incorporated substances, *Macromolecules,* 25, 125, 1992.
56. **Shimm, D. S., Hynynen, K., Anhalt, D. P., Roemer, R. B., and Cassady, J. R.,** Scanned focused ultrasound hyperthermia: initial clinical results, *Int. J. Rad. Oncol. Biol. Phys.,* 15, 1203, 1988.
57. **Hynynen, K.,** Demonstration of enhanced temperature elevation due to non-linear propagation of focused ultrasound in dog's thigh *in vivo, Ultrasound Med. Biol.,* 13, 85, 1987.
58. **Paaske, W. P., Hovind, H., and Sejrsen, P.,** Influence of therapeutic ultrasonic irradiation on blood flow in human cutaneous, subcutaneous and muscular tissues, *Scand. J. Clin. Lab. Invest.,* 31, 389, 1973.
59. **Gersten, J. W.,** Non-thermal neuromuscular effects of ultrasound, *Am. J. Phys. Med.,* 37, 235, 1958.
60. **Hadgraft, J., McElnay, J. C., and Murphy, T. M.,** Phonophoresis as an enhancer of skin absorption, in *Proc. Int. Conf. Prediction of Percutaneous Penetration,* Manchester, U.K., 1989, 67.
61. **Bommannan, D., Menon, G. K., Okuyama, H., Elias, P. M., and Guy, R. H.,** Sonophoresis. II. Examination of the mechanism(s) of ultrasound-enhanced transdermal drug delivery, *Pharm. Res.,* 9, 1043, 1992.
62. **Bartek, M. J., Labudde, J. A., and Maibach, H. I.,** Skin permeability *in vivo*: comparison in rat, rabbit, pig and man, *J. Invest. Dermatol.,* 58, 114, 1972.
63. **Wester, R. C. and Maibach, H. I.,** Rhesus monkey as an animal model for percutaneous absorption, in *Animal Models in Dermatology,* Churchill Livingstone, Edinburgh, 1975, 133.
64. **Julian, T. N. and Zenter, G. M.,** Ultrasonically mediated solute permeation through polymer barriers, *J. Pharm. Pharmacol.,* 38, 871, 1986.
65. **Hagiwara, S.,** Decomposition of anionic surface active agents by ultrasonic waves in aqueous solution, *Kyoto Furitsu Daigaku Gakujutsu Hokoku: Rigaku, Seikatsu Kagaku,* 23, 49, 1972.
66. **Kirsten, E. B., Zinsser, H., and Reid, J. M.,** Effect of IMC ultrasound on the genetics of mice, *IEEE Trans. Ultrasonic Eng.,* 112, 1963.
67. **Cowden, J. W. and Abell, M. R.,** Some effects of ultrasonic radiation on normal tissues, *Exp. Mol. Pathol.,* 2, 367, 1963.

Chapter 15.3

Delipidization of the Cutaneous Permeability Barrier and Percutaneous Penetration

Efraim Menczel

CONTENTS

I. INTRODUCTION

In an earlier publication[1] the classical studies on the enhanced effects of skin delipidization on percutaneous penetration of chemicals were reviewed. An observation in an earlier *in vitro* investigation,[2] as well as the results of a more recent clinical trial,[3] indicated that the accelerated permeation following lipid removal from the skin was counteracted by presumably intrinsic lipogenesis. In the past decade the infrastructure of the cutaneous barrier was elaborated by applying delipidization extraction techniques, as lipids play a predominant role in the overall protection of the human interior milieu. Reproducible and considerable percutaneous penetration of chemicals can be attained by overcoming the complexities of this protective apparatus through appropriate depletion of its lipids.

II. CUTANEOUS PERMEABILITY BARRIER

A. LIPOIDAL CHARACTERISTICS OF THE CUTANEOUS BARRIER

The principal barrier between the internal milieu and the external environment is the stratum corneum (SC) of the epidermis. It is composed of fibrous protein-enriched corneocytes embedded in lipid-enriched intercellular membrane bilayers.[4] The biosynthesis of lipids occurs in the keratinocytes in all nucleated layers of the epidermis.

0-8493-2605-2/95/$0.00+$.50

The newly synthesized lipids are delivered by lamellar bodies to the interstices of the SC during epidermal differentiation.

The homeostatic pattern of the lipids (range and concentrations) in the intercellular membrane bilayers is essential for the lipoidal cutaneous barrier in the various body areas. The epidermal lipids amount to about 4.4% of epidermis dry weight,[5] whereas the isolated SC contains about 10% lipids of total weight, 80% of which are within the intercellular matrix.[6]

Sphingolipids are predominant, comprising 35 to 45% of the intercellular domain of the SC.[4] Sphingolipids are fatty acid amides linked to sphingosine and these are known as ceramides of several types and as glycosylceramide where the sugar moiety is glucose. Analysis of the fatty acids of ceramides has shown that linoleic acid, an essential unsaturated fatty acid, is most commonly found in their structure.[7] Gangliosides detected in human epidermis are also linked to ceramides.[8] A recent study revealed age- and sex-dependent changes in ceramides.[9] Only in females, after reaching maturity, does the percentage of ceramide 2 decrease and of ceramide 3 increase with age. These findings complement levarometry tests on human skin.[10]

The other main lipids are sterols and fatty acids; these, together with ceramides, account for nearly all the SC lipids.[8] The sterols include cholesterol, cholesteryl sulfate, and cholesteryl glycoside. Evidence has accumulated to indicate that cholesterol, accounting for 20 to 25% of total lipid weight, has a critical role for barrier function.[11] Mention should be made of the presence of 7-dehydrocholesterol, the photochemical precursor of the essential vitamin D_3.[12] The free fatty acids account for about 25% of the lipid present and consist mainly of palmitic, stearic, oleic, and docosanoic acids.[8]

In addition, the lipoidal cutaneous barrier contains phospholipids, wax esters, and hydrocarbons,[8] as well as triglycerides.[11] The phospholipids account for <5% of SC lipids, but they are essential for the maintenance of the membrane bilayers.[11]

Intensive studies have indicated that the cutaneous barrier is composed of two lipid-related barriers.[4,13] The first level of barrier function is subserved by highly nonpolar lipids such as free fatty acids, triglycerides, etc. The second level of barrier integrity is more resilient and mediated by the polar sphingolipids, synergistic with the polar cholesterol.

Maibach's study group[14] in the 1960s pointed out regional variations of human body skin in the percutaneous absorption of chemicals. These reflect differences in the lipid composition of the human SC cutaneous permeability barrier at various sites which, correspondingly, influences the rate of permeation of the permeants.[15]

The dermal tissue contains substantial amounts of cholesterol and nonsaponifiable lipids. In hairless mice about 77 and 73% of total cutaneous cholesterol and nonsaponifiable lipids, respectively, are synthesized in the dermis.[16] These findings substantiate studies on the dermal retention of certain chemicals in the process of percutaneous penetration;[17–19] evidence indicating protein binding in the dermis of some chemical moieties also has been reported.[20]

B. DELIPIDIZATION OF THE CUTANEOUS BARRIER

Absolute acetone is the most common solvent for delipidization of SC sheets obtained from excised animal skin in investigations on the permeability functioning of the cutaneous barrier.[4,13,21–31] The outer skin surface is scrubbed with acetone-soaked cotton balls for about 10 min. The amount of lipids extracted depend upon the intensity of the acetone treatment, whether gentle or vigorous. Compared to intact SC by weight, the percentage of the extracted lipid profile is:[27]

	Sphingolipids	Cholesterol	Fatty acids	Triglycerides	Sterol esters
Gentle	12	9	10	14	48
Vigorous	19	12	10	3	41

The main difference between gentle and vigorous acetone treatments is in the amounts of sphingolipids and cholesterol extracted. The appreciable amount of the highly nonpolar sterol esters extracted by either treatment represents only 33% of the total lipids in the whole SC.[27]

The delipidization procedure by acetone produced a marked disruption of the cutaneous barrier. This disruption, measured by transepidermal water loss, was superior to that attained by tape stripping of the skin slices.[31]

In one study petroleum ether delipidization was carried out prior to the acetone treatment.[13] The purpose of this sequential delipidization procedure was to differentiate between polar and nonpolar lipids, and to assess which type of lipid is essential for the proper function of the cutaneous barrier. The highly nonpolar organic solvent, petroleum ether extracted nonpolar lipids (triglycerides, free fatty acids, sterol esters, alkanes) and the remaining polar lipids (sphingolipids, free sterols) were extracted by acetone. The depletion of nonpolar lipids per se by this procedure caused only a modest level of barrier dysfunction, while removal of the polar lipids led to a profound barrier perturbation.[13]

In an *in vivo* trial with volunteers, the delipidization process was carried out in two phases[32] using a mixture of acetone:ether (1:1). At the initial phase (10 min), mostly sebaceous lipids were removed. The fraction of SC lipids was extracted during the subsequent second phase (30 min); this extract consisted of ceramides, free fatty acids, cholesterol, cholesterol esters, and glycolipid. It should be noted that the cutaneous barrier may also be abrogated by a surfactant solution (5 to 10% sodium dodecyl sulfate).[21,23,28,29,33] Cutaneous barrier perturbation stimulates accelerated biosynthetic processes for the production of lipids (equal to lipogenesis) and DNA synthesis.[4,21–23,25,26,28,29,31] The increased transepidermal water loss appears to act as a signal for the enhanced lipogenesis[30] of sphingolipids, sterols, and fatty acids[23] linked to the barrier function homeostasis. The epidermal — but not dermal — sterol and fatty acid biosynthesis was 2.9 and 2.5 times higher, respectively, at 1 to 4 h following barrier abrogation, returning to normal by 12 h.[21,29] On the other hand, sphingolipid biosynthesis is delayed, peaking at 6 h and returning to normal by 12 to 24 h.[22,26] The activated lipogenesis results in complete restoration of barrier structure and function (Figure 1).[22,30] The distorted barrier function also induces DNA synthesis,[4,31] which also occurred in abnormal barrier function of the diseased state.[34]

These delipidization studies were interpreted to mean that the cutaneous barrier requirements regulate epidermal lipids and DNA synthesis.[4]

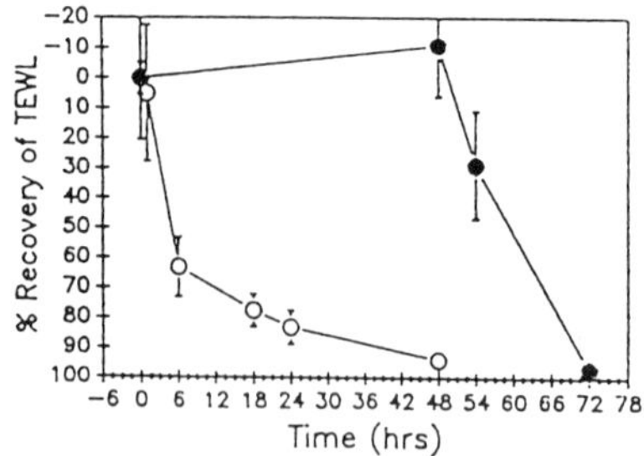

Figure 1 Recovery of cutaneous barrier function after acetone treatment (open circles) within 48 h. In animals covered with a vapor-impermeable membrane following acetone treatment (solid circles), no recovery; after 48 h the vapor-impermeable membrane is removed and barrier recovery ensues. Mean ± S.E.M. TEWL, transepidermal water loss. (From Grubauer, G. et al., *J. Lipid Res.*, 30, 323, 1989. With permission.)

C. EXOGENOUS LIPIDAL REPLENISHMENT FOR RESTORATION OF THE CUTANEOUS BARRIER

Many cellular functions and responses are affected when the membrane lipid composition is modified.[35] The removal of the lipidal components of the cutaneous barrier results in perturbation of the barrier functions. Recovery of the barrier is achieved by intrinsic accelerated processes of lipogenesis; it also may be attained by topical application of an exogenous mixture of lipids.[24] However, the application of single components of SC or an incomplete mixture of two components delays the restoration of the barrier function. Replenishment of the three major components of SC, ceramides, cholesterol, and fatty acids, by topical application allows barrier recovery to occur normally.[24] The same holds true upon topical application of SC lipids extracted by delipidization of human volunteer skin with an acetone:ether (1:1) mixture.[32]

Chromatographic separation of the components of these lipids and subsequent topical application of each of the fractions proved that only the fractions of sphingolipids and cholesterol esters restore the barrier function.[32,33] This finding confirms previous reports on the critical role of sphingolipids in establishing and maintaining the cutaneous barrier function.[11,13]

III. SKIN LIPIDS AND PERCUTANEOUS PENETRATION

A. SKIN LIPIDS CONTENT

The differences in percutaneous penetration of chemicals through various skin sites[14] were correlated to the lipid content in the respective areas. Elias et al.[15] found greater permeation of water and salicylic acid through isolated sheets of SC from leg skin as compared to that of abdominal skin; the leg skin was obtained from patients undergoing amputation and the abdominal skin was autopsy tissue. Compared to abdominal SC, that of the leg skin was more permeable: the fluxes of water and salicylic acid through the leg skin were 200 and 100% greater, respectively (Figure 2).

Remarkably, the percentage lipid weights of these tissues differed distinctively: means of 3 and 6% for leg and abdominal skin, respectively. These results indicate that the degree of percutaneous penetration in various body areas is inversely related to the percentage of lipid weights of the respective SC tissues.

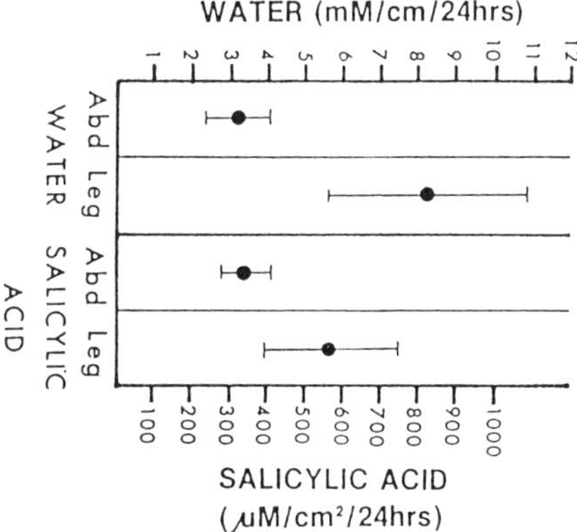

Figure 2 SC permeability to water and salicylic acid; abdomen (Abd) vs. leg. Mean ± S.E.M. (From Elias, P.M. et al., *J. Invest. Dermatol.,* 76, 297, 1981. With permission.)

B. DELIPIDIZATION

Two recent studies illustrate the novel approaches in evaluating the enhancing effects of skin delipidization on the overall processes of percutaneous penetration.

1. Effect on Chemicals with Low Lipophilicity

Several studies have indicated that ionized forms of acid or basic organic compounds which exhibit only slight lipophilicity are impermeable through the cutaneous route. On the other hand, considerable permeation is effected by the distinct lipophilic nonionized forms of these compounds.[17,20] *In vitro* studies on excised skins of human mamma and shed snake (*Python reticulatus*) have shown measurable diffusion values of ionized salicylic acid achieved by skin delipidization prior to the percutaneous penetration experiments.[36] The delipidizing agent was a mixture of chloroform:methanol (2:1 v/v). The same methodology was utilized to assess the permeation of compounds with various degrees of lipophilicity. Whereas the diffusion rates of highly lipophilic chemicals was not influenced by the delipidization procedure, a pronounced difference in the cutaneous permeation was effected with compounds exhibiting low lipophilicity. Delipidization had no effect on the percutaneous penetration of the highly lipophilic dinitrochlorobenzene; in contrast, an appreciable enhancement of the percutaneous permeation was demonstrated for the low lipophilic salicylamide (Figure 3).

The investigators of this study deduced from the amount of lipids extracted from the skins that these were not completely delipidized. Obviously, some lipids remained to allow uninhibited permeation of the highly lipophilic compounds. No interference of lipogenesis was observed in percutaneous penetration during these experiments. The pH buffering could have affected the enzymatic biosynthetic processes.

The main conclusion of this investigation is the significance of lipid depletion in increasing the extent of percutaneous penetration of chemicals of low lipophilicity.

2. Effect on Rapid Onset of Anesthesia

To prevent intense pain from dermal puncture, an aqueous gel was developed for topical application containing the effective local anesthetic lidocaine (10%), combined

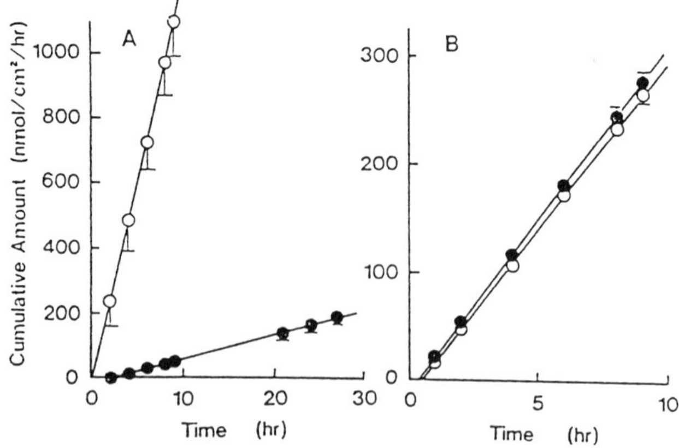

Figure 3 Cumulative amounts percutaneously penetrated vs. time for salicylamide (A) and dinitrochlorobenzene (B). Pretreatment with chloroform:methanol (2:1) (open circles) and untreated (solid circles). Mean ± S.E.M. (From Harada, K. et al., *J. Invest. Dermatol.*, 99, 278, 1992. With permission.)

with an "absorption promoter" (3% glycyrrhetinic acid monohemiphthalate). Reduction of anesthesia onset time was attempted by three pretreatments intended to attenuate the cutaneous barrier. The three pretreatments were stripping with adhesive tape, surface scrubbing, and delipidization with benzine (petroleum ether), a nonpolar organic solvent used for cleansing the area.[37] In contrast to previously reported investigations,[2,3] in this comparative clinical trial no interference by lipogenesis could have been expected; the maximum time span for anesthesia onset was set within 60 min, whereas the biosynthesis of lipids starts 1 to 6 h after distorting the cutaneous barrier by delipidization.[22,26,29] Moreover, lidocaine per se has no direct effect on the cutaneous lipids,[38] and any abrogation of the barrier is attributable only to the pretreatments.

The best results were achieved with the stripping pretreatment. The delipidizing effect of benzine (petroleum ether) was second best, but the anesthesia onset is still distinctly more rapid than that of the control (Figure 4). The delipidization by petroleum ether, being a nonpolar organic solvent, is limited and hence the cutaneous barrier is modestly affected.[13]

Skin delipidization enhancing percutaneous penetration of low lipophilic short acting pharmacologic agents is definitely rational, provided the duration of activity falls short of the peak time of sphingolipids biosynthesis (6 h).[22,26]

C. MILD LIPIDAL DEPLETION

The high permeability of ethanol for epidermis was reported in many reviews.[39] Among the alcohols, the permeability of methanol is the highest, but because of its toxic properties, any practical application in medicine is prohibitive. Ethanol was successfully utilized in developing Estraderm® (Ciba-Geigy), an estradiol transdermal device which consists of an ethanol-based estradiol reservoir with a rate-controlling membrane.

In an *in vitro* investigation with human cadaver skin it was found that at moderate concentrations (50 to 75%) of ethanol, estradiol is cotransported across the cutaneous

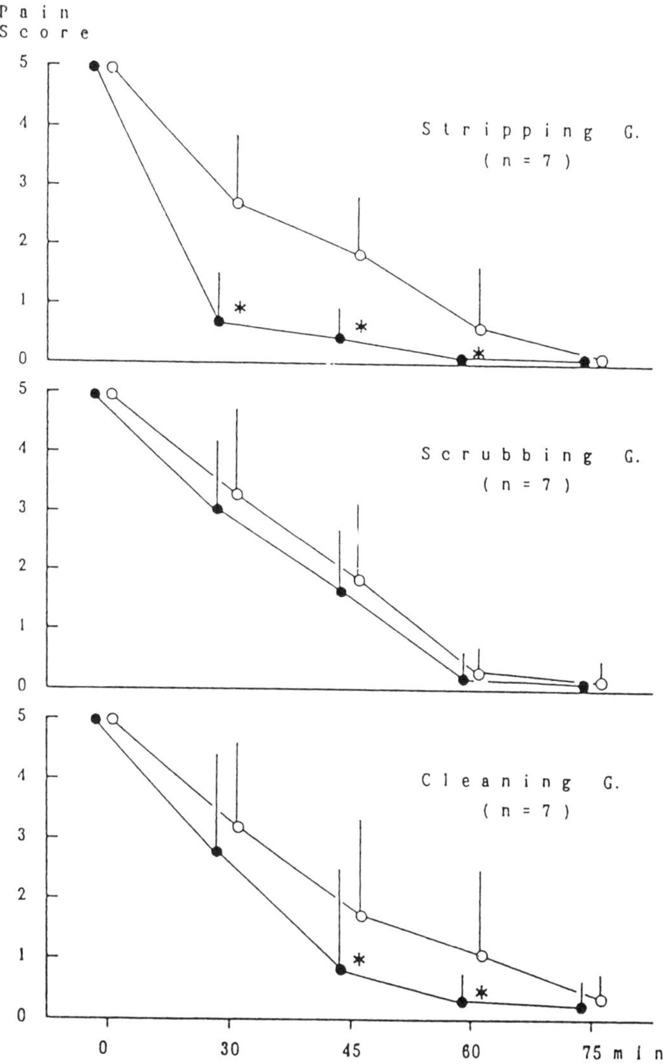

Figure 4 Comparison of pain scores between pretreated (solid circles) and unpretreated (open circles) after initiation of dermal patch anesthesia. G., Study group; Cleaning, with benzine (petroleum ether). *, Significantly lower compared to unpretreated (p <0.05). (From Kano, T. et al. *Anesth. Analg.*, 75, 555, 1992. With permission.)

barrier, with enhanced permeation of both estradiol and ethanol.[40] A further observation, using male hairless mice permeation experiments, indicated a double effect of ethanol even at lower concentrations (≤25%); the transport of estradiol across the lipoidal pathway is accelerated and concomitantly the enzymatic conversion of estradiol to estrone is inhibited.[41] In another recently reported study Williams and Barry[42] implied that the principle of "cotransport of ethanol with the permeant" is not the crucial enhancing factor of this type of percutaneous penetration. This *in vitro* investigation was designed to assess the rate of estradiol permeation across excised human skin, keeping the concentration of ethanol constant (about 50%) at both donor and receptor sites; nevertheless, the enhancement of estradiol permeation persisted.[42] An ethanol–water mixture also proved to increase nitroglycerin flux across human epidermis five- to tenfold.[43] In a recent screening study both methanol and ethanol showed the highest permeation fluxes of ketoprofen across excised hairless mice skin.[44]

Controversial reports were published on the exact mechanism of the enhancement of percutaneous penetration of permeants by ethanol and other short-chain alcohols. Convincingly, Guy's group of investigators ascertained, by attenuated total reflectance infrared (ATR-IR) spectroscopy, that ethanol causes (at least in part) extraction of lipids from the SC intercellular matrix; the mild lipidal depletion may lower skin barrier function and render the cutaneous membrane more permeable.[45,46]

IV. CONCLUSIONS

1. Skin delipidization became an invaluable research tool for the elucidation of the structure, composition, and the biological mechanisms maintaining the cutaneous barrier functions.
2. In-depth skin investigations both *in vitro* and *in vivo* unfold the conditions for enhancement of percutaneous penetration of suitable permeants (such as low lipophilic chemicals) by delipidization using appropriate agents (polar and nontoxic solvents).
3. Lipogenesis does not counteract the accelerated percutaneous permeation by delipidization of short-acting pharmacologic agents, such as local anesthetics, etc.
4. Mild depletion of intercellular lipids of SC by ethanol effectively enhances percutaneous absorption of many chemical moieties.

ACKNOWLEDGMENT

The editorial assistance of Ms. Shani Hanft is gratefully acknowledged.

REFERENCES

1. **Menczel, E.,** Skin delipidization and percutaneous absorption, in *Percutaneous Absorption,* Bronaugh, R. L. and Maibach, H. I., Eds., Marcel Dekker, New York, 1985, 133.
2. **Blank, I. H., Scheuplein, R. J., and MacFarlane, D. J.,** Mechanism of percutaneous absorption. III. The effect of temperature on the transport of non-electrolytes across the skin, *J. Invest. Dermatol.,* 49, 582, 1967.
3. **Bucks, D. A. W., Maibach, H. I., Menczel, E., and Wester, R. C.,** Percutaneous penetration of hydrocortisone in humans following skin delipidization by 1:1:1 trichlorethane, *Arch. Dermatol. Res.,* 275, 242, 1983.
4. **Proksch, E., Holleran, W. M., Menon, G. K., Elias, P. M., and Feingold, K. R.,** Barrier function regulates epidermal lipid and DNA synthesis, *Br. J. Dermatol.,* 128, 473, 1993.
5. **Reinertson, R. P. and Wheatley, V. R.,** Studies on the chemical composition of human epidermal lipids, *J. Invest. Dermatol.,* 32, 49, 1959.
6. **Grayson, S. and Elias, P. M.,** Isolation and lipid biochemical characterization of SC membrane complexes: implication for the cutaneous permeability barrier, *J. Invest. Dermatol.,* 78, 128, 1982.
7. **Wright, S.,** Essential fatty acids and the skin, *Br. J. Dermatol.,* 125, 503, 1991.
8. **Yardley, H. I. and Summerly, R.,** Lipid composition and metabolism in normal and diseased epidermis, *Pharm. Ther.,* 13, 357, 1981.
9. **Denda, M., Koyama, J., Hori, J., Horii, I., Takahashi, M., Hara, M., and Tagami, H.,** Age and sex dependent change in SC sphingolipids, *Arch. Dermatol. Res.,* 285, 415, 1993.

10. **Lanir, Y., Manny, V., Zlotogorski, A., Shafran, A., and Dikstein, S.,** Influence of ageing on the *in vivo* mechanics of the skin, *Skin Pharmacol.,* 6, 223, 1993.
11. **Schurer, N. Y. and Elias, P. M.,** The biochemistry and function of SC lipids, *Adv. Lipid Res.,* 24, 27, 1991.
12. **Holick, M. F., MacLaughlin, J. A., Clark, M. B., Holick, S. A., Potts, J. T., Anderson, R. R., Blank, I. H., and Parrish, J. A.,** Photosynthesis of previtamin D_3 in human skin and the physiologic consequences, *Science,* 210, 203, 1980.
13. **Grubauer, G., Feingold, K. R., Harris, R. M., and Elias, P. M.,** Lipid content and lipid type as determinants of the epidermal permeability barrier, *J. Lipid Res.,* 30, 89, 1989.
14. **Feldmann, R. J. and Maibach, H. I.,** Regional variations in percutaneous penetration of C^{14} cortisol in man, *J. Invest. Dermatol.,* 48, 181, 1967.
15. **Elias, P. M., Cooper, E. R., Korc, A., and Brown, B. E.,** Percutaneous transport in relations to SC structure and lipid composition, *J. Invest. Dermatol.,* 76, 297, 1981.
16. **Feingold, K. R., Brown, B. E., Lear, S. R., Moser, A. H., and Elias, P. M.,** Localization of de novo sterologenesis in mammalian skin, *J. Invest. Dermatol.,* 81, 365, 1983.
17. **Menczel, E. and Goldberg, S.,** pH effect on the percutaneous penetration of lignocaine hydrochloride, *Dermatologica,* 156, 8, 1978.
18. **Reifenrath, W. G., Hawkins, G. S., and Kurtz, M. S.,** Percutaneous penetration and skin retention of topically applied compounds: an *in vitro-in vivo* study, *J. Pharm. Sci.,* 80, 526, 1991.
19. **Guy, R. H. and Maibach, H. I.,** Drug delivery to local subcutaneous structures following topical administration, *J. Pharm. Sci.,* 72, 1375, 1983.
20. **Menczel, E. and Touitou, E.,** Cutaneous permeation of lipophilic molecules; effects of enhancers, in *Percutaneous Absorption,* 2nd ed., Bronaugh, R. L. and Maibach, H. I., Eds., Marcel Dekker, New York, 1989, 121.
21. **Menon, G. K., Feingold, K. R., Moser, A. H., Brown, B. E., and Elias, P. M.,** De novo sterologenesis in the skin. II. Regulation by cutaneous barrier requirements, *J. Lipid Res.,* 26, 418, 1985.
22. **Holleran, W. M., Feingold, K. R., Mao-Qiang, M., Gao, W. N., Lee, J. M., and Elias, P. M.,** Regulation of epidermal sphingolipid synthesis by permeability barrier function, *J. Lipid Res.,* 32, 1151, 1991.
23. **Grubauer, G., Feingold, K. R., and Elias, P. M.,** Relationship of epidermal lipogenesis to cutaneous barrier function, *J. Lipid Res.,* 28, 746, 1987.
24. **Mao-Qiang, M., Feingold, K. R., and Elias, P. M.,** Exogenous lipids influence permeability barrier recovery in acetone treated murine skin, *Arch. Dermatol.,* 129, 728, 1993.
25. **Feingold, K. R., Mao-Qiang, M., Menon, G. K., Cho, S. S., Brown, B. E., and Elias, P. M.,** Cholesterol synthesis is required for cutaneous barrier function in mice, *J. Clin. Invest.,* 86, 1738, 1990.
26. **Holleran, W. M., Feingold, K. R., Mao-Qiang, M., Brown, B. E., and Elias, P. M.,** Sphingolipid synthesis in murine epidermis is regulated by permeability barrier requirements, *Clin. Res.,* 38, 635A, 1990.
27. **Grubauer, G., Feingold, K. R., and Elias, P. M.,** Importance of non-polar SC lipids for barrier function in hairless mice, *Clin. Res.,* 35, 688A, 1987.
28. **Proksch, E., Elias, P. M., and Feingold, K. R.,** Regulation of 3 hydroxy-3 methylglutaryl-coenzyme A reductase activity in murine epidermis, *J. Clin. Invest.,* 85, 874, 1990.
29. **Grubauer, G., Feingold, K. R., and Elias, P. M.,** Cutanous barrier requirements regulate the biosynthesis of sterols and fatty acids in mouse skin, *J. Invest. Dermatol.,* 87, 142, 1986.
30. **Grubauer, G., Elias, P. M., and Feingold, K. R.,** Transepidermal water loss: the signal for recovery of barrier structure and function, *J. Lipid Res.,* 30, 323, 1989.
31. **Proksch, E., Feingold, K. R., Mao-Qiang, M., and Elias, P. M.,** Barrier function regulates epidermal DNA synthesis, *J. Clin. Invest.,* 87, 1668, 1991.
32. **Imokawa, G., Akasaki, S., Hattori, M., and Joshizuka, N.,** Selective recovery of deranged water-holding properties by SC lipids, *J. Invest. Dermatol.,* 87, 758, 1986.
33. **Imokawa, G., Akasaki, S., Minematsu, G., and Kawai, M.,** Importance of intercellular lipids in water retention properties of the SC: induction and recovery study of surfactant dry skin, *Arch. Dermatol. Res.,* 281, 45, 1989.
34. **Fisher, L. B. and Maibach, H. I.,** Physical occlusion controlling epidermal mitosis, *J. Invest. Dermatol.,* 59, 106, 1972.

35. **Spector, A. A. and Yorek, M. A.,** Membrane lipid composition and cellular function, *J. Lipid Res.,* 26, 1015, 1985.
36. **Harada, K., Murakami, T., Yata, N., and Yamamoto, S.,** Role of intercellular lipids in SC in the percutaneous permeation of drugs, *J. Invest. Dermatol.,* 99, 278, 1992.
37. **Kano, T., Nakamura, M., Hashiguchi, A., Sadanaga, M., Morioka, T., Mishima, M., and Nakano, M.,** Skin pretreatments for shortening onset of dermal patch anesthesia with 3% GA MHPh 2 Na-10% lidocaine gel mixture, *Anesth. Analg.,* 75, 555, 1992.
38. **Simmonds, A. C. and Halsey, M. J.,** General and local anaesthetics perturb the fusion of phospholipid vesicles, *Biochim. Biophys. Acta,* 813, 331, 1985.
39. **Scheuplein, R. J. and Blank, I. H.,** Permeability of the skin, *Physiol. Rev.,* 51, 702, 1971.
40. **Liu, P., Kurihara-Bergstrom, T., and Good, W. R.,** Cotransport of estradiol and ethanol through human skin *in vitro:* understanding the permeant/enhancer flux relationship, *Pharm. Res.,* 8, 938, 1991.
41. **Liu, P., Higuchi, W. I., Song, W., Kurihara-Bergstrom, T., and Good, W. R.,** Quantitative evaluation of ethanol effects on diffusion and metabolism of beta-estradiol in hairless mouse skin, *Pharm. Res.,* 8, 865, 1991.
42. **Anon.,** Drug delivery systems: *in vitro* studies, (1993 Annual Meeting of the British Pharmaceutical Society), *Pharm. J.,* 251, 414, 1993.
43. **Berner, B., Mazzenga, G. C., Otte, J. H., Stephens, R. J., Juang, R.-H., and Ebert, C. D.,** Ethanol: water mutually enhanced transdermal therapeutic system. II. Skin permeation of ethanol and nitroglycerin, *J. Pharm. Sci.,* 78, 402, 1989.
44. **Goto, S., Uchida, T., Lee, C. K., Yasutake, T., and Zhang, J.-B.,** Effect of various vehicles on ketoprofen permeation across excised hairless mouse skin, *J. Pharm. Sci.,* 82, 959, 1993.
45. **Bommannan, D., Potts, R. O., and Guy, R. H.,** Examination of the effect of ethanol on human SC *in vivo* using infrared spectroscopy, *J. Control. Rel.,* 16, 299, 1991.
46. **Potts, R. O., Mak, V. H., Guy, R. H., and Francoeur, M. L.,** Strategies to enhance permeability via SC lipid pathways, *Adv. Lipid Res.,* 24, 173, 1991.

Chapter 15.4

Electroporation

Mark R. Prausnitz, Vanu G. Bose, Robert Langer, and James C. Weaver

CONTENTS

I. INTRODUCTION

Transdermal drug delivery offers many potential advantages over conventional methods of drug administration.[1–4] However, very few drugs can be administered transdermally at therapeutic levels, due to the low permeability of human skin. The remarkable barrier properties of skin are attributed primarily to the stratum corneum (SC), the skin's outer layer. The SC is a dead tissue composed of flattened cells filled with cross-linked keratin and an extracellular matrix made up of lipids arranged largely in bilayers.[5,6] Intercellular pathways are generally believed to be the most important routes for transdermal transport. Therefore, permeabilization of the lipid bilayers occupying these intercellular pathways would be expected to increase transdermal transport.

A number of chemical, electrical, and other approaches to enhance transport across skin have found varied success, as discussed elsewhere in this book. This chapter presents a novel approach to enhancement involving electroporation, an electrical phenomenon known to dramatically and reversibly alter lipid bilayer permeability. We examined the possibility of electroporating the intercellular lipid bilayers of the SC to enhance transdermal drug delivery. In a recent paper[7] we discussed skin electroporation in detail. Here, we provide a review of this topic, as well as more recent developments.

II. ELECTROPORATION OVERVIEW

Electroporation, which includes electropermeabilization, involves the creation of aqueous pathways in lipid bilayer membranes by the application of a brief electric

0-8493-2605-2/95/$0.00+$.50

field pulse.[8–12] Permeability and electrical conductance of lipid bilayers, such as cell membranes, are increased by many orders of magnitude. Moreover, the associated local electric field can contribute to transmembrane molecular transport by electrophoresis and/or electroosmosis. These membrane changes can persist for up to hours, but are reversible or irreversible, depending mainly on pulse magnitude and duration. Electroporation has been demonstrated in many different mammalian, plant, yeast, bacterial, and other cells, as well as in artificial planar and spherical membranes. Thus, electroporation appears to be universal in lipid bilayers, with onset largely independent of their exact composition or structure. Although the creation of transient aqueous pathways, or electropores, is the proposed mechanism by which electroporation occurs, the exact physical nature of an electropore and the possibility of imaging them by any form of microscopy remain unresolved.[8,10,11,13,14]

Electrical exposures typically involve square wave or exponential electric field pulses which generate transmembrane potentials of approximately 1 V and last 10 μs to 10 ms.[8–12] For lipid bilayers on the order of 10 nm thickness, this corresponds to a local field strength within the membrane of 10^6 V/cm. Based largely on electrical measurements, electropores are thought to be created on the submicrosecond time scale.[15–18] They then continue to grow in size for the duration of the electrical exposure. Maximum pore diameters are believed to occur up to 10 nm, although a distribution in sizes is expected.[19] After the pulse, pores are believed to shrink to a metastable state over a characteristic time of milliseconds.[20,21] These long-lived metastable pores are thought to be ~1 nm in radius.[22,23] Having lifetimes from subseconds to hours, these pores eventually disappear completely under reversible conditions. The onset of electroporation has been shown to occur largely independent of exact membrane composition and experimental conditions. However, the time scale of recovery is a strong function of conditions, especially temperature, where low temperature (i.e., 4°C) increases pore lifetimes.[8,10]

Although electroporation has been demonstrated under a variety of conditions, a range of electrical parameters exists for which electroporation is known to occur, and a smaller range exists for which electroporation is reversible. Both the magnitude and duration of the induced transmembrane voltage are important to the occurrence of electroporation. For example, electroporation generally occurs for short pulses (0.1 to 10 μs) which generate a transmembrane voltage slightly greater than 1 V, medium-length pulses (10 to 100 μs) of 0.5 to 1 V, and long pulses (≥1 ms) of 0.2 to 0.5 V.[24,25] Less work has been done on pulses shorter than 0.1 μs.

While electrical characterization of electroporation is important to mechanistic understanding, most applications have emphasized the ability of electroporation to increase molecular transport across lipid bilayers. Many different molecules have been transported across membranes by electroporation, ranging progressively in size from small ions to sugars to oligonucleotides to proteins to DNA to virus particles.[11] Electroporation has found widespread application in molecular biology as a method to introduce DNA into cells in suspension for gene transfection.[8,10] More recently, electroporation of cells in monolayers[26,27] and cells which are part of intact tissues[28–32] also was demonstrated. For example, electroporation of tumors as a method of increasing local cellular uptake of chemotherapeutic agents was applied recently to humans as part of a phase I trial in France.[33] The studies discussed in this chapter also deal with electroporation of tissue, namely skin.[7,34–38] However, in distinct contrast with other tissues in which cell membranes are electroporated, electroporation of skin appears to involve electroporation of the multilamellar, intercellular lipid bilayers of the SC.

III. SKIN ELECTROPORATION

This chapter discusses whether electroporation of the SC is possible, and whether it can be distinguished from conventional iontophoresis. Although both electroporation and iontophoresis involve electric fields, the two phenomena are fundamentally different. Iontophoresis acts primarily on the drug, moving molecules across skin by electrophoresis and/or electroosmosis. Any skin structural changes are a secondary effect. In contrast, electroporation is expected to cause transient, but large changes in tissue permeability, involving significant structural changes in the skin. The electric field is believed to cause transport by a combination of two mechanisms during electroporation: (1) electropores are created and (2) as pores appear, molecules are moved through the pores by electrophoresis and/or electroosmosis due to the local field.

A. MOLECULAR FLUX

To determine whether electroporation of the SC occurs, we subjected human cadaver epidermis under physiological conditions to electric pulses which cause electroporation in other systems. The experimental methods used were described previously.[7,38] Briefly, heat-stripped cadaver epidermis was loaded into side-by-side permeation chambers, exposed to well-stirred phosphate-buffered saline (PBS, pH 7.4), and allowed to hydrate fully (12 to 18 h, 4°C). The temperature was raised to 37°C and fresh PBS containing 1 m*M* fluorescent compound (calcein, Lucifer Yellow, or erythrosin derivative) was added to the outer, SC side. After a few hours, electric pulsing was applied with Ag/AgCl electrodes. An exponential pulse (decay time constant, τ=1.0 to 1.3 ms) was applied every 5 s for 1 h, with the negative electrode on the SC side unless otherwise noted. In presenting results we reported voltages across the skin rather than voltages across the electrodes because they are more relevant. The receptor compartment was sampled periodically by emptying its contents and replacing it with fresh PBS. Analysis by calibrated spectrofluorimetry allowed measurement of receptor compartment fluorescent compound concentrations, and thereby, calculation of time-average transdermal fluxes.

Quantitative measurements of transdermal molecular fluxes and electrical measurements are consistent with the three characteristic features of electroporation:[8–12] (1) large increases in molecular flux and ionic conductance, (2) reversibility over a range of voltages, where recovery has two time constants (millisecond and minute), and (3) structural changes in the membrane barrier.

First, transdermal fluxes of calcein (623 Da, – 4 charge), a moderate-sized, highly polar, fluorescent molecule which does not normally cross skin in detectable quantities, were measured during application of low duty cycle electric field pulses. Fluxes before pulsing were below the detection limit (imposed by background fluorescence), while fluxes during pulsing were up to 10,000-fold greater. Figure 1 shows that flux increased nonlinearly with increasing pulse voltage; i.e., the flux increased strongly with increasing voltage below ~100 V and increased weakly with

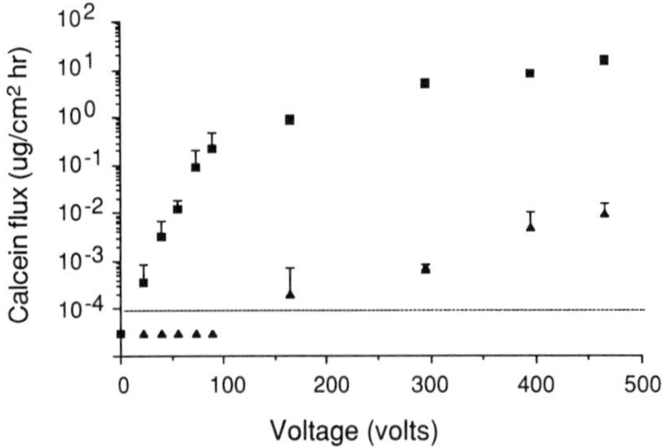

Figure 1 Transdermal fluxes of calcein due to exposure of human skin to different electrical conditions. Calcein flux during application of "forward-polarity" pulses (■) and approximately 1 h after pulsing in the "reverse" direction (see text) (▲). This figure suggests that a transition point may exist at ~100 V, below which flux increases as a strong function of voltage and flux increases are reversible, and above which flux increases only weakly with voltage and effects are only partially reversible. Standard deviation bars are shown. Fluxes below the calcein flux detection limit of 10^{-4} μg/cm²/h are indicated below the dashed line. (From Prausnitz, M. R. et al., *Proc. Natl. Acad. Sci. U.S.A.*, 90, 10504, 1993. With permission.)

increasing voltage at higher voltages. Supporting electrical measurements also showed increases in skin conductance of one to three orders of magnitude (see below).

Second, reversibility was assessed. Following electrical pulsing for 1 h, transdermal fluxes generally decreased by ~90% within 30 min and >99% within 1 or 2 h, consistent with significant reversibility. Electrical conductance measurements also showed recovery (see below). However, elevated postpulsing fluxes could be caused not only by irreversible alterations of skin structure, but also by the efflux of calcein "loaded" into the skin during high fluxes caused by pulsing.

The results of an additional, and possibly better, test of reversibility are also shown in Figure 1. Skin was pulsed with the electrode polarity reversed, leaving the transtissue voltage magnitude during pulsing the same. However, the reversed polarity electrophoretic driving force associated with the pulse should have moved calcein away from the skin, significantly reducing transdermal transport during pulsing. By measuring fluxes ~1 h after such reversed pulsing, long-lived changes in skin permeability can be assessed independently (Figure 1). These data suggest that pulses below ~100 V caused no detectable long-lived changes in skin permeability. However, higher voltage pulses appear to have caused lasting changes. Figure 1 also suggests that a transition region may exist at ~100 V, below which flux increased as a strong function of voltage, and flux increases were reversible; above which flux increased only weakly with voltage and effects were only partially reversible. The exact mechanism underlying this transition is presently unclear. However, for applications it is potentially important that up to 1000-fold flux increases which appear to be fully reversible can be achieved using pulses below ~100 V. The longer-lived changes associated with up to 10,000-fold flux increases may limit application of higher-voltage electroporation.

Third, changes in skin structure cannot be expected to be revealed by microscopy, for reasons discussed below. However, demonstrating that increased fluxes caused

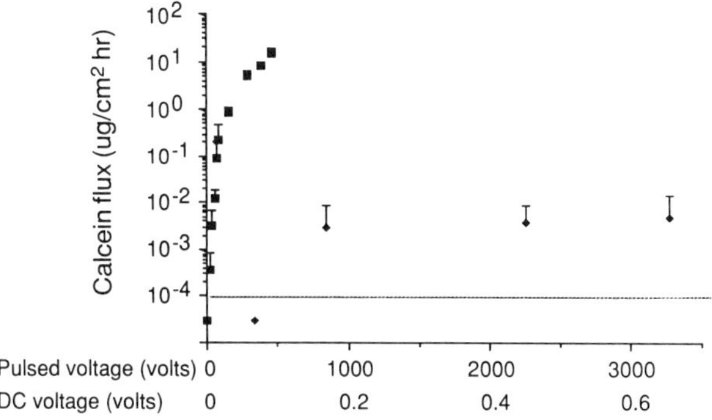

Figure 2 Transdermal fluxes of calcein during pulsing (■) and during application of DC iontophoresis (♦). Upper axis indicates pulsing voltages electrically "equivalent" to continuous DC voltages on lower axis (see text), suggesting that skin structural changes may be needed to explain the high fluxes caused by electroporation. Standard deviation bars are shown. Fluxes below the calcein flux detection limit are indicated below the dashed line. (From Prausnitz, M. R. et al., *Proc. Natl. Acad. Sci. U.S.A.*, 90, 10504, 1993. With permission.)

by pulsing cannot be explained by electrophoresis alone suggests that changes in skin structure are necessary to explain our results. We therefore compared fluxes caused by low duty cycle high-voltage pulsing to fluxes caused by the continuous low-voltage DC current which would provide the same total electrophoretic transport contribution if no changes in skin structure occurred. For example, if the skin were unaltered (i.e., same conductance), then constant application of 0.1 V would transfer the same amount of charge across the skin as the pulsed application of 500 V for 1 ms every 5 s, making these conditions "equivalent" electrophoretically. As seen in Figure 2, application of continuous voltages caused fluxes three orders of magnitude smaller than pulsing under "equivalent" conditions, suggesting that skin structural changes are needed to explain these results.

To appropriately characterize electroporation, we believe that measurement of changes in molecular flux and electrical properties is the best approach, because these measures are widely used in the electroporation literature. Upon initial consideration, electron microscopy might also appear to be an appropriate tool for visualizing the pores created by electroporation. However, currently no satisfactory electron micrographs of electropores in any membrane exist, primarily because electropores are believed to be small (<10 nm), sparse (<0.1% of surface area), and generally short-lived (μs to s). Thus, visualization of electropores by any form of microscopy is not expected.[14] Moreover, although the name "electroporation" suggests the creation of physical pores, all that has been experimentally established is that transiently elevated transport and electrical conductance occur. We therefore did not employ electron microscopy to look for pores in the complex multilaminate structures of the skin, as they have not been imaged in simpler systems.

Enhanced transport of two other polar molecules across the skin was achieved by electroporation: Lucifer Yellow (457 Da, –2 charge) and an erythrosin derivative (1025 Da, –1 charge), a small macromolecule, neither of which normally crosses skin at detectable levels. These molecules were selected because they are fluorescent and have different physical properties than calcein. As seen in Figure 3, pulsing can cause

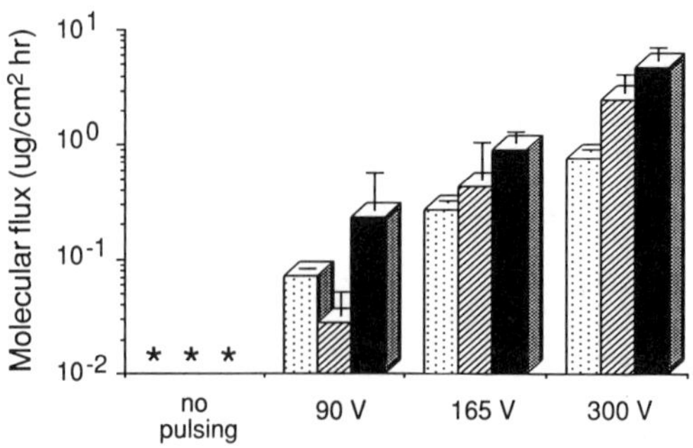

Figure 3 Transdermal fluxes of (▫) an erythrosin derivative (1025 Da, –1 charge), (▨) Lucifer Yellow (457 Da, –2 charge), and (▪) calcein across human skin *in vitro.* This figure demonstrates that electroporation increases the flux of a number of polar molecules having different molecular characteristics. Standard deviation bars are shown. The (*) symbol indicates a flux below the detection limit: 10^{-2} μg/cm²/h for the erythrosin derivative and 10^{-3} μg/cm²/h for Lucifer Yellow. (From Prausnitz, M. R. et al., *Proc. Natl. Acad. Sci. U.S.A.,* 90, 10504, 1993. With permission.)

fluxes of both molecules similar to those caused for calcein under the same conditions. This suggests that electroporation-enhanced transport may be broadly applicable to many molecules, possibly including those of larger molecular weights.

Finally, electroporation *in vivo* was performed on anesthetized hairless rats. Using protocols similar to those employed *in vitro,* electroporation at voltages ranging from 30 to 300 V caused transport of 10 to 20 μg/cm²/h.[7,38] No calcein was detected in the serum of unpulsed rats. That the *in vivo* fluxes did not increase with voltage suggests that a rate-limiting step other than transport across the SC existed, perhaps uptake of calcein from a skin depot into the bloodstream. No visible skin damage was observed after pulsing at voltages <150 V; erythema and edema were evident at higher voltages. Long-term biochemical and pathological studies are needed.

Together these results have implications for understanding mechanisms of skin electroporation and for applications to transdermal drug delivery. First, the three characteristic features of electroporation were found in pulsed skin, suggesting that electroporation is the mechanism of flux enhancement. Moreover, for applications, the marked flux increases which are reversible over a range of voltages could make possible the therapeutic delivery of many drugs across skin.

B. ELECTROPORATION AND IONTOPHORESIS

Studies have been performed by Tamada, Bommannan, and co-workers to assess flux increases due to iontophoresis following a single electroporation pulse and to compare them to fluxes by iontophoresis alone.[35,36] The experimental apparatus used was similar to that discussed above, involving heat-stripped human cadaver epidermis in side-by-side permeation chambers with saline buffered at pH 7.4. For electroporated samples, a single exponential-decay electric field pulse was applied (300 to 400 V, τ = 5 to 9 ms), followed by 10 to 60 min constant-current iontophoresis using Ag/AgCl electrodes. Passive flux was measured before and after electrical exposures. For iontophoresis-only control samples, the identical protocol was followed, except the high-voltage pulse was omitted.

The results of a study with luteinizing hormone-releasing hormone (LHRH, 1182 Da, +1 net charge) are shown in Figure 4. For iontophoresis-only samples, the flux

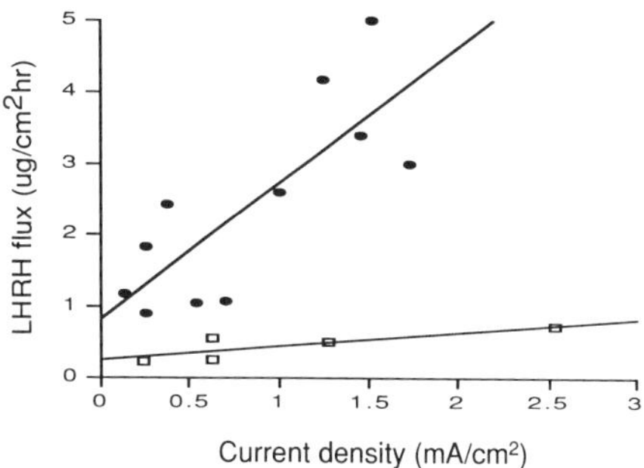

Figure 4 Transdermal transport of LHRH due to iontophoresis following a single electroporation pulse (•) and iontophoresis alone (□). See text for experimental protocols. Linear regressions are shown. This figure shows that application of a single electroporation pulse before iontophoresis can significantly increase the flux of LHRH relative to iontophoresis alone. (Data from Bommannan, D. et al., *Proc. Int. Symp. Control. Rel. Bioact. Mater.*, 20, 97, 1993.)

increased with increasing current density. However, for the samples exposed to iontophoresis at the same current density, following a single electroporation pulse, LHRH was transported to a significantly greater extent. Moreover, within several hours after the electrical exposure, fluxes decreased substantially and were close to pretreatment levels. Similar results have been shown for [arg^8]-vasopressin (1084 Da, +2 net charge) and neurotensin (1693 Da, +1 net charge), in which flux increases due to electroporation followed by iontophoresis were three to eight fold greater than iontophoresis alone.

These results demonstrate that the enhancement due to electroporation and iontophoresis can be combined, making an even more powerful approach to transdermal drug delivery than either one alone. Moreover, the additional enhancement of peptide transport across the skin due to electroporation may lead to noninvasive, controlled delivery of peptides at therapeutic levels. These results show that a single electroporation pulse increased the effects of iontophoresis for many minutes after the pulse, but appeared to reverse after hours. This indicates that a lasting change in skin properties occurred and is consistent with transient structural changes.

C. ELECTRICAL ANALYSIS

Skin electrical properties have been extensively characterized.[39–42] Changes in skin impedance have been reported in response to a wide range of physical and emotional stimuli, exhibiting significant intersubject variability. The most commonly used electrical model for skin is the parallel combination of a resistor (~100 kΩ cm^2) and a capacitor (~10 nF/cm^2). More complicated models were proposed in which the choice of model is determined by the skin substructures of interest and the relevant frequency range. However, these linear models are valid only over a small voltage range (<1 V), above which the electrical properties of skin are nonlinear.[43–45]

To study changes in skin impedance due to electroporation, skin was prepared and loaded into permeation chambers as in the molecular flux experiments. Measurement and analysis of skin electrical properties were done as described previously.[37] Briefly, an exponential voltage pulse was applied across the chamber. Current during the pulse was obtained by measuring the voltage across a 5-Ω sampling resistor placed in series with the chamber, while the voltage across the skin was measured using two

Ag/AgCl electrodes placed near the skin. Impedance spectra were measured before and after pulsing by applying current steps ranging from 0.1 to 2 μA to the outer electrodes of a four-electrode measurement system. The voltage developed at the inner electrodes was measured by a high impedance differential amplifier and digitized by a PC-based data acquisition system. The data were later analyzed to determine the skin impedance as a function of frequency. The impedance spectra were then fit to the most statistically significant electric circuit model, which consisted of the typical parallel R-C circuit, modified by placing a series R-C circuit in parallel with it. The series R-C is a lumped approximation of the high-frequency properties of skin. This approximation provides a more accurate representation of skin electrical properties over the relevant frequency range (less than a few kilohertz).[37] Impedance measurements were made before the pulse and at several times >20 ms after the pulse.

The saline on either side of the chamber had a resistance on the order of 100 Ω. Thus, the nominal charging time of the system (in the absence of nonlinear effects) would be on the order of 1 μs (i.e., charging time, $\tau = RC = 100\ \Omega \times 10\ nF = 1\ \mu s$). If skin electrical properties remained unchanged during a pulse (i.e., $R = 10^5\ \Omega$ and $C = 10\ nF$), current after the microsecond charging time would be 1 to 5 mA for typical pulses of 100 to 500 V across the skin. However, currents of 500 to 4000 mA were measured under these conditions (data not shown). The three order of magnitude difference between predicted and measured currents suggests that skin electrical properties underwent dramatic changes on the time scale of a microsecond. This result is supported by measurements made near the end of the pulse, where effective skin resistances on the order of 100 Ω were determined. This was done by assuming a linear circuit model is valid because the voltage is nearly constant at the end of the pulse.

For transdermal voltages <100 V, the impedance spectrum measured 20 ms after the pulse was identical to the prepulsing impedance. This suggests that within milliseconds the skin had recovered fully from the changes induced during pulsing. At higher voltages a threshold appeared, above which lasting changes in impedance were evident. This threshold was between 200 and 300 V, depending on the particular sample. Figure 5A shows the impedance of a representative skin sample before pulsing, and at three different times after pulsing. The most significant change in the impedance was the resistance (impedance at 0 Hz), which was determined by evaluating the DC impedance of the fitted model. Resistance after a pulse is plotted as a function of time in Figure 5B. This curve has three characteristic time constants: one <20 ms (between the pulse and the first impedance measurement), one between 5 and 20 s, and the third between 50 and 200 s. Resistance returned to 5 to 100% of its prepulse value, depending on pulsing voltage and the sample used. Incomplete recovery indicates that some permanent changes in skin structure occurred.

These results are consistent with three important features of electroporation:

1. Changes in skin electrical properties of several orders of magnitude occurred on a time scale of microseconds. Although changes in skin electrical properties also occur in iontophoresis (i.e., exposure at a few volts over longer times), skin resistance decreases by only up to one order of magnitude on the time scale of minutes. This is a seven order of magnitude difference in time scale.

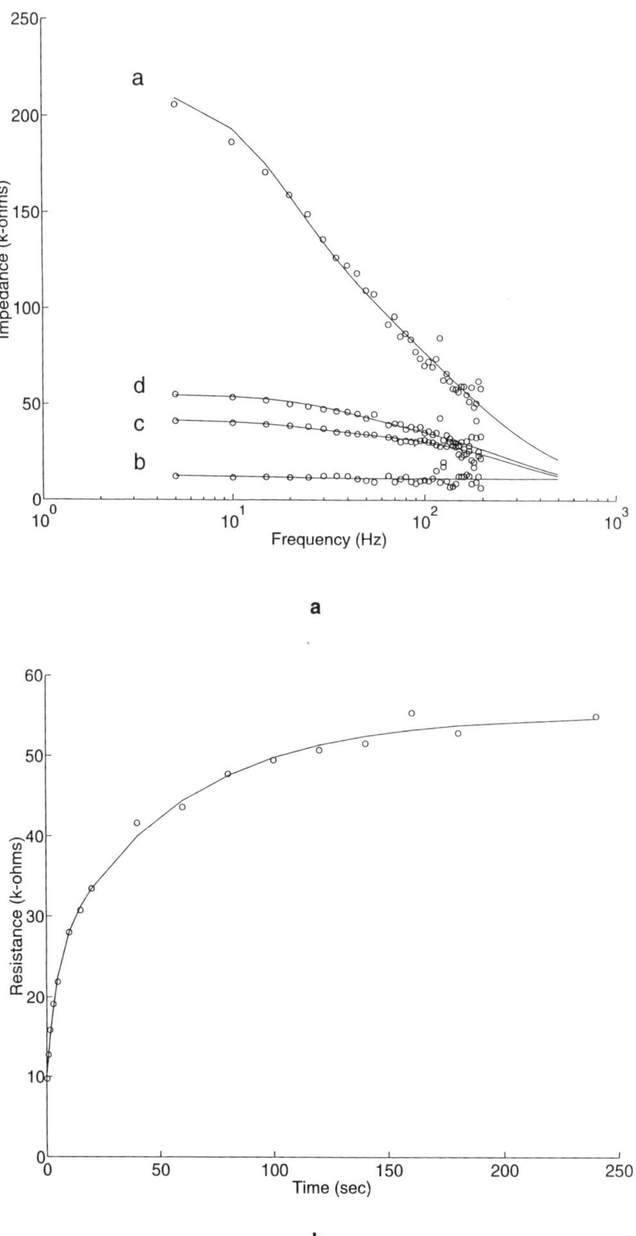

Figure 5 (A) Impedance spectra of a representative skin sample before pulsing at 210 V (a), and at 800 ms (b), 40 s, (c) and 4 min (d) after pulsing. The impedance "recovered" toward its prepulse value over time. (B) Resistance of the skin after pulsing, calculated from impedance spectra. Prepulse resistance was 220 kΩ; 20 ms postpulse the resistance was 20-fold lower. The resistance recovery was characterized by three time constants: <20 ms (between the pulse and the first impedance measurement), 5 s, and 57 s for the data shown.

2. Apparently, a threshold of a few hundred volts exists, below which long-lasting electrical changes in skin are not seen. Assuming a few hundred bilayers lie in a cross-section of SC, the observed electroporation threshold of a few hundred volts would be expected because the literature shows that the electroporation threshold for a single lipid bilayer is on the order of 1 V.[8–12]
3. A range of voltages exists over which changes in electrical properties are fully reversible and above which the changes are only partially reversible. The existence of these two ranges is consistent with electroporation in other systems.[8–12]

IV. DISCUSSION

A. ELECTROPORATION MECHANISM

It is well established that the SC is the primary barrier to transdermal transport;[1–4] thus, our interpretation is that changes in the SC account for the observed increases in flux due to electroporation. Although studied mainly in the context of living cells, electroporation also has been investigated widely in artificial planar bilayer membranes and liposomes.[8–12,23] Because electroporation is a physical process based on electrostatic interactions and thermal fluctuations within fluid membranes, no active transport processes are involved.[8–12] Thus, electroporation could occur in the SC, even though it does not contain living cells.

"Proving" that electroporation occurs in skin cannot be done. In the literature electroporation is described experimentally as characteristic behavior (e.g., very large increases in molecular transport and conductance in lipid bilayers), occurring at characteristic voltages (e.g., approximately 1 V across a bilayer), and over characteristic times (e.g., submicrosecond onset and biphasic recovery over milliseconds and minutes). Although the mechanisms by which these events occur (e.g., creation of aqueous pores, called electropores) are plausible, these mechanisms are hypotheses; electropores have not been experimentally observed by imaging. Therefore, an experimental investigation of skin electroporation should establish whether phenomena similar to those observed in cell electroporation occur in skin as well.

The above experiments demonstrate very large increases in transdermal flux, which are reversible over a range of conditions and appear to be associated with structural changes. These results were seen with six different molecules having molecular weights up to approximately 1700 Da. Similar results were observed *in vivo* with animal skin. Electrical analysis showed dramatic electrical changes occurring within 1 μs and recovery with millisecond and second time constants. Our interpretation is that these experimental results exhibit the characteristic behavior of electroporation. We therefore conclude that electroporation of skin has occurred.

B. DRUG DELIVERY APPLICATIONS

Although electroporation causes large flux increases across the SC, deeper viable tissue may be essentially unaffected. This localization is expected because the SC has a much higher electrical resistance than other regions of the skin. As a result, an electric field applied to the skin will concentrate in the SC, resulting in other, viable tissues being exposed to much lower fields. Therefore, an electric field sufficient to cause electroporation could exist in the SC, while a significantly lower field exists in viable tissues, insufficient to cause electroporation. An implicit targeting mechanism results in which the greatest electric fields are generated where the largest resistivities exist, thereby protecting the already-permeable viable parts of the skin and deeper tissues.

It is presently difficult to state with certainty which electrical conditions will be acceptable for clinical use. Many features, including pulse voltage/current/energy, pulse length, pulse frequency, duration of total exposure, and electrode size, site, and design, will be important. A complete consideration of the safety of electroporation of skin is beyond the scope of this study. However, that the electrical exposures used were fully reversible over a range of voltages is a strong indication that the procedure is not damaging and may be safe. Moreover, a clinical precedent has been set for safely applying electric pulses to skin with voltages up to hundreds of volts and durations up to milliseconds. Such diagnostic and therapeutic applications include transcutaneous electrical nerve stimulation, functional electrical stimulation, electromyography, and somatosensory evoked potential testing.[46,47]

Because of the overall hydrophobic character and net negative charge of the SC, transdermal transport of negatively charged hydrophilic molecules is especially challenging.[1–4] Calcein, with eight charge sites and a net charge of –4,[48] is therefore considerably more difficult to transport across the skin than many other molecules. Approaches to transdermal flux enhancement involving chemical enhancers have been successful with some lipophilic and moderately polar molecules, but limited in applicability to highly polar and charged molecules. Iontophoresis was employed successfully with some polar and charged molecules. For many drugs, delivery rates in the microgram per square centimeter per hour range could be therapeutic, while significantly higher rates of delivery may be required for other drugs. In general, a 10-fold increase in flux caused by an enhancement method is impressive, while a 100-fold increase is of great interest. Thousand-fold increases are rarely found. The up to 10,000-fold increases in flux caused by electroporation are therefore potentially very significant and could make possible transdermal delivery of many drugs at therapeutic levels.

Finally, transdermal flux enhancement has been demonstrated with other techniques, including chemical, iontophoretic, and ultrasonic methods. Because electroporation is mechanistically different, involving temporary alterations of skin structure, it could be used in combination with these or other enhancers. Together, these results suggest that electroporation of skin occurs and may be useful to enhance transdermal drug delivery.

ACKNOWLEDGMENT

This work was supported in part by Cygnus Therapeutic Systems (M. R. P., V. G. B., and J. C. W.), Army Research Office Grant DAAL03-90-G-0218 (V. G. B. and J. C. W.), and National Institutes of Health Grants GM34077 (J. C. W.) and GM44884 (R. L.).

REFERENCES

1. **Bronaugh, R. L. and Maibach, H. I., Eds.,** *Percutaneous Absorption, Mechanisms Methodology Drug Delivery,* Marcel Dekker, New York, 1989.
2. **Hadgraft, J. and Guy, R. H., Eds.,** *Transdermal Drug Delivery: Developmental Issues and Research Initiatives,* Marcel Dekker, New York, 1989.

3. **Champion, R. H., Burton, J. L., and Ebling, F. J. G., Eds.,** *Textbook of Dermatology,* Blackwell Scientific, London, 1992.
4. **Cullander, C. and Guy, R. H.,** Transdermal delivery of peptides and proteins, *Adv. Drug Deliv. Rev.,* 8, 291, 1992.
5. **Bouwstra, J. A., Vries, M. A. D., Gooris, G. S., Bras, W., Brussee, J., and Ponec, M.,** Thermodynamic and structural aspects of the skin barrier, *J. Control. Rel.,* 15, 209, 1991.
6. **Elias, P. M.,** Epidermal barrier function: intercellular lamellar lipid structures, origin, composition and metabolism, *J. Control. Rel.,* 15, 199, 1991.
7. **Prausnitz, M. R., Bose, V. G., Langer, R., and Weaver, J. C.,** Electroporation of mammalian skin: a mechanism to enhance transdermal drug delivery, *Proc. Natl. Acad. Sci. U.S.A.,* 90, 10504, 1993.
8. **Neumann, E., Sowers, A. E., and Jordan, C. A., Eds.,** *Electroporation and Electrofusion in Cell Biology,* Plenum Press, New York, 1989.
9. **Tsong, T. Y.,** Electroporation of cell membranes, *Biophys. J.,* 60, 297, 1991.
10. **Chang, D. C., Chassy, B. M., Saunders, J. A., and Sowers, A. E., Eds.,** *Guide to Electroporation and Electrofusion,* Academic Press, New York, 1992.
11. **Orlowski, S. and Mir, L. M.,** Cell electropermeabilization: a new tool for biochemical and pharmacological studies, *Biochim. Biophys. Acta,* 1154, 51, 1993.
12. **Weaver, J. C.,** Electroporation: a general phenomenon for manipulating cells and tissues, *J. Cell. Biochem.,* 51, 426, 1993.
13. **Chang, D. C. and Reese, T. S.,** Changes in membrane structure induced by electroporation as revealed by rapid-freezing electron microscopy, *Biophys. J.,* 58, 1, 1990.
14. **Weaver, J. C.,** Electroporation: a dramatic nonthermal electric field phenomenon, in *Electricity and Magnetism in Biology and Medinine,* Blank, M., Ed., San Francisco Press, San Francisco, 1993, 95.
15. **Benz, R. F., Beckers, F., and Zimmermann, U.,** Reversible electrical breakdown of lipid bilayer membranes: a charge-pulse relaxation study, *J. Membr. Biol.,* 48, 181, 1979.
16. **Serpersu, E. H., Kinosita, K., and Tsong, T. Y.,** Reversible and irreversible modification of erythrocyte membrane permeability by electric field, *Biochim. Biophys. Acta,* 812, 770, 1985.
17. **Hibino, M., Shigemori, M., Itoh, H., Nagayama, K., and Kinosita, K., Jr.,** Membrane conductance of an electroporated cell analyzed by submicrosecond imaging of transmembrane potential, *Biophys. J.,* 59, 209, 1991.
18. **Neumann, E., Werner, E., Sprafke, A., and Kruger, K.,** Electroporation phenomena. Electrooptics of plasmid DNA and of lipid bilayer vesicles, in *Colloid and Molecular Electro-optics 1992,* Jennings, B. R. and Stoylov, S. P., Eds., IOP Publishing, Bristol, U.K., 1992.
19. **Barnett, A. and Weaver, J. C.,** A unified, quantitative theory of reversible electrical breakdown and rupture, *Bioelectrochem. Bioenerg.,* 25, 163, 1991.
20. **Chernomordik, L. V., Sukharev, S. I., Abidor, I. G., and Chizmadzhev, Y. A.,** Breakdown of lipid bilayer membranes in an electric field, *Biochim. Biophys. Acta,* 736, 203, 1983.
21. **Kinosita, K., Jr., Hibino, M., Itoh, H., Shigemori, M., Hirano, K., Kirino, Y., and Hayakawa, T.,** Events of membrane electroporation visualized on a time scale from microsecond to seconds, in *Guide to Electroporation and Electrofusion,* Chang, D. C., Chassy, B. M., Saunders, J. A., and Sowers, A. E., Eds., Academic Press, New York, 1992, 29.
22. **Glaser, R. W., Leikin, S. L., Chernomordik, L. V., Pastushenko, V. F., and Sokirko, A. I.,** Reversible electrical breakdown of lipid bilayers: formation and evolution of pores, *Biochim. Biophys. Acta,* 940, 275, 1988.
23. **Abidor, I. G., Arakelyan, V. B., Chernomordik, L. V., Chizmadzhev, Y. A., Pastushenko, V. F., and Tarasevich, M. R.,** Electric breakdown of bilayer membranes. I. The main experimental facts and their qualitative discussion, *Bioelectrochem. Bioenerg.,* 6, 37, 1979.
24. **Benz, R. and Zimmermann, U.,** Relaxation studies on cell membranes and lipid bilayers in the high electric field range, *Bioelectrochem. Bioenerg.,* 7, 723, 1980.
25. **Neumann, E.,** The relaxation hysteresis of membrane electroporation, in *Electroporation and Electrofusion in Cell Biology,* Neumann, E., Sowers, A. E., and Jordan, C. A., Eds., Plenum Press, New York, 1989, 61.
26. **Kwee, S., Nielsen, H. V., and Celis, J. E.,** Electropermeabilization of human cultured cells grown in monolayers, *Bioelectrochem. Bioenerg.,* 23, 65, 1990.

27. **Raptis, L. and Firth, K. L.,** Electroporation of adherent cells in situ, *DNA Cell Biol.,* 9, 615, 1990.
28. **Okino, M. and Mohri, H.,** Effects of a high voltage electrical impulse and an anticancer drug on *in vivo* growing tumors, *Jpn. J. Cancer Res.,* 78, 1319, 1987.
29. **Powell, K. T., Morgenthaler, A. W., and Weaver, J. C.,** Tissue electroporation: observation of reversible electrical breakdown in viable frog skin, *Biophys. J.,* 56, 1163, 1989.
30. **Mir, L. M., Orlowski, S., Belehradek, J., and Paoletti, C.,** Electrochemotherapy: potentiation of antitumor effect of bleomycin by local electric pulses, *Eur. J. Cancer,* 27, 68, 1991.
31. **Titomirov, A. V., Sukharev, S., and Kistanova, E.,** *In vivo* electroporation and stable transformation of skin cells of newborn mice by plasmid DNA, *Biochim. Biophys. Acta,* 1088, 131, 1991.
32. **Salford, L. G., Persson, B. R. R., Brun, A., Ceberg, C. P., Kongstad, P. C., and Mir, L. M.,** A new brain tumour therapy combining bleomycin with *in vivo* electropermeabilization, *Biochem. Biophys. Res. Commun.,* 194, 938, 1993.
33. **Mir, L. M., Belehradek, M., Domenge, C., Orlowski, S., Poddevin, B., Belehradek, J., Schwaab, G., Luboinski, B., and Paoletti, C.,** Electrochemotherapy, a novel antitumor treatment: first clinical trial, *C. R. Acad. Sci. Ser. III,* 313, 613, 1991.
34. **Prausnitz, M. R., Bose, V. G., Langer, R., and Weaver, J. C.,** Transdermal drug delivery by electroporation, *Proc. Int. Symp. Control. Rel. Bioact. Mater.,* 19, 232, 1992.
35. **Bommannan, D., Leung, L., Tamada, J., Sharifi, J., Abraham, W., and Potts, R.,** Transdermal delivery of luteinizing hormone releasing hormone: comparison between electroporation and iontophoresis *in vitro, Proc. Int. Symp. Control. Rel. Bioact. Mater.,* 20, 97, 1993.
36. **Tamada, J., Sharifi, J., Bommannan, D. B., Leung, L., Azimi, N., Abraham, W., and Potts, R.,** Effect of electroporation on the iontophoretic delivery of peptides *in vitro, Pharm. Res.,* 10, S-257, 1993.
37. **Bose, V. G.,** Electrical Characterization of Electroporation of Human SC, M.S. thesis, Massachusetts Institute of Technology, Cambridge, 1994.
38. **Prausnitz, M. R., Seddick, D. S., Kon, A. A., Bose, V. G., Frankenburg, S., Klaus, S. N., Langer, R., and Weaver, J. C.,** Methods for *in vivo* tissue electroporation using surface electrodes, *Drug Deliv.,* 1, 125, 1993.
39. **Horton, J. W. and Ravenswaay, A. C. V.,** Electrical impedance of the human body, *J. Franklin Inst.,* 220, 557, 1935.
40. **Yamamoto, T. and Yamamoto, Y.,** Non-linear electrical properties of skin in the low frequency range, *Med. Biol. Eng. Comput.,* 19, 302, 1981.
41. **Rosell, J., Colominas, J., Riu, P., Pallas-Areny, R., and Webster, J. G.,** Skin impedance from 1 Hz to 1 MHz, *IEEE Trans. Biomed. Eng.,* 35, 649, 1988.
42. **Geddes, L. A. and Baker, L. E.,** *Principles of Applied Biomedical Instrumentation,* 3rd ed., John Wiley & Sons, New York, 1989.
43. **Stephens, W. G. S.,** The current-voltage relationship in human skin, *Med. Electron. Biol. Eng.,* 1, 389, 1963.
44. **Kasting, G. B. and Bowman, L. A.,** DC electrical properties of frozen, excised human skin, *Pharm. Res.,* 7, 134, 1990.
45. **Sims, S. M., Higuchi, W. I., and Srinivasan, V.,** Skin alteration and convective solvent flow effects during iontophoresis. II. Monovalent anion and cation transport across human skin, *Pharm. Res.,* 9, 1402, 1992.
46. **Webster, J. G., Ed.,** *Encyclopedia of Medical Devices,* John Wiley & Sons, New York, 1988.
47. **Reilly, J. P.,** *Electrical Stimulation and Electropathology,* Cambridge University Press, New York, 1992.
48. **Furry, J. W.,** Preparation, Properties and Applications of Calcein in a Highly Pure Form, Ph.D. thesis, Iowa State University, Ames, 1985.

Chapter 15.5

The Use of Ion Pairing to Facilitate Percutaneous Absorption of Drugs

Sybille Matschiner, Reinhard Neubert, and Wolfgang Wohlrab

CONTENTS

I. INTRODUCTION

Ion pairing has long been known to facilitate the transport of charged drugs through lipophilic barriers such as artificial or biological membranes. The concept of ion pairing was first introduced by Bjerrum[1] in 1926 to explain the decrease in electrical conductance of sodium chloride in liquid ammonia. It was developed further by Sadek and Fuoss,[2] Winstein et al.,[3] and Diamond.[4] Since that time, ion pairing, or the complexation between cations and anions, has been widely used in analytical chemistry as an extraction method,[5] in chromatography,[6] and as a tool to study the penetration of ionized molecules through artificial and biological membranes.[7] Lippold,[8] Jonkman and Hunt,[9] and Neubert[10] reviewed the literature on ion pair transport and made important contributions to the pharmaceutical application of ion pairs. Jonkman and Hunt[9] questioned the validity of the ion pair concept for the gastrointestinal absorption of drugs.

In this chapter the ion pair hypothesis with respect to the topical route of drug delivery is discussed. This includes dermal and transdermal administration.

It is evident that the penetration through the lipophilic regions of the stratum corneum (SC) is the main route for percutaneous absorption of drugs. Therefore, only drugs with lipophilic properties can penetrate the SC. However, it is generally accepted that drugs in their nonionized form have better transport properties through biological membranes as compared to their more hydrophilic, ionized forms.[11] One way to overcome this adverse effect of ionization is the use of lipophilic counterions to form facilitate partitioning into and through the biological membranes. Schanker[12] proposed a hypothesis on ion pair absorption of ionized drugs. Special structural and solvation requirements are necessary for oppositely charged compounds to form a new species, the ion pair.[9] These ion pairs of interest are electrically neutral and usually have measurable lipid properties.[9] However, all investigations on the field of ion pairing emphasize that the ability of ion pair formation to influence the behavior of drugs depends strongly on the physicochemical properties of both: drug and counterion. Therefore, counterions with the following properties are needed:

0-8493-2605-2/95/$0.00+$.50

- high lipophilicity
- sufficient stability
- physiological compatibility
- metabolic stability

The possibility of improving the absorption and the pharmacokinetics of hydrophilic drugs as a result of ion pair formation and increased lipophilicity is still controversially discussed in the literature. Some authors reported that the transport of certain drugs was not affected by ion pair formation.[13] In contrast, the concept of ion pair transport was still not extensively used in the field of dermal and transdermal administration. However, the use of ion pair transport in this field has some advantages in comparison to oral administration. Both ions can be administered together in the vehicle so they can diffuse to the vehicle–skin interface. On the other hand, the SC can be pretreated with the counterion. Then the drug applied onto the skin can form ion pairs on the vehicle–skin interface. In both cases the ion pair is present at the interface and can diffuse through the skin down its concentration gradient.

II. ION PAIR TRANSPORT ACROSS ARTIFICIAL MEMBRANES

Several studies on ion pairing to facilitate percutaneous absorption of drugs were carried out using various *in vitro* models with artificial membranes and different lipids. The main model used was the rotating diffusion cell (RDC) introduced by Albery et al.[14] The lipophilic barrier in the RDC are membranes impregnated with isopropyl myristate (IPM). Baker and Hadgraft[15] used this model to show that the transport of methyl orange can be enhanced by some alkanol amines. Of the amines synthesized, a C_{18} alkyl chain length was found to be the optimum. The counterion was incorporated in the membrane.

In further studies Hadgraft and Wotton[16] investigated the Ethomeens, a group of ethoxylated tertiary amines derived from natural fats and oils, for their ability to facilitate percutaneous absorption of the model substance sodium salicylate. They used a pH gradient of 6 to 7.4, according to the physiological conditions for the topical administration and to provide the driving force. From a series of amines the authors identified Ethomeen S12 (bis-(2-hydroxyethyl)oleylamine) to be the best promoter for the transport of sodium salicylate.

On the other hand, Green et al.[17] investigated long-chain fatty acids for their use as counterions to facilitate the transdermal absorption of cationic drugs. Several β-adrenoreceptor blocking agents served as model drugs. The driving force in this investigation was a pH gradient in a direction opposite to that described above. The pH value of the donor was >7.4 and lay between the pK_a values of the drug and the counterion. Ion pairs could be formed on the donor–membrane interface and diffuse down their concentration gradient to the membrane–acceptor interface. The pH of the acceptor was about 7.4 so that the ion pair could dissociate into the single ions. The mechanism is shown in Figure 1.

Using the same mechanism, Azone® (1-dodecylazacycloheptan-2-one) was found to be capable of enhancing the transport of salicylate anions.[18] Even though Azone® is recognized as a penetration enhancer, the authors concluded that the effect on artificial membranes indicates the ability of Azone® to form ion pairs.

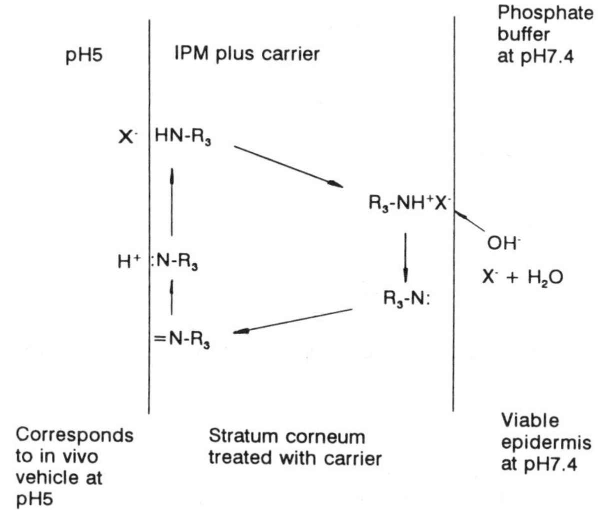

Figure 1 Proposed facilitated transport scheme. (From Hadgraft, H. et al., *J. Pharm. Pharmacol.*, 37, 725, 1985. With permission.)

Another possible mechanism for the ion pair transport is to administer both ions together in the vehicle (see Figure 2). Matschiner et al.[19] studied the dermal penetration of erythromycin in combination with various counterions into a lipophilic acceptor of a multilayer membrane system.[20] The top layer of the membranes was acidic, simulating the acid layer of the skin. Table 1 shows that long-chain alkylsulfonates increase the penetration into the lipophilic acceptor as they did for dodecylsulfate and hexylsalicylate. No effect was found with the counterions desoxycholate and octansulfonate. This is possibly due to a sterically or thermodynamically induced hindrance in the formation of ion pairs. Another expression might be that the lipophilicity of the ion pair with octansulfonate is too low for an enhancement in the penetration.

Gasco et al.[21] described the effect of carboxylic acids on the penetration of chlorpromazine through a dimethylpolysiloxane nonpolar membrane and found a possible ion pair formation. The effect varied among carboxylic acids, whereas oxaloacetic acid had the highest enhancement. The increase of the diffusion of substituted phosphonium salts in combination with chloramphenicol succinate through polyethylene membranes impregnated with buffer-saturated *n*-octanol was explained as ion pair diffusion.[22] In contrast, Ahmed et al.[13] investigated the influence of some bile salts on the transport of mequitazine across IPM membranes using RDC. The hypothesis that ion pairing may increase the transport of drugs is not supported by Ahmed et al.[13] Only by using the ion pair mequitazine–deoxycholate did they observe an increase in the transport rate. This is determined as an “anomalous increase” and explained by steric factors. Furthermore, they found that concentrations below the critical micelle concentration (CMC) of the bile salt slowly decreased the transport through the membrane. On the other hand, concentrations above the CMC decreased it markedly (Figure 3). They explained these results with the formation of unabsorbable or slowly absorbable ion pairs or complexes. Above the CMC of the bile salt the

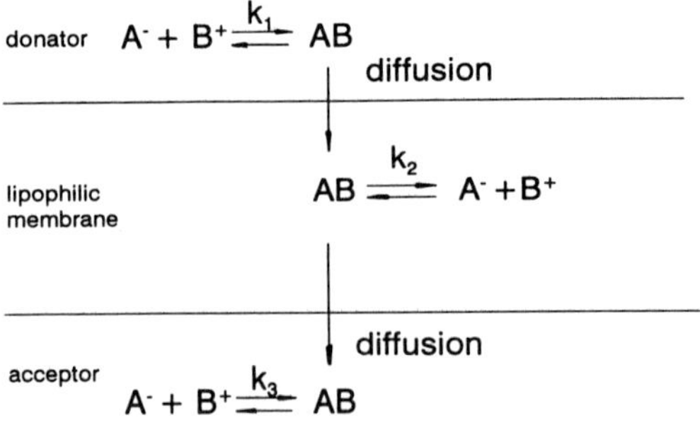

Figure 2 Possible scheme for ion-pair transport through membranes — application of drug and counterion.

Table 1 Penetration of Different Ion Pairs with Erythromycin into the Multilayer Membrane System

Counterion	Penetrated amount of erythromycin (%)
Octanesufonate	9.3 ± 2.1
Dodecansulfonate	14.7 ± 1.7
Tetradecansulfonate	21.2 ± 1.9
Octadecansulfonate	22.5 ± 4.4
Hexylsalicylate	17.2 ± 3.4
Dodecylsulfate	25.4 ± 5.8
Dehydrocholate	8.9 ± 1.9
Erythromycin	11.1 ± 2.8

Note: t = 60 min, mean ± S.D., n = 6, vehicle: 15% macrogolstearate, 10% propylene glycol, 75% glycerol.

decrease in the flux may be due to a formation of mixed micelles. The different complexes were not determined within this study.

Chen et al.[23] studied the effect of various inorganic ions on the partitioning of dyclonine ion pairs into phosphatidylcholine liposomes. They found an increase in the octanol–water partition coefficient and in the liposome uptake with increasing chain length of the alkane sulfonate used as a counterion. Lee et al.[24] carried out a study to determine the effect of taurodeoxycholate on the encapsulation efficiency of isopropamide iodide in large unilamellar liposomes. They concluded that the increased partitioning of isopropamide iodide into octanol and the increased encapsulation of the liposomes are due to ion pair formation of the substance with taurodeoxycholate and a solubilization of ion pairs in the phospholipid bilayer of liposomes.

To prove the results observed in artificial membranes, many investigators used excised human and animal skin. Only a marked change in drug properties upon ion pair formation measured can be expected to improve the penetration of hydrophilic ionizible drugs into and across skin.

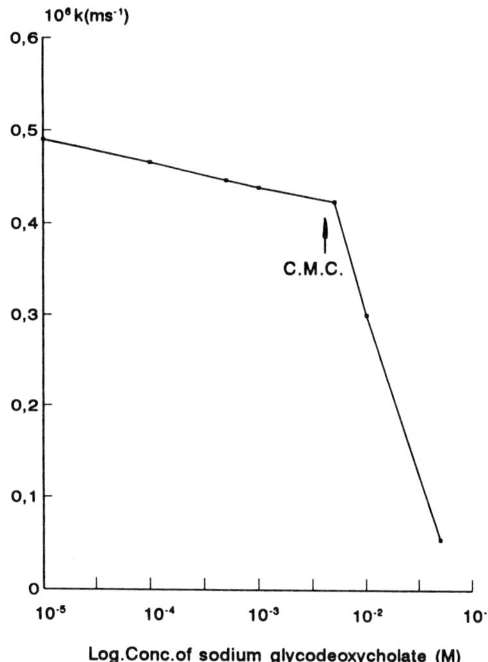

Figure 3 The effect of bile salt concentration on the transport rate of mequitazine hydrochloride across IPM. (From Ahmed, M. et al., *Int. J. Pharm.*, 12, 219, 1982. With permission.)

III. ION PAIR TRANSPORT ACROSS EXCISED SKIN

To evaluate the results on artificial membranes various studies were carried out on excised living skin, especially excised human skin. Oakley et al.[25] investigated the effects of ionization on the percutaneous absorption of drugs using the model compound nicotine. The partition of nicotine as a function of pH was studied in excised human SC, *n*-butanol, *n*-octanol, IPM and miglyol 812. A partitioning of ion pairs into the organic liquids and the SC was suspected. The counterion trichloracetate caused a ninefold increase in the lipophilicity with the organic lipids but not with the SC. The authors concluded that this suggests a fundamental difference in the partitioning of ion pairs into organic lipids and the SC. Another reason may be the low lipophilicity of the counterion in comparison to the lipids of the SC. Using van't Hoff plots for characterizing the partitioning of nicotine it was found that the nonionized form was in the lipid regions of the SC and the ionized form was in the aqueous region. Binding studies indicated that neither the nonionized nor the ionized species is bound significantly in the SC.

Kurihara-Bergstrom et al.[26] found an increased skin permeation of salicylate caused by ethanol–water systems. They explain it with alternations involving the polar pathway. Polar pathway alternations may occur in either or both the lipid polar head and proteinaceous regions of the SC. The authors also considered ion pair formation as making a contribution to increased permeation.

In further investigations[27] sulfate was demonstrated to enhance the terbutalin flux through human skin *in vitro*. It is proposed that this enhancement result is the combination of two actions: the isopropanol effects as penetration enhancer and the formation of ion pairs between terbutalin and sulfate. The overlapping of the two effects was described by Green et al.[28] They observed a more dramatic enhancement in the penetration of neutral caffeine and anionic salicylate through excised human skin with fatty acids. Because both molecules are unable to form ion pairs, the fatty acids are probably capable of exerting a disruptive influence on the skin. On the other hand, cationic drugs appeared to pass excised human skin more rapidly than predicted by the model membrane data. This may be due to ion pairing with free fatty acids or other anionic drugs within the skin or an effect on the membrane structure. The authors concluded that only a low enhancing ability of fatty acids could be found for neutral or anionic penetrants and that this indicates the ion pairing hypothesis. In further *in vitro* and *in vivo* investigations Green et al.[29] showed that oleic and linoleic acid increased the permeability of naphazoline, caffeine, and sodium salicylate through the SC. They concluded that fatty acids had a disruptive effect on the structure of the SC. Naphazoline penetration enhancement may additionally be caused by ion pair formation.

Hadgraft et al.[30] studied the enhancing effect on percutaneous absorption of Ethomeen S12-pretreated SC. (Ethomeen S12 is an amine found to be suitable for this purpose after investigations on artificial membranes.[16]) A significant increase in the permeation of salicylate could be achieved following pretreatment with the counterion. However, caffeine penetration was also enhanced by Ethomeen S12, indicating a nonspecific permeation. Although the enhancement of salicylate transport was much greater than that of caffeine, this result also indicates the overlapping of an ion pairing and a penetration-enhancing effect.

Nash et al.[31] studied the percutaneous absorption of lidocaine-*n*-alcanoate ion pairs through excised hairless mouse skin. Figure 4 indicates that the differences in flux between lidocaine and various ion pairs were significant.

Young et al.[32] found that *in vitro* percutaneous absorption of isopropamide iodide through hairless mouse skin was increased by sodium salicylate.

Investigations on the topical absorption of levobunolol, coupled to octanoic acid as lipophilic ion pair, through hairless mouse skin was shown to be higher than that of levobunolol alone.[33]

Studies on the penetration of indomethacin through hairless mouse skin at different pH values indicate ion pair formation as a mechanism for penetration of ionized indomethacin.[34,35] Benzalkonium chloride was shown to enhance the skin permeation rate of indomethacin significantly. Tan et al.[35] concluded that the differences in the rate of enhancement of several cationic agents were due to special structural and solvation requirements.

Langguth and Mutschler[36] measured the flux of tropsium chloride with and without sulfates and sulfonates as counter ions through human abdominal epidermis. Figure 5 indicates that the ion pair formation increases the flux significantly. The authors found that the lipophilicity of both series of ion pairs increased with the number of carbon ions, showing a maximum of seven carbon atoms in the alkyl chain length of the counterion. However, the relationship between lipophilicity and solubility of the ion pairs in the skin must be taken into consideration, especially for transdermal administration. The behavior of tropsium octansulfonate (Trsp.-8-SO_3 in Figure 5) is explained by the authors as an exception to the rule.

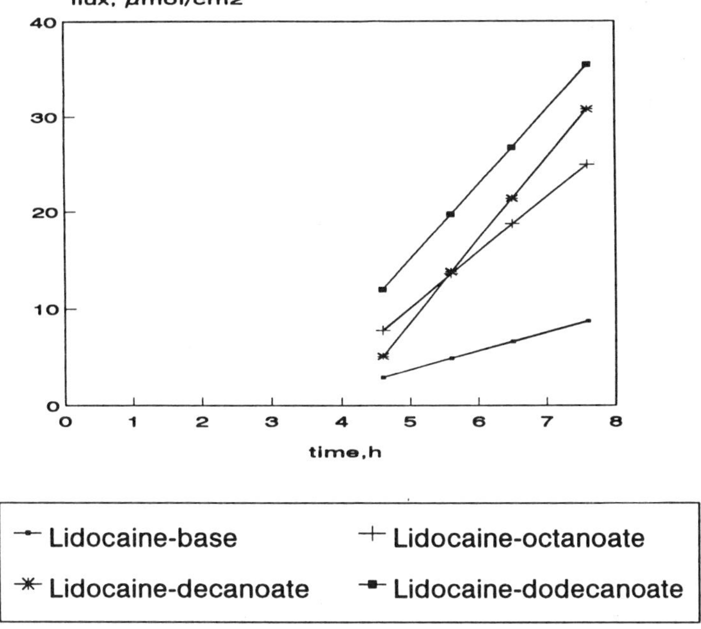

Figure 4 Percutaneous absorption of lidocaine base and lidocaine-*n*-alcanoate ion pairs from ethanolic solution under steady-state conditions through excised hairless mouse skin using normal saline as receptor fluid. The unidirectional vertical bars represent the standard deviation of each point. (From Nash, R. A. et al., *Skin Pharmacol.,* 5, 160, 1992. With permission.)

A study of the dermal penetration of erythromycin with octadecansulfonate as an ion pair into the sebaceous glands of excised human skin was carried out by Matschiner et al.[37] In this special case the sebaceous glands are the center of activity for erythromycin. The penetration of erythromycin into sebaceous glands can be doubly enhanced using the ion pair instead of the erythromycin-base alone (see Figure 6). Additionally, sufficient correlation was found between the results obtained on an adjusted multilayer membrane system and on excised human skin.

Young et al.[38] showed increased penetration of isopropamide iodide in combination with sodium salicylate through hydrated SC. They explained this effect with a possible ion pair formation between the two compounds.

All these investigations indicate that other than all the factors that influence percutaneous absorption using excised skin, damage to the membrane structure caused either by the drug or the counterion may play an important role. It would be greatly advantageous to separate this effect from the effect of ion pairing.

IV. ION PAIR TRANSPORT *IN VIVO*

Only a few studies were carried out to prove ion pair transport *in vivo* after topical administration. Ishikura et al.[39] measured the bioavailability of diltiazem hydrochloride after topical administration in rabbits with and without the counterion disodium chromoglycate. Increased bioavailability was found after combined application of both ions. The authors postulated that ionizable water-soluble drugs are absorbed

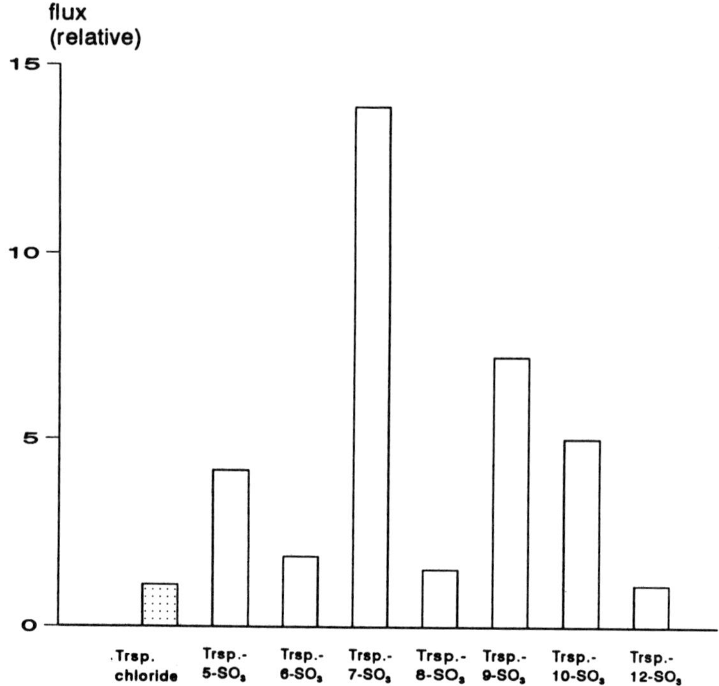

Figure 5 Transepidermal permeation of tropsium chloride and tropsium ion pairs through human epidermis at +32°C. The fluxes of the ion pairs are relative expressions (tropsium chloride = 1). (From Langguth, P. and Mutschler, E., *Arzneim. Forsch. Drug Res.,* 37, 1362, 1987. With permission.)

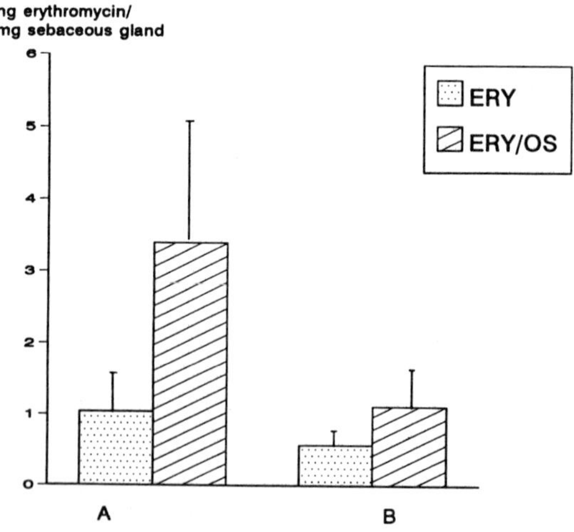

Figure 6 Penetration of erythromycin and the ion pair erythromycin–octadecansulfonate into the sebaceous glands of excised human skin. (A) Vehicle: 15% macrogolstearate, 10% propylene glycol, 75% glycerol. (B) Vehicle: 15% macrogolstearate, 10% propylene glycol, 3% zinc oxide, 72% glycerol. Mean ± S.D., n = 3. ERY = erythomycin, ERY/OS = ion pair between erythomycin and octadecansulfonate.

through the skin by forming fat-soluble ion pairs. Additionally, a decrease in the barrier function of the skin against absorption was found after the administration of nonelectrolytes. The nonelectrolytes must not hinder the formation of ion pairs.

Green et al.[29] investigated the effect of fatty acids on the skin permeation of different molecules and suggested that the enhanced flux of cationic naphazoline could be accounted for by an increase in lipophilicity through ion pairing. Disruptive changes in the structure of the SC were also taken into account.

Other *in vivo* studies of the enhancement of percutaneous absorption were confined to measurements of corneal penetration. An analysis of the aqueous humor of rabbits receiving topical timolol with octanoic acid as a lipophilic ion pair in a solution and in an oil-in-water microemulsion showed that the bioavailability of these drugs was 3.5 to 4.2 times higher in comparison to the oral administration of timolol alone (Gallarate et al.)[40]

Wilson et al.[41] investigated the absorption of sodium chromoglycate alone and in combination with dodecylbenzyl-dimethylammonium chloride in rabbits after corneal administration. For the ion pair system it was found that both ions were in the aqueous humor at 30 min in an approximately 10:1 ratio of dodecylbenzyl-dimethylammonium chloride:sodium chromoglycate. Neither ion could be found after single dosing of the ions.

V. DISCUSSION

All the examples above indicate the general possibility of ion pairing to facilitate the percutaneous absorption of drugs. Three methods explain the mechanism of this process:

1. Administration of the drug together with the counterion (see Figure 2)
2. Pretreatment of the SC with the counterion (see Figure 1)
3. Administration of only the drug and use of native substances in the SC for counterions

The problem in the first method is that the counterions used in these studies (e.g., fatty acids and alkylsulfonates) are mostly known to be penetration enhancers.[42] This means that these substances also influence the structure of the membrane in a way that the drug ion can better penetrate the SC. Thus, when a surfactant is considered for use as a counterion the following possibilities occur:[41]

The surfactant can act on the drug ion, leading to the formation of a ion pair
Micelles can be formed
The membrane system used can be modified in a way that permits passage of the drug (penetration enhancer)

Therefore, the key to the further application of the ion pair concept will be the search for specific lipophilic counterions for dermal as well as transdermal administration. Counterions necessary for dermal use must be able to interact with skin lipids in order to transport the drugs to the required location in the skin and to prevent transdermal absorption. In contrast, counterions to facilitate transdermal absorption of drugs should have well-defined hydrophilic/lipophilic properties to permit passage to the blood system.

One problem in most of the investigations of ion pair transport is that possible damage to the skin was not measured. Therefore, it cannot be exactly divided into the ion pairing effects and effects caused by changes in the SC structure. The decrease in absorption found by Ahmed et al.,[13] using mequitazine in combination with different surfactants, could be due to micelle formation. On the other hand, in order to explain the mechanism of ion pair transport it is necessary to measure the penetration of both drug and counterion. Wilson et al.[41] studied the penetration of both, and found an ratio of 10:1 counterion:drug 30 min after penetration. They concluded that either the extent or the rate of penetration (or both) is altered, or that the ocular clearance is affected by ion pair formation.

Nevertheless, to apply the advantages of ion pair transport to dermal and transdermal absorption of drugs, the physicochemical background of all connected processes must be investigated more deeply.

REFERENCES

1. **Bjerrum, N.,** *Kong. Danske Vidensk. Selk., Mat.-Fys. Medd.,* 7, 9, 1926, cited by Giebelmann, G., Ionenpaaranylytik. I., *Pharmazie,* 40, 507, 1985.
2. **Sadek, H. and Fuoss, R. M.,** Electrolyte-solvent interaction, *J. Am. Chem. Soc.,* 76, 5905, 1954.
3. **Winstein, S., Clippinger, F., Fainberg, A. M., and Robinson, G. C.,** Salt effects and ion-pairs in solvolysis, *J. Am. Chem. Soc.,* 76, 2597, 1954.
4. **Diamond, R. M.,** The aqueous solution behaviour of large univalent ions, *J. Phys. Chem.,* 77, 2513, 1963.
5. **Giebelmann, R.,** Ionenpaaranalytik. II., *Pharmazie,* 41, 748, 1986.
6. **Giebelmann, G.,** Ionenpaaranalytik. III., *Pharmazie,* 42, 44, 1987.
7. **Ritschel, W. A.,** *Handbook of Basic Pharmacokinetics,* 4th ed., Drug Intelligence Publications, Hamilton Press, Illinois, 1992, 62.
8. **Lippold, B. C.,** Ionenpaare — ihre Bildung, Bestimmung und Bedeutung, *Pharmazie,* 28, 713, 1973.
9. **Jonkman, J. H. G. and Hunt, C. A.,** Ion pair absorption of ionized drugs — fact or fiction, *Pharm. Wkbl. Sci. Ed.,* 5, 41, 1983.
10. **Neubert, R.,** Ion pair transport across membranes, *Pharm. Res.,* 6, 743, 1989.
11. **Cools, A. and Jansen, L.,** Influence of sodium ion-pair formation on transport kinetics of warfarin through octanol impregnated membranes, *J. Pharm. Pharmacol.,* 35, 689, 1983.
12. **Schanker, L. S.,** Physiological transport of drugs, in *Advances in Drug Research,* Harper, N. J. and Simmons, A. B., Eds., Academic Press, London, 1964, 71.
13. **Ahmed, M., Hadgraft, J., and Kellaway, I. W.,** The effect of bile salts on the interfacial transport of phenothiazines, *Int. J. Pharm.,* 12, 219, 1982.
14. **Albery, W. J., Bruke, J. F., Leffler, E. B., and Hadgraft, J.,** Interfacial transfer studies with a rotating diffusion cell, *J. Chem. Soc. Faraday Trans. I,* 72, 1618, 1976.
15. **Baker, N. and Hadgraft, J.,** Facilitated percutaneous absorption, a model system, *Int. J. Pharm.,* 8, 193, 1981.
16. **Hadgraft, J. and Wotton, P. K.,** Facilitated transport of anionic drugs across artificial lipid membranes, *J. Pharm. Pharmacol.,* 36, 22P, 1984.
17. **Green, P. G., Hadgraft, J., and Ridout, G.,** Enhanced *in vitro* skin permeation of cationic drugs, *Pharm. Res.,* 6, 628, 1989.
18. **Hadgraft, J., Walters, K. A., and Wotton, P. K.,** Facilitated transport of sodium salicylate across an artificial lipid membrane by Azone®, *J. Pharm. Pharmacol.,* 37, 725, 1985.
19. **Matschiner, S., Neubert, R., and Wohlrab, W.,** Optimisation of topical erythromycin formulations using ion pairing, accepted for publication.
20. **Neubert, R. and Wohlrab, W.,** *In vitro* methods for the biopharmaceutical evaluation of topical formulations, *Acta Pharm. Technol.,* 36, 197, 1990.
21. **Gasco, M. R., Trotta, M., and Carlotti, M. E.,** Effect of carboxylic acid on permeation of chlorpromazine through dimethyl polysiloxane membrane, *J. Pharm. Sci.,* 71, 239, 1982.
22. **Davis, S. S., Kinkel, K. F. M., Olejnik, O., and Tomlinson, E.,** Enhancement of drug transport by ion pair formation, *J. Pharm. Pharmacol.,* 3, 104, 1981.

23. **Chen, C. R., Zatz, J. L., and Reilly, E.,** Ion pairing of dyclonine with dyes, *Drug Dev. Ind. Pharm.,* 19, 1265, 1993.
24. **Lee, J. H., Shim, C. K., Lee, M. H., and Kim, S. K.,** Enhanced entrapment of isopropamide iodide in liposomes by ion pairing with sodium taurodeoxycholate, *Drug Dev. Ind. Pharm.,* 14, 451, 1988.
25. **Oakley, D. M. and Swarbrick, J.,** Effects of ionization on the percutaneous absorption of drugs: partitioning of nicotine into organic liquids and hydrated SC, *J. Pharm. Sci.,* 76, 866, 1987.
26. **Kurihara-Bergstrom, T., Knutson, K., De Nolte, L. J., and Goates, C. Y.,** Percutaneous absorption enhancement of ionic molecules by ethanol-water systems in human skin, *Pharm. Res.,* 7, 762, 1990.
27. **Kurihara-Bergstrom, T. and Liu, P.,** Enhanced *in vitro* skin transport of ionized terbutaline using its sulfate salt form in aqueous isopropanol, *S.T.P. Pharm. Sci.,* 1, 52, 1991.
28. **Green, P. G., Hadgraft, J., and Ridout, G.,** Enhanced *in vitro* skin permeation of cationic drugs, *Pharm. Res.,* 6, 628, 1989.
29. **Green, P. G., Guy, R. H., and Hadgraft, J.,** *In vitro* and *in vivo* enhancement of skin permeation with oleic and lauric acid, *Int. J. Pharm.,* 48, 103, 1988.
30. **Hadgraft, J., Green, P. G., and Wotton, P. K.,** Facilitated percutaneous absorption of charged drugs, in *Percutaneous Absorption,* 2nd ed., Bronaugh, R. L. and Maibach, H. I., Eds., Marcel Dekker, New York, 1989, 555.
31. **Nash, R. A., Metha, D. B., Matias, J. R., and Orentreich, N.,** The possibility of lidocaine ion pair absorption through excised hairless mouse skin, *Skin Pharmacol.,* 5, 160, 1992.
32. **Young, C. S., Shim, C. K., Lee, M. H., and Kim, S. K.,** Effects of sodium salicylate on *in vitro* percutaneous penetration of isopropamide iodide through mouse skin, *Int. J. Pharm.,* 45, 59, 1988.
33. **Gallarate, M., Gasco, M. R., Trotta, M., Chetoni, P., and Saettone, M. F.,** Preparation and evaluation *in vitro* of solutions and o/w microemulsions containing levobunolol as ion pair, *Int. J. Pharm.,* 100, 219, 1993.
34. **Tan, E. L., Liu, J. C., and Chien, W.,** Transdermal delivery of indomethacin. I. Permeation of ionized species, *Pharm. Res.,* 6, S-171, 1989.
35. **Tan, E. L., Liu, J. C., and Chien, W.,** Transdermal delivery of indomethacin. II. Involvement of an apparent ion pairing phenomenon, *Pharm. Res.,* 6, S-168, 1989.
36. **Langguth, P. and Mutschler, E.,** Lipophilisation of hydrophilic compounds, *Arzneim-Forsch. Drug Res.,* 37, 1362, 1987.
37. **Matschiner, S., Neubert, R., Wohlrab, W., and Matschiner, F.,** Influence of ion pairing on the penetration of erythromycin into sebaceous glands, *Br. J. Dermatol.,* in preparation.
38. **Young, C. S., Shim, C. K., Lee, M. H., and Kim, S. K.,** Effect of sodium salicylate on *in vitro* percutaneous penetration of isopropamide iodide through mouse skin, *Int. J. Pharm.,* 45, 59, 1988.
39. **Ishikura, T., Nagai, T., Sasai, Y., and Shishikura, T.,** Enhanced percutaneous absorption of ionizable water-soluble drugs, *Drug Des. Deliv.,* 1, 285, 1987.
40. **Gallarate, M., Gasco, M. R., and Trotta, M.,** Influence of octanoic acid on membrane permeability of timold from solutions and from microemulsions, *Acta. Pharm. Technol.,* 34, 102, 1988.
41. **Wilson, C. G., Tomlinson, E., Davis, S. S., and Oleijnik, O.,** Altered ocular absorption and disposition of sodium chromoglycate upon ion pair and complex cocervate formation with dodecylbencyldimethylammonium chloride, *J. Pharm. Pharmacol.,* 31, 749, 1981.
42. **Barry, B. W.,** Mode of action of penetration enhancers in human skin, *J. Control. Rel.,* 6, 85, 1989.

Chapter 16.1

Raman Spectroscopy

Adrian C. Williams and Brian W. Barry

CONTENTS

I. INTRODUCTION

The molecular basis for the barrier nature of stratum corneum (SC) is attracting much interest. Powerful analytical techniques including electron spin resonance spectroscopy[1] and X-ray diffractometry[2,3] have been employed recently to probe the nature of the SC. Some of the most useful data on the molecular composition and organization of SC constituents have been provided by Fourier transform (FT) infrared (FTIR) spectroscopy.[4–10] However, as a naturally hydrated tissue the SC can present difficulties for IR spectroscopic studies because water itself strongly absorbs IR radiation. In contrast, the Raman spectrum of water is weak, and hence Raman spectroscopy has been a technique of choice for the molecular characterization of a wide variety of biological systems.

II. THE RAMAN EFFECT

The Raman effect takes its name from the Indian scientist C. V. Raman, who, with his student, K. S. Krishnan, first obtained evidence for the modified scattering of light in February 1928. For his work, Raman received the Nobel Prize for Physics in 1930 and sparked an explosion of academic interest in the Raman effect. These early studies employed mercury arc lamps as the source of the exciting radiation, and the experimental techniques available dictated that severe limitations were placed on the samples that were suitable for analysis. However, over the last 30 years a renaissance in the use of the technique has been seen, mainly because of advances in instrumentation. In particular, lasers now provide a source of high energy monochromatic radiation which can be focused to a spot, computers permit repetitive scanning, and improvements in detector technology allow greater sensitivity of measurement. More recently, the advent of FT-Raman spectrometers and their commercialization provides

0-8493-2605-2/95/$0.00+$.50

relatively easy to use systems in benchtop forms. In addition to the well-known advantages of an interferometer-based system (as opposed to a dispersive instrument), FT-Raman systems excite samples via a laser operating at 1064 nm (in the near-IR region of the spectrum), which avoids some problems of sample fluorescence that may be encountered when employing a visible laser for sample excitation.

III. THEORETICAL ASPECTS OF RAMAN SPECTROSCOPY

When monochromatic radiation illuminates a compound, most of the radiation transmits unchanged, but a small portion scatters. If this scattered component passes into a spectrometer, a strong line is detected at the unmodified frequency of the radiation used to excite the sample (the Rayleigh line). The scattered radiation also contains frequencies arrayed above and below the frequency of the Rayleigh line. The differences between the Rayleigh line and these weaker Raman line frequencies correspond to the vibrational frequencies present in the excited molecules. The frequencies of these molecular vibrations are typically around 10^{13} Hz; a more convenient unit for analysis is the wavenumber (cm^{-1}), which is proportional to frequency.

The Raman lines are generally weak in intensity and hence their detection and measurement is difficult. Raman bands at wavenumbers less than the Rayleigh line are called Stokes lines and those at wavenumbers higher than the incident radiation are anti-Stokes lines. The Stokes lines are usually more intense than the anti-Stokes lines and so the Stokes portion of the spectrum is generally analyzed. The abscissa of the spectrum is usually labeled the wavenumber shift (cm^{-1}) and the negative sign (for Stokes shift) is usually dispensed with. A typical spectrum of sulfur, often employed as a standard for calibration in Raman studies, is shown in Figure 1, illustrating both the Stokes and anti-Stokes lines.

IV. A COMPARISON OF INFRARED AND RAMAN SPECTROSCOPIES

A. THEORETICAL CONSIDERATIONS

Both IR and Raman are vibrational spectroscopic techniques, and the IR absorption spectrum and Raman scattering spectrum for a given species may often be quite similar. However, sufficient differences exist in the types of chemical groups that are IR and Raman active to make the techniques complementary rather than competitive. In order to discern fully the vibrational modes of a molecule it is necessary to examine both types of spectra. This procedure is illustrated in Figure 2, in which FTIR and FT-Raman spectra of human SC are compared.

The selection rules for IR and Raman activity of a molecular vibration differ. Briefly, a vibrational mode is IR active when the dipole moment changes during a vibration, whereas the Raman process is a scattering effect resulting from an induced dipole moment which depends on the molecular polarizability altered during a vibration. The complementary nature of the two techniques is emphasized by the rule of mutual exclusion; for a molecule with a center of symmetry (such as benzene), vibrational transitions in the IR and Raman spectra are mutually exclusive. Thus, a

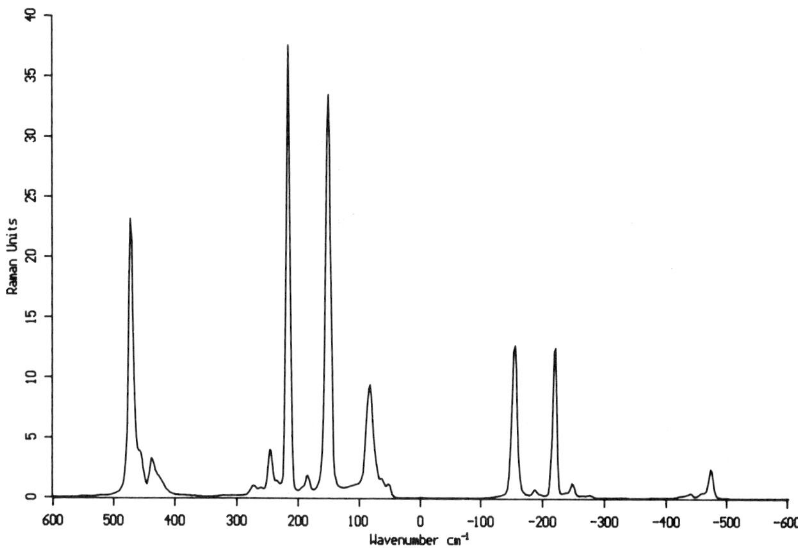

Figure 1 A typical FT-Raman spectrum of sulfur showing both Stokes and anti-Stokes lines.

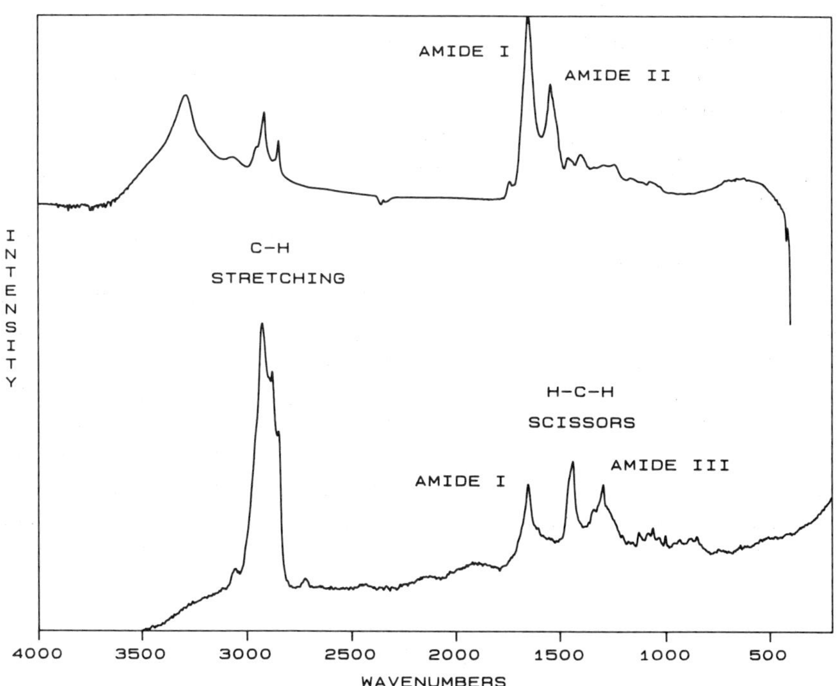

Figure 2 Typical FTIR (top) and FT-Raman (bottom) spectra of human SC.

Table 1 Assessment of Differences in Data Acquisition and Analysis Between IR and Raman Spectroscopy

	IR	Raman
Polar bonds (C=O)	Good	Bad
Homopolar bonds (C=C)	Bad	Good
Water as a solvent	Bad	Good
Glass accessories	Bad	Good
Low concentrations	Good	Bad
Spectral range	OK	Good
Fluorescence	Good	?
Linearity of response	?	Good
Availability	Good	Bad

molecule may show an IR absorption band for a particular vibration, but not a Raman band, or vice versa, depending on molecular symmetry. Other noncenter symmetric molecules often exhibit important intensity differences between the Raman and IR bands.

B. PRACTICAL CONSIDERATIONS

Some of the practical implications of the differences in the two types of vibrational spectroscopy are listed in Table 1.

Asymmetrical modes and vibrations arising from polar groups (such as carbonyl stretching) tend to be strongly IR active and weak Raman scatterers, whereas symmetrical modes and homopolar bonds (such as a disulfide bridge) are usually strongly Raman active. As a consequence, water provides a weak Raman spectrum (weak O-H stretching modes) as does glass. The practical considerations are that glass accessories can be used for sampling and water is a good solvent for Raman studies. Sample preparation is therefore simple using the Raman technique, which, as a surface phenomenon, merely requires the sample to be placed in the laser beam. However, as previously noted, the Raman effect is relatively weak, and hence a material needs to be present at a level of at least 1% in a sample for high precision work. Fluorescence can also be problematic in Raman studies, although near-IR laser excitation has helped to reduce this effect. The spectral range from the Raman effect is generally greater than is easily obtained from the IR, with a spectrum from 3500 to 10 cm^{-1} typically being collected, and the intensity of the Raman scattering is proportional to the concentration of the scattering species. Each Raman band is usually characterized by its intensity, shape, half-width, and polarizability characteristics, and these features provide good structural information about a compound.[11] The factors governing the intensities of Raman bands differ from those for IR bands, and modes that are both IR and Raman active tend to be sharper in the Raman spectrum, as is seen for biological macromolecules.[12]

V. RAMAN INSTRUMENTATION

As previously indicated, a variety of instruments are available for Raman spectroscopic studies. Briefly, dispersive instruments use a visible laser source (typically an Ar ion or HeNe laser) to excite the samples. Such systems may be adjusted macroscopically, with the laser focused to a spot of 100 μm diameter, or microscopically, with a spot diameter of around 10 μm. Traditionally, these types of instruments are relatively slow and somewhat difficult to operate, but may be valuable for some specialized studies. However, recent advances in detector technology and, in particular, the improvements in charge-coupled detectors have allowed the commercialization of fast spectral acquisition visible laser-excitation Raman spectrometers. Problems with sample fluorescence from such systems, particularly with biological samples, persist.

Fourier transform-Raman spectrometers now provide easy to operate and versatile benchtop systems. The near-IR laser (usually Nd:YAG) which excites the sample reduces some of the fluorescence problems associated with the visible laser systems, and the interferometer allows rapid spectral collection and averaging, thus improving spectral quality. The well-established advantages obtained from an interferometer (Jacquinot, Felgett, and Connes advantages) are also evident in the FT-Raman systems. As with the visible laser-excited spectrometers, the FT systems can be used macroscopically and microscopically, although spatial resolution is not as great in the FT instruments. A detailed description of the various instruments available and of the advantages of using FT-Raman spectrometers can be found in the literature.[13]

VI. RAMAN SPECTROSCOPY OF HUMAN AND ANIMAL SKINS

The FT-Raman spectrum of human SC was compared to that from FTIR in a study that demonstrated the main differences between the two techniques.[14] Vibrational modes from water in the naturally hydrated tissue (O-H stretching at around 3250 cm^{-1} and H-O-H bending at around 1620 cm^{-1}) were clearly evident in the IR spectrum, with the potential for interference with vibrations from endogenous molecules. These interfering features were not evident in the FT-Raman spectrum. Clear differences in band intensities were evident between the two vibrational spectroscopic techniques, as, for example, with the carbonyl stretching motion of the amide I peak, which is a strong IR feature, but is somewhat weaker in the Raman. Band positions were, however, remarkably consistent between the two spectroscopies. Other spectral features showed considerable variations between the techniques, such as the strongly Raman active H-C-H scissoring mode (around 1300 cm^{-1}) and the amide II band (N-H bending at around 1550 cm^{-1}), which is strong in the IR spectrum, but very weak in the Raman spectrum. This example illustrates the complementary nature of the spectroscopies; for a full description of the vibrational modes of a system both Raman and IR data are required.

Assignments consistent with the FT-Raman vibrations have been made for human SC, and have been compared with comprehensive band assignments from the FTIR spectrum.[15] This study revealed that from the FT-Raman spectrum nearly 40 spectral features were evident, whereas in the FTIR spectrum approximately 20 features were assigned. Water again had a role to play in the spectral information available, with no clear IR bands assignable below about 1000 wavenumbers because water strongly absorbs IR radiation (particularly at lower wavenumbers), causing a gradual decline in the quality of the IR spectrum. This characteristic is especially important for studies on lipid backbone conformational order and modifications induced by chemical, electrical, or thermal means, which are clearly discernible features in the Raman spectrum at around 1000 to 1150 cm^{-1}. Other features at (relatively) low wavenumbers include C-S-S-C conformational data (at around 526 cm^{-1}) and C-S stretching modes at around 623 and 644 wavenumbers.

A comparison of some experimental techniques for obtaining Raman spectra of human skin was published recently.[16] Using a variety of spectrometers, Raman spectra were recorded from human SC using visible or near-IR laser excitation under microscopic and macroscopic sampling conditions. Inter- and intrasample variation was assessed, as was the effect of water on the quality of the Raman spectra. The stability of the samples to laser excitation was monitored by multiple long-term spectral analysis and, by using a fiberoptic probe, spectra were also obtained *in vivo,* an advantage associated with FTIR analysis, for which attenuated total reflectance techniques have proved valuable. Spectra were reproducible within and between samples of human SC. While peak positions were consistent, some minor differences in the intensities of spectral features were evident between cadavers, possibly correlating with differences that have been reported in the composition of SC constituents between individuals.[17] The spectral features were also relatively insensitive to the water content of the tissue, indicating that the technique may be valuable for studies involving aqueous donor phases. Spectral analysis showed the tissue to be stable to near-IR laser excitation for at least 1 h with power at the sample of approximately 350 mW. We subsequently analyzed human SC for 8-h periods using a low-power IR laser and found no evidence for tissue degradation under these conditions. *In vivo* spectra revealed some minor differences to the *in vitro* data, although bands attributable to lipid and protein vibrations were invariant between spectra from excised and *in vivo* tissues. The comparison of instruments employed to compare Raman spectra from human SC *in vitro* illustrated some interesting discrepancies in the data obtained. The peak positions derived from the different instruments were again reasonably consistent, but marked changes in the relative peak intensities arose. These alterations are attributed to orientation effects of the sample alignment in the laser beam which can affect the polarizability of a given bond, thus modifying peak intensity. With the sample oriented at the same angle in the laser, both visible and near-IR laser-excited samples provided similar spectra, although the quality of the spectrum from the FT-Raman system was superior for the reasons previously outlined.

The linearity of response of Raman scattering with concentration of species has been valuable in studies of penetration enhancer interactions with human skin.[18–20] The terpenes 1,8-cineole and D-limonene were shown to be effective penetration enhancers for model polar (5-fluorouracil) and nonpolar (estradiol) drugs.[21,22] Despite using a range of analytical techniques,[23,24] the modes of action of these enhancers in human skin remain unclear. Recently we included FT-Raman spectroscopy in probing the interactions of these enhancers with constituents of human SC.[18] Because the Raman spectra of the terpenes possess distinct features not found in SC (such as a C-O-C bending motion from the structure of cineole), we can employ these vibrational modes as "internal standards" for normalization and subtraction of the enhancer signal from the tissue spectrum. This procedure allows an assessment of molecular interactions without interference from the exogenous materials spectrum; i.e., we can isolate the motions attributable to the SC. Infrared studies usually require the use of isotopically substituted enhancers for this type of study (typically deuterated compounds), whose availability is somewhat restricted.

We also applied FT-Raman spectroscopy to study potential interactions of the more widely investigated permeation enhancer dimethylsulfoxide (DMSO) with human SC.[19,20] While IR spectroscopy has shown that DMSO interacts with the protein component of the tissue, its mechanism of action is unclear. The weak Raman scattering of water has allowed us to probe interactions in aqueous solutions of the aprotic solvent; DMSO was clearly shown to disrupt the water structure, indicating that this effect may be partially responsible for a conformational change in the protein fraction of the naturally hydrated corneocytes.

Animal skins have been examined by Raman spectroscopy using both visible and near-IR laser excitation.[25–27] The complementary nature of IR and Raman spectroscopies was again demonstrated for snake skin; vibrational modes were assigned for the two techniques.[25] Snake skin posed problems for analysis using "conventional" Raman spectroscopic techniques because of the considerable sample fluorescence; indeed, some fluorescence was also obtained when FT-Raman analysis was employed. The molecular nature of three different types of snake skin were compared in a subsequent study which found that the reptilian tissue was remarkably consistent between species.

A molecular comparison of snake skin to that of human and pig SC was recently published.[27] The mammalian tissues were similar in their components, although some variations were noted in the relative amounts of SC constituents. Porcine skin also possessed a greater sulfur content than the human material, a feature which was not related to the hairy nature of the pig tissue. In contrast, the snake skin differed markedly in its molecular composition, most notably because of the additional β-keratin layer present in the tissue.

In summary, it is clear that Raman spectroscopy, especially the FT instruments, can offer good quality fundamental information as to the molecular nature of the SC and may be the technique of choice for some purposes such as when aqueous donor solutions are present. More specialized applications of the technique, for example, using a visible laser for sample excitation or polarizing the incident radiation, can provide unique molecular data which are unavailable from the more widely used spectroscopic techniques.

REFERENCES

1. **Rehfeld, S. J., Plachy, W. Z., Hou, S. Y. E., and Elias, P. M.,** Localisation of lipid microdomains and thermal phenomena in murine SC and isolated membrane complexes: an electron spin resonance study, *J. Invest. Dermatol.*, 95, 217, 1990.
2. **Bouwstra, J. A., Gooris, G. S., van der Spek, J. A., and Bras, W.,** Structural investigations of human SC by small angle x-ray scattering, *J. Invest. Dermatol.*, 97, 1005, 1991.
3. **Cornwell, P. A., Barry, B. W., Bouwstra, J. A., and Gooris, G. A.,** Small angle x-ray diffraction investigations of terpene enhancer actions on the lipid barrier in human skin, in *Prediction of Percutaneous Penetration, Methods, Measurements, Modelling,* Vol. 36, Brain, K. R., James, V. J., and Walters, K. A., Eds., STS Publishing, Cardiff, U.K., 1993, 18.
4. **Potts, R. O.,** *In vivo* measurement of water content of the SC using infrared spectroscopy: a review, *Cosmet. Toilet.*, 100, 27, 1985.
5. **Golden, G. M., Guzek, D. B., Harris, R. R., McKie, J. E., and Potts, R. O.,** Lipid thermotropic transitions in human SC, *J. Invest. Dermatol.*, 86, 255, 1986.
6. **Knutson, K., Krill, S. L., Lambert, W. J., and Higuchi, W. I.,** Physicochemical aspects of transdermal permeation, *J. Control. Rel.*, 6, 59, 1987.

7. **Golden, G. M., McKie, J. E., and Potts, R. O.,** Role of SC lipid fluidity in transdermal drug flux, *J. Pharm. Sci.,* 76, 25, 1987.
8. **Mak, V. H. W., Potts, R. O., and Guy, R. H.,** Percutaneous penetration enhancement *in vivo* measured by attenuated total reflectance spectroscopy, *Pharm. Res.,* 7, 835, 1990.
9. **Bommannan, D., Potts, R. O., and Guy, R. H.,** Examination of SC barrier function *in vivo* by infrared spectroscopy, *J. Invest. Dermatol.,* 95, 403, 1990.
10. **Mak, V. H. W., Potts, R. O., and Guy, R. H.,** Does hydration affect intercellular lipid organisation in the SC?, *Pharm. Res.,* 8, 1064, 1991.
11. **Long, D. A.,** Linear and non-linear Raman effects: the principles, *Chem. Br.,* 25, 589, 1989.
12. **Tu, A. T.,** *Raman Spectroscopy In Biology: Principles and Applications,* John Wiley & Sons, New York, 1982.
13. **Hendra, P., Jones, C., and Warnes, G.,** *Fourier Transform Raman Spectroscopy: Instrumental and Chemical Applications,* Ellis Horwood, New York, 1991.
14. **Williams, A. C., Edwards, H. G. M., and Barry, B. W.,** Fourier transform Raman spectroscopy; a novel application for examining human SC, *Int. J. Pharm.,* 81, R11, 1992.
15. **Barry, B. W., Edwards, B. W., and Williams, A. C.,** Fourier Transform Raman and infrared vibrational study of human skin: assignment of spectral bands, *J. Raman Spectrosc.,* 23, 641, 1992.
16. **Williams, A. C., Barry, B. W., Edwards, H. G. M., and Farwell, D. W.,** A critical comparison of some Raman spectroscopic techniques for studies of human SC, *Pharm. Res.,* 10, 1642, 1993.
17. **Elias, P. M., Cooper, E. R., Korc, A., and Brown, B. E.,** Percutaneous transport in relation to SC structure and lipid composition, *J. Invest. Dermatol.,* 76, 297, 1981.
18. **Anigbogu, A. N. C., Williams, A. C., Barry, B. W., and Edwards, H. G. M.,** Fourier transform Raman spectroscopy in the study of interactions between terpene penetration enhancers and human SC, in *Prediction of Percutaneous Penetration; Methods, Measurements, Modelling,* Vol. 3b, Brain, K. R., James, V. J., and Walters, K. A., Eds., STS Publishing, Cardiff, U.K., 1993, 27.
19. **Anigbogu, A. N. C., Williams, A. C., Barry, B. W., and Edwards, H. G. M.,** Human skin-penetration enhancer interactions: an FT-Raman spectroscopic study of the effects of dimethylsulphoxide, *J. Pharm. Pharmacol.,* 45(Suppl 1.2)1123, 1993.
20. **Barry, B. W., Anigbogu, A. N. C., and Williams, A. C.,** FT-Raman study of DMSO interactions with human skin, *Pharm. Res.,* 10(Suppl.), 239, 1993.
21. **Williams, A. C. and Barry, B. W.,** Terpenes and the lipid-protein-partitioning theory of skin penetration enhancers, *Pharm. Res.,* 8, 17, 1991.
22. **Williams, A. C. and Barry, B. W.,** The enhancement index concept applied to terpene penetration enhancers for human skin and model lipophilic (oestradiol) and hydrophilic (5-fluorouracil) drugs, *Int. J. Pharm.,* 74, 157, 1991.
23. **Williams, A. C. and Barry, B. W.,** Permeation, Fourier transform infrared spectroscopy and differential scanning calorimetry investigations of terpene penetration enhancers in human skin, *J. Pharm. Pharmacol.,* 41(Suppl.), 12P, 1989.
24. **Williams, A. C. and Barry, B. W.,** Differential scanning calorimetry does not predict the activity of terpene penetration enhancers in human skin, *J. Pharm. Pharmacol.,* 42(Suppl.), 156P, 1990.
25. **Barry, B. W., Edwards, H. G. M., and Williams, A. C.,** Fourier transform Raman and infrared spectra of snake skin, *Spectrochim. Acta,* 49A, 801, 1993.
26. **Edwards, H. G. M., Farwell, D. W., Williams, A. C., and Barry, B. W.,** Raman spectroscopic studies of the skins of the Sahara sand viper, the carpet python and the American black rat snake, *Spectrochim. Acta,* 49A, 913, 1993.
27. **Williams, A. C., Edwards, H. G. M., and Barry, B. W.,** A comparison of FT-Raman of mammalian and reptilian skin, *Analyst,* 119, 563, 1994.

Chapter 16.2

Electronic Spin Resonance

Danyi Quan and Howard I. Maibach

CONTENTS

I. INTRODUCTION

A major barrier to diffusion of chemicals through the skin is its outermost layer, the stratum corneum (SC). The SC is composed of corneocytes embedded in lipid domains consisting of alternately hydrophilic and lipophilic layers.[1,2] In order to extend the variety of drugs that might be administrated via the skin and to increase the percutaneous absorption of drugs, considerable attention has been focused on the mechanism of action of skin penetration enhancers.[3,4]

Many skin penetration enhancers have been proven to interact in some way with SC lipid structure, generally by increasing the fluidity of the intercellular lipid bilayers.[5,6] In the lipid regions at least two types of disorder can be distinguished, namely the disorder of the alkyl chains inside one lipid bilayer (a shorter-range disorder) and the disorder in the lipid bilayer arrangement (a longer-range disorder).[7] Over the past few years several physical techniques, such as differential scanning calorimetry (DSC), X-ray diffraction (XRD), Fourier transform infrared (FTIR) spectroscopy, nuclear magnetic resonance (NMR), and electron spin resonance (ESR) spectroscopy have been used to gain more information on the interaction of penetration enhancers with the skin.[8–16]

Electron spin resonance spectroscopy of the nitroxide spin label was introduced as a valuable method in the study of the structure of biological membranes, membrane properties, and drug–membrane interaction.[17,18] Spin labels are specifically incorporated with the lipid or the lipid part of biological membranes. Thus, each label reflects the properties of a different membrane region. Electron spin resonance spectra of membrane-incorporated spin labels are sensitive to the rotational mobility

0-8493-2605-2/95/$0.00+$.50

of the spin labels, the polarity of the environment surrounding the spin labels, and the orientation of the spin labels. These effects have been used to advantage in numerous studies of membranes and skin. Some physical conditions (e.g., temperature) and chemicals can perturb biological membranes to yield characteristic changes in their respective ESR spectra.[19–21]

Although many substances are known as penetration enhancers, a detailed knowledge of the mechanism of action of enhancers is currently developing. Recently, an ESR study of the effect of a skin penetration enhancer on lipid fluidity in 5-doxyl stearic acid-labeled human SC was conducted by Quan and Maibach.[22] This chapter investigates the model of action of laurocapram (1-dodecylazacycloheptan-2-one, Azone®) on the human skin. Four doxyl stearic acids (DSAs; 5-DSA, 7-DSA, 12-DSA, and 16-DSA) were used as spin labels. In the skin bilayers this type of spin label interposes itself into the lipid bilayers.[17,20] Because the orientation of labels in bilayers must reflect the local molecular structure and should serve as delicate indicators of conformational changes in bilayers, we approached the action of Azone® on the human skin by studying ESR spectra so as to gain more insight into its mechanism of action.

II. METHODS

A. PREPARATION OF EPIDERMIS AND STRATUM CORNEUM

Human abdominal skin was obtained from fresh cadavers with a dermatome. The dermatomed skin was immersed in a 60°C water bath for 2 min, and then the epidermis was separated from the dermis by mechanical removal. The dry epidermal skin was stored in a desiccator at –20°C until further use. The epidermis (before dry) was placed, SC side up, on filter paper and floated on 0.5% trypsin (type II, Sigma), in a tris-HCl buffer solution (pH 7.4) for 2 h at 37°C. After incubation any softened epidermal parts were removed by mild agitation of the SC sheets. Samples were dried and stored in a desiccator at –20°C.

B. SPIN-LABELING PROCEDURES AND PRETREATMENT WITH THE SKIN PENETRATION ENHANCER

5-, 7-, 12-, and 16-Doxyl stearic acid were used as lipid spin labels in this study. The dry SC sheets (a slice of 0.4 cm^2) were incubated in the tris buffer solution (pH 7.4) of each spin label (10 µg/ml) for 2 h at 37°C, and then dried under a flow of nitrogen gas for 1 h at 37°C over silica gel. For a pretreatment, 5 µl of ethanol containing 25, 100, and 250 µg of Azone®, respectively, was spread on the SC side of the previously prepared SC sheets. Similar treatment with ethanol alone was performed as a control sample. After evaporating the ethanol, all samples were incubated at 37°C for 1 h, and were then followed by the procedure described above to label with four spin labels.

C. ELECTRON SPIN RESONANCE MEASUREMENT

Three slices of SC sheets previously treated and labeled were mounted on the flat surface of a modified quartz cell (Wilmad Glass Co., Buena, NJ). The cells allow thermostated mineral oil to be passed behind the sample throughout the experiment; the temperature is controlled at 37°C. First derivative microwave absorption spectra were recorded using an ER/200D ESR spectrometer (IBM Instruments, CT). Spectra

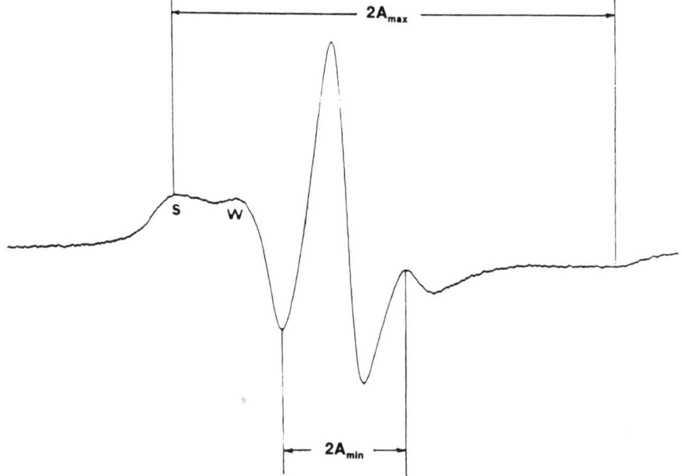

Figure 1 The calculation of order parameter *(S)*: $2A_{max}$, outer maximum hyperfine splitting, $2A_{min}$, inner minimum hyperfine splitting, S, strongly binding, and W, weakly binding.

were collected and averaged on the PC/AT using software written in PC/FORTH (Version 3.2, Laboratory Microsystems, CA). The hyperfine splittings of labeled skin samples were determined with a 100-gauss scan width, 4×10^{-5} receiver gain, and 10 ms time constant. A microwave power setting of 25 mW was used for all samples, and temperatures were controlled to 37°C ± 0.5°C. Each sample was scanned three times and the ESR parameters from each spectrum were averaged to give a single estimate for that sample.

The order parameters *(S)* were calculated according to Griffith and Jost,[23] Hubbell and McConnell,[24] and Marsh.[25]

$$S = \left(A_{\parallel} - A_{\perp}\right) / \left[A_{zz} - 1/2\left(A_{xx} + A_{yy}\right)\right]\left(a_0'/a_0\right) \tag{1}$$

where $2A_{\parallel}$ is identified with the outer maximum hyperfine splitting, $2A_{max}$, and $A_{\perp}$ is obtained from the inner minimum hyperfine splitting, $2A_{min}$ (Figure 1), using the following corrections:

$$A_{\perp} = A_{min}(G) + 1.4\left[1 - \left(A_{max} - A_{min}\right) / \left(A_{zz} - A_{xx}\right)\right]$$

a_0' is the isotropic hyperfine splitting coupling constant for nitroxide molecule in the crystal state:

$$a_0' = 1/3\left(A_{xx} + A_{yy} + A_{zz}\right) \tag{2}$$

The values used to describe the rapid anisotropic motion of membrane-incorporated probes of fatty acid type are

$$\left(A_{xx}, A_{yy}, A_{zz}\right) = (6.1,\ 6.1, 32.4)\text{ gauss}$$

Similarly, the isotropic hyperfine splitting coupling constant for the spin label in the membrane (a_0) is given by:

$$a_0 = 1/3\left(A_{\|} + 2A_{\perp}\right) \tag{3}$$

a_0 values are sensitive to the polarity of the environment of the spin label because increases in the a_0 value reflect an increase in the polarity of the medium.

The S provides a measure of the flexibility of the spin label in the membrane. It follows that $S = 1$ for highly ordered systems and $S = 0$ for completely isotropic motion. Increases in the order parameter reflect decreases in the segmental flexibility of the spin label and, conversely, decreases in the order parameter reflect increases in the flexibility.

III. RESULTS AND DISCUSSION

A. EFFECT OF AZONE® ON 5-DSA LABELED HUMAN STRATUM CORNEUM

The ESR spectra of 5-DSA-labeled SC treated without or with ethanol were recorded from 5 to 24 h after labeling. Figure 2 gives the spectra of 5-DSA-labeled SC without treatment (control). Two spectral components can be seen: the bound components (arrows b) and the fluid components (arrows f). The fluid components are especially clear at 5 to 8 h after labeling, and the line width of the fluid component is narrow. These spectra indicate that 5-DSA partitioned between a nonpolar (immobilized) environment and an aqueous (fluid) environment. With the diffusion of 5-DSA into the SC, the fluid components became smaller, while bound components were more prominent. In addition, more bound components were present as observed in the ESR spectra of untreated SC.

Table 1 gives the ESR parameters as a function of labeling time. Small increases in the S of 5-DSA-labeled SC (control sample) indicate that 5-DSA took time to enter the SC. The polarities (a_0) of both untreated and ethanol-treated SC were almost unchanged, suggesting that 5-DSA did not change the polarity of the environment of lipid bilayers during its partition into the SC. Results show that ethanol reduced the order parameter by 10 and 1% at 5 and 24 h, respectively. The difference in binding (spin label bound to lipids) between ethanol-treated and untreated samples is also included in Table 1. The binding extent of 5-DSA in these two different skin environments was obviously different between 5 and 8 h ($p < 0.02$). The bound peaks in untreated SC slightly increased (increase index: 13.6%) with increasing time; while the bound peaks in ethanol-treated SC greatly increased from 5 to 24 h (increase index: 80%). At 24 h, the binding ratio of ethanol-treated samples reached the same value as the untreated sample. Ethanol-induced changes in ESR spectra were shown as a weakening of the bound components and a delay of bindings.

5-Doxyl stearic acid is used as a lipid spin label and is known to provide information about the physical state of membrane lipids. Lipids in a fluid bilayer (or

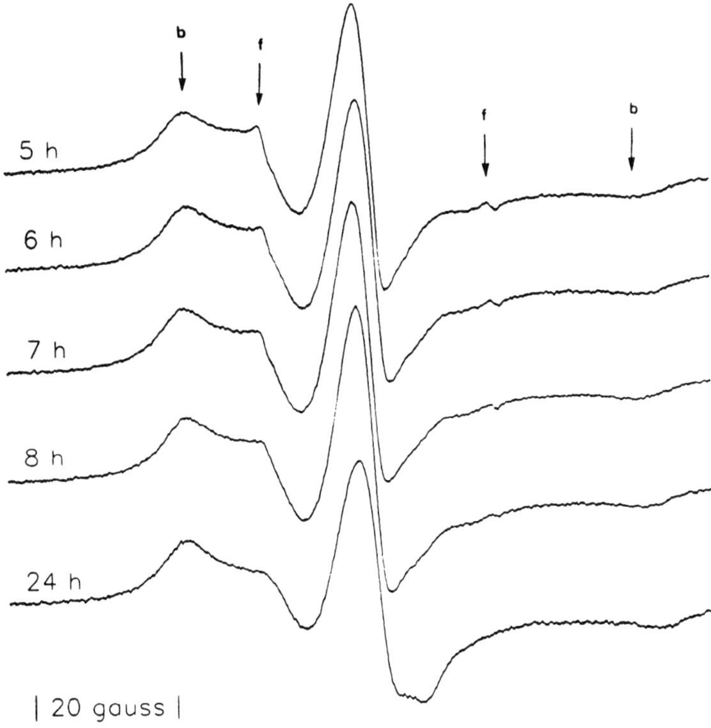

Figure 2 ESR spectra of the 5-DSA-labeled human SC at 37°C, recorded from 5 to 24h after labeling. The binding spectral components are indicated by arrows b, and the "fluid" spectral components are indicated by arrows f.

Table 1 ESR Parameters of 5-DSA-Labeled Human Stratum

Time	Polarity, a_0 (gauss)[a]		Order Parameter (S)[b]		Binding Ratio[c]	
(h)	No treatment	Ethanol	No treatment	Ethanol	No treatment	Ethanol
5	16.16	16.16	0.80	0.78	1.29	1.25
6	16.16	16.16	0.82	0.80	1.50	1.22
7	16.20	16.16	0.82	0.82	1.60	1.33
8	16.16	16.16	0.84	0.84	1.56	1.35
24	16.10	15.98	0.87	0.86	2.00	2.00

[a] Calculated by Equation 3. Values ±0.05.
[b] Calculated by Equation 1. Estimated uncertainty is values ± 0.02.
[c] Binding ratio is the ratio of the height of peak S to peak W, which represents a rough estimate of the overall mobility of all the spin label sites.

monolayer) environment can be distinguished from lipids bound to protein by using the 5-DSA spin label.[26,27] The ESR spectra of 5-DSA-incorporated human SC show two spectral components: the bound component (b) is characteristic of lipid associated with the hydrophobic surfaces of proteins, and the fluid component (f) is a fluid bilayer-like component.[28,29] Especially noteworthy is that the binding of 5-DSA to SC and S are a function of labeling time. When the ESR parameters are used to estimate the membrane properties, it is important to record the time when the spectra are taken as different values may be obtained at different times. Ethanol had an obvious effect on the behavior of spin label bound to lipid bilayers (less immobilization). Decreases in S could be related to an increase in the freedom of motion of the spin label, greater freedom being associated with the fluidity of local lipid layer environments surrounding the spin label. However, an obvious increase in bound components and order parameters of ethanol-treated SC at 24 h demonstrates that the influence of ethanol on lipids of SC decreased with time. Therefore, the ethanol-induced change in lipid bilayers of SC can be considered significant, and this effect diminishes with time, which might be responsible for ethanol dissolving some of the lipids from the upper layers of the SC and causing a temporary perturbation in the interior of the SC.

Three Azone® concentrations were applied in this study. The ESR spectra of Azone®-treated human SC were measured at 37°C as a function of labeling time, and totally different from those of 5-DSA labeled SC and ethanol-treated SC. No fluid components and only a little bound component could be seen. The spin label still showed a weak binding to lipid bilayers, even at 24 h.

The corresponding parameters obtained from the ESR spectra at three concentrations of Azone® are summarized in Table 2. The molecular freedom of motion is related to S as defined by Equation 1. The isotropic splitting parameter a_0 reflects the polarity of the local surroundings of the spin label in a membrane, and the parameter increases with increasing polarity. When a low Azone® concentration was used (25 µg), S and a_0 values showed a slight decrease as a function of time. In the case of higher concentrations, although the S values still showed an decreasing trend, these values were obviously smaller than that at a low concentration. Azone® reduced the S by as much as 54% at a low applied concentration (25 µg), and by 78 and 80% at higher concentrations (100 and 250 µg, respectively). These results suggest that Azone® led to a fluid environment in the SC, and this action increased as the concentration increased.

The present results show that Azone® caused a conversion of the strongly immobilized labels (bound components) to weakly immobilized labels. This suggests that Azone® caused a change in the conformation of 5-DSA that was buried within the lipid bilayer matrix. Compared with control samples, an obvious decrease in S, even at 25 µg Azone®, indicates that Azone® caused an increase in the flexibility of the local lipid bilayer in the SC. Clearly, at a high concentration (250 µg), decreased S values indicate that 5-DSA was surrounded by a more flexible lipid environment. Because the orientation of the spin label in the lipid bilayer must reflect the conformational changes of local molecular structure, one of the effects of Azone® was to cause a conformational change in lipid bilayers of SC. Although it is impossible to directly compare the effect of Azone® on a_0, the ESR spectra show that the polarities surrounding 5-DSA in the treated skin system differed greatly from those in the untreated skin system. In addition, concentration effects on the ESR spectra of SC demonstrate that proportionality to the amount applied was not direct. In other words, the flexibility of 5-DSA significantly increased from 25 to 100 µg Azone®, and then showed a small change from 100 to 250 µg Azone®. Such a saturation of the enhancement effect has been observed in some permeation experiments in which Azone® was used as an enhancer.[30]

Table 2 ESR Parameters of 5-DSA-Labeled Human SC Treated with Azone

Treatment[a]	Time[b] (h)	Polarity a_0[c] (gauss)	Order Parameter (S)[d]	S:W[e]
25 μg Azone	5	15.17	0.41	0.33
	24	14.68	0.39	0.44
100 μg Azone	5	14.07	0.18	—
	24	13.77	0.19	—
250 μg Azone	5	14.19	0.15	—
	24	13.95	0.17	—

[a] The SC was treated with the indicated amount of Azone®.

[b] ESR spectra were recorded at the indicated time after labeling.

[c] Calculated by Equation 3. Estimated uncertainty is ± 0.2.

[d] Calculated by Equation 1. Values ± 0.02 gauss.

[e] S:W ratio is the ratio of the height of peak S to peak W shown in Figure 1, which represents a rough estimate of the overall mobility of all spin label sites.

B. EFFECT OF AZONE® ON 5-DSA-LABELED HUMAN EPIDERMIS

Considering epidermal lipids play important roles in the formation [illegible] a permeability barrier,[2,31] an experimental design com[illegible] man epidermis treated with Azone®. The [illegible] epidermis in the absence or presence of increasing amounts of Azone® were recorded from 5 to 24 h after labeling. No fluid component and a larger bound peak were observed at 5 h. This type of spectra was characteristic of anisotropic motion within an ordered structure. The results suggest that the spin label was strongly immobilized within lipid bilayers in the epidermis. Although Azone® treatment led to a decrease in spin label binding to epidermal lipids, the binding behavior differed greatly from that of Azone®-treated SC. Regardless of the concentration of Azone® applied, an obvious bound peak could be detected at 5 h, and the molecular motion of the spin label could be considered to be a typical anisotropic motion. As time increased (24 h), the low-concentration treatment (25 μg) resulted in a marked increase in the bindings (43%), while the high-concentration treatment showed a small change. Such a change in binding was not found in the treated SC. Therefore, combining these two skin compartments, it is helpful to comprehend the state of the epidermis after enhancer treatment. Figure 3 compares the order parameters in these two skin systems. Apparently, the S value of treated epidermis was more than two times greater than the corresponding S value of the treated SC, indicating that Azone® mainly altered the permeation function of the SC and showed a weakened effect on the epidermis.

Because the ESR spectra of 5-DSA-labeled epidermis treated with 25 μg Azone® showed a good recovery process (Figure 4), a detailed discussion is given. The spectra were recorded from 5 to 24 h after labeling. Obviously, the molecular motion of 5-DSA under this condition varied from comparatively minimal anisotropy to typical anisotropy. The order parameter S was changed from 0.61 to 0.87, further suggesting that the effect of a low Azone® concentration on the epidermal lipids was small and decreased as time increased. Note that the spectrum recorded at 8 h was

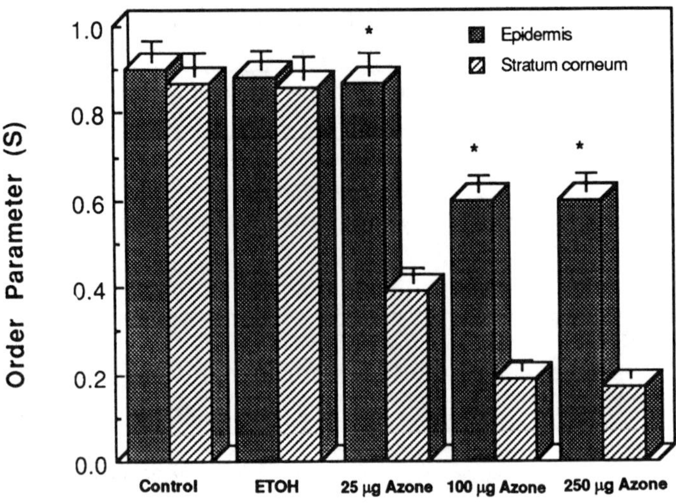

Figure 3 Comparison of the effect of Azone® on order parameters in two skin systems: 5-DSA-[illegible]man epidermis or SC, recorded at 24 h. * represents $p < 0.0001$. Mean ± S.E.M. ($n = 3$).

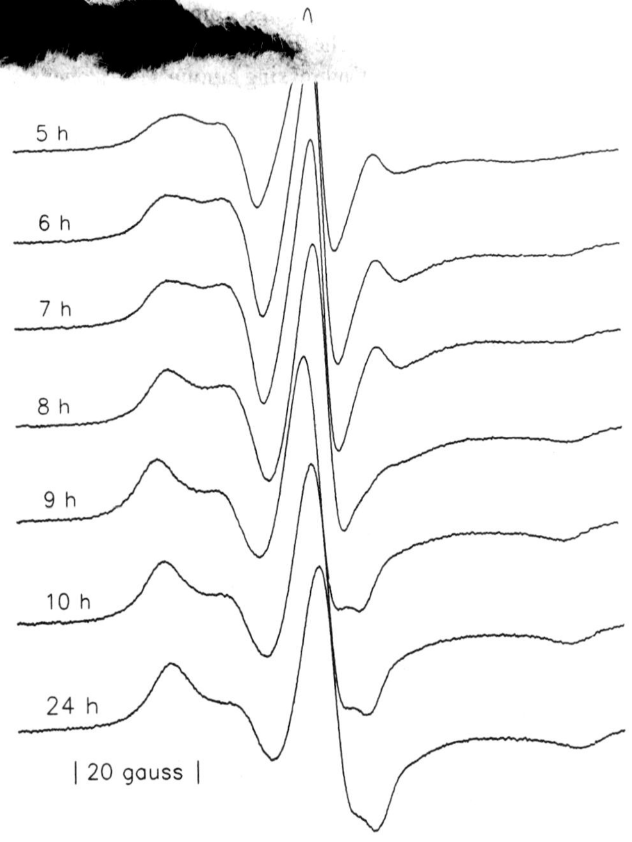

Figure 4 Time-dependence ESR spectra of 5-DSA-labeled human epidermis treated with 25 µg Azone® recorded from 5 to 24 h after labeling.

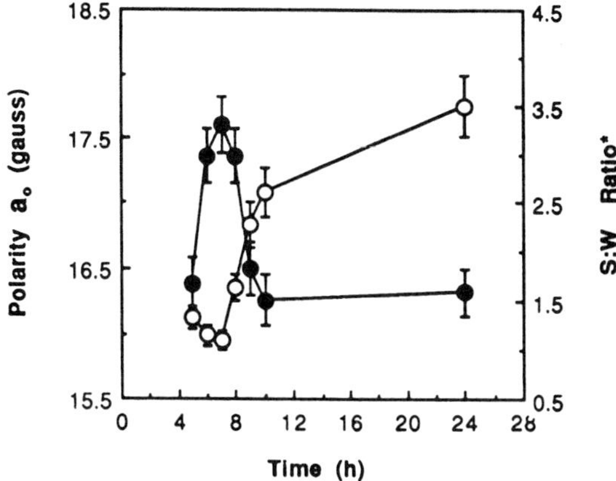

Figure 5 Time dependence of polarity (a_0) and S:W ratio, of 5-DSA-labeled human epidermis treated with 25 μg Azone®. * The ratio of the height of the peak S to peak W represents a rough estimate of overall mobility of the spin label sites. Mean ± S.E.M. (n = 3).

a turning point. From this point, the treated epidermis gradually recovered from the temporary disorder induced by Azone® with increasing time. The relationship between changes in the a_0 or S:W peak ratio caused by 25 μg Azone® and the labeling time is shown in Figure 5. The a_0 values were calculated as defined in Equation 3, and the ratio of the height of the peak S to peak W represents an estimate of overall mobility of the spin label sites.[27,32] S and W represent the strongly immobilized and weakly immobilized spin label, respectively (Figure 1). The time-dependent changes in both polarity and S:W ratio showed a maximum and a minimum value. This fact may be explained in two ways. First, when the epidermis was treated with Azone®, with permeation of the enhancer into the SC, the polarity of the local environment surrounding the spin label increased and reached a maximum value; i.e., a major polar environment formed. Further permeation of the enhancer led to a decrease in polarity, and almost remained a constant after 10 h, which was close to the polarity of the untreated SC. Second, the S:W ratio reflects the extent of spin label binding to the lipid bilayers, and its change can be considered to be a conformational modification in the epidermal lipids. With the permeation of the enhancer into the SC, the bound peaks became smaller, and reached a minimum value at 7 h. After 7 h, the S:W ratio continued to increase. The epidermal lipids might undergo the following changes: ordered system → temporary conformational modifications → ordered system, suggesting that Azone® induced a temporary effect on lipids. The overall effects of Azone® were an increasing fluidity of the lipid bilayers (small S value) and causing a major polar environment (large a_0 value), which resulted in a temporary conformational modification in the lipid bilayers (changes in S/W values). No significant changes were seen in the S of 25 μg Azone®-treated SC from 5 to 24 h (S: 0.41 to 0.39). However, the corresponding S of 25 μg Azone®-treated epidermis were changed from 0.61 to 0.87. Clearly, the S value in the treated epidermis was greater than that in the treated SC, even at 5 h. Therefore, the action of a low concentration on the epidermis decreased as the enhancer permeated. In other words, a low Azone® concentration induced a temporary disorder in the epidermis, especially in the SC. Such an effect on the epidermis was reversible. Following these

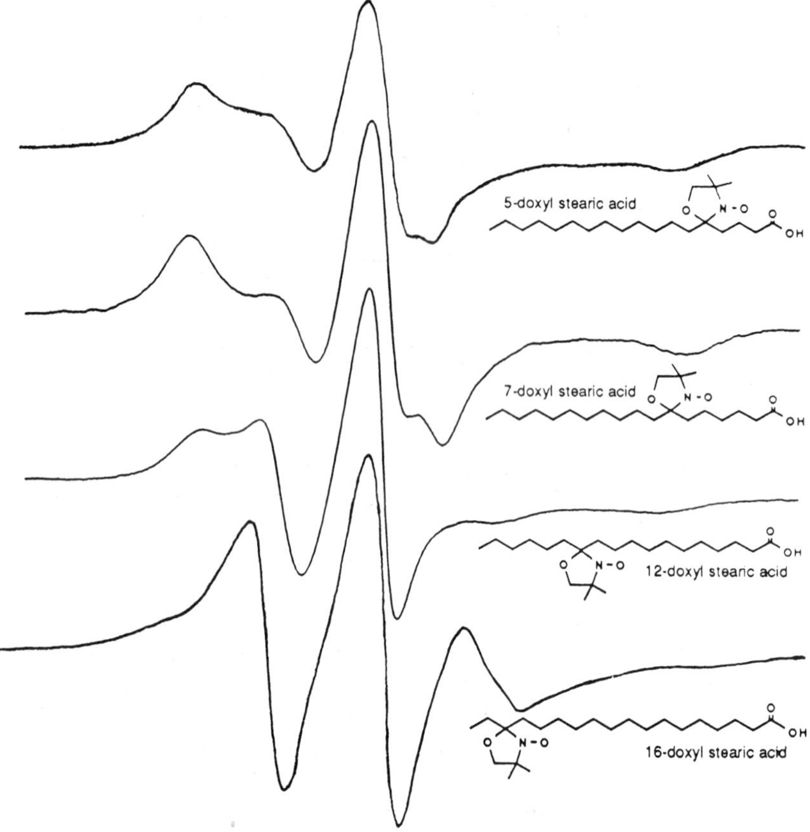

Figure 6 The structures of four stearic acid spin labels and their typical ESR spectra in human SC.

results, we can differentiate two effects, one on the lipids of the SC and one on the epidermis.

C. EFFECT OF AZONE® ON THE DEPTH OF LIPID BILAYERS

In order to localize the effect of Azone®, we measured ESR parameters of human SC labeled with a set of doxyl fatty acids: 5-, 7-, 12-, and 16-DSA. Their structures and typical ESR spectra are given in Figure 6. These spectra show that outmost lines move in and linewidths become narrower as the doxyl group is translated from the C5 to the C7, the C12, and finally the C16 position. This result is due to the different flexibility profiles of lipid bilayers because these spin labels diffused into the SC and bound to different regions in the bilayers. Each spin label served as an indicator and reflected the order in the different sites which was bound to the spin label. For the control sample, the S of 5-DSA, 7-DSA, 12-DSA, and 16-DSA at 24 h are 0.87 0.87, 0.60, and 0.41, respectively. The data indicate that the mobility in lipid bilayers gradually increased from the surface to the inside. Three concentrations of Azone® were also used in this study. Note that Azone® showed less effect on 7-DSA-labeled SC, even at a high concentration applied (S=0.5). Figure 7 gives a clear comparison of S or a_0 value changes in different regions labeled with four stearic acids. The

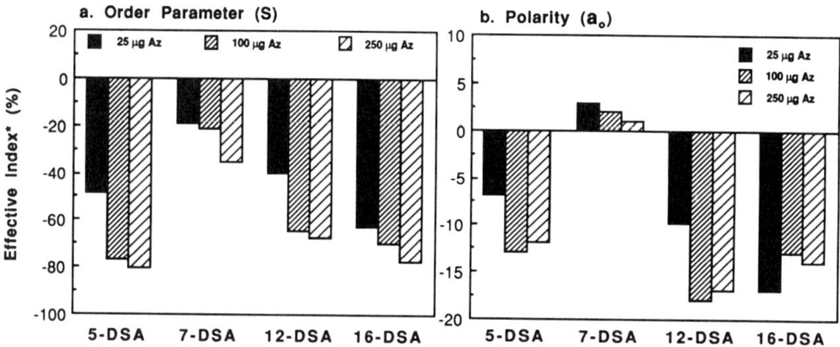

Figure 7 Effective index of Azone® on the order parameter (S) and polarity (a_0) of human SC. * All data were calculated from ESR spectra recorded at 5 h after labeling and compared to the corresponding control sample.

effective index was calculated from ESR spectra recorded at 5 h after labeling and compared to the corresponding control sample. After being treated with Azone®, the S for each spin-labeled region showed a decrease, and the polarity also decreased, except for a small increase in 7-DSA-labeled SC. At a low Azone® concentration, the extend of the disorder from surface to inside of lipids follows: 45, 20, 40, and 60%, which were 5-DSA, 7-DSA, 12-DSA, and 16-DSA labeled SC, respectively. Obviously, the disordering action of Azone® on lipid bilayers is greater deep in the lipid bilayer because 16-DSA-labeled SC showed the smallest S value. In addition, the higher S of 5-DSA-labeled SC might be contributed to the residual amount of Azone® on the surface of the SC. The S in this case should be included: (1) 5-DSA in Azone® resided on the surface of the SC; (2) 5-DSA bound to lipid bilayers which were changed by Azone®. That is why the S value was higher than that of 7-DSA-labeled SC.

Previous studies have shown that the structural features of compounds that induce changes in the skin permeability include an alkyl chain of around 8 to 16 carbon atoms and a polar head group.[33,34] Azone®, which has a polar head group and a long alkyl side chain, is thought to incorporate into structured lipids, with the ring structure lying in the plane of polar head groups. The presence of such a seven-membered ring forces apart the alkyl chains of the skin lipids in order to have more free space in which to move, hence inducing the disorder and change in skin permeability.[35] The current result is in accordance with this explanation. In general, the action of Azone® on the lipid bilayers showed a greater disorder in the deep (lipophilic) region. This phenomenon might be due to its long alkyl side chain inserts into the lipid bilayer and reaches to the deep lipophilic region after it permeates into the SC.

IV. CONCLUSIONS

1. The effect of ethanol on the ESR spectra of the SC is significant but small. Ethanol affects the spin label binding to the lipid bilayers in the SC and causes a small increase in the flexibility of the local bilayer around the spin label. However, this effect decreases with increasing time; thus, it may be associated with dissolving some of lipids and causing a temporary perturbation in lipid bilayers.

2. Azone® produced a significant change in the ESR spectra of 5-DSA-labeled human SC — from a strongly immobilized spectrum to a weakly immobilized spectrum. This suggests that Azone® induces a change in the conformation of 5-DSA that is buried within lipid bilayers. It can be regarded as a conformational modification of the lipid bilayer. In addition, it is also found that effect of Azone® on both flexibility and polarity of the spin label is not in direct proportion with the amount of Azone® used.
3. A set of stearic acid spin labels which have C_{18} atoms chain length and different positions of labeling (C_5, C_7, C_{12}, and C_{16}) were used. The results show that the flexibility of the fatty acid chains in the lipid bilayers of the SC increases considerably as soon as the chain length becomes shorter (labeling position is far from the -COOH group), suggesting that various fatty acid spin labels can reflect the property of different regions in the lipid bilayers.
4. Azone® leads to greater effects on the deeper region of lipid bilayers because S values obviously increase from the 7- to the 16-DSA-labeled SC, indicating its action on the more lipophilic region in the SC.

REFERENCES

1. **Barry, B. W.,** *Dermatological Formulations.* Marcel Dekker, New York, 1983, 160.
2. **Elias, P. M.,** Epidermal lipids, barrier function, and desquamation, *J. Invest. Dermatol.,* 80, 44, 1983.
3. **Goodman, M. and Barry, B. W.,** Lipid-protein-partitioning (LPP) theory of skin enhancer activity: finite dose technique, *Int. J. Pharm.,* 57, 29, 1989.
4. **Potts, R. O., Golden, G. M., Francoeur, M. L., Mak, V. H. W., and Guy, R. H.,** Mechanism and enhancement of solute transport across the SC, *J. Control. Rel.,* 15, 249, 1991.
5. **Barry, B. W.,** Model action of penetration enhancers in human skin, *J. Control. Rel.,* 6, 85, 1987.
6. **Barry, B. W.,** Lipid-protein-partitioning theory of skin penetration enhancement, *J. Control. Rel.,* 15, 237, 1991.
7. **Blaurock, A. E.,** Evidence of bilayer structure and of membrane interactions from X-ray diffraction analysis, *Biochim. Biophys. Acta,* 650, 167, 1982.
8. **Bouwstra, J. A., de Vries, M. A., Gooris, G. S., Bras, W., Brussee, J., and Ponec, M.,** Thermodynamic and structural aspects of the skin barrier, *J. Control. Rel.,* 15, 209, 1991.
9. **Friberg, S. E., Kayali, I. H., Margosiak, M., Osborne, D. W., and Ward, A. J. I.,** SC and transport properties, in *Topical Drug Delivery Formulations — Drugs Pharmaceutical Sciences,* Vol. 42, Osborne, D. W. and Aman, A., Eds., Marcel Dekker, New York, 1990, 29.
10. **Gay, C. L., Murphy, T. M., Hadgraft, J., Kellaway, I. W., Evans, J. C., and Rowlands, C. C.,** A electron spin resonance study of skin penetration enhancers, *Int. J. Pharm.,* 49, 39, 1989.
11. **Gay, C. L., Hadgraft, J., Kellaway, I. W., and Rowlands, C. C.,** The effect of skin penetration enhancers on human SC lipids: an electron spin resonance study, in *Prediction of Percutaneous Penetration,* Scott, R. C., et al., Eds., IBC Technical Services, London, 1990, 322.
12. **Golden, G. M., Guzek, B., McKie, J. E., and Potts, R. O.,** Role of SC lipid fluidity in transdermal drug flux, *J. Pharm. Sci.,* 76, 25, 1987.
13. **Goodman, M. and Barry, B. W.,** Differential scanning calorimetry of human SC: effects of penetration enhancers azone and dimethyl sulphoxide, *Anal. Proc.,* 23, 397, 1986.
14. **Mak, V. H. W., Potts, R. O., and Guy, R. H.,** Percutaneous penetration enhancement *in vivo* measured by attenuated total reflectance infrared spectroscopy, *Pharm. Res.,* 8, 835, 1990.
15. **Takeuchi, Y., Yasukawa, H., Yamaoka, Y., Morimoto, Y., Nakao, S., Fukumori, Y., and Fukuda, T.,** Destabilization of whole skin lipid bio-liposomes induced by skin penetration enhancers and FT-IR/ATR (Fourier transform infrared/attenuated total reflection) analysis of SC lipids, *Chem. Pharm. Bull.,* 40, 484, 1992.
16. **Ward, A. J. I. and du Reau, C.,** The essential role of lipid bilayers in the determination of SC permeability, *Int. J. Pharm.,* 74, 137, 1991.
17. **Curtain, C. C. and Gorden, L. M.,** ESR spectroscopy of membranes, in *Membranes, Detergents, and Receptor Solubilization,* Venter, J. C. and Harrison, L. C., Eds., Alan R. Liss, New York, 1984, 177.

18. **Sauerheber, R. D., Gordon, L. M., Crosland, R. D., and Kuwahara, M. D.,** Spin-label studies on rat liver and heart plasma membranes: do probe interactions interfere with the measurement of membrane properties?, *J. Membr. Biol.,* 31, 131, 1977.
19. **Cannon, B., Polnaszek, C., Butler, K., Eriksson, L., and Smith, I. C. P.,** The fluidity and organization of mitochondrial membrane lipids of the brown adipose tissue of cold-adapted rats and hamsters as determined by nitroxide spin probes, *Arch. Biochem. Biophys.,* 167, 550, 1975.
20. **Hubbell, W. L. and McConnell, H. M.,** Orientation and motion of amphiphilic spin labels in membranes, *Proc. Natl. Acad. Sci. U.S.A.,* 64, 20, 1969.
21. **Seelig, J.,** Spin label studies of oriented smectic liquid crystals (a model system for bilayer membranes), *J. Am. Chem. Soc.,* 92, 3881, 1970.
22. **Quan, D. Y. and Maibach, H. I.,** An electron spin resonance study. I. Effect of Azone® on 5-doxyl stearic acid-labeled human SC, *Int. J. Pharm.,* 104, 61, 1994.
23. **Griffith, O. H. and Jost, P. C.,** Lipid spin labels in biological membranes, in *Spin Labeling. Theory and Applications,* Berliner, L. J., ed., Academic Press, New York, 1976, 453.
24. **Hubbell, W. L. and McConnell, H. M.,** Molecular motion in spin-labeled phospholipids and membranes, *J. Am. Chem. Soc.,* 93, 314, 1971.
25. **Marsh, D.,** Electron spin resonance: spin labels, in *Membrane Spectroscopy,* Grell, E., Ed., Springer-Verlag, Berlin, 1981, 51.
26. **Birrell, G. B., Anderson, P. B., Jost, P. C., Griffith, O. H., Banaszak, L. J., and Seelig, J.,** Lipid environments in the yolk lipoprotein system. A spin-labeling study of the lipovitellin/phosvitin complex from *Xenopus laevis, Biochemistry,* 21, 2444, 1982.
27. **Sinha, B. K. and Chignell, C. F.,** Interaction of antitumor drugs with human erythrocyte ghost membranes and mastocytoma P815: a spin label study, *Biochem. Biophys. Res. Commun.,* 86, 1051, 1979.
28. **Jost, P. C. and Griffith, O. H.,** The lipid-protein interface in biological membranes, *Ann. N.Y. Acad. Sci.,* 348, 391, 1980.
29. **Jost, P. C., Nadakavukaren, K. K., and Griffith, O. H.,** Phosphatidylcholine exchange between the boundary lipid and bilayer domains in cytochrome oxidase containing membranes, *Biochemistry,* 16, 3110, 1977.
30. **Lambert, W. J., Higuchi, W. I., Knutson, K., and Krill, S. L.,** Dose-dependent enhancement effects of Azone® on skin permeability, *Pharm. Res.,* 6, 798, 1989.
31. **Wertz, P. W.,** Epidermal lipids, *Semin. Dermatol.,* 2, 106, 1992.
32. **Rigaud, J. L., Gary-bobo, C. M., and Taupin, C.,** Effect of chemical modifiers of passive permeability on the conformation of spin-labeled erythrocyte membranes, *Biochim. Biophys. Acta,* 373, 211, 1974.
33. **Quan, D. Y., Higuchi, R. I., Takayama, K., Higashiyama, K., and Nagai, T.,** Promoting effect of 2-*n*-alkylcyclohexanones on the percutaneous absorption of indomethacin, *Drug Design Deliv.,* 5, 149, 1989.
34. **Quan, D. Y., Higuchi, R. I., Takayama, K., Higashiyama, K., and Nagai, T.,** Enhancing effect of piperidone derivatives on the percutaneous absorption of indomethacin, *Drug Design Deliv.,* 6, 61, 1990.
35. **Hadgraft, J., Walters, K. A., and Guy, R. H.,** Epidermal lipids and topical drug delivery, *Semin. Dermatol.,* 2, 139, 1992.

Chapter 16.3

X-Ray Fluorescence

J. David Robertson and Michael Jay

CONTENTS

I. INTRODUCTION

X-ray fluorescence (XRF) is an emission spectroscopic technique which can be used for both quantitative and qualitative elemental analysis. In XRF the atoms in a sample are excited to emit their characteristic X-rays by exposing the sample to a source of low-energy ionizing radiation. The energy of the emitted X-ray identifies the element and the number of X-rays of a given energy is a measure of the concentration of that element in the sample matrix.

As a tool for *in vivo* elemental analyses, XRF has been applied to a number of medical tracer studies. For example, the technique has been used to investigate the lead (Pb) content in childrens teeth,[1] to measure the mercury (Hg) content of blood, urine, and kidney tissue,[2] and to determine hepatic iodine (I) concentrations.[3] The most common clinical use of XRF is the determination of the distribution and/or content of I in the thyroid gland.[4,5] Recently, we demonstrated that radioisotope-induced XRF could be used as a simple, noninvasive technique for monitoring percutaneous absorption *in vivo* by the surface disappearance method.[6] In this chapter we outline the basic analytical methodology for these measurements and describe the use of XRF to investigate the penetration-enhancing effects of ethyl acetate (EtAc), *N*-methyl-2-pyrrolidinone (NMP), and dimethylsulfoxide (DMSO) on the percutaneous absorption of 2-iodobenzoic acid and 2-bromobenzoic acid.

II. THEORY

In radioisotope-induced XRF the X- and/or γ-rays from a radioactive source interact with the electrons in the atom in such a manner that an electron is ejected from one of the inner shells (K or L), as shown in Figure 1. The incident photons can only interact with the atom by the photoelectric effect mechanism if the energy of the

0-8493-2605-2/95/$0.00+$.50

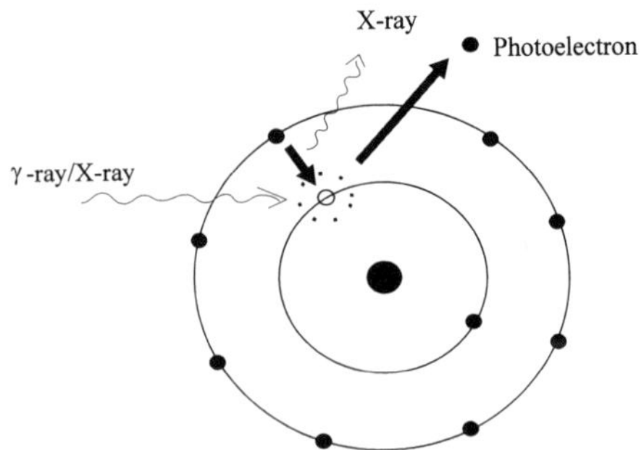

Figure 1 An illustration of photoinduced X-ray fluorescence.

photon is greater than the binding energy of the electron in the bombarded atom. When this occurs, the loss of the inner shell photoelectron leaves the atom in an excited state and the atom can return to its original state by emitting either Auger electrons or X-rays. In the second case, X-rays are emitted when an outer-shell electron in the atom fills the vacancy left by the ejected photoelectron. For qualitative analysis, the emitted X-ray is characteristic of the target atom in that its energy is equal to the energy difference between the initial and final states of the transferred electron. For quantitative analysis, the number of emitted X-rays of a specific energy can be related to the concentration of the element in the sample.

Consider, for example, our use of radioisotope-induced XRF to measure the percutaneous absorption of 5-iodouracil by monitoring the number of I K_α X-rays from the absorption site as a function of time.[6] An I K_α X-ray is emitted when a 60-keV γ-ray from the radioactive ^{241}Am source first interacts with an I atom in the sample matrix to eject an electron from the innermost (K) shell of the electron cloud (binding energy of 33.2 keV), and this vacancy is then filled by an electron from the adjacent (L) shell. The I K_α X-ray at 28.5 keV can, with current energy-dispersive X-ray spectrometers, be distinguished easily from the X-rays from any other element. The number of I K_α X-rays registered in the detector per unit time *(Y)* can, in this case, be estimated by the "thin target" formula:

$$Y = F(E_0) \cdot N_z \cdot \Omega \cdot \varepsilon_z \cdot \omega_z \cdot \sigma(E_0)_z \tag{1}$$

where $F(E_0)$ is the flux of 60 keV photons on the target (photons per second)
N_z is the number of I atoms per square centimeter in the target
Ω is the solid angle subtended by the X-ray detector
ε_z is the intrinsic efficiency of the detector for I K_α X rays
ω_z is the K-shell fluorescence yield for I
$\sigma(E_0)_z$ is the I K-shell photoelectric cross-section for 60 keV photons (per square centimeter)

Equation 1 can be used for the *in vivo* surface disappearance measurements because the sample layer, a drug or compound applied to the skin surface, is thin enough so that the photon flux ($F(E_0)$) is not significantly attenuated in passing through the layer and the I K_α X-rays are not reabsorbed by the sample layer. When these two conditions are not satisfied, a more detailed calculation is required.[7]

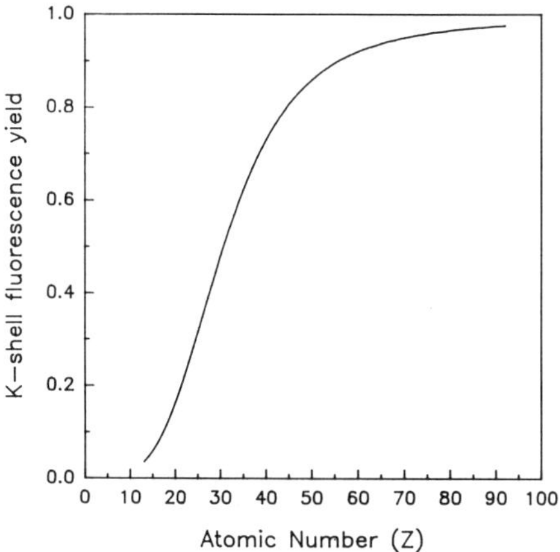

Figure 2 The variation in the K-shell fluorescence yield (ω_z) with atomic number. (Data from Lederer, C. M. and Shirley, V. S., *Table of Isotopes,* Vol. 7, John Wiley & Sons, New York, 1978, A10.)

Ideally, XRF could be used to measure the percutaneous absorption rate of any compound that contains elements that are found in only minor or trace levels in the skin. Practically, X-ray fluorescence is well suited for measuring the absorption of compounds that contain, or can be labeled with, elements with an atomic number ≥20. As can be seen from Figure 2, the K-shell fluorescence yield (ω_z), or probability of photon emission following the creation of a vacancy in the K-shell, increases with increasing atomic number and is near zero below atomic number 20.[8] Likewise, the intrinsic detector efficiency (ε_z) of most detectors, while near unity for X-rays in the energy range between 5 to 15 keV, falls off rapidly for X-rays from elements below atomic number 20 whose X-ray energies are below 5 keV because of severe absorption in the window on the detector. Finally, as seen in Figure 3, the photoelectric cross-section is at a maximum just above the absorption edge of an element and falls off rapidly as the photon energy increases above this value.[9] Because most isotopic X-ray sources provide principal radiations well above the K-shell binding energy of calcium, the probability of producing X-rays from elements below atomic number 20 is small.

While Equation 1 provides a reasonable estimate of the X-ray yield for a percutaneous absorption measurement, it must be kept in mind that the XRF technique is not a "true" surface analysis technique. The XRF signal does not disappear when the compound leaves the skin surface. Instead, the decrease in the X-ray yield with time will be due to both the attenuation of the X-rays as the marker atom migrates through the skin and the decrease in the X-ray yield as the marker atom is taken up by the blood and lymph vessels.[6] For a higher energy X-ray (e.g., 28.5 keV I K_α), a 3-mm thick skin layer would attenuate the X-ray yield by only 5%. If absorption is defined as the combination of permeation and resorption, this difference will have no affect upon absorption rate measurements at a given site. This difference could, however, lead to site-to-site absorption rate variations that are simply due to the change in X-ray yield with skin thickness. Given that the lower energy X rays are more readily absorbed by the skin matrix, the magnitude of any such site-to-site variations will increase as the energy of the X-ray, or corresponding atomic number of the marker atom, decreases.

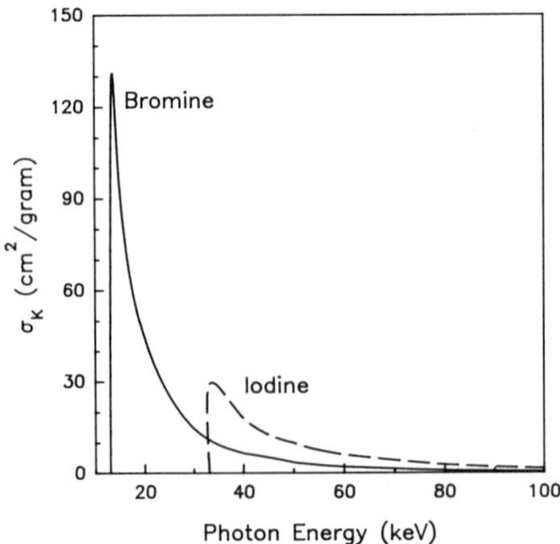

Figure 3 The K-shell photoelectric cross-section (σ_K) for Br and I as a function of incident photon energy. (Data from Storm, E. and Harvey, I. L., *Nucl. Data Tables,* A7, 565, 1970.)

III. EXPERIMENTAL SYSTEM

A schematic diagram of the XRF system employed in our *in vivo* absorption studies is shown in Figure 4. In this system the 60-keV γ-rays and 17-keV Np L X-rays from a sealed (Be window) 500 mCi ^{241}Am annular source are used as the fluorescence source. A 30-mm^2 Si(Li) detector, with a full-width-half-maximum resolution of 165 eV for the Mn K_α line, is used to measure the X-rays from the skin surface. The detector is mounted vertically in a tripod assembly with the endcap pointing down; the end of the detector is 20 cm from the bottom of the tripod. The Pb annular source holder, which is attached to the endcap of the detector (Figure 4), is designed in such a way that the XRF source irradiates an area of 3.1 cm^2 on a sample that is placed 2.0 cm from the front surface of the holder.

All of the XRF percutaneous absorption measurements in our laboratory have, thus far, been performed on female Sprague-Dawley albino rats. Details of how the absorption site is prepared and the compounds are applied can be found in Reference 6. An example of an XRF spectrum of the skin area immediately following the application of 40 µl of a 2-iodobenzoic acid/DMSO solution is given in Figure 5a. The large background in the center of the spectrum is present in all the XRF spectra and is due to the coherent and incoherent scattering of the excitation photons from the rat. It is corrected for by subtracting an initial "background" spectrum of the subject, taken prior to the application of any compound, from each subsequent fluorescence spectrum. The corresponding background corrected spectrum for the 2-iodobenzoic acid (2-IBA)/DMSO solution is shown in Figure 5b. No dead time correction is required in the background subtraction procedure, as the dead time of the XRF counting system for a given animal remains constant.

The practical application of XRF as a simple, noninvasive means to measure percutaneous absorption will depend upon the X-ray yields from the XRF system employed. For a given element, the measured X-ray yield, *Y,* is simply the number of counts in the X-ray peak divided by the counting time, *t,* used to accumulate the XRF spectrum. An estimate of the X-ray yields *(Y)* in our system for five different marker atoms or labels, all at an areal concentration of 1 mg/cm^2, is given in Table 1.

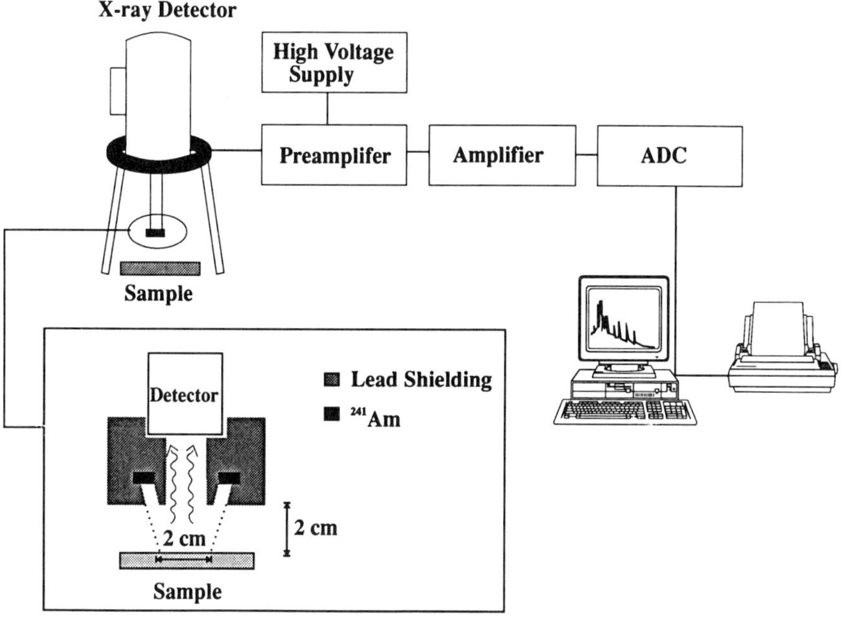

Figure 4 A schematic illustration of the system used for the *in vivo* X-ray fluorescence measurements.

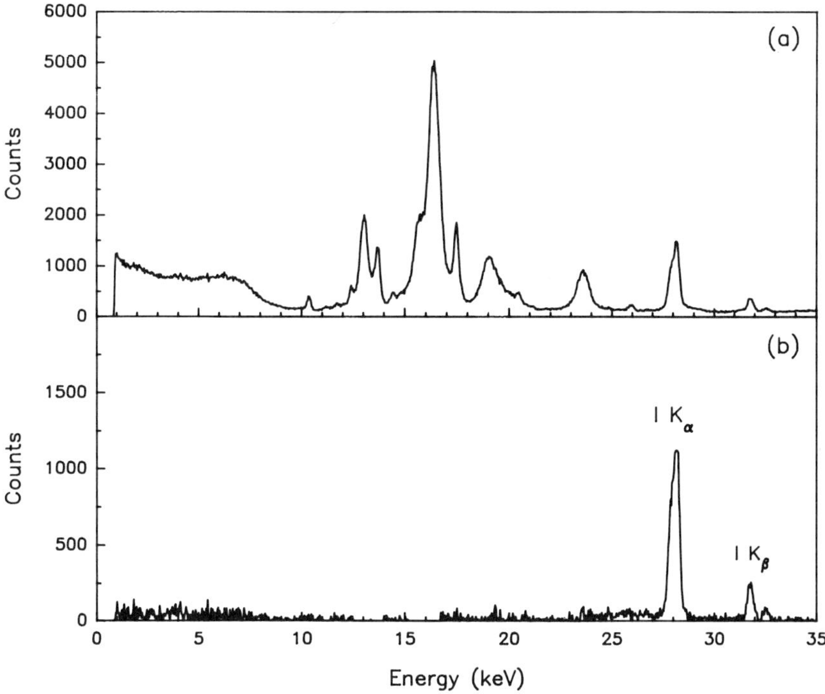

Figure 5 The original (a) and background-subtracted (b) XRF spectra of the skin of a rat immediately following the topical application of 10.5 mg/cm² of 2-IBA acid.

Table 1 An Estimate of the X-ray Yields (Y) that Would Be Obtained with Our XRF System for Elements Applied to the Skin at a Concentration of 1 mg/cm^2

Element	X-ray Yield (counts per second)
I[a]	11
Ag	11
Br	240
Zn	220
Cl	8

[a] Measured X-ray yield.

These values were calculated using Equation 1 and the measured X-ray yield from 1 mg/cm^2 of I on the skin surface. The large increase in the yields for Br and Zn is due to the high photoelectric cross-section in the interaction of the 17 keV Np L X-rays from the ^{241}Am source with these two elements; the K-shell binding energies of Br and Zn at 13.5 and 9.7 keV, respectively, are close to the energies of the Np L X rays. Because the X-ray yields are directly proportional to the areal concentration of an element, the values in Table 1 or similar calculations with Equation 1 can be used to determine the concentration ranges that can be examined with the XRF system. For example, consider a compound that contains Zn as the marker atom. The initial fluorescence yield Y_0 (counts per second) in our system for this compound would be equal to

$$Y_0 = W \cdot A_0 \cdot 220 \tag{2}$$

where W is the weight percentage of Zn in the compound and A_0 is the initial areal concentration (milligrams per square centimeter) of the compound applied to the skin. Because the statistical uncertainty of an individual XRF yield measurement is given by

$$\sigma_y = \sqrt{\frac{Y}{t}} \tag{3}$$

the precision of the X-ray yield measurement at low concentrations can be improved by increasing the counting time t. An increase in counting time will, however, result in a larger radiation dose for the subject.

IV. PENETRATION ENHANCEMENT MEASUREMENTS

A. BACKGROUND

As an example of the use of XRF as a simple, noninvasive means to investigate percutaneous absorption *in vivo,* we present briefly our investigation of the penetration-enhancing effects of EtAc, NMP, and DMSO on female Sprague-Dawley rats with 2-IBA and 2-bromobenzoic acid (2-BrBA) as the model compounds.

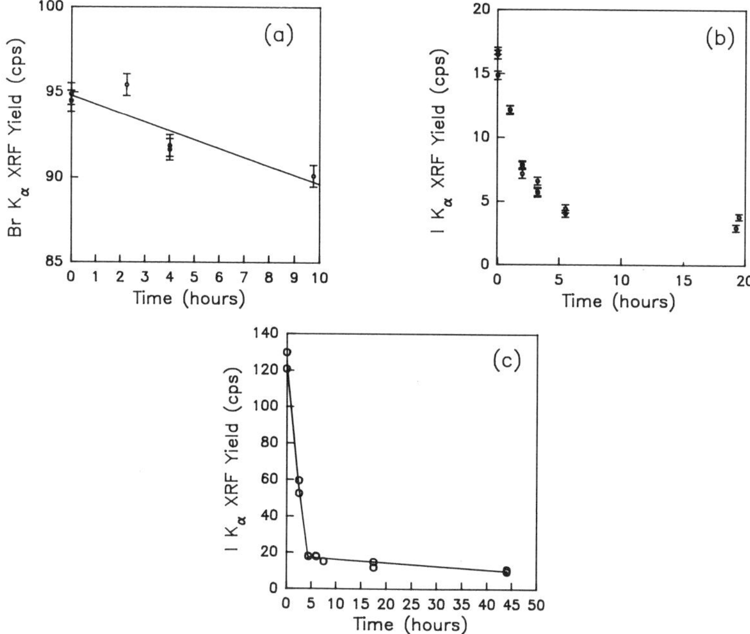

Figure 6 The variation of the K_α XRF yields (Y) with time from rats treated with (a) 2-BrBA in EtAc, (b) 2-IBA in NMP, and (c) 2-IBA in DMSO.

B. EXPERIMENTAL PROCEDURE

2-Iodobenzoic acid was dissolved in EtAc at a concentration of 76 mg/ml, in NMP at concentrations of 40 and 79 mg/ml, and in DMSO at concentrations of 104 and 212 mg/ml. 2-Bromobenzoic acid was dissolved in EtAc at a concentration of 76 mg/ml, in NMP at a concentration of 84 mg/ml, and in DMSO at a concentration of 78 mg/ml. Because of the photosensitive nature of these compounds, the 2-IBA and 2-BrBA powder and solutions were stored in the dark at all times. In accordance with state and federal regulations the use of female Sprague-Dawley albino rats in these experiments was approved by the Institutional Animal Care and Use Committee at the University of Kentucky. Details of how the absorption site is prepared and how the compounds are applied can be found in Reference 6.

The absorption of the 2-IBA and 2-BrBA solutions was followed by periodically accumulating 5-min XRF spectra of the applied site over a maximum period of 48 h. Between each measurement, the rat was removed from the XRF system and the plastic platform, and allowed food and water *ad libitum* in the cage. During this time, the drug site was protected from scratching or bathing by wrapping the rat with cling gauze in a figure-eight fashion around the front legs and over the body. After the initial XRF measurement, the rat was reanesthetized as needed before being placed back in the XRF system.

C. RESULTS AND DISCUSSION

The variation of the Br K_α X-ray yield with time for a rat treated with the 2-BrBA in EtAc solution is shown in Figure 6a. The XRF measurements on this subject

Table 2 Solutions that Exhibited Zero-Order Absorption

Rat # no.	Initial Conc (mg/cm²)	Absorption Rate Constant k_0 (μg/cm²/h)	Correlation Coefficient	Norm
		2-IBA in EtAc (76 mg/ml)		
1	3.88	68 ± 30	0.70	3.1
2	3.88	51 ± 17	0.77	3.8
3	3.88	41 ± 12	0.88	0.9
		2-BrBA in EtAc (76 mg/ml)		
4	3.88	43 ± 15	0.82	8.0
5	3.88	21 ± 6	0.88	2.3
		2-BrBA in NMP (84 mg/ml)		
14	4.28	245 ± 24	0.98	15.1
15	4.28	283 ± 15	0.99	5.0

indicate that the absorption of the 2-BrBA/EtAc solution follows zero-order kinetics with an absorption rate constant, k_0, of 21 ± 6 μg/cm²/h. The rate constant is obtained from:

$$k_0 = \left(\frac{A_0}{Y_0}\right) \cdot m \tag{4}$$

where A_0 is the initial areal concentration of 2-BrBA, Y_0 is the Br K_α X-ray yield at time $t = 0$, and m is the slope of the line fit to the data in Figure 6a. X-ray fluorescence measurements on a second animal treated with the 2-BrBA/EtAc solution yielded similar results. Likewise, a study of animals treated with the 2-IBA in EtAc and 2-BrBA in NMP solutions revealed that the absorption of these solutions also follow zero-order kinetics. The absorption rates obtained from the *in vivo* measurements on animals treated with the 2-BrBA/EtAc, 2-IBA/EtAc, and 2-BrBA/NMP solutions are summarized in Table 2.

In marked contrast to the results for 2-BrBA in NMP, the absorption of the 2-IBA/NMP solution does not follow zero-order kinetics. As can be seen from Figure 6b, the I K_α X-ray yield from a rat treated with 40 μl of the 40 mg/ml 2-IBA/NMP solution does not decrease linearly with time. Similar XRF yield curves were obtained from *in vivo* measurements on five other animals treated with the 40 mg/ml 2-IBA/NMP solution and four animals treated with a 79 mg/ml 2-IBA/NMP solution.

N-Methyl-2-pyrrolidinone has been shown in previous studies to increase the transport of, for example, steroids,[10,11] caffeine,[12] and aspirin.[13] It is not surprising, therefore, that in this study NMP increases, in comparison to EtAc, the percutaneous absorption of both 2-BrBA and 2-IBA. The observed difference in the absorption kinetics between the 2-IBA/NMP and 2-BrBA/NMP solutions was, on the other hand, wholly unexpected. In order to determine whether a chemical reaction between the two benzoic acid analogues and the solvent was responsible for this observed difference, the NMP solutions were analyzed by capillary gas chromatography. No evidence for a chemical reaction between the benzoic acids and NMP was observed. Moreover, a comparison of the gas chromatographic analysis of freshly prepared NMP solutions to those used in the percutaneous absorption measurements indicated that the benzoic acid compounds used in the *in vivo* studies had not undergone a photochemical reaction. This leads us to conclude that in the case of the halogenated benzoic acid compounds the marker Br and/or I atom alters the chemistry of the compounds in such a way that different absorption kinetics are observed when NMP is used as the solvent.

An example of the variation of the I K_α XRF yield with time for a rat treated with the 2-IBA in DMSO solution (212 mg/ml) is shown in Figure 6c. Similar absorption curves were obtained for the 104 mg/ml 2-IBA/DMSO solution and the 78 mg/ml 2-BrBA/DMSO solution. The model that we use to describe these data separates the absorption of 2-IBA and 2-BrBA in DMSO into two zero-order components. From the time of application to time t_1, the absorption of the benzoic acid compounds from the skin surface is allowed to proceed rapidly at a rate constant k_1. After time t_1, the compound is absorbed at a slower rate defined by a rate constant k_2. The change in the permeability of the stratum corneum (SC) at time t_1 in the model is attributed to the absorption of the enhancer such that the concentration of DMSO in the SC falls below some critical level. The XRF yield in this case is modeled as:

$$Y = \left(\frac{Y_0}{A_0}\right) \cdot \left(A_0 - k_1 t\right) \qquad t \le t_1 \tag{5}$$

and

$$Y = \left(\frac{Y_0}{A_0}\right) \cdot \left(\left(A_0 - k_1 t\right) - k_2 t\right) \qquad t > t_1 \tag{6}$$

where k_1 and k_2 are the two zero-order rate constants. A summary of the model parameters obtained from a regression (Marquardt-Levenberg algorithm) analysis of the XRF data from rats treated with the 2-IBA/DMSO and 2-BrBA/DMSO solutions is given in Table 3. In this treatment of the data the rate constant for the absorption of the benzoic acid compound after time t_1 (k_2) is comparable to the rate constant with EtAc as the solvent.

The idea that the two-component curve shown in Figure 6c results from the absorption of the model compounds at two different rates from the surface because of solvent depletion was tested in a stripping experiment. As noted above, the XRF technique is not a "true" surface analysis technique in that the signal does not disappear when the compound leaves the skin surface. Instead, the decrease in the fluorescence yield with time is due to both the attenuation of the X-ray yield as the compound migrates through the skin and the decrease in the X-ray yield as the compound is taken up by the blood and lymph vessels. Hence, the two-component curve could also arise from the rapid migration of the 2-IBA/DMSO solution from the surface into a reservoir and the slow absorption of the compound from the subsurface reservoir. In the stripping experiment 40 μl of the 212 mg/ml 2-IBA in DMSO solution was applied and allowed to absorb for 20 h. The I K_α XRF yield at this time was 22 ± 0.2 counts per second. The application site was then "stripped"

Table 3 The Parameters Obtained from the Two-Component Zero-Order Model Used to Describe the Absorption of the DMSO Solutions

Rat no.	Initial Conc (mg/cm²)	Absorption Constant k_1 (mg/cm²/h)	Absorption Constant k_2 (mg/cm²/h)	t_1 (h)	Norm
		2-IBA in DMSO (212 mg/ml)			
16	10.8	2.4 ± 0.07	0.02 ± 0.01	3.9 ± 0.1	9.0
17	10.8	1.5 ± 0.1	0.06 ± 0.03	3.1 ± 0.4	5.5
18	10.8	1.5 ± 0.08	0.04 ± 0.04	4.9 ± 0.4	22
		2-IBA in DMSO (104 mg/ml)			
19	5.3	1.9 ± 0.1	0	2.0 ± 0.1	11
19	5.3	2.4 ± 0.2	0.01 ± 0.01	1.5 ± 0.1	3.7
19	5.3	1.0 ± 0.4	0.01 ± 0.01	4.3 ± 0.2	4.6
20	5.3	0.5 ± 0.02	0.01 ± 0.01	6.6 ± 0.4	12
21	5.3	0.7 ± 0.01	0.02 ± 0.01	3.8 ± 0.4	16
22	5.3	0.4 ± 0.04	0.03 ± 0.01	5.0 ± 0.7	16
23	5.3	0.7 ± 0.1	0.03 ± 0.01	2.8 ± 0.4	4.0
		2-BrBA in DMSO (78 mg/ml)			
24	4.0	1.2 ± 0.02	0	2.4 ± 0.1	5.1

with ten pieces of tape in order to remove the SC[14] and a fluorescence spectrum was accumulated. Because the I K_α XRF yield fell to zero after the stripping, we concluded that the model compound is being absorbed from the skin surface or SC and not from a subsurface reservoir.

The ability of DMSO to accelerate skin permeation has been attributed to the extraction of SC lipids,[12,15] the displacement of bound water and loosening of the polymeric structure within the corneocyte,[16,17] and osmotically inducing delamination of the SC.[18] The idea that a critical concentration of DMSO in the SC is required for rapid absorption is supported by the steady-state, *in vitro* diffusion studies of Kurihara-Bergstrom et al.[19] Their work demonstrated that while the activity-adjusted permeability coefficients of the permeants methanol, 1-butanol, and 1-octanol were invariant to DMSO concentrations of 50% strength, they increased systematically and profoundly when the DMSO percentage strength was raised to >75%. According to the results presented in Table 3, 40 µl of DMSO induces this severe barrier impairment in the nonstationary case for an average of 4 h. While these results do not establish a "critical concentration" of DMSO for the altered barrier permeability, they do demonstrate that the barrier impairment induced by the application of DMSO persists for only a short time. Moreover, given the fact that DMSO is rapidly absorbed through the skin, it is reasonable to attribute this sudden change in permeability to the depletion of the solvent.

V. SUMMARY

Radioisotope-induced XRF can be used as a simple, noninvasive means to measure percutaneous absorption *in vivo* by the surface disappearance method. The chief advantage of the technique is that it does not rely upon the use of radiolabeled compounds and does not, as a result, expose the individual to a whole-body radiation dose. The technique is, however, not totally benign as it does require that the subject be exposed to an external, localized radiation dose.

X-ray fluorescence is practically well suited for measuring the absorption of compounds that contain, or can be labeled with, elements with an atomic number ≥20. The difference in absorption kinetics observed between two nearly identical compounds, 2-BrBA in NMP and 2-IBA in NMP, indicates, however, that consideration should be given to the effect that the addition of a heavy atom label would have on the percutaneous absorption of a compound. On the other hand, this difference and the two-component absorption curve observed with DMSO for these two model compounds does illustrate the importance of being able to investigate the nonstationary effect of penetration enhancers *in vivo* with a rapid and simple technique such as XRF.

This technique can also be applied to other drug delivery systems, e.g., controlled release of drugs following IM or subdermal administration, and release of compounds impregnated in artificial skin preparations. Because it is a noninvasive technique, XRF can be used to quantify the absorption of compounds through damaged skin (wounds, burns, etc.) and is applicable to human use due to its acceptable external and localized radiation dose.

REFERENCES

1. **Bloch, P., Garanoglie, G., Mitchell, G., and Shapiro, I. M.,** Measurement of lead content of children's teeth in situ by X-ray fluorescence, *Phys. Med. Biol.,* 20, 56, 1976.
2. **Walsh, P., Hamrick, P., and Underwood, N.,** Application of X-ray emission spectrometry to the determination of mercury in biological samples, *Rev. Sci. Instrum.,* 44, 1019, 1973.
3. **Meignan, M. and Galle, P.,** Exploration thyroidienne partition rescence. X., *Nouv. Presse Med.,* 7, 13, 1978.
4. **Patton, J. A. and Brill, A. B.,** Simultaneous emission and fluorescent scanning of the thyroid, *J. Nucl. Med.,* 19, 464, 1978.
5. **Fragu, P., Schlumberger, M., Davy, J. M., Slama, M., and Berdeaux, A.,** Effects of amiodarone therapy on thyroid iodine content as measured by X-ray fluorescence, *J. Clin. Endocrinol. Metab.,* 66, 762, 1988.
6. **Robertson, J. D., Ferguson, E., Jay, M., and Stalker, D. J.,** Noninvasive *in vivo* percutaneous absorption measurements using X-ray fluorescence, *Pharm. Res.,* 9, 1410, 1992.
7. **Tinney, J. F.,** *In vivo* X-ray fluorescence analysis — concepts and equipment, in *Semiconductor Detectors in the Future of Nuclear Medicine,* Hoffer, P. B., 1971, 214.
8. **Lederer, C. M. and Shirley, V. S.,** *Table of Isotopes,* Vol. 7, John Wiley & Sons, New York, 1978, A10.
9. **Storm, E. and Harvey, I. L.,** Photon cross sections from 1 keV to 100 MeV for elements Z=1 to Z=100, *Nucl. Data Tables,* A7, 565, 1970.
10. **Bennett, S. L., Barry, B. W., and Woodford, R.,** Optimization of bioavailability of topical steroids: non-occluded penetration enhancers under thermodynamic control, *J. Pharm. Pharmacol.,* 37, 298, 1984.
11. **Barry, B. W., Wouthwell, D., and Woodford, R.,** Optimization of bioavailability of topical steroids: penetration enhancers under occlusion, *J. Invest. Dermatol.,* 82, 49, 1984.
12. **Southwell, D. and Barry, B. W.,** Penetration enhancement in human skin; effect of 2-pyrrolidone, dimethylformamide and increased hydration on finite dose permeation of aspirin and caffeine, *Int. J. Pharm.,* 22, 291, 1984.
13. **Embery, G. and Dugard, P. H.,** The isolation of dimethyl sulfoxide soluble components from human epidermal preparations. A possible mechanism of action of dimethyl sulfoxide in effecting percutaneous migration phenomena, *J. Invest. Dermatol.,* 57, 308, 1971.
14. **Rougier, A., Dupuis, D., Lotte, C., Roguet, R., Wester, R. C., and Maibach, H. I.,** Regional variation in percutaneous absorption in man: measurement by the stripping method, *Arch. Dermatol. Res.,* 278, 465, 1986.

15. **Allenby, A. H., Creasey, N. H., Edginton, J. A. G., Fletcher, J. A., and Schock, C.,** Mechanism of action of accelerants on skin penetration, *Br. J. Dermatol.,* 81, 47, 1969.
16. **Montes, L. F., Day, J. L., Ward, C. J., and Kennedy, L.,** Ultrastructural changes in the horny layer following local application of DMSO to guinea pig skin, *J. Invest. Dermatol.,* 48, 184, 1967.
17. **MacGregor, W. S.,** The chemical and physical properties of DMSO, *Ann. N.Y. Acad. Sci.,* 141, 3, 1967.
18. **Chandrasekaran, S. K., Campbell, P. S., and Michaels, A. S.,** Effect of dimethyl sulfoxide on drug permeation through human skin, *AIChE J.,* 23, 810, 1977.
19. **Kurihara-Bergstrom, T., Flynn, G. L., and Higuchi, W. I.,** Physicochemical study of percutaneous absorption enhancement by dimethyl sulfoxide: kinetic and thermodynamic determinants of dimethyl sulfoxide mediated mass transfer of alkanols, *J. Pharm. Sci.,* 75, 479, 1986.

Chapter 16.4

Assessing Penetration Enhancers for Topical Corticosteroids

Eric W. Smith and John M. Haigh

CONTENTS

I. INTRODUCTION

Topical corticosteroids have been used for a wide range of dermatological conditions for the last 4 decades.[1] For many years the topical delivery system was a relatively simple cream or ointment base, with little thought given to improving the formulation as far as drug delivery was concerned. The main emphasis in the initial stages of development was on the alteration of the corticosteroid molecule, in an attempt to produce moieties with a higher intrinsic topical effect with lower mineralocorticoid side effects. Once this avenue of research was exhausted, attention was placed on the lipophilicity of the molecule with the production of various types of esters in an attempt to produce molecules which would pass through the stratum corneum (SC) with reasonable ease.

In recent years the nature of the semisolid drug delivery base has received considerable attention.[2–5] The nature of the vehicle has a profound effect on the rate of release of the topical corticosteroid from the formulation and its passage through the SC. One of the most important aspects of the formulation of the base is the inclusion of substances which aid this trans-SC diffusion, the so-called penetration enhancers.[6] The modes of action of the various different types of penetration enhancers are reviewed elsewhere in this book.

The best method for the assessment of the release of corticosteroids from topical formulations is obviously the clinical trial. Clinical trials, however, are laborious, costly, and difficult to mount. Patients suffering from dermatological complaints are not ideal subjects for the testing of topical corticosteroid formulations as it is difficult to obtain standardized lesions which are necessary for the comparison of results between formulations.[7] Alternatively, a number of *in vitro* models exist for this type of assessment, but it is often problematic to obtain correlation with the *in vivo* situation.

Of all the *in vivo* methods available for the assessment of topical corticosteroid formulations, the human skin blanching assay is one of the most reliable. The production of blanching in human skin is a side effect of topical corticosteroid

0-8493-2605-2/95/$0.00+$.50

application and was first observed in 1950.[8] In 1962[9] it was postulated that this blanching might be utilized as a measure of the percutaneous absorption of corticosteroids from topical formulations. The test has been improved considerably over the years[10–14] and it now provides a reliable and precise method for the assessment of the release of topical corticosteroids from their delivery formulations. For many years this test was (and sometimes still is) referred to as the vasoconstriction test. The exact mechanism of induced blanching has not been fully elucidated, and because the measurement performed during the test is the estimation of the degree of blanching produced, we believe that the best terminology for this test is the human skin blanching assay.

A number of publications[15–17] questioned the validity of the human skin blanching assay. While it must be appreciated that this assay procedure is highly subjective, this problem can be minimized by utilizing large numbers of application sites for the same formulation, a group of volunteers numbering no less than 12, and visual assessments of blanching made by at least two, and preferably three, observers.[11] However, we do not believe that this is the reason for recent criticism of this technique. Some researchers have made their comments based on the apparent nonequivalence of some generic products.[16,17] This seems to us to be nonsense. It is hardly scientific to question the technique because it produces unexpected results! In our opinion one of the main problems with regard to the use of the human skin blanching assay is that many researchers still attempt to make comparisons between formulations based on a single reading of topical corticosteroid-induced blanching. For several years we have advocated the use of multiple readings over a period of time (normally on the order of 36 h) after application of the steroid.[11] In this way time-response curves can be generated which produce much more meaningful results.

A number of instrumental (mainly reflectance) methods for the objective determination of corticosteroid-induced blanching have been available for many years. Several years ago we advanced the opinion[11] that these were cumbersome, expensive, and time consuming, and that no real advantages over the visual method of determination had been demonstrated by their use. These methods have been the subject of debate in the recent literature, many researchers again insisting that the instrumental methods are superior even though they have themselves demonstrated that the instrumental results obtained agree closely with those obtained by visual determinations. The superiority was defined on the basis of producing absolute numbers by the instrumental method and numerical gradings by visual assessments. It is of interest to us that antagonists of the use of visually scored data in the human skin blanching assay reported recently[18] that the human observer method is unlikely to be replaced by a spectrophotometric assessment method in the near future. We previously mentioned that instrumental techniques that measure one aspect of the blanching phenomenon do not seem to have the same reproducibility and discriminating potential as that of the human eye, which assimilates the global appearance of the skin at the application site and surrounding tissue. We have documented[19] exceptional reproducibility using visual data which, to our knowledge, has not been paralleled using instrumental techniques.

Because the human skin blanching assay can be used to assess the release of topical corticosteroids from semisolid bases, it stands to reason that it can also be useful in the assessment of the efficacy of penetration enhancers. A number of publications give details of the optimized methodology for this assay procedure.[11,12] Provided the protocol of this method is strictly adhered to by experienced workers, the assay has been shown to be sensitive, accurate, and reproducible.[10] Some of the advantages of using this assay procedure are that healthy normal skin is used, it is not painful to the volunteers and several preparations can be compared simultaneously. Another great advantage of the use of the human skin blanching assay is that it has been conclusively proven that the degree of observed corticosteroid-induced blanching in normal human skin is directly proportional to the clinical efficacy of the formulation.[20]

II. *IN VIVO* ASSESSMENT OF TOPICAL CORTICOSTEROID FORMULATIONS

We were involved recently in the efficacy assessment of the excipients urea, resorcinol, oleic acid, and propylene glycol in an extemporaneous oil-in-water cream delivery system containing 0.12% betamethasone 17-valerate, in order to ascertain whether, in this particular delivery system, they act as penetration enhancers.

All four of the compounds mentioned above were investigated previously and found to act as penetration enhancers for various topical corticosteroids in a number of different semisolid formulations, but their effects on the release of betamethasone 17-valerate from an oil-in-water cream base were not previously reported. The corticosteroid-induced blanching produced by the formulations was measured over 32 h using the human skin blanching assay and the scores were plotted as a function of the percentage of the total possible score (%TPS) vs. time. The blanching assessment experiments were all conducted in the unoccluded mode only. Occlusion causes hydration of the SC, thus aiding the passage of the corticosteroid through the SC (discussed elsewhere in this book). The occluded mode would therefore tend to mask any effects that the other compounds may have on the rate and extent of the release of betamethasone 17-valerate from the formulation. The unoccluded mode is also the most commonly utilized therapeutic application procedure. All the formulations were assayed by high-performance liquid chromatography[21] and found to contain the equivalent concentrations of betamethasone 17-valerate.

As can be seen from Figures 1 and 2, it is quite clear that only propylene glycol acts as a penetration enhancer for betamethasone 17-valerate from this particular formulation. Oleic acid, resorcinol and urea all reduce the amount of betamethasone 17-valerate penetrating the SC. Therefore, the formulations containing these excipients would be expected to be less efficacious than the formulations containing propylene glycol or that containing no penetration enhancer. The three excipients that do not act as penetration enhancers for betamethasone 17-valerate in this particular formulation clearly cause a reduction in the partitioning potential of the steroid from the semisolid base. Thus, less drug will be released from the delivery system to the SC. Propylene glycol, which does act as a penetration enhancer in this particular system is thought to act by perturbing the multilammelar bilayers of the SC intracellular lipids which consist mainly of cholesterol, ceramides, and free fatty acids.

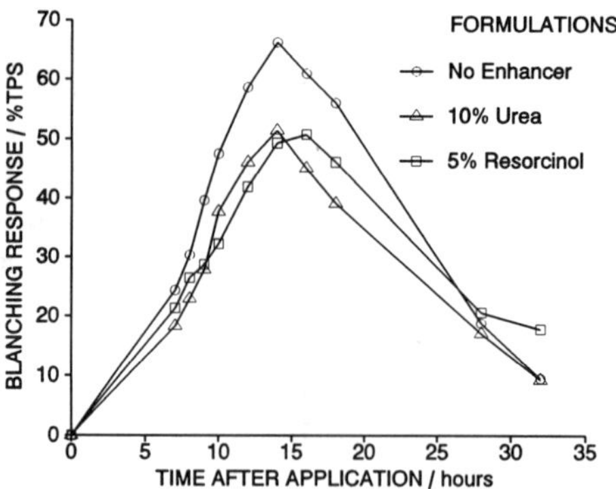

Figure 1 Human skin blanching response vs. time after application profiles for an oil-in-water cream formulation containing 5% resorcinol, 10% urea, and no enhancer.

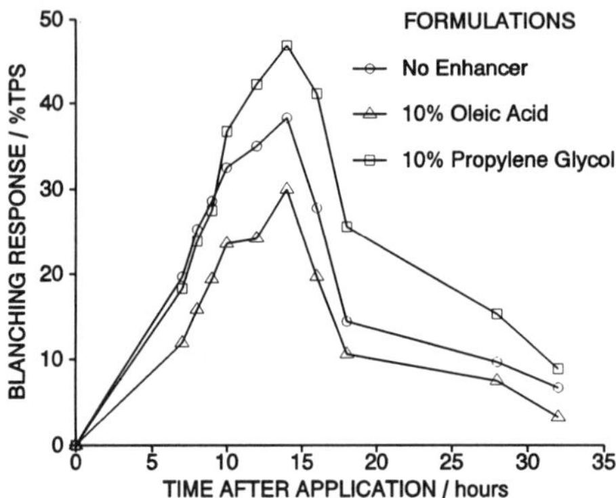

Figure 2 Human skin blanching response vs. time after application profiles for an oil-in-water cream formulation containing 10% oleic acid, 10% propylene glycol, and no enhancer.

III. CONCLUSIONS

Of interest is the fact that some compounds act as penetration enhancers in certain systems with particular corticosteroids and not in others. We have preliminary results showing that resorcinol acts as a penetration enhancer with betamethasone 17-valerate in a different semisolid cream base. It is obvious, therefore, that generalizations cannot be made with respect to which enhancer will be the most useful for a particular steroid in a particular formulation. Each individual system is required to be assessed for topical availability, preferably utilizing a reliable *in vivo* method.

From the above results it can be seen that the human skin blanching assay is a particularly useful method for assessing the effects of possible penetration enhancers in identical topical formulations containing the same concentration of a particular corticosteroid. While the foregoing discussion is concerned primarily with the assessment of the effect of penetration enhancers on the topical availability of corticosteroids from semisolid formulations it is clear that the arguments will apply to any molecule designed for release from a topical formulation to the SC.

REFERENCES

1. **Sulzberger, M. B. and Witten, V. H.,** Effect of topically applied compound F in selected dermatoses, *J. Invest. Dermatol.,* 19, 101, 1952.
2. **Meyer, E., Haigh, J. M., and Kanfer, I.,** Comparative bioavailability of some locally manufactured betamethasone valerate containing preparations, *S. Afr. Pharm. J.,* 50, 445, 1983.
3. **Meyer, E., Kanfer, I., and Haigh, J. M.,** Comparative blanching activities of some topical corticosteroid containing lotions, *S. Afr. Pharm. J.,* 48, 551, 1981.
4. **Smith, E. W., Meyer, E., and Haigh, J. M.,** Blanching activities of betamethasone formulations: the effect of dosage form on topical drug availability, *Drug Res.,* 40, 618, 1990.
5. **Haigh, J. M., Smith, E. W., Meyer, E., and Fassihi, R.,** Influence of the oil phase dispersion in a cream base on the *in vivo* release of betamethasone 17-valerate, *S.T.P. Pharm. Sci.,* 2, 259, 1992.
6. **Barry, B. W., Southwell, D., and Woodford, R.,** Optimization of bioavailability of topical steroids: penetration enhancers under occlusion, *J. Invest. Dermatol.,* 82, 49, 1984.
7. **Baker, H. and Sattar, H. A.,** The assessment of four new fluocortolone analogues by a modified vasoconstriction assay, *Br. J. Dermatol.,* 80, 46, 1968.
8. **Hollander, J. L., Stoner, E. K., Brown, E. M., and De Moor, P.,** The use of intra-articular temperature measurement in the evaluation of anti-arthritic agents, *Ann. Rheum. Dis.,* 9, 401, 1950.
9. **McKenzie, A. W. and Stoughton, R. B.,** Method for comparing percutaneous absorption of steroids, *Arch. Dermatol.,* 86, 608, 1962.
10. **Barry, B. W. and Woodford, R.,** Activity and bioavailability of topical steroids. *In vivo/in vitro* correlations for the vasoconstrictor test, *J. Clin. Pharmacol.,* 3, 43, 1978.
11. **Haigh, J. M. and Kanfer, I.,** Assessment of topical corticosteroid preparations: the human skin blanching assay, *Int. J. Pharm.,* 19, 245, 1984.
12. **Smith, E. W., Meyer, E., Haigh, J. M., and Maibach, H. I.,** The human skin blanching assay as an indicator of topical corticosteroid bioavailability and potency: an update, in *Percutaneous Absorption,* 2nd ed., Bronaugh, R. L. and Maibach, H. I., Eds., Marcel Dekker, New York, 1989, 443.
13. **Smith, E. W., Meyer, E., Haigh, J. M., and Maibach, H. I.,** The human skin blanching assay for comparing topical corticosteroid availability, *J. Dermatol. Treat.,* 2, 69, 1991.
14. **Meyer, E. W., Smith, E. W., and Haigh, J. M.,** Sensitivity of different areas to the flexor aspect of the human forearm to corticosteroid-induced skin blanching, *Br. J. Dermatol.,* 127, 379, 1992.
15. **Shah, V. P., Peck, C. C., and Skelly, J. P.,** Vasoconstriction-skin blanching assay for glucocorticoids: a critique, *Arch. Dermatol.,* 125, 1558, 1989.
16. **Stoughton, R. B.,** Are generic formulations equivalent to trade name topical glucosteroids?, *Arch. Dermatol.,* 123, 1312, 1987.
17. **Guin, J. D., Wallis, M. S., Walls, R., Lehman, P. A., and Franz, T. J.,** Quantitative vasoconstrictor assay for topical corticosteroids: the puzzling case of fluocinolone acetonide, *J. Am. Acad. Dermatol.,* 29, 197, 1993.
18. **Conner, D. P., Zamani, K., Almirez, R. G., Millora, E., Nix, D., and Shah, V. P.,** Use of reflectance spectrophotometry in the human corticosteroid skin blanching assay, *J. Clin. Pharmacol.,* 33, 707, 1993.
19. **Smith, E. W., Meyer, E., and Haigh, J. M.,** Accuracy and reproducibility of the multiple-reading skin blanching assay, in *Topical Corticosteroids,* Maibach, H. I. and Surber, C., Eds., S. Karger, Basel, 1992, 65.
20. **Cornell, R. C. and Stoughton, R. B.,** Correlation of the vasoconstriction assay and clinical activity in psoriasis, *Arch. Dermatol.,* 121, 63, 1985.
21. **Smith, E. W., Haigh, J. M., and Kanfer, I.,** A stability-indicating HPLC assay with on-line clean-up for betamethasone 17-valerate in topical dosage forms, *Int. J. Pharm.,* 27, 185, 1985.

Chapter 16.5

Fluorescence Spectroscopy

William Abraham

CONTENTS

I. INTRODUCTION

The phenomenon of fluorescence is described briefly followed by examples from the literature on the various membrane properties that have been investigated using fluorescence spectroscopy. The barrier to percutaneous penetration is reviewed briefly and then the use of fluorescence spectroscopy in studying the effect of penetration enhancers on the skin barrier is described. Most of the work on using this powerful technique in understanding the effect of penetration enhancers is still in its infancy. The objective of this chapter is to stimulate interest in this area and facilitate research in understanding the mechanism of action of penetration enhancers in reducing the barrier property of skin. A second objective is to facilitate development of a suitable biophysical correlate to flux enhancement caused by penetration enhancers.

The phenomenon of fluorescence is the emission of photons from an electronic excited state of a molecule. This occurs typically in the time scale of 10^{-8} s after excitation. This process can be followed by monitoring three important fluorescence parameters, Stokes shift, fluorescence lifetime, and anisotropy which give information about the environment around the molecule that is emitting the photons.

Upon excitation, the electrons from the ground electronic state occupy higher vibrational levels of excited electronic states. The electrons relax back to the ground vibrational level of the first excited electronic state, giving off the excess energy in a nonradiative fashion known as internal conversion. The phenomenon of fluorescence is the emission of the excited state electron from the first excited electronic state to the different vibrational levels of the ground electronic state as shown in Figure 1. Due to the loss of energy by internal conversion, the emission spectrum is

0-8493-2605-2/95/$0.00+$.50

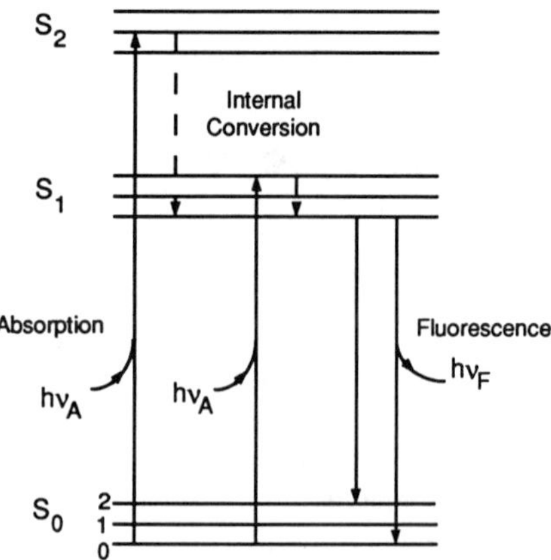

Figure 1 Jablonski diagram showing the absorption and emission of light.

at a lower energy or longer wavelengths as compared to the excitation spectrum. This difference in energy is known as the Stokes shift. In addition, there is solvent relaxation wherein the increased dipole of the excited state causes the surrounding solvent molecules to respond, creating a lower energy excited state of the fluorophore. Also possible are specific interactions with the solvent molecules such as hydrogen bonding. Thus, the Stokes shift depends on the polarity and the hydrogen-bonding ability of the solvent.[1] Lifetime is defined as the average time that the molecule spends in the excited state between excitation and emission. Any factor that affects the excited state of the fluorophore will affect the lifetime of the probe. Fluorescence lifetimes provide useful information about the environment of the probe.[2]

The excitation phenomenon occurs only in those molecules whose absorption moment is parallel to the electric vector of the incident photons. Any angular displacement of the fluorophore between absorption and emission would depolarize the emission. The anisotropy is a measure of these angular displacements and therefore the microviscosity of the medium. This has led to numerous applications of anisotropy measurements in membrane dynamics.[3] In addition to steady-state anisotropy, one could also measure the time-dependent decay of the anisotropy which provides considerable information about the diffusional motion of the fluorophore in a given medium.[4]

II. FLUORESCENCE IN LIPID BILAYERS

Fluorescence spectroscopy has been used extensively to study the structural and motional properties of lipids in model lipid bilayers and in biological membranes.[4,5] The structural aspects include the organizational aspects such as the distribution of lipids in bilayers, i.e., phase separation, as well as the structural constraint on the reorientation of the lipids. The dynamic aspects include the rotational diffusion of the acyl chains as well as the *trans*-gauche isomerization along the acyl chains of the lipids. These aspects collectively represent the fluidity of the lipid bilayer, which directly reflects the barrier property of the membrane.

A. STEADY-STATE MEASUREMENTS

Fluorescence parameters such as Stokes shift, anisotropy, and fluorescence quenching can be measured under steady-state conditions. The Stokes shift observed in steady-state emission spectra has been used to determine the polarity gradient in lipid bilayers.[6] Other fluorescent parameters such as the steady-state anisotropy and the depth-dependent fluorescence quenching in lipid bilayers also have been used to investigate biomembranes.[7,8] A series of anthroyloxy fatty acid (AF) probes where the fluorophore 9-anthracene carboxylic acid is esterified to 2, 6, 9, 12, 16, or other positions along the acyl chain of a fatty acid have been used widely to investigate the fluidity and polarity gradients in the lipid bilayers.[6] Steady-state anisotropy of probes such as the AF, *N*-phenyl naphthylamine, diphenylhexatriene (DPH) have been used to detect the gel to liquid crystalline phase transition and the effect of cholesterol on the organization of lipids in bilayers.[6] Temperature dependence of fluorescence anisotropy of head group-labeled fluorophores has been used to study lamellar to hexagonal phase transition in phosphatidylethanolamine systems.[9]

B. DYNAMIC MEASUREMENTS

The dynamic measurements fall under two categories: lifetime and time-resolved anisotropy measurements. Fluorescence lifetime has been used to study the phase transitions and phase separation of lipids into domains in model systems.[10,11] Diphenylhexatriene, parinaric acids, and AF probes have been used in lifetime experiments.[10,12,13] Diphenylhexatriene and *cis*-parinaric acid have been shown to partition equally between different lipid phases while *trans*-parinaric acid and AF probes have been shown to partition preferentially into the gel and liquid crystalline phases, respectively.[12,14]

More recently, the conventional analysis of the lifetime data in terms of discrete exponential decays with pre-exponential weight factors has been compared to a distribution model. In the later approach the lifetime data are analyzed in terms of distribution of lifetimes around the values obtained from the discrete analysis. This approach has been more effective in investigating a variety of natural membranes as well as model systems made up of lipid mixtures.[15] The general conclusion from the distributional approach for DPH probes was that DPH was in a variety of distinct lipid environment as seen by the wider distribution in natural membranes and model systems containing a mixture of unsaturated acyl chains.[15]

Time-resolved anisotropy provides insight into the rotational motion in lipid bilayers. The rotational motion has a structural component and a dynamic component. The structural component provides information on the rotational constraint in response to a thermal and/or a chemical perturbation. For example, the effect of a membrane protein or a drug molecule on the lipid rotational motion can be monitored by time-resolved anisotropy. The dynamic component provides information on the rate of rotation of the lipid components in membranes. Time-resolved anisotropy data in lipid bilayers are generally analyzed in terms of two models: a two-component model described by:[4]

$$r(t) = a_1 \exp(-t/\phi_1) + a_2 \exp(-t/\phi_2) \qquad (1)$$

where $r(t)$ is the anisotropy, and ϕ_1 and ϕ_2 are the rotational correlation times. Usually, ϕ_2 is very large as compared to ϕ_1. When ϕ_2 is long compared to the fluorescence lifetime, then Equation 1 may be replaced by:

$$r(t) = a_1 \exp(-t/\phi_1) + r_{inf} \quad (2)$$

where, $a_1 = r_0 - r_{inf}$; r_0 is the anisotropy that would be observed in the absence of rotational diffusion, and r_{inf} is the limiting anisotropy observed at times that are long compared to the fluorescence lifetime.

The limiting anisotropy has been used to calculate an order parameter S, where $S = (r_{inf}/r_0)^{1/2}$.[4] For example, order parameters were obtained for parinaric acid in phosphatidylcholine bilayers that were close to that obtained by deuterium nuclear magnetic resonance (NMR).[16] It should be noted that the order parameter is specific to the fluorophore.

III. INVESTIGATION OF PENETRATION ENHANCEMENT

The extraordinary barrier property of mammalian skin has been localized to the stratum corneum (SC). The highly ordered extracellular lipid bilayers of the SC constitute this barrier.[17,18] The extracellular membranous structures consist of saturated, nonpolar lipids that are arranged as multiple lamellae.[19] Also, these lipids are in the rigid gel phase at physiological temperature.[20] Attempts to overcome this barrier in transdermal drug delivery include the use of chemical penetration enhancers that would perturb this barrier.[21,22] A variety of penetration enhancers have been investigated in recent years, and are described in great detail in several of the chapters in this book.

A. PHYSICAL METHODS

In addition to determining the flux enhancement of drug molecules across skin treated with penetration enhancers, attempts have been made using physical methods such as differential scanning calorimetry (DSC),[20,23,24] electron spin resonance (ESR),[25] Fourier transform infrared (FTIR),[26,27] Raman,[28] and fluorescence spectroscopy[29–31] to understand the mode of action of these chemical enhancers on the epidermal barrier function.

Differential scanning calorimetry has been widely used to investigate the effect of penetration enhancers on the thermal phase transition of the lipid and protein components of the SC.[20,23,24] Results from different laboratories have shown two transitions occurring between 60 and 80°C in the SC and have been assigned to the intercellular lipid lamellae and the covalently attached lipids of the corneocyte cell envelope. The higher temperature transition occurring at 95°C was irreversible and was assigned to protein denaturation. The effect of penetration enhancers on these phase transitions have been used to determine the mode of their action. For example, DSC thermal profiles of the SC treated with a variety of fatty acids showed that *cis*-unsaturated fatty acids affected the lipid-associated transition and did not alter the protein transition. It was also shown that the lipid phase transition was shifted to lower temperatures and that this shift was inversely correlated to the flux enhancement.[23] The effect of azones and alkyl sulfoxides on thermal transitions showed a similar effect.[24] These studies led to the conclusion that these enhancers acted by disrupting the packing of the lipids in the intercellular bilayers of the SC.

The reader is referred to Chapters 16.1 and 16.2 on Raman and ESR spectroscopy for details on these techniques. Another physical technique that has been used widely to study the effect of ethanol, alkyl sulfoxides, and *cis*-monounsaturated fatty acids on the SC is FTIR spectroscopy.[26,27,32] The C-H symmetric and asymmetric stretching occurring around 2850/cm^{-1} have been used to monitor the lipid-associated changes in the SC in response to a chemical perturbant. Deuterium NMR has been used to investigate the packing order of the SC lipids *in vitro.*[33,34] Bilayer (L_α) to nonbilayer (H_{II}) transition was observed at high temperatures and it was proposed that the SC lipids could be induced to form the more permeable H_{II} phase by the addition of molecules (enhancers) of suitable geometry.[33,34]

B. FLUORESCENCE METHODS

1. Alkanols

Recently, fluorescence spectroscopy has been used to investigate the interaction of short-chain alkanols with the SC lipids.[29,30] Model systems made up of SC lipid liposomes (SCLL) and distearoylphosphatidylcholine/distearoylphosphatidic acid liposomes (DSPL) were used to study the mode of action of alkanols. In this study fluorescence parameters such as the emission maxima, fluorescence quantum yields, lifetimes, and steady-state anisotropy were measured for a variety of probes in the vesicles treated with short-chain alkanols. The amounts of different alkanols used in these experiments were 30% ethanol, 10% *n*-propanol, 2% *n*-butanol, or 1% *n*-pentanol. These produced an enhancement of 10 over the passive flux of lipophilic permeants and were defined as iso-enhancement concentrations. The fluorescence emission maxima and lifetimes which are sensitive to the polarity of the environment (cf. Section II) did not show any significant effect in liposomes that were treated with varying amounts of alkanols. This led to the conclusion that no change occurred in the polarity of the microenvironment at different depths in the bilayers upon alcohol treatment.[29,30] In the same study the authors showed some interesting changes in the steady-state anisotropy (r_{ss}) of ANS, DPH, and AF probes in DSPL and SCLL. ANS and DPH were used to probe the head group and the hydrophobic regions, respectively, and AF probes were used to investigate the depth-dependent effects.

The results from the SCLL are summarized in Table 1 and in Figure 2. The percent change in r_{ss} for the HAF and DPH which probe the head group and the hydrocarbon regions, respectively, showed changes that were comparable to that observed in the DSPL.[29] However, the depth-dependent effects of alkanols under iso-enhancement concentrations were quite different in the SCLL. Significant increases in fluidity were detected around carbons 2 and 9, while no change occurred around carbon 16. Largest increase in fluidity around carbon 2 was caused by 30% ethanol while the largest increase around carbon 9 was caused by 1% *n*-pentanol.

Using the r_{ss} values of AF probes and the Perrin equation,[1] average correlation times were calculated in the same study.[29,30] The average correlation time $\langle\phi\rangle$ is defined as

$$\langle\phi\rangle = \langle\tau\rangle / \{(r_0/r_{ss}) - 1\} \tag{3}$$

Table 1 Percent Change in the Steady-State Anisotropy (r_{ss} %) of DPH and HAF Induced By *n*-Alkanols Under Iso-enhancement Concentrations in SCLL

	r_{ss} (%)	
Alkanols	**HAF**	**DPH**
30% ethanol	70.8	9.3
10% *n*-propanol	28.5	10.5
2% *n*-butanol	6.9	5.2
1% *n*-pentanol	5.6	12.0

[a] From Kim, Y. H. et al., *Biochim. Biophys. Acta,* 1148, 139, 1993.

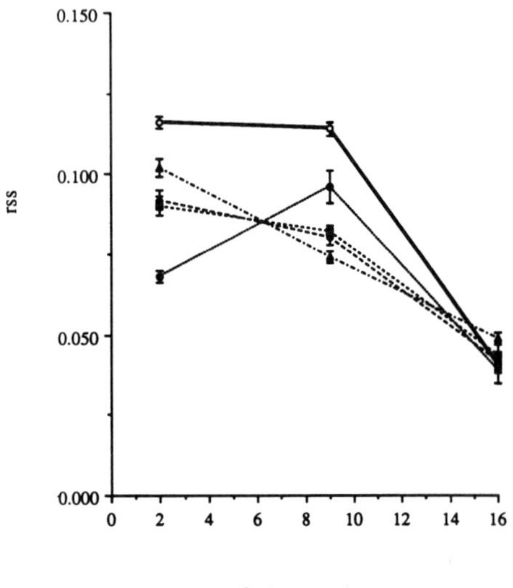

Figure 2 Depth-dependent effects of *n*-alkanols under iso-enhancement concentrations on the steady-state anisotropy (r_{ss}) obtained with 2-AS, 9-AS, and 16-AP in SCLL. Symbols: open circles (buffer); closed circles (30% ethanol); closed squares (10% *n*-propanol); closed diamonds (2% *n*-butanol); closed triangles (1% *n*-pentanol). (From Kim, Y. H., Ph.D. thesis, University of Utah, Salt Lake City, 1992. With permission.)

where r_0 is the anisotropy in the absence of rotational diffusion and was determined to be 0.23.[29] $\langle\tau\rangle$ is the average lifetime and is defined as

$$\langle\tau\rangle = f_1\tau_1 + f_2\tau_2 \tag{4}$$

where τ_1 and τ_2 are the two lifetimes measured for AF probes with fractional contributions f_1 and f_2. Figure 3 shows the rotational correlation times for 2-AS, 9-AS, and 16-AP (AS = anthroyloxy stearic acid; AP = anthroyloxy palmitic acid) in SCLL treated with different alkanols at iso-enhancement concentrations. The authors

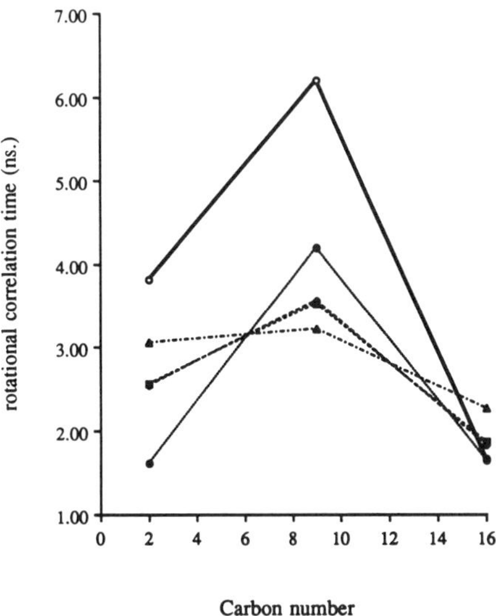

Figure 3 Effects of *n*-alkanols under iso-enhancement concentrations on the average rotational correlation time (<ϕ>) obtained with 2-AS, 9-AS, and 16-AP in SCLL. Symbols: open circles (buffer); closed circles (30% ethanol); closed squares (10% *n*-propanol); closed diamonds (2% *n*-butanol); closed triangles (1% *n*-pentanol). (From Kim, Y. H., Ph.D. thesis, University of Utah, Salt Lake City, 1992. With permission.)

suggested that the regions of intermediate depth in SCLL were more ordered than the region near the bilayer center based on the rotational correlation times. However, it should be noted that 16-AP may not probing the center of the bilayer in the SC as the average chain length of the lipids of the SC is C_{24}.[35] The higher ordering in the region between carbon 2 and 9 could be due to the high cholesterol content of the SC. The rigid rings of the cholesterol extend up to carbon 9 in lipid bilayers.[36] Also, the rotational correlation time showed the largest drop around carbon 2 with 30% ethanol, and around carbon 9 with 1% *n*-pentanol. This was interpreted as due primarily to the increased rotational rate of the fluorophore caused by the alkanols. It should be noted that no concomitant increase occurred in the polarity in the hydrocarbon region as the lifetimes remained fairly constant upon alkanol treatment.[29,30]

Phase-modulated fluorescence spectroscopy is being used in the author's laboratory to investigate the phase transition of SC lipids in epidermis as well as the effects of a variety of penetration enhancers on these membranous structures. Studies using AF probes have shown that these probes are sensitive to changes in the polarity and H-bonding ability of the solvents.[37] The gel to liquid crystalline phase transitions were detected in DSPC liposomes, pig SC, and human epidermis at temperatures established by other physical methods.[31] Also, it was shown that the lipid bilayers of the SC were in a rigid anhydrous environment, even in a fully hydrated tissue based on the comparison of lifetimes of AF probes in hexane, DSPC aqueous suspensions, oriented bilayers, pig SC, and human epidermis.[38] This is consistent with the relatively nonpolar nature of the predominant lipid constituents of the SC such as the ceramides and cholesterol.[35]

One approach to studying the polarity or fluidity changes at different depths in the lipid bilayers of the SC is to monitor the quenching efficiency of the AF probes in lipid bilayers by a penetrating fluorescence quencher such as iodide.[8] This approach is being investigated in human epidermis in the author's laboratory. Anthroyloxy fatty acid probes incorporated in human epidermis showed a quenching efficiency that is depth dependent. The quenching efficiency showed the trend 2-AS > 6-AS > 9-AS ~ 12-AS > 16-AP (unpublished observation). This approach could be used to determine the site of perturbation or fluidization in SC lipid bilayers by a given class of enhancers.

2. Oleic Acid

Fluorescence lifetimes and time-resolved anisotropy data for DPH in heat-separated human epidermis treated with different amounts of oleic acid will be described here to highlight the potential of this approach in studying the effect of penetration enhancers on skin. It should be noted that these results are part of an ongoing investigation in the author's laboratory and preliminary results are included in this chapter to stimulate interest in this area of research.[39]

The lifetimes for DPH in skin treated with different amounts of oleic acid showed a gradual decrease with increasing amounts of oleic acid in the donor vehicle, as shown in Figure 4. This suggested a gradual increase in the polarity and the dielectric of the medium with increasing uptake of oleic acid into the SC presumably due to the increased access of the disordered hydrocarbon core of the lipid bilayers to water. The time-resolved anisotropy data were analyzed using a hindered rotor model. The order parameter *(S)* was calculated using the r_{inf} values determined from the anisotropy measurements. *S* decreased with increasing oleic acid in the donor vehicle.[39] Thus, the overall packing order of the SC lipids was decreased with oleic acid uptake. It should be noted that DPH partitions uniformly between different lipid phases. The information obtained from DPH is averaged over the rigid gel and the fluid lipid phases in the SC. An interesting feature of this study was that the oleic acid uptake into skin was shown to be fairly linear with the amount of oleic acid in the donor vehicle, up to 0.5%. The effect of oleic acid on the flux of a model compound, benzoic acid, and the fluorescence parameters as well as the uptake into skin were saturated beyond 0.5% oleic acid in the donor formulation.

3. Surfactants

The effects of a series of pure dodecyl ether ethoxylates of single ethoxyl chain length ($C_{12}E_1$ to $C_{12}E_8$) upon the fluidity of a model bilayer system, DSPC multilamellar vesicles, was investigated by fluorescence polarization spectroscopy.[40] These surfactants are part of the "Brij" surfactant series, which have been shown to enhance percutaneous penetration.[41] These were steady-state anisotropy measurements of DPH, *cis*-parinaric acid, and ANS incorporated in DSPC vesicles. Based on the onset temperature of the gel to liquid crystalline phase transition, as monitored by steady-state anisotropy, the authors implied that more hydrophobic surfactants $C_{12}E_2$ to $C_{12}E_5$ were more effective fluidizers than the surfactants of higher hydrophile-lipophile balance (HLB), $C_{12}E_6$ and $C_{12}E_7$. Also, $C_{12}E_4$ caused the largest drop in the steady-state anisotropy of DPH, $C_{12}E_5$ was the most effective for *cis*-parinaric acid, and $C_{12}E_6$ caused the maximum drop in anisotropy of ANS in DSPC bilayers

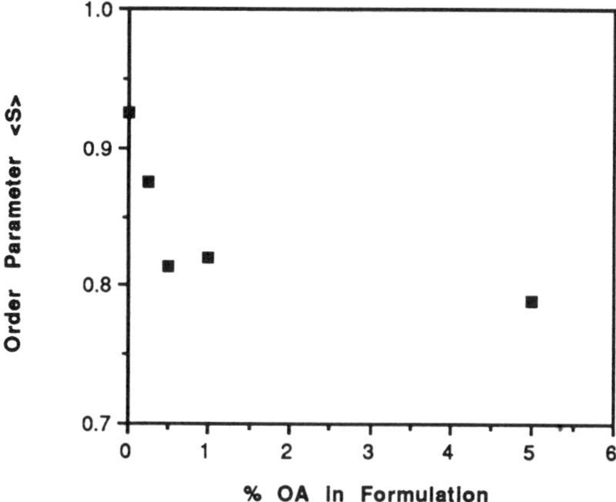

Figure 4 Fluorescence lifetimes of DPH in human epidermis at different oleic acid concentrations in the donor formulation.

containing 50 mol% of the surfactant at 30°C. The authors concluded that surfactants of intermediate HLB ($C_{12}E_4$ to $C_{12}E_6$) would be the best fluidizers of lipid bilayers and therefore the best enhancers of percutaneous penetration. Also, such fluorescence measurements with model membranes could be used as quick and easy screens for potential penetration enhancers. The conclusions drawn from such model systems should be treated with caution as DSPC bilayer systems may not be relevant models for the SC membranes.

IV. CONCLUSION

Fluorescence spectroscopy is a well-established tool used in the investigation of lipid bilayers in model systems and in biomembranes. This method offers a very high selectivity and sensitivity. Also, the phenomenon of fluorescence occurs in 10^{-8} s, which is a favorable time scale to study the dynamics of rotational diffusion in membranes. The state-of-the-art time- and frequency-domain instruments provide very high resolution of fluorescence intensity and anisotropy decays on the picosecond scale.

The SC, with its extracellular membranous structures, which provide the major barrier to percutaneous penetration, is an ideal tissue for fluorescence investigation. However, a solid tissue such as the SC is a highly scattering medium and offers a unique set of problems in terms of sample handling, data acquisition, and data analysis. Nevertheless, the mode of action of different classes of enhancers can be studied in skin using fluorescence spectroscopy. Only limited work has been done with alkanols, surfactants, and oleic acid using model bilayer systems and human epidermis. The different fluorescence approaches described in this chapter offer a wide choice of methods to investigate the mechanism of penetration enhancement and resolve the site of action at a molecular level. In addition, the response of the SC lipids to chemical and physical perturbation could be correlated to flux enhancement in terms of fluorescence parameters. Thus, establishing a biophysical correlate to flux enhancement would be a facile way to investigate penetration enhancement.

REFERENCES

1. **Lakowicz, J. R.,** *Principles of Fluorescence Spectroscopy,* Plenum Press, New York, 1983, chap. 1 and 7.
2. **Lakowicz, J. R.,** *Principles of Fluorescence Spectroscopy,* Plenum Press, New York, 1983, chap. 3.
3. **Cogen, U., Shinitzky, M., Weber, G., and Nishida, T.,** Microviscosity and order in the hydrocarbon region of phospholipid and phospholipid-cholesterol dispersions determined with fluorescent probes, *Biochemistry,* 12, 521, 1973.
4. **Stubbs, C. D. and Williams, B. W.,** Fluorescence in membranes, in *Topics in Fluorescence Spectroscopy,* Vol. 3, *Biochemical Applications,* Lakowicz, J. R., Ed., Plenum Press, New York, 1991.
5. **Lentz, B. R.,** Membrane fluidity as detected by diphylhexatriene probes, *Chem. Phys. Lipids,* 50, 171, 1989.
6. **Thulborn, K. R., Tilley, L. M., Sawyer, W. H., and Treloar, E. R.,** The use of n-(9-anthroyloxy) fatty acids to determine fluidity and polarity gradients in phospholipid bilayers, *Biochim. Biophys. Acta,* 558, 166, 1979.
7. **Lentz, B., Barenholz, Y., and Thompson, T. E.,** Fluorescence depolarization studies of phase transitions and fluidity in phospholipid bilayers. I. Single component phosphotidylcholine liposomes, *Biochemistry,* 15, 4521, 1976.
8. **Chaplin, D. B. and Kleinfeld, A. M.,** Interaction of fluorescence quenching with the n-(9-anthroyloxy) fatty acid membrane probes, *Biochim. Biophys. Acta,* 731, 465, 1983.
9. **Han, X. and Gross, R. W.,** Nonmonotonic alterations in the fluorescence anisotropy of polar head group labeled fluorophores during the lamellar to hexagonal phase transition of phospholipids, *Biophys. J.,* 63, 309, 1992.
10. **Parassassi, T., Conti, F., Glaser, M., and Gratton, E.,** Detection of phospholipid phase separation. A multifrequency phase fluorimetry study of 1,6-diphenyl-1,3,5-hexatriene fluorescence, *J. Biol. Chem.,* 259, 14011, 1984.
11. **Barrow, D. A. and Lentz, B. R.,** Membrane structural domains, *Biophys. J.,* 48, 221, 1985.
12. **Sklar, L. A.,** The partition of cis-parinaric acid and trans-parinaric acid among aqueous fluid lipid and solid lipid phases, *Biochemistry,* 32, 169, 1980.
13. **Matayoshi, E. D. and Kleinfeld, A. M.,** Emission wavelength-dependent decay of the 9-anthroyloxy-fatty acid membrane probes, *Biophys. J.,* 35, 215, 1981.
14. **Huang, N., Casteel, K. F., Feigenson, G. W., and Spink, C.,** Effect of fluorophore linkage position of n-(9-anthroyloxy) fatty acids on probe distribution between coexisting gel and fluid phospholipid phases, *Biochim. Biophys. Acta,* 939, 124, 1988.
15. **Williams, B. W. and Stubbs, C. D.,** Properties influencing fluorophore lifetime distributions in membranes, *Biochemistry,* 27, 7994, 1988.
16. **Wolber, P. K. and Hudson, B. S.,** Fluorescence lifetime and time-resolved polarization anisotropy studies of acyl chain order and dynamics in lipid bilayer, *Biochemistry,* 20, 2800, 1981.
17. **Michaels, A. S., Chandrasekaran, S. K., and Shaw, J. E.,** Permeation through human skin: theory and *in vitro* experimental measurement, *AIChE J.,* 21, 985, 1975.
18. **Elias, P. M. and Friend, D. S.,** The permeability barrier in mammalian epidermis, *J. Cell Biol.,* 65, 180, 1975.
19. **Lavker, R. M.,** Membrane coating granules: the fate of the discharged lamellae, *J. Ultrastruct. Res.,* 55, 79, 1976.
20. **Van Duzee, B. F.,** Thermal analysis of human SC, *J. Invest. Dermatol.,* 65, 404, 1975.
21. **Barry, B. W.,** Mode of action of penetration enhancers in human skin, *J. Control. Rel.,* 6, 85, 1987.
22. **Walters, K. A. and Hadgraft, J.,** *Pharmaceutical Skin Penetration Enhancement,* Marcel Dekker, New York, 1993.
23. **Francoeur, M. L., Golden, G. M., and Potts, R. O.,** Oleic acid: its effects on SC in relation to (trans)dermal drug delivery, *Pharm. Res.,* 7, 621, 1990.
24. **Goodman, M. and Barry, B. W.,** Action of skin penetration enhancers, Azone®, oleic acid, and decylmethyl sulfoxide: permeation and differential scanning calorimetry (DSC) studies, *J. Pharm. Pharmacol.,* 38, 71, 1986.
25. **Quan, D. and Maibach, H. I.,** Electron spin resonance, Chapter 16.2 in this book.

26. **Ongpipattanakul, B., Burnette, R. R., Potts, R. O., and Francoeur, M. L.,** Evidence that oleic acid exists in a separate phase within SC lipids, *Pharm. Res.,* 8, 350, 1991.
27. **Kai, T., Mak, V. H. W., Potts, R. O., and Guy, R. H.,** Mechanism of percutaneous penetration enhancement: effect of n-alkanols on the permeability barrier of hairless mouse skin, *J. Control. Rel.,* 12, 103, 1990.
28. **Williams, A. C. and Barry, B. W.,** Raman spectroscopy, Chapter 16.1 in this book.
29. **Kim, Y. H., Higuchi, W. I., Herron, J. N., and Abraham, W.,** Fluorescence anisotropy on the interaction of the short chain n-alkanols with SC lipid liposomes (SCLL) and distearoyl-phosphatidylcholine (DSPC)/distearoylphosphatidic acid (DSPA) liposomes, *Biochim. Biophys. Acta,* 1148, 139, 1993.
30. **Kim, Y. H.,** Studies of Mechanisms of Action of Short Chain Normal-Alkanols as Skin Transport Enhancers, Ph.D. thesis, University of Utah, Salt Lake City, 1992.
31. **Garrison, M. D., Potts, R. O., and Abraham, W.,** Frequency-domain fluorescence spectroscopy of human SC, in *Proc. SPIE, Time-Resolved Laser Spectroscopy in Biochemistry IV,* Lakowicz, J. R., Ed., Bellingham, WA, 1994.
32. **Oertel, R. P.,** Protein conformational changes induced in human SC by organic sulfoxides: an infrared spectroscopic investigation, *Biopolymers,* 16, 2329, 1977.
33. **Abraham, W. and Downing, D. T.,** Deuterium NMR investigation of polymorphism in SC lipids, *Biochim. Biophys. Acta,* 1068, 189, 1991.
34. **Abraham, W. and Downing, D. T.,** Lamellar structures formed by SC lipids *in vitro*: a deuterium nuclear magnetic resonance (NMR) study, *Pharm. Res.,* 9, 1415, 1992.
35. **Wertz, P. W. and Downing, D. T.,** Ceramides of pig epidermis: structure determination, *J. Lipid Res.,* 24, 759, 1983.
36. **Yeagle, P. L.,** Cholesterol and the cell membrane, *Biochim. Biophys. Acta,* 822, 267, 1985.
37. **Garrison, M. D., Doh, L. M., Potts, R. O., and Abraham, W.,** Fluorescence spectroscopy of 9-anthroyloxy fatty acids in solvents, *Chem. Phys. Lipids,* 70, 155, 1994.
38. **Garrison, M. D., Doh, L. M., Pechtold, L. A. R. M., Potts, R. O., and Abraham, W.,** Fluorescence spectroscopic evaluation of SC lipids and related model systems, in *Proc. Prediction of Percutaneous Penetration Conference,* Vol. 3B, Brain, K. R., James, V. J., and Walters, K. A., Eds., STS Publishing, Cardiff, U.K., 1993, 1.
39. **Garrison, M. D., Doh, L. M., Potts, R. O., and Abraham, W.,** Effect of oleic acid on human epidermis: Fluorescence spectroscopic investigation, *J. Control. Rel.,* 31, 263, 1994.
40. **French, E. J.,** The Enhancement of Percutaneous Absorption by Nonionic Surfactants, Ph.D. thesis, University of Bath, Bath, U.K., 1991.
41. **Walters, K. A., Walker, M., and Olejnik, O.,** Nonionic surfactant effects on skin permeability characteristics, *J. Pharm. Pharmacol.,* 40, 525, 1988.

Chapter 17.1

Some New Approaches to Understanding and Facilitating Transdermal Drug Delivery

Philip S. Magee

CONTENTS

I. INTRODUCTION

Permeation enhancement of a dermally applied drug by one or more copenetrants is a dramatically sophisticated process at the molecular level. As such, it demands and is receiving intensive study from both academic and industrial researchers, as recently reviewed by Ghosh and Banga,[1] and by Santus and Baker.[2] This is a many-layered problem with perhaps an order of magnitude in complexity over the general problem of solvation which is slowly emerging in molecular detail after a century of study.[3] All vehicles and permeation enhancers will display complex solvent behavior with both the transported drug and any structures modified within the stratum corneum (SC). While useful permeation enhancers span the molecular range from water[4,5] to phospholipids,[6] it is well to remember that the molecular behavior of water is, and may always be, an ongoing field of research. When overlaid with the complexity of "ordinary" transdermal transport[7] it is perfectly clear that permeation enhancement by copenetrants will be an ongoing research problem well into the next century.

Meanwhile, those who sit and wait for enlightenment are soon left behind by those who take the positive approach and do it anyway. The art of formulation has a long history of delivering pesticides, drugs, and cosmetics with stubborn physical properties to their assigned target by methods that mix science with intuition and experience.[8–10] The transdermal delivery of drugs at rates controlled in part by carefully selected penetration enhancers is both an investigational science and a patentable art form. One of the formulators that I know describes her very best products as "Picasso's", and knowing the intense effort and constant experimentation that went into her work, I fully agree. That is why this chapter addresses a combination of new ideas about permeation at the molecular level and a very practical device for assisting formulators in the art of selecting reasonable enhancers.

0-8493-2605-2/95/$0.00+$.50

II. PERMEATION AND PERMEATION BARRIERS

In the simplest reasonable pharmacokinetic model, we show the penetrant piercing the SC into the viable epidermis with one rate constant going and back-partitioning into the SC by another rate constant. Single rate constants also describe metabolism and further penetration into the dermis for capillary clearance. Such models are readily computed by adjusting the constants and provide good matches with experimental measures of penetration.[11] No molecular scientist would be surprised to find 100 or more actual rate processes in operation as the penetrant flirts with local domains in the SC, diffuses through the varying cellular morphologies of the viable epidermis down through the basal layer, and finally enters the acellular dermis layer in search of a capillary while reversibly binding with multitudes of fixed and humoral structures along the way. The immensity of the problem is exactly why we invoke simple models to "explain" what we see experimentally. Nearly all QSAR expressions are vastly simpler than the bioprocesses they model. An illustrative case in point is the minimum concentration of C_1 to C_{10} normal alcohols required to cause narcosis in tadpoles.[12] The plot of log(1/MIC) vs. log*P*(octanol/water) is perfectly bilinear with optimum narcosis at *n*-hexanol and a line-splitting correlation of r = 1.000. Nothing could be simpler except the need for at least five kinetically separate processes to move the alcohol from the aqueous phase to the neural target site within the animal. Why, then, do these simple models work so well? One reason is an averaging process that allows a complex event to be perceived and measured as a single rate constant as, for example, the skin permeability constant, K_p or P, from Fick's first law. The drug and vehicle are placed on the SC side of the cell with the sink fluid on the receptor side and simply measured that way. The interior processes are restricted to the black box of unobserved events. Another important reason in dermal studies and in all areas of QSAR is the concept of rate-limiting barriers; that is, the observed rate is actually the slowest step or steps of a complex process. It is widely accepted, for example, that the SC is the rate-limiting layer for most drugs,[7] although very lipophilic compounds may experience the viable epidermis and dermis as limiting due to the aqueous content of these layers.[13] This comes as a mixed blessing, depending on the level of interest in the molecular process. It certainly simplifies and renders possible all problems at the practical level such as how much goes through and at what rate.

Potts and Guy[14] took the *in vitro* data set assembled by Flynn[15] to develop a global expression for logK_p, the dermal permeability constant. The expression is surprisingly simple, with only two dominant factors, log*P*(octanol/water) and either molecular weight (MW) or molecular volume (MV). A slight modification that I prefer uses MR (molar refraction) to model polarizable volume or London forces. The equation is quite strong and predicts well across an enormous range of polarity (log*P* = –1.38 to 5.49).

$$\log K_p = 0.801\ \log P - 0.0260\,\mathrm{MR} - 2.71$$

$$\text{cofficient } T \text{ values} = 11.62, 11.42$$

$$n = 91 \qquad r = 0.820 \qquad s = 0.699 \qquad F = 89.94 \tag{1}$$

While log$P$ is the dominant descriptor of layer partitioning and reversible binding, MR serves as a molecular friction which increases with the size and polarizability of the permeants. Although MW correlates equally well, this number is a nuclear descriptor having little to do with the induced dipole moments responsible for London forces. Correlation among MW, MV, and MR is fortuitous. Like K_p itself, this extremely useful global equation conceals a wealth of local information. On factoring the data into log$P$ ranges or into chemical classes, it becomes clear that nothing as simple as partitioning and London forces is occurring throughout the set, although these factors represent the average behavior.[16] London forces are strongly supported only for polar compounds (log$P$ = –1.38 to 1.96) that one would expect to invade the SC protein domain.[17] For example, Anderson and Raykar[18] find that 4-methylphenol (log$P$ = 1.95) and methyl 4-hydroxyphenylacetate (log$P$ = 1.63) partition identically from water into normal and delipidized SC. The lipid domain does not participate in the process. Aliphatics and steroids correlate simply, but differently, with log$P$ while phenols exhibit complex behavior.

Aliphatics and water:

$$\log K_p = 0.474 \;\log P - 2.88$$

$$\text{cofficient } T \text{ values} = 11.01$$

$$n = 21 \qquad r = 0.930 \qquad s = 0.283 \qquad F = 121.25 \tag{2}$$

Steroids:

$$\log K_p = 0.953 \;\log P - 5.97$$

$$\text{cofficient } T \text{ values} = 8.88$$

$$n = 28 \qquad r = 0.867 \qquad s = 0.533 \qquad F = 78.80 \tag{3}$$

Phenols:

$$\log K_p = 1.73 \;\log P - 0.199 \log P^2 - 0.0355\,\text{MR} - 0.301\,\sigma(-) - 1.01$$

$$\text{cofficient } T \text{ values} = 4.32, 2.71, 3.33, 4.60$$

$$n = 18 \qquad r = 0.962 \qquad s = 0.110 \qquad F = 40.64 \tag{4}$$

Each of these equations predicts substantially better within their class than the general Potts-Guy equation (compare s values). All are expressions of rate-limiting behavior that is customized for each chemical class. While it is not currently possible to indicate the contribution of each barrier, various sources of evidence[7] suggest the following:

- Up to log$P$ = 2.0, SC protein domain is rate limiting
- From about 2.0 to 5.0, SC lipid domain is progressively dominant
- >4.0, the rate-limiting barrier shifts to the epidermis/dermis

Of singular note is the fact that $\log K_p$ for water, the supporter of life and the smallest permeation enhancer, is well predicted by the Potts-Guy equation and by the set of simple aliphatics correlated above. In permeation studies of water plus homologous alcohols, K_p for water falls close to that of methanol.[19] This very ordinary performance of nonorganic water has profound implications for the transport of polar drugs through the SC.

III. DOMAINS OF THE STRATUM CORNEUM

While it is correct to describe the SC lipid domain as the only obligatory barrier, it is not correct to view it as the only SC pathway. As stated above, water behaves in simple accordance with its physical properties in crossing the lipid barrier. Moreover, the SC can absorb water into the protein domain until the completely hydrated tissue contains five to six times its weight of strongly bound water resulting in a several-fold increase in SC thickness.[20] It does not require much imagination to realize that the initially contiguous lipid domain will rupture in the process to accelerate access to the hydrating cells. Thus, we have free access of water and other polar substances into the protein domain despite the lipid barrier. One of the purposes of a good penetration enhancer is to loosen the highly structured lipid phase to facilitate SC transport. Passage through the protein domain should reflect transport through ordinary proteinaceous tissue in the body, the differences being the degree of hydration and the presence of keratin and lipoproteins that may retard permeation by offering multiple sites for reversible binding. A probable mode of action for some penetration enhancers is to saturate these protein sites and present a less retarding surface to the penetrant. If one views SC penetration as a chromatography, the softening of these binding sites is analogous to reversed-phase chromatography. The observation by Guy et al.[21] of radial diffusion in the epidermal layers makes the analogy more credible.

Some of the features of the two SC domains have an impact on both ordinary and assisted percutaneous absorption. The wide range of skin permeability from different parts of the body[22,23] is fully consistent with a similar variation in human SC lipids.[24] The variation occurs both in location and in the vertical strata of the skin in progressing upward from the basal layer through the stratum granulosum to the inner and outer layers of the SC.[24,25] Thus, there is no definite composition of SC lipids, though neutral lipids (sterols, fatty acids, triglycerides and HC's) comprise about 78%, ceramides about 18%, with polar lipids and cholesteryl sulfate as the remainder.[25] As a percentage of the SC, the lipid domain fluctuates from about 9% (abdomen)[26] down to about 2% in the palmar–plantar regions.[24] Thus, the contiguous lipid envelope of the interlocking cornified cells representing the 91 to 98% protein domain of the SC is quite thin. This is readily visualized by cytochemical techniques developed by Nemanic and Elias.[27] The interstitial lipids appear irregular under the microscope,[27] but are known to be highly organized, perhaps even crystalline, at the molecular level. Four endothermic transitions are detectable in the SC between 40° and 100°C by differential scanning calorimetry.[28] These endotherms identify transitions from ordered to disordered states, and this technique has achieved major importance in assessing the effect of permeation enhancers on the SC domains. In sum, the lipid barrier is responsible for controlling transepidermal water loss (TEWL), permitting us to live safely in a nonaqueous environment. It is interesting to note that both neutral and polar lipids play a complementary role. Delipidization with nonpolar solvents does not remove the barrier, while extraction with both acetone and hexane removes it completely.[29] Thus, the removal of both classes of lipids is required to destroy the protective barrier. The relation of TEWL to percutaneous absorption is shown clearly in the work of Dupuis et al.[31] For six locations on the human body, TEWL is in linear correlation with the percutaneous absorption of benzoic acid (r = 0.97). As water behaves normally in percutaneous absorption (see previous section), it is very likely that the K_p of water and TEWL are simply reverse measures of the same barrier. Correlation with other compounds is therefore expected via the Potts-Guy equation.

The protein domain is the tandem pathway for polar and moderately lipophilic compounds. It certainly should play a role in the transport of all systemic drugs and chemicals (log$P$ = –0.5 to 3.5), although not a dominant role at the more lipophilic end (2.5 to 3.5). At 10- to 50-fold the mass of the lipid domain and considering the large difference in structural polarity, the capacity of the cellular protein domain for strong hydrogen bonding and relatively strong London forces far outweighs that of the lipid domain. Moreover, it is always partially hydrated and capable of generating a large sponge domain through further hydration.[17] Both random and hydrophobically organized waters are present to interact with penetrants. The cellular material of the protein domain contains organized keratin filaments, 60 to 80 Å in diameter, which present likely regions for nonspecific binding of polar drugs.[30] It is these structures that provide the most likely sites for both hydrogen bonding and strong London forces (MR) described in the previous section.

IV. MODIFYING THE STRATUM CORNEUM

In principle, we could take an average polarity value based on SC lipid analyses[24,25] and by comparing it with the average polarity of the polypeptides in the protein domain, work out the distribution of a given drug between the two. This is premature and thus it is necessary to speak of modifying the phases separately while realizing that some penetration enhancers will do both. Based on the polarity of the penetration enhancer, we can guess rather easily which phase is being strongly impacted. As one peruses the compounds described in the CTFA dictionary[32] and in *McCutcheons,*[33] it is clear that many of these cannot be described by measures or calculations of log$P$(octanol/water). Many of the structures lie outside the rules of calculation and many others are clearly candidates for micelle formation, wherein no real concentration in water can be measured. To facilitate this problem and place small polar enhancers (solvents) on the same polarity scale with large lipophilic nonionic surfactants, the following definition is proposed:

$$\text{Polarity (POL)} = \text{MW (polar structures)/MW compound} \qquad (5)$$

The polar structures are defined as all heteroelements, with any closely associated carbons or hydrogens. Thus, a carboxamide group would be counted as $CONH_2$, the remainder being entirely lipophilic C, H, and sometimes S and halogen; i.e., all fragments having a positive lipophilic contribution in the ordinary calculation of log*P*. This simple definition provides a number ranging from 0.00 to 1.00 that crudely classifies the probable destination of each compound. Now we can discuss modification of the lipid and protein domains by selected examples.

Differential scanning calorimetry clearly shows the destruction (melting) of three of the endotherms in the SC following treatment with Azone® (1-dodecylaza-cycloheptan-2-one) (POL = 0.15).[28] The fourth endotherm, near 100°C, is thought to represent the organization of intercellular keratin. The other three are clearly in the lipid domain. Azone® is clearly targeted to disrupt the bilayer structures by interposing its polar head and bulky seven-membered ring among the tightly packed head groups, effectively lowering the melting point and liquifying the layer. Many other penetration enhancers with bulky polar head groups (pentaerythritol dioleate, lauramide DEA) or those with long POE groups (polyethyleneglycol-10 laurate, nonoxynol-10) can totally disrupt an organized packing. The principle is simply the lowering of the melting point (or transition point) by random introduction of a strongly associated, but poorly packed intruder. Hydrogen bonding may be a factor in localizing the head groups in some cases, but not in all. The fluidized lipid domain is certainly a lower energy pathway for lipophilic drugs and, for polar compounds, it may lower the penetration barrier to the cellular domain of the SC.

Compounds capable of modifying the cellular domain are urea,[1] water,[4,5] propylene glycol,[34] dimethylsulfoxide,[35] and other enhancers with POL values >0.5. Recent work with powdered human SC shows a positive correlation between log*P*(SC/water) and log*P*(octanol/water) for lipophilic compounds, a negative slope for polar compounds, and a relatively flat relation in between, where both domains participate.[17] This is in perfect agreement with separate and combined enhancement of the two domains as a function of penetration enhancer polarity. Urea, water, propylene glycol, and dimethylsulfoxide have log*P*(octanol/water) values of –2.11, –1.38, –0.92, and –1.35. Like acetone (log*P*(octanol/water) = –0.24), dimethylsulfoxide is amphiphilic with miscibility in both domains. Its passage through the SC is quite destructive, with swelling, distortion, and intercellular delamination.[35]

Granting the invasion of polar enhancers into the cellular (protein) domain, we need to consider likely mechanisms that would increase the K_p of a copermeating drug. At least two effects can be exerted by the protein domain to retard the passage of a polar drug. One is the molecular friction of London forces as modeled by MR (polarizable volume); the other is the capacity to form strong hydrogen bonds. Both of these events are in the low kilocalorie per mole range and, while fully reversible, can exert strong effects on protein domain penetration. Activation energies for transdermal penetration can be high for polar drugs such as sulfanilamide (E^* = 30.4 kcal/mol) and ibuprofen (E^* = 41.4) as compared to lipid domain permeants such as 4-bromophenol (E^* = 8.8).[36] Most of this energetic effect is attributable to strong multiple hydrogen bonding. The most likely structure for strong polar binding in the cellular domain is the highly organized keratin filaments, as previously stated.[30] Moreover, the most likely mechanism for inhibiting this event is the saturation binding of polar penetration enhancers. Through binding at the most energetic sites, the enhancer both neutralizes the protein hydrogen bonds and presents a surface that expresses weaker London forces to facilitate drug penetration.

These effects for both domains are not directly supported by experimental results, but represent the best current thinking based on sound physicochemical principles. It would be very surprising to find completely different mechanisms in operation.

V. A RATIONAL APPROACH TO SELECTING ENHANCERS

As the lipid domain of the SC forms an obligatory barrier for all penetrants, the transport of both polar and lipophilic drugs may be assisted by enhancers (e.g., Azone) that loosen the organized structures. For drugs with POL >0.5, the incorporation of a second enhancer to penetrate and modify the cellular domain could provide a synergistic effect, e.g., propylene glycol. Aside from these considerations, there is the problem of drug/penetration enhancer compatibility in the formulation. Ideally, penetration enhancers need to be selected in some way that relects both the SC target and compatibility with the permeant drug. Phase separation within the formulation or by a chromatography effect within the SC layers can only reduce the efficacy of enhancement. One approach to rational selection by the author is now described.

By careful selection of types and polarity, a Quattro Pro spreadsheet was assembled with 139 penetration enhancers drawn from the CTFA dictionary.[32] Twenty-one drugs were also entered as experimental matching candidates. The following fields were entered and all cells were filled with simple and calculated values:

CASE	sequential number to restore order by sorting
DRUG/VEHICLE	name of drug or vehicle
CODE	drug (D), vehicle (V)
FORMULA	empirical formula, Azone® = $C_{18}H_{35}NO$
FORMPOL	polar substructures, Azone® = CNO
MW	molecular weight of drug or vehicle
MWH	molecular weight of polar substructures
POL	MWH/MW
HBA	count of acceptor electron pairs (N and O)
HBD	count of donor N-H and O-H groups

The table can be sorted on any numerical entry for rapid assessments, and, more profitably, it can be searched for a range of characteristics matching any known drug. Most effective is a search that combines POL with the hydrogen-bonding counts. As an example, to match minoxidil with a compatible and potentially useful enhancer.

$$\text{Minoxidil} - C_9H_{15}N_5O\ (209.25) \qquad \text{FORMPOL} - N_5OH_2\ (88.07)$$

$$\text{POL} = 0.42 \qquad \text{HBA} = 6 \qquad \text{HBD} = 4$$

$$\text{Search Range: POL} = 0.36 \text{ to } 0.48 \qquad \text{HBA} = 4 \text{ to } 8 \qquad \text{HBD} = 2 \text{ to } 6 \tag{6}$$

For the search, simply expand the range about the values for minoxidil. These can be expanded until a reasonable match is found or one can drop the hydrogen-bond restrictions (one or both) and base the search purely on polarity. In the present case our database found the following penetration enhancers for minoxidil:

	POL	HBA	HBD
Diethylene glycol	0.47	6	2
Dipropylene glycol	0.37	6	2
1,2,6-Hexanetriol	0.38	6	3
bis-Hydroxyethylglycol ether	0.44	8	2
Propylene glycol	0.45	4	2
Triethylene glycol	0.44	8	2

These selections at least provide a logical starting point for formulation research. A searchable database of this type requires <1 week to assemble and can be highly personalized by inclusion of favorite penetration enhancers and solvents.

In summary, most of the ideas presented in this chapter will be richly modified by future research but, for the most part, they are immediately useful as mental tools and should largely stand the test of time.

REFERENCES

1. **Ghosh, T. K. and Banga, A. K.,** Methods of enhancement of transdermal drug delivery, in *Pharmaceutical Technology,* Part I, Physical and biochemical approaches, March, 72–98, Part IIA, Chemical permeation enhancers, April, 62–90, Part IIB, Chemical permeation enhancers, May, 68–80, 1993.
2. **Santus, G. C. and Baker, R. W.,** Transdermal enhancer patent literature, *J. Control. Rel.,* 25, 1, 1993.
3. **Reichardt, C.,** *Solvents and Solvent Effects in Organic Chemistry,* VCH, Weinheim, 1988.
4. **Ward, A. J. I. and Osborne, D. W.,** Hydrotropy and penetration enhancement, in *Pharmaceutical Skin Penetration Enhancement,* Walters, K. A. and Hadgraft, J., Eds., Marcel Dekker, New York, 1993, chap. 17.
5. **Roberts, M. S. and Walker, M.,** Water. The most natural penetration enhancer, in *Pharmaceutical Skin Penetration Enhancement,* Walters, K. A. and Hadgraft, J., Eds., Marcel Dekker, New York, 1993, chap. 1.
6. **Martin, G. P.,** Phospholipids as skin penetration enhancers, in *Pharmaceutical Skin Penetration Enhancement,* Walters, K. A. and Hadgraft, J., Eds., Marcel Dekker, New York, 1993, chap. 3.
7. **Magee, P. S.,** Percutaneous absorption: critical factors in transdermal transport, in *Dermatotoxicology,* 4th ed., Marzulli, F. N. and Maibach, H. I., Eds., Hemisphere Publishing, New York, 1991, chap. 1.
8. **Scher, H. B., Ed.,** *Advances in Pesticide Formulation Technology,* ACS Symp. Ser. No. 254, American Chemical Society, Washington, DC, 1984.
9. **Scher, H. B., Ed.,** *Controlled Release Pesticides,* ACS Symp. Ser. No. 53, American Chemical Society, Washington, DC, 1977.
10. *Pharmaceutical Skin Penetration Enhancement,* Walters, K. A. and Hadgraft, J., Eds., Marcel Dekker, New York, 1993.
11. **Carver, M. P., Williams, P. L., and Riviere, J. E.,** The isolated perfused porcine skin flap. III. Percutaneous absorption pharmacokinetics of organophosphates, steroids, benzoic acid and caffeine, *Toxicol. Appl. Pharmacol.,* 97, 324, 1989.
12. **Hansch, C., Steward, A. R., Isawa, J., and Deutsch, E. W.,** The use of a hydrophobic bonding constant for QSAR, *Mol. Pharmacol.,* 1, 205, 1965.
13. **Scott, R. C. and Ramsay, J. D.,** Comparison of the *in vivo* and *in vitro* percutaneous absorption of a lipophilic molecule (cypermethrin), *J. Invest. Dermatol.,* 89, 142, 1987.
14. **Potts, R. O. and Guy, R. H.,** Predicting skin permeability, *Pharm. Res.,* 9, 663, 1992.
15. **Flynn, G. L.,** Physicochemical determinants of skin absorption, in *Principles of Route-to-Route Extrapolation for Risk Assessment,* Gerrity, T. R. and Henry, C. J., Eds., Elsevier, New York, 1990, 93.
16. **Magee, P. S.,** current research studies, PM608 to PM613, 1993. Available on request.

17. **Hui, X., Wester, R. C., Magee, P. S., and Maibach, H. I.,** Partitioning of chemicals from water into powdered human SC, *In Vitro Toxicology,* in press.
18. **Anderson, B. D. and Raykar, P. V.,** Solute structure-permeability relationships in human SC, *J. Invest. Dermatol.,* 93, 280, 1989.
19. **Scheuplein, R. J.,** Percutaneous absorption after twenty-five years, *J. Invest. Dermatol.,* 67, 31, 1976.
20. **Scheuplein, R. J. and Blank, I. H.,** Permeability of the skin, *Physiol. Rev.,* 51, 702, 1971.
21. **Guy, R. H., Maibach, H. I., and Hadgraft, J.,** Radial transport in the dermis, in *Percutaneous Absorption,* Bronaugh, R. L. and Maibach, H. I., Eds., Marcel Dekker, New York, 1985, chap. 25.
22. **Maibach, H. I.,** *In vivo* percutaneous penetration of corticoids and unresolved problems in their efficacy, *Dermatologica,* 152(Suppl. 1), 11, 1976.
23. **Southwell, D., Barry, B. W., and Woodford, R.,** Variations in permeability of human skin within and between specimens, *Int. J. Pharm.,* 18, 299, 1984.
24. **Lampe, M. A., Burlingame, A. L., Whitney, J., Williams, M. L., Brown, B. E., Roitman, E., and Elias, P. M.,** Human SC lipids: characterization and regional variations, *J. Lipid Res.,* 24, 120, 1983.
25. **Lampe, M. A., Williams, M. L., and Elias, P. M.,** Human epidermal lipids: characterization and modulations during differentiation, *J. Lipid Res.,* 24, 131, 1983.
26. **Schurer, N. Y. and Elias, P. M.,** The biochemistry and function of SC lipids, in *Advances in Lipid Research,* Vol. 24, Skin Lipids, Elias, P. M., Havel, R. J., and Small, D. M., Eds., Academic Press, New York, 1991, 27.
27. **Nemanic, M. K. and Elias, P. M.,** *In situ* precipitation: a novel cytochemical technique for visualization of permeability pathways in mammalian SC, *J. Histochem. Cytochem.,* 28, 573, 1980.
28. **Barry, B. W.,** Mode of action of penetration enhancers in human skin, *J. Control. Rel.,* 6, 85, 1987.
29. **Onken, H. D. and Moyer, C. A.,** The water barrier in human epidermis. Physical and chemical nature, *Arch. Dermatol.,* 87, 584, 1963.
30. **Stuttgen, G.,** Drug absorption by intact and damaged skin, in *Dermal and Transdermal Absorption,* Brandau, R. and Lippold, B. H., Eds., Wissenschaftliche Verlagsgesellschaft mbH, Stuttgart, 1982, chap. 2.
31. **Dupuis, D., Rougier, A., Lotte, C., Wilson, D. R., and Maibach, H. I.,** *In vivo* relationship between percutaneous absorption and transepidermal water loss according to anatomic site in man, *J. Soc. Cosmet. Chem.,* 37, 351, 1986.
32. **Nikitakis, J. M., McEwen, G. N. and Wenninger, J. A., Eds.,** *CTFA International Cosmetic Ingredient Dictionary,* 4th ed., The Cosmetic Toiletry and Fragrance Association, Washington, DC, 1991.
33. *McCutcheon's 1993, Volume 1, Emulsifiers & Detergents,* MC Publishing Company, Glen Rock, NJ, 1993.
34. **Zatz, J. L. and Dalvi, U. G.,** Evaluation of solvent-skin interaction in percutaneous absorption, *J. Soc. Cosmet. Chem.,* 34, 327, 1983.
35. **Chandrasekaran, S. K., Campbell, P. S., and Michaels, A. S.,** Effect of dimethyl sulfoxide on drug permeation through human skin, *AIChE J.,* 23, 810, 1977.
36. **Ito, Y., Ogiso, T., and Iwaki, M.,** Thermodynamic study on enhancement of percutaneous penetration of drugs by azone, *J. Pharmacobiodyn.,* 11, 749, 1988.

Chapter 17.2

Future Perspectives for Penetration Enhancers

Eric W. Smith and Howard I. Maibach

CONTENTS

I. INTRODUCTION

The foregoing chapters elegantly portray the current status in our knowledge of transdermal penetration enhancement. There can be no dispute that the understanding of enhancer mechanisms of action, and the analytical tools that we can employ to research this field, have advanced greatly in the past few years, or that there is still much to discover before comprehension of this phenomenon is complete. Each chapter has clearly concentrated on a particular aspect of this diverse field and has provided an in-depth description and analysis of that focus. As a closing chapter for this book it is appropriate for the editors to make some global comment to summarize the current strengths and shortcomings in the field.

II. CURRENT PERSPECTIVES

On reading the foregoing chapters, a number of aspects of this research field are apparent. Most penetration enhancement studies are concerned with the intercellular route of drug permeation. While it is generally believed that this is the major absorption pathway for lipophilic drugs, it must be borne in mind that the transcellular and appendageal routes may be used extensively by penetrating moieties. It is also clear that most analytical techniques for studying penetration enhancement have, understandably, focused on determining changes that take place in the intercellular lipid bilayer region, and few researchers have as yet expanded their research to include the corneocytes, sweat glands, and hair follicles. It is improbable that enhancer methods would modify the lipid domains exclusively without also affecting the intracellular environments and appendages.

Many of the other observations regarding the research presented in this volume have been stated and repeated several times in the past regarding experiments in transdermal drug delivery. Several of the studies have been conducted under conditions that are not physiological. The relevance of the data obtained under these circumstances to the *in vivo* situation, therefore, must be assessed by the reader. Many studies employ dosages of drug or enhancer that are higher than applicable in clinical practice. If the same experiment was attempted *in vivo,* the potential for

0-8493-2605-2/95/$0.00+$.50

toxicity, from drug or enhancer, would be much greater. Similarly, research to date has not made sufficient distinction between the skin of different species, or of different anatomical sites of the same species, as far as penetration enhancement is concerned. It is still unclear to what extent penetration enhancement methods affect the stratum corneum (SC) of different species, different races, and different sites of application. Having established that a difference in the biochemical composition of the SC exists between species and at different anatomical sites,[1,2] it would be naive to assume that penetration enhancement methods would affect all these locations equally.

Finally, some comment must be made about the analytical techniques that are currently being employed for researching transdermal penetration enhancement. It is undisputed that many of these analytical techniques are very powerful in their ability to aid in visualizing or deciphering what is occurring in the SC during penetration enhancement. What remains uncertain at this stage is our interpretation of the data, bearing in mind our current knowledge of the topic. For example, several studies appeared in the literature in which microscopic techniques are used to visualize penetrants.[3,4] What remains uncertain in many of these studies is the interpretation of exactly what is being visualized by the technique being used. Permeants that are tagged in some way by chemically adding a fluorescent portion to the penetrating molecule, for example, may have this additive cleaved once the complex enters the SC. Any fluorescence visualization technique, therefore, would only locate the position of the fluor in the skin; it offers no guarantee that the fluor and permeant are still linked.

In addition, fluorescence techniques were used recently to investigate the route followed by permeant molecules penetrating the skin under iontophoresis. Micrographs of such a study typically show diffuse fluorescence in the upper strata of the skin, which diminishes in intensity in the deeper layers, but remains concentrated around the hair follicles. The immediate assumption is that penetration (of the permeant-fluor complex) under iontophoresis is taking place via the hair follicles. It is equally possible that penetration via the SC is rapid and that specific adsorption of the complex takes place in the vicinity of the hair follicles; the definitive answer can only be obtained if mass transfer studies to a distal receptor are conducted simultaneously. It is probable that scientists are making the correct assumptions about the data that they generate simply because they are the most experienced in the particular field; however, at face value the conclusions drawn in many studies are open to varied interpretation.

III. FUTURE PERSPECTIVES

Currently the main criteria for investigation in screening potential penetration enhancers are: adequate improvement in the rate of permeant delivery, a lack of toxicity, and a lack of permanent disruption or destruction of the stratum corneum barrier. It is clear that this field is still in its infancy — in spite of several years of research in this field, we have yet to see commercial delivery vehicles on the market which contain penetration enhancers. The exception to this would be the inclusion of alcohol or propylene glycol into formulations where their purpose may be "disguised" as solubilizers rather than declared as penetration enhancers for registration purposes. Is it possible that the impact on transdermal delivery that once was associated with these techniques may not be fully realized simply because of the costs associated with regulatory registration formalities? The situation will undoubtedly improve as greater understanding of the mechanisms by which chemical penetration enhancement is achieved, and the longer-term effects of enhancer usage are unfolded with continued research in this field. It will especially be interesting to assess the results from extensive investigations into intra-cellular and appendageal modifications following enhancer usage, in light of our current knowledge of the intercellular domain modifications. Similarly, analytical techniques used to study this topic will continue to improve; however studies will need to concentrate on specific details so that ambiguities in interpretation of results are avoided.

Advances in physical enhancement methods will undoubtedly lead to commercially viable devices that are simple for the patient to use. Devices currently available for iontophoresis are relatively large when compared to simple transdermal patches, although more compact iontophoretic units capable of delivering the controlled potential difference to the skin have been developed recently. The great advantage in this technique is the ability to deliver large proteins and peptides across the skin and it offers hope that life sustaining compounds such as insulin may possibly be administered via this route. In contrast, the widespread use of phonophoresis to enhance transdermal permeation does not seem equally promising at this stage — there has simply not been enough research as yet into this enhancement mechanism.

Related studies in this discipline will continue to improve our knowledge of penetration enhancement: the metabolic processes within the skin, for example, may provide several mechanisms by which drug delivery and clinical outcomes could be improved. The concept of using prodrugs to enhance drug delivery has been explored relatively poorly to date but offers a potential solution for administering certain drug classes.[5,6] Alternatively, the possibility of delaying the biological regeneration of the SC barrier following enhancer application may provide a synergistic mechanism for enhancing penetration. It is now understood that the SC will rapidly respond to the disruptive molecular effects of chemical enhancers. If the metabolic regeneration of the barrier may be delayed by co-administration of a retarder then the penetration window may be held patent for a longer period and more drug could, theoretically, be delivered through this reduced barrier. This technique has the potential for reducing the total dose of enhancer chemical needed in the formulation, but requires the metabolic retarder to have an acceptable safety profile.

The possibilities seem endless as we begin to scratch the surface of enhanced drug delivery. It is interesting to reflect on these new ideas in light of the commonly-held belief 20 years ago that the SC was simply a layer of dead cells, and to wonder what secrets of the skin barrier will be unveiled in the next 20 years.

REFERENCES

1. **Elias, P. M., Goerke, J., and Friend, D. S.,** Mammalian epidermal barrier layer lipids: composition and influence on structure, *J. Invest. Dermatol.*, 69, 535, 1977.
2. **Elias, P. M. and Menon, G. K.,** Structural and lipid biochemical correlates of the epidermal permeability barrier, *Adv. Lipid Res.*, 24, 1, 1991.

3. **de Haan, F. H. N., Boddé, H. E., de Bruijn, W. C., Ginsel, L. A., and Junginger, H. E.,** Visualizing drug transport across SC: cryotechniques, vapour fixation, autoradiography, *Int. J. Pharm.,* 56, 75, 1989.
4. **Robertson, J. D., Ferguson, E., Jay, M., and Stalker, D. J.,** Noninvasive *in vivo* percutaneous absorption measurements using X-ray fluorescence, *Pharm. Res.,* 9, 1410, 1992.
5. **Seki, T., Kawaguchi, T., and Juni, K.,** Enhanced delivery of zidovudine through rat and human skin via ester prodrugs, *Pharm. Res.,* 7, 948, 1990.
6. **Sloan, K. B., Getz, J. J., Beall, H. D., and Prankerd, R. J.,** Transdermal delivery of 5-fluorouracil (5-FU) through hairless mouse skin by 1-alkylaminocarbonyl-5-FU prodrugs: physicochemical characterization of prodrugs and correlations with transdermal delivery, *Int. J. Pharm.* 93, 27, 1993.

INDEX

A

B

C

D

E

F

G

H

I

K

L

M

N

O

P

R

S

T

U

V

W

X